Manual for Pharmacy Technicians

THIRD EDITION

LINDA FRED, R.PH.

DIRECTOR OF INPATIENT PHARMACY SERVICES
CARLE FOUNDATION HOSPITAL

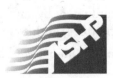

American Society of Health–System Pharmacists®

Bethesda, Maryland

Any correspondence regarding this publication should be sent to the publisher, American Society of Health-System Pharmacists, 7272 Wisconsin Avenue, Bethesda, MD 20814, attn: Special Publishing. Produced in conjunction with the ASHP Publications Production Center.

The information presented herein reflects the opinions of the contributors and reviewers. It should not be interpreted as an official policy of ASHP or as an endorsement of any product.

This book is not sponsored or endorsed by the Pharmacy Technician Certification Board (PTCB). Although every effort has been made on behalf of the authors, editor, and publisher to provide an extensive manual, comprehension of the material included in this text and the practice exam does not guarantee successful completion of the PTCB national certification examination or any other examination.

The authors, editor, and publisher of this work have made a conscientious effort to provide the reader with accurate and up-to-date information, but the nature of the information is evolving, and may be subject to change due to the dynamic nature of drug information and drug distribution systems. This information should be used solely in preparation for the certification exam or other academic purposes. No information contained in this text should be used to provide patient care.

Acquisitions Editor: Cynthia Reilly

Editorial Project Manager: Dana Battaglia

Production Manager: Johnna Hershey

Page composition: David Wade

ISBN: 1-58528-090-9

Table of Contents

continued

Preface

In the process of planning this new edition of **Manual for Pharmacy Technicians** we discussed many goals, including improved visual interest and expanded and updated content, but the underlying principle remained the same—to produce a book that would continue to serve well the purposes of the many and varied users. I believe we have made considerable improvements in what was already a good text.

One of the first things you will notice when you thumb through the book is an increased use of color. We have also made a concerted effort to include more graphics—drawings in the physiology chapter, for example. There is a general increase in the use of figures and tables throughout the material.

The ordering of the chapters has been revised to improve the flow of the content. We've added chapters on medical terminology, physiology, and biopharmaceutics. These new chapters, while they may not be directly related to the jobs of many technicians, do provide a great deal of additional context for understanding both the Manual's content as well as the technician's roles in supporting the pharmacist and serving the patients.

Many chapters have additional content. The calculations chapter, for example, now covers some basic statistics to aid technicians involved in quality improvement activities. The pharmacology chapter is updated for new drugs. The practice site-specific chapters have updated content to reflect the changing focus of those areas. Even content as "old" as interpreting a prescription is "new" in that more electronic transmission is happening and things aren't as simple as the patient handing you a piece of paper.

We had many goals and aspirations for this book. I believe we've been successful in meeting the majority of them. What you still see, however, is a great book with a lot of potential uses. It is terrific for new employee training. It is fantastic for preparing for the certification exam. It is a phenomenal tool for the educator in a pharmacy technician certificate program.

I hope you find it indispensable (and the pun wasn't intended, but I do like it).

Linda Fred, Editor
2004

Acknowledgments

Many of the same individuals were involved in producing the third edition of the **Manual for Pharmacy Technicians** who shared their talents the last time around. It is such a great honor to have been associated with this work and with the gifted group of people who have volunteered their time and their knowledge to make this project not simply a reality, but a product we can be proud of and which can serve many functions.

As with the previous edition, there are many to thank. Obviously, I am grateful to the authors who were the direct contributors and to the reviewers who provided thoughtful commentary on our work—helping us refine each chapter. There has been a terrific support staff at ASHP—especially Cynthia Reilly, Dana Battaglia, and Johnna Hershey. You were tremendously helpful in keeping me on task when my full-time life threatened to intrude on my secret identity as an editor.

I have been allowed a great deal of flexibility in my schedule by my employer and I wish to acknowledge those people at Carle Foundation Hospital who contributed by supporting my "extracurricular" activity—especially John Snyder and Mary Ingram. And always, my love and my gratitude to my wonderful husband Michael and my lovely daughter Ellen who allowed me to devote time to this project (again) that I might have spent with them.

Linda Fred

2004

ASHP and Linda Fred again gratefully acknowledge the Illinois Council of Health-System Pharmacists (ICHP) for their support in the development of this publication.

Contributors

Bonnie S. Bachenheimer, Pharm.D.
Drug Information Clinical Specialist
Advocate Lutheran General Hospital
Park Ridge, Illinois

Karen E. Bertch, Pharm.D., FCCP
Director, Pharmacy Services, Product Planning,
Premier, Incorporated
Oak Brook, Illinois
Per Diem Clinical Pharmacist
Coram Healthcare
Mt. Prospect, Illinois

Linda Y. Fred, R.Ph.
Director of Inpatient Pharmacy Services
Carle Foundation Hospital
Urbana, Illinois

Alice J.A. Gardner, Ph.D.
Assistant Professor of Pharmacology and Toxicology
Department of Pharmaceutical Sciences
Massachusetts College of Pharmacy & Health Sciences
School of Pharmacy -Worcester
Worcester, Massachusetts

Douglas C. Higgins, R.Ph.
Doug's Pharmacy
Paxton, Illinois

Rebecca Kentzel, CPhT
Manager of Project Management Office
OSF Healthcare System
Mackinaw, Illinois

Jacqueline Z. Kessler, M.S., R.Ph., FASHP
Clinical Specialist
Advocate Lutheran General Hospital
Park Ridge, Illinois

Tanya C. Knight-Klimas, Pharm.D., CGP, FASCP
Clinical Assistant Professor of Pharmacy
Temple University School of Pharmacy
Clinical Geriatric Pharmacist
Living Independently For Elders (LIFE)
Saint Agnes Medical Center
Philadelphia, PA

Connie Larson, Pharm.D.
Medication Safety Officer
Assistant Director, Safety and Quality
Hospital Pharmacy Services
University of Illinois Medical Center at Chicago
Chicago, Illinois

Richard K. Lewis, Pharm.D., MBA
Continuing Education Administrator
ProCE, Incorporated

Steven Lundquist, Pharm.D.
Clinical Director
Cardinal Health
Pharmacy Management
Marco Island, Florida

Scott M. Mark, Pharm.D., M.S., M.Ed., CHE, FASHP
Director of Pharmacy
Children's National Medical Center
Washington, District of Columbia

continued

Contributors

continued

Jerrod Milton, BScPharm
Adjunct Assistant Clinical Professor
University of Colorado Health Sciences Center,
School of Pharmacy
Director, Pharmacy Services
The Children's Hospital
Denver, Colorado

Diane F. Pacitti, Ph.D., R.Ph.
Assistant Professor of Pharmaceutical Sciences
Massachusetts College of Pharmacy and Health
Sciences
Worcester, Massachusetts

Michele F. Shepherd, Pharm.D., M.S., FASHP, BCPS
Clinical Specialist
Department of Medical Education
Abbott Northwestern Hospital
Minneapolis, Minnesota

Sheri Stensland, Pharm.D.
Assistant Professor of Pharmacy Practice
Shared Faculty for Walgreens
Midwestern University Chicago College of Pharmacy
Downers Grove, Illinois

Gerald A. Storm, R.Ph.
Director of Pharmacy
OSF-Saint Francis Medical Center
Peoria, Illinois

Philip R. Torf, R.Ph., J.D.
Attorney-at-Law
Torf Law Firm
Northbrook, Illinois
Administrator
Institute for Pharmacy Law
Northbrook, Illinois

Reviewers

Renee Acosta, R.Ph., M.S.

Katrin Fulginiti, R.Ph., MGA

David Hendrick

Lisa K. Linn, R.Ph.

Barbara Limburg Mancini, Pharm.D., BCNSP

Janet Montgomery, Pharm.D.

Anna Nowobilski-Vasilios, Pharm.D., MBA, FASHP, BCNSP

Bonnie L. Senst, R.Ph., M.S.

Introduction to Pharmacy

MICHELE F. SHEPHERD

The primary responsibility of any employee in the profession of pharmacy is to ensure that patients receive the proper drug therapy for their specific medical conditions. To achieve this goal, pharmacy personnel in hospitals, community pharmacies, and other health care settings perform a variety of duties designed to deliver the correct drug in the correct amount to all patients at all times in a timely manner. These duties range from ordering medications from suppliers to distributing drugs to patients to monitoring patients. Pharmacists are assisted by pharmacy technicians in several capacities to fulfill these obligations.

The pharmacy profession has roots dating back thousands of years and is based in the sciences of mathematics, chemistry, and medicine. Knowledge from these sciences is applied to the development and the study of drugs (pharmacology), how they are affected by the body (pharmacokinetics), and how the body is affected by the drugs (pharmacodynamics). Pharmacists and pharmacy technicians must be honest and ethical and protect the rights and privacy of patients. To establish and maintain a profession consistent with these goals, state boards of pharmacy enforce pharmacy laws and regulations and require practicing pharmacists to meet minimum education and experience standards. Some state boards of pharmacy also require that pharmacy technicians be registered or certified.

This chapter emphasizes the differences between the duties and responsibilities of pharmacy technicians and pharmacists and introduces technician competency expectations.

Pharmacy Training and Education

A *profession* is an occupation or vocation that requires advanced training in a liberal art or science. *Technicians* are persons skilled in the practical or mechanical aspects of a profession. Technicians assist professionals in

Learning Objectives

After completing this chapter, the technician should be able to

1. Outline the differences in responsibilities of pharmacy technicians and licensed pharmacists.

2. State the purpose of a policies and procedures manual.

3. Define differences between licensing and certification.

4. List four settings in which pharmacy is practiced.

5. List five functions that pharmacy technicians perform in various pharmacy settings.

6. Define pharmaceutical care.

7. Explain why the use of outpatient pharmacy and medical services is increasing.

routine, day-to-day functions that do not require professional judgment. Although technicians may be capable of functioning efficiently and safely without supervision, professionals are ultimately responsible for the technicians' activities and performance. Legally, professionals, such as pharmacists, are held liable for the performance of technicians; therefore, pharmacists must approve the technicians' work.

Pharmacy Technicians

Pharmacy technicians assist licensed pharmacists by completing tasks that do not require the professional judgment of a pharmacist and that can be reviewed by a licensed pharmacist to ensure accuracy. The assistance of technicians allows pharmacists to spend more time engaged in activities that require their professional judgment, such as patient care.

Training prerequisites for pharmacy technicians vary from state to state and from employer to employer, but most employers require pharmacy technicians to have at least a high school diploma. As the level of technician responsibility increases, so does the amount of required training or experience. Many employers have established criteria to classify technicians on the basis of their training or experience. For instance, a pharmacy technician 1 (PT-1) may be a newly hired technician who is responsible only for filling hospital unit-dose medication carts. A pharmacy technician 2 (PT-2) in that same hospital may have 5 years of job experience and be able to fill unit-dose medication carts, charge and credit patient accounts, compound (mix) intravenous (IV) solutions, and inventory narcotics. Similar classifications may exist in community pharmacies: A PT-1 might receive prescriptions as patients come to have them filled and check patients out at the cash register when they are ready to leave, whereas a PT-2 may be able to enter data in computerized patient profiles, label and fill prescriptions, or review patient insurance information. Technicians may be trained on the job or by completing a formal program, such as an associate degree program or course work at a community or technical college.

On-the-Job Training

Employers often offer on-the-job training to technicians. Technicians are trained to perform tasks specific to the job or position for which they were hired. Usually, technicians are taught only those skills they need to perform the particular job. For example, a technician may be trained on the job to fill prescriptions or unit-dose medication carts, compound IV solutions or medications, or enter prescription information into a computer database. When this type of training is very informal, another technician familiar with the job instructs the trainee; when it is more structured, the trainee participates in a training course developed by the employer. Some practice sites may offer training courses that consist of classroom teaching combined with hands-on experience that last from 1 week to 6 months. In addition to covering general pharmacy topics such as aseptic technique, pharmaceutical calculations, technician responsibilities, and pharmacy rules and regulations, these courses cover job-related issues such as patient confidentiality, organizational policies and procedures, and employee responsibilities.

Formal Programs

Community and technical college programs are broader in scope. These programs may be completed in 6 to 24 months and are more rigorous than on-the-job training. They cover all the technical duties related to pharmacy plus such topics as medical terminology, pharmaceutical calculations, drug distribution systems, IV admixture procedures, and medication packaging techniques. In these programs, student technicians gain skills, knowledge, and experience by attending classes and completing clerkships at local hospitals or community pharmacies. After completion of many of these programs, students will have earned an associate of science degree or a pharmacy technician certificate. Most programs offer full-time, part-time, and night classes plus financial assistance to those who qualify. Some may even be available as on-line distance learning programs.

Pharmacists

Pharmacists are professionals who have had advanced training in the pharmaceutical sciences. In all states, pharmacists must be licensed by the state's board of pharmacy before they can practice pharmacy and must follow the board of pharmacy regulations as they practice. In all states, licensed pharmacists supervise the activities of technicians and are held accountable for the technicians' performance.

Pharmacists must earn a college or university degree in pharmacy to become eligible to take the licensing examination offered by their state board of pharmacy. They learn how to use medical information to evaluate health care–related situations safely and effectively. Often, the answers are not black and white, so pharmacists must rely on their education and professional judgment to make the best decision. Two types of entry-level degrees, two main types of post-graduate degrees, and a number of postgraduate training opportunities are available for pharmacists.

To be eligible for enrollment in an entry-level pharmacy degree program, students must have completed a minimum of 2 years of college course work. The first professional college degree that pharmacists usually earn is either a bachelor of science (B.S.) in pharmacy or a doctor of pharmacy (Pharm.D.). Pharmacists with B.S. degrees have completed 5 years of college—2 years of general college courses followed by 3 years of pharmacy courses.

In the past, a pharmacist would have earned a Pharm.D. degree by attending 6 years of pharmacy school or by completing a 5-year B.S. program followed by an additional 2-year program. Currently, most schools of pharmacy are offering only a 6-year Pharm.D. degree. Many schools also offer "external Pharm.D." programs. Pharmacists with B.S. degrees who wish to earn a Pharm.D. degree may enroll in one of these programs. Using advanced communication technology such as videoconferencing and Internet Web sites, pharmacists can take classes from a school of pharmacy located any distance away, continue to work a full-time job, and maintain their family lives while fulfilling the requirements of a Pharm.D. degree. Pharmacists who choose this option are often those who have several years of experience working as pharmacists and desire to advance their education but have other obligations that make it impractical for them to return to college full-time. After earning an entry-level degree, many pharmacists elect to pursue a postgraduate degree, such as a master's in science (M.S.), which emphasizes the pharmaceutical sciences, or a master's in business administration (M.B.A.), which stresses the business aspects of pharmacy. Generally, an M.S. or M.B.A. requires 2 years of full-time study and production of a thesis. By completing 2 additional years of course work and another thesis, pharmacists with a master's degree can earn a doctor of philosophy (Ph.D.) degree in the pharmaceutical sciences or in social and administrative pharmacy. Some pharmacists combine their pharmacy degree with other degrees, such as law (J.D.) or medicine (M.D.).

Many pharmacists have also completed a 1- or 2-year postgraduate training program, called a residency. Residencies provide the opportunity to gain clinical experience, usually in a hospital setting, after earning a degree. Fellowships, usually 2 or 3 years in length, also provide postgraduate training, but they focus on pharmacy research rather than clinical pharmacy practice.

When filling prescriptions or physician orders, pharmacists must rely on their education and professional judgment to determine if the prescription is appropriate for each patient. They must verify that the medication is appropriate for the patient's condition, the dosage is correct, the patient is not allergic to the drug, and the prescribed medication will not interact with other medications the patient is taking. They must also counsel and educate the patient on how to take the medication properly and alert the patient to possible side effects of the drug. Pharmacists perform these functions every time a prescription or order is filled.

Policies and Procedures

Technicians must observe the policies and procedures (P&P) established by their practice sites and the pharmacy departments. P&P documents give guidance concerning the employer's expectations of the employees. They are compiled in a reference manual readily available for all employees. Many accrediting organizations, such as the Joint Commission on Accreditation of Healthcare Organizations (JCAHO), require that pharmacy departments develop P&P manuals.

P&P manuals cover broad areas, such as hiring requirements and employee benefits, relevant to all employees working for the organization. Departmental P&P are developed by individual departments and give direction on issues specific to those departments. P&P help coordinate the activities, for example, of the many departments in a hospital or stores in a corporate pharmacy chain. When each department or store knows what it can expect from the others, use of resources is more efficient, duplication of services may be reduced, and patient care is improved. Some P&P may be applicable to more than one department or store. For example, the pharmacy, nursing, and laboratory departments in a hospital may all share the same policy on disposal of used needles.

P&P manuals provide a guide for consistent orientation, training, and evaluation of personnel. These manuals set expectations for all employees so they know how to perform their jobs and how their job performance will be evaluated. Managers who evaluate employees use these written standards and expectations to measure employee performance so that they can identify personnel who are not performing up to the standard as well as recognize employees who are surpassing job expectations. Managers can evaluate the performance of individuals and the pharmacy as a whole by comparing the performance with the criteria set forth by the P&P.

Pharmacy department P&P address issues concerning the delivery of efficient, quality drug therapy, such as the following:

- Correct aseptic (sterile) technique when compounding IV admixtures or compounded medications
- Monitoring of patients for drug allergies
- Proper handling of cancer chemotherapeutic agents
- Distribution and control of all drugs used in the organization
- Ensuring that patients receive the correct drugs
- Use of investigational (experimental) drugs
- Management of toxic or dangerous drugs
- Provision for pharmacy services in the event of a disaster
- Identification of medications brought into the organization by patients
- Management of drug expenditures and the pharmacy budget

Pharmacy P&P are developed by the director or manager of pharmacy services with input from pharmacists, appropriate physicians, and other health care professionals. After the P&P are written, a committee reviews them before they are implemented. P&P are usually revised and updated annually. Most often, pharmacy P&P are reviewed by the Pharmacy and Therapeutics Committee, but other committees may also review the P&P that are pertinent to them. For example, the Infection Control Committee may review the pharmacy P&P on disposal of needles used to compound IV solutions, or the Oncology Committee may review the P&P on cleaning up spilled chemotherapy drugs. **Figures 1-1** and **1-2** show examples of a preface to a pharmacy P&P manual and a table of contents, respectively.

Position Descriptions

The P&P manual includes position, or job, descriptions. Position descriptions define the functions and tasks for which employees are responsible. They outline the authority of the positions, that is, who reports to the employee and to whom the employee reports. Other information, such as dress code, work schedule,

and the physical requirements of the position, may be included. Every position in the pharmacy, from director or manager to staff pharmacist to pharmacy technician, has a written position description. Two sample pharmacy technician position descriptions are shown in **Figures 1-3** and **1-4**. As the examples show, position descriptions vary from organization to organization and may even vary within an organization. A pharmacy often has several different technician position descriptions, each with its own set of duties and expectations.

A PT-1 may be responsible for such duties as entering medication orders into the pharmacy computer system, filling medication orders or prescriptions, stocking medication storage shelves, and maintaining automated unit-dose dispensing systems. As the PT-1 gains more experience and demonstrates competence in that position, he or she may move into a PT-2 position, which requires more responsibility and skill. An example of a PT-2 position is an IV admixture or compounding technician position, which requires the technician to be comfortable with mathematical calculations, have manual dexterity, and be able to follow sterile (aseptic) technique. Medications may be costly or may pose some risk to the technician if not stored, handled, and prepared properly, so it is very important that the technician be well trained for such a position. Technicians should be familiar with the description for the position(s) they fill in a pharmacy because they are often expected to perform in a number of positions, each with its own set of required skills and duties.

Licensure and Certification

The American Society of Health-System Pharmacists (ASHP) Task Force on Technical Personnel in Pharmacy has compiled definitions of the following terms:

- *Accreditation*—The process of granting recognition or vouching for conformance with established criteria (usually refers to recognition of an *institution*).[1]
- *Certification*—A voluntary process by which a nongovernmental agency or association grants recognition to an *individual* who has met certain predetermined qualifications specified by that agency or association. This recognition demonstrates to the public that the certified individual has achieved a certain level of knowledge, skill, or experience.[1]

PREFACE

I. PURPOSE

The purpose of a policy and procedure manual is to provide an authoritative source of official organizational policies, procedures, and practices, as well as to define operational responsibilities and the line of authority in the various areas within a department. The departmental *Policy and Procedure Manual* will serve:

A. As a means of standardizing and coordinating procedures
B. As a reference and guide for daily operations
C. As a means of orientation for new pharmacy personnel
D. As a central record of the departmental policies

II. MATERIALS INCLUDED IN THE MANUAL

The *Policy and Procedure Manual* is divided into five main areas:

  DIVISION 01 General
  DIVISION 02 Drug Distribution Division
  DIVISION 03 Administration and Technology Division
  DIVISION 04 Drug Information Division
  DIVISION 05 Clinical Services, Education, and Research Division

The divisions are subdivided into various chapters as listed in the table of contents to cover the topics included in each division.

III. AUTHORITY OF THIS MANUAL

A. The instructions contained in this manual are official and shall be relied upon as the basis for the performance of work. It is the responsibility of each employee to be thoroughly familiar with each policy and procedure covered in the manual that affects the scope of responsibility of that employee. Questions about any specific policy or procedure should be referred to the employee's supervisor for clarification. Since all conceivable work situations cannot be anticipated by an instruction, the policies and procedures set forth in this manual shall be regarded as guides to performance under related or analogous conditions.
B. Situations may arise where conformance with the instructions in this manual may not be possible. This may be because the original instructions may not have anticipated additional factors that may be present in a given situation. Whenever such a situation arises, the supervisor is expected to exercise judgment as to whether the instruction shall be suspended pending review by the director of pharmacy or in emergency situations whether other action is required, provided there is no violation of law or fixed hospital policy. This does not mean that the supervisor may, at will, suspend the effect of instruction with which he or she may not be in agreement. This shall be regarded as an emergency authority only, and in every case of the exercise of this authority, a full written report shall be made to the director of pharmacy. This report shall justify why emergency exception to the rules was taken without prior authorization.

IV. OTHER GENERAL PUBLISHED INSTRUCTIONS

A. Other general published instructions of the Department of Pharmacy shall be within the framework of the policies and procedures of this manual or shall be supplementary to it. In the event of conflict between other published instructions and this manual, the manual shall take precedence, unless otherwise specified.
B. Occasionally, it may be necessary to issue temporary instructions that will take precedence over materials in the manual. When this is done, the temporary instruction shall clearly state the exceptions and shall include a time limit for the temporary instructions.
C. If a supervisor should issue oral or written instructions in conflict with this manual, such superseding instructions shall be followed, but it is the responsibility of the person receiving them to point out the conflict with the manual. This shall be regarded as an emergency authority only, and in every case of the exercise of this authority, a full report shall be made to the director of pharmacy. This report shall justify why emergency exception to the rules was taken without prior authorization.

V. HOW TO FIND MATERIAL

The material covered by this manual has been organized into divisions, chapters, sections, parts, and subparts. All subdivisions are numbered with Arabic numerals. A typical section designation, therefore, would be 01-20-15:

  DIVISION 01 General
  CHAPTER 20 Policy and Procedure Manual
  SECTION 15 Distribution

When more than one page is required for a particular part or subpart, a dash and the letter "A" shall follow the first page number. The second page would be "B" and so on, as necessary. Through reference to the table of contents, one may ordinarily find all related material together. Sample forms will appear at the end of each division and will be numbered consecutively within each division.

VI. NEW MATERIAL AND REVISIONS

Chapters, sections, parts, and subparts are numbered so that additional information may be inserted without altering the numbering system; that is, originally every fifth digit was used. In most cases, a draft of proposed new material will be sent to all concerned individuals so that suggestions and recommendations can be made. All new material, as well as revisions of old material, will be placed in each volume of the manual by the secretarial staff, at which time a copy, under cover of a transmittal memorandum, where necessary, will be sent to each employee concerned, stating that the attached policy and procedure has been placed in the manuals. A copy of the *Policy and Procedure Manual* will be located in each area of the Department of Pharmacy and will be available to any departmental employee.

Figure 1-1. Preface to pharmacy policies and procedures manual.

Source: Hethcox JM. The policy and procedure manual. In: Handbook of institutional pharmacy practice. 3rd ed. Brown TR, ed. Bethesda, MD: American Society of Hospital Pharmacists; 1992:60.

Figure 1-2. Portion of a table of contents of a pharmacy department policies and procedures manual, illustrating content organization based on departmental management responsibilities.

Source: Ginnow WK, King CM Jr. Revision and reorganization of a hospital pharmacy policies and procedures manual. *Am J Hosp Pharm.* 1978; 35:698–704.

JOB DESCRIPTION: SUPPORTIVE PERSONNEL

REPORTS TO: Director of pharmacy and staff pharmacist(s)

SUPERVISES: N/A

EDUCATION/
TRAINING: High school diploma or equivalent preferred; typing skills required

EXPERIENCE: Institutional pharmacy experience preferred

WORK SCHEDULE: May be required to work rotating shifts, including weekends and holidays

PHYSICAL
REQUIREMENTS: May require standing for long periods; may require lifting of heavy boxes

OCCUPATIONAL
HAZARDS: May be exposed to potentially hazardous and toxic substances

APPEARANCE: Neat, professional appearance required

ATTITUDE: Courteous, cooperative attitude required

Responsibilities and Duties

Responsibilities of pharmacy supportive personnel include compliance with all applicable policies, procedures, codes, and standards of the facility. Supportive personnel work under the direct supervision of a licensed pharmacist and do not perform duties that can legally be performed only by a licensed pharmacist.

The following duties are *representative* of the position. Additional duties and projects may be assigned.

- Assist pharmacists in providing effective, appropriate, and safe pharmacy services.
- Participate in pharmacy orientation programs, training programs for pharmacy supportive personnel, pharmacy staff meetings, and inservice educational programs.
- Assist in maintaining the cleanliness and orderliness of the pharmacy.
- Maintain records.
- Issue supplies to other departments.
- Assist in stock control (inventorying, stocking, pricing, and monitoring usage).
- Pick up and deliver drug orders.
- Participate in activities that resolve unsafe and unsanitary practices.
- Attend and participate in other programs, committees, meetings, and functions required by the facility or the pharmacy.

Reviewed and accepted:

_____   _____
Supportive Staff Member   Date

_____   _____
Supervisor   Date

Figure 1-3. Example of a position description for a pharmacy technician.

Source: Ploetz PA, Woller TW. Pharmacy technicians. In: Handbook of institutional pharmacy practice. 3rd ed. Brown TR, ed. Bethesda, MD: American Society of Hospital Pharmacists; 1992:401.

POSITION DESCRIPTION OF A PHARMACY TECHNICIAN

DIVISION	01	General
CHAPTER	10	Department of Pharmaceutical Services
SECTION	15	Position Description
PART	05	Drug Distribution
SUBPART	30	Pharmacy Technician

Immediate Superior: Appropriate Section Supervisor or Pharmacist on duty during Supervisor's absence

Immediate Subordinate: None

Authority: Proceed within the expressed limits of established policies and procedures securing approval from the Supervisor or Pharmacist on duty for deviations from same.

Responsibilities

1. Be familiar with, understand, and comply with all policies and procedures affecting the scope of responsibility as compiled in the Department of Pharmaceutical Services Policy and Procedure Manual.
2. Respond to the Hospitals' Disaster Call at any time of day or night.
3. Work cooperatively with all Hospitals and Health Science Center employees and promote and maintain good interpersonal and interdepartmental relationships.
4. Maintain good relationships with the public in behalf of the Department of Pharmaceutical Services and the University of Minnesota Hospitals.
5. Advise Supervisor of malfunctioning equipment and unsafe equipment.
6. Make recommendation to the Supervisor as to how methods and procedures can be improved.
7. Observe and report to the Supervisor any unusual situations, occurrences, conditions, or complaints including those related to drugs, drug requests, drug usage, or security within the Pharmacy or the Hospitals.
8. Perform other related duties as assigned by authorized personnel or as may be required to meet emergency situations.
9. Keep work area in a clean and orderly manner.
10. Perform oral and/or written requests given by the Supervisor or other Pharmacists. Conflicting instructions should be resolved by the Supervisor or in his (or her) absence, the Administrative Pharmacy Officer.
11. Be accountable for the time period in which scheduled to work in dispensing area to the Supervisor or to the Pharmacist in charge. Notify the Supervisor or Pharmacist in charge when leaving the area assigned for breaks or meals.
12. Have all work checked by a Pharmacist.
13. When assigned to Inpatient area, perform duties according to Policy and Procedure on Inpatient Responsibility of Personnel (02-10-10-20). The ratio of technicians to pharmacists in this area shall not exceed 1 to 1.
14. When assigned to unit dose activities in the pharmacy satellites, perform duties according to Policy and Procedure on Technician Daily Procedures (02-20-10). The ratio of technicians to pharmacists in this area shall not exceed 3 to 1.
    a. Maintain adequate supplies of controlled substances on all nursing areas served by the satellite.
    b. Change unit dose medication cassettes.
    c. Periodically inventory the area and reorder additional supplies of drugs from Central Pharmacy as needed.
    d. Restock shelves in the dispensing areas upon receipt of stock replacement.
    e. Fill unit dose medication drawers.
    f. Prepare IV admixture solutions as required.
    g. Prepare extemporaneous package injectable and oral dosage forms.
    h. Fill new medication orders.
    i. Enter new medication orders into the computer.
    j. Type accurate and legible labels for IV admixtures, packaged doses, and pass/self meds.
15. When assigned to the Outpatient area, perform duties according to Policy and Procedure on Outpatient Responsibilities to Personnel (02-15-10).
16. When assigned to the IV Admixture Sterile Prep Packaging Service:
    a. Prepare IV Admixtures, Total Parenteral Nutrition Solutions (TPN), Antilymphocytic Globulin Solutions (ALG, ATG, IGG), skin test antigens, antibiotic piggybacks and syringes, and other sterile products as requested.
    b. Perform all clerical work associated with the IV Admixture Service such as calculations, computer processing, typing, coordinating, and workload statistics.
    c. Monitor credits returned, reissuing appropriate preparations and discarding expired ones.
    d. The ratio of technicians to pharmacists in this area shall not exceed 3 to 1.
17. When assigned as the Controlled Substance Courier, maintain adequate supplies of controlled substances on all nursing areas' maintained controlled substance floorstock.
18. Answer the telephone in assigned areas as per Departmental Policy and Procedures on Telephone Communications (01-45-05).

Figure 1-4. Example of a position description for a pharmacy technician.

Source: Coe CP. Elements of quality in pharmaceutical care. Bethesda, MD: American Society of Hospital Pharmacists; 1992:219.

- *Credentialing*—The process of formally verifying and assessing professional or technical competence.[1]

- *Licensure*—The process by which an agency of government grants permission to an individual to engage in a given occupation upon finding that the applicant has attained the minimal degree of competency necessary to ensure that the public health, safety, and welfare will be reasonably well protected.[1]

- *Registration*—The process of making a list or being enrolled in an existing list. Registration may be required to legally carry out some functions.[2]

Technicians

Certain professional organizations, including ASHP, the American Pharmaceutical Association (APhA), the American Association of Colleges of Pharmacy (AACP), and the National Association of Boards of Pharmacy (NABP), became jointly involved with the Scope of Pharmacy Practice Project. The objective of the project was to perform a validated task analysis of the functions, responsibilities, and tasks of pharmacists and technicians. This analysis documented what pharmacy technicians do and what knowledge they need to effectively perform those activities.

Participants in the Scope of Pharmacy Practice Project recognized the need for a national technician certification program for credentialing, accrediting, certifying, licensing, or registering technicians, to replace the various state programs that now exist. In 1995, APhA, ASHP, the Illinois Council of Hospital Pharmacists (ICHP), and the Michigan Pharmacists Association (MPA) established the Pharmacy Technician Certification Board (PTCB). The PTCB was created to develop a voluntary national pharmacy technician certification program.[3] Previously, the pharmacy profession had not established standardized technician training programs or licensing procedures to the extent it had for pharmacists.

Some states, such as Texas, now require certification of pharmacy technicians; others are considering it.[4] The NABP also supports a national program to assess technician compentency.[5] Technicians who wish to become certified may take the National Pharmacy Technician Certification Examination offered by the PTCB. The first such examination was held in 1995. To take the examination, candidates must have a high school diploma or a graduate equivalency diploma

(GED), must never have been convicted of a felony, and must submit the appropriate application form, fees, and supporting documents. This 3-hour, closed-book examination consists of 125 multiple-choice questions plus an additional 15 nonscored questions. The nonscored questions are pretest questions and are not used in calculating the candidate's score, but provide information for possible use on future examinations. Each question has four possible answers to choose from, with only one being the correct or best answer. The score is based on the number of correctly answered questions.

The questions are written to assess the knowledge and skills that are deemed necessary to perform the work of pharmacy technicians. The exam divides these activities into three function areas:

I. *Assisting the pharmacist in serving patients,* including activities related to dispensing prescriptions, distributing medications, and collecting and organizing information

II. *Maintaining medication and inventory control systems,* pertaining to activities related to purchasing medications and supplies, controlling inventory, and storing, preparing, and distributing medications according to policies and procedures

III. *Participating in the administration and management of pharmacy practice,* including administrative activities that deal with such issues as operations, human resources, facilities and equipment, and information systems

Sixty-four percent of the examination tests the candidate on topics in function I, 25 percent in function II, and the remaining 11 percent in function III. Candidates who have passed the exam may use the designation *CPhT* (certified pharmacy technician) after their names. To maintain the certification, technicians must recertify every 2 years by completing at least 20 hours of continuing education. A maximum of 10 hours may be earned at the technician's workplace under the direct supervision of a pharmacist. These credits must be special assignments or training; regular work hours do not apply. At least 1 hour of continuing education must be related to pharmacy law. Several references are available to assist candidates preparing for the examination. More information about the exam can be obtained from the Pharmacy Technician Certification Board at 2215 Constitution Avenue, NW, Washington, DC 20037-2985, (202) 429-7576, or on its Web site at www.ptcb.org.

Currently, ASHP accredits pharmacy technician training programs. Most of these programs are offered by vocational, technical, and community colleges. Accreditation standardizes the formal training that pharmacy technicians receive; it also provides institutions that offer a technician training program with guidelines on how to train competent pharmacy technicians. Pharmacy technician training programs must meet the minimum criteria set by ASHP to earn accreditation.[6]

Pharmacists

After earning a B.S. degree or Pharm.D. degree, candidates must pass an examination administered by their state's board of pharmacy. The board of pharmacy includes pharmacists and members of the public who have been appointed to the board by the state governor. The members of a state board of pharmacy are responsible for protecting the citizens of their state. The board does so by passing pharmacy rules and regulations to be followed in addition to the laws enacted by the state legislature.[7] Once candidates have passed their state's board of pharmacy examination, they become registered pharmacists (R.Ph.) and are allowed to practice pharmacy in that state.[2]

Some pharmacists choose to become certified as pharmacotherapy specialists. After passing a day-long certification examination, they earn the title of Board Certified Pharmacy Specialist and may add the initials BCPS to their credentials. These pharmacists must still comply with the requirements of their state's board of pharmacy. There are also certification examinations in nutrition support, nuclear pharmacy, psychiatric pharmacy, and oncology. Other specialty certification examinations are under development.

Pharmacy Practice Settings

Pharmacy is practiced in many environments, which are commonly divided into *ambulatory care* and *institutional* settings. Ambulatory care settings are those, such as community, home care, and mail order, that serve patients living in their own homes or similar situations. Institutional settings are those in which patients receive long- or short-term care by health professionals. The two primary institutional settings are long-term care and hospitals. Other pharmacy practice settings include ambulatory clinics, managed care, hospice care, research facilities, educational centers, and the pharmaceutical industry.

Although the specific pharmacy activities of practice settings may vary, the primary goal of each remains the same: to ensure that patients receive the proper drug therapy for their medical conditions.

Community Pharmacy

The community pharmacy is the corner drugstore or the local retail or grocery store pharmacy; the average person is probably most familiar with this practice site. Community pharmacies can be members of a chain of pharmacies or can be independently owned. Usually, patients are customers who are being treated by doctors as outpatients and come into the store with prescriptions. Generally, these patients live in their own homes under their own care.

Technicians in community settings often prepare prescription labels to be checked by a pharmacist, order and maintain drug inventory, process insurance claims, and operate a cash register.

Mail Order Pharmacy

Pharmacists and technicians also work in mail order facilities, where patients may have their prescriptions filled and refilled through the mail. A major difference between mail order pharmacies and community pharmacies is the lack of face-to-face contact with the patients. Mail order pharmacists, however, must use the same degree of professional judgment that is used in community or institutional settings. Technicians' duties in a mail order pharmacy are similar to those in the community setting.

Managed Care

A managed care program is simply a type of health insurance program that allows patients to pay a blanket fee for their health care services rather than the traditional fee for service. Managed care programs attempt to improve the quality of health care delivery and patient outcomes. One definition of a managed care prescription program is "the application of management principles to achieve maximum health outcomes at the lowest cost."[8] Pharmacists who work in managed care environments may not have direct patient contact but may instead manage drug therapy on a global basis by collecting information from patients' computerized medication profiles and pooling it into a large database. Prescription drug use and physician prescribing patterns are then analyzed for trends that indicate optimal or suboptimal medication therapy. Pharmacists subsequently try to minimize drug costs and improve patient outcomes or results through the development of drug formularies and disease-specific drug therapy guidelines.

Technicians in a managed care setting may collect data, research information, or assist pharmacists in writing reports.

Hospital Pharmacy

Patients are admitted to hospitals for short-term supervised medical care by health care professionals in a structured, formal manner. Pharmacists are directly involved with patient care and have daily interactions with physicians, nurses, and other caregivers. They develop plans of pharmaceutical care and, with the other caregivers, monitor the patients' drug therapy. Depending on the size of the hospital, some pharmacists provide specialized services in areas such as pediatrics, oncology, infectious diseases, nutrition support, and drug information. In addition to providing direct patient care, pharmacists evaluate trends in medication use and physician prescribing, develop guidelines for medication use, educate patients and health care professionals, and implement and maintain drug distribution systems. They also work with nurses, physicians, and other members of hospital committees and work groups, both within and outside of the pharmacy department.[9]

Technicians who work in hospitals work with pharmacists to accomplish many of the pharmacy's goals. Generally, technicians spend time entering physician medication orders into a computer, preparing IV drug admixtures, repackaging and labeling unit dose medications, delivering medications, and completing paperwork for quality assurance or billing purposes.

Long-Term Care

Long-term facilities are those where patients stay for extended periods. They include nursing homes, mental or psychiatric institutions, intermediate-care facilities for mentally retarded patients, and skilled nursing facilities. Patients in these settings require professional care but not to the same degree that hospitalized patients do. Pharmacists and technicians in long-term care practices perform many of the same activities as those in hospital settings.

Home Health Care

Home health care is defined as "physician ordered services provided to patients at their residences, be it their own homes or any other setting in which the patients live."[10] Such services may include personal care; respite care; shopping assistance; drug and infusion therapy; or

speech, physical, or occupational therapy.[10, 11] Home care pharmacists assess the patient for the appropriateness of home medication administration, and if they find it is appropriate, go on to develop a pharmaceutical care plan to monitor and educate the patient. Medications administered in the home setting may be as simple as oral tablets or capsules or as complex as drug therapy administered intravenously.

Technician duties in a home care setting may include preparing IV and sterile products, maintaining computerized patient profiles, and accompanying a pharmacist to a patient's home.

Expansion of Technician Responsibilities

Table 1-1 lists some of the functions that pharmacy technicians perform in pharmacy settings around the country. Some of the functions listed are not routinely performed by technicians in most inpatient or outpatient pharmacies but are viewed by some pharmacists as appropriate for the future if training is provided and current limitations are removed.

Trends in Pharmacy Practice

Focus on Providing Pharmaceutical Care

The concept of pharmaceutical care was introduced in the early 1990s. *Pharmaceutical care* is defined as "the direct, responsible provision of medication-related care for the purpose of achieving definite outcomes that improve a patient's quality of life."[21]

Pharmaceutical care involves cooperation between a pharmacist, patient, and other health care professionals in designing, implementing, and monitoring a therapeutic medication plan. It consists of three major functions: (1) identification of potential and actual drug-related problems, (2) resolution of actual drug-related problems, and (3) prevention of potential drug-related problems. Pharmaceutical care makes the pharmacist directly responsible to the patient for the quality of that care. The basic goals, processes, and relationships of pharmaceutical care are the same regardless of practice setting.[21]

Increasing Impact of Technology

Technical advances are changing the practice of pharmacy. New machines and systems have been developed to help dispense medications and monitor medication use more accurately, timely, and cost-effectively. Because advanced computer systems collect and store patient information, that information is more

TABLE 1-1.[12-20] **FUNCTIONS OF PHARMACY TECHNICIANS**

Information Management

- Assist with drug use evaluations and quality improvement activities
- Collect data for drug therapy monitoring activities
- Collect data for pharmacokinetic activities
- Enter orders into a computer or patient profile
- Maintain patient medication profiles
- Provide drug information (e.g., available dosage forms and strengths, costs, or package size) to patients, nurses, and physicians

Medication Preparation

- Compound and reconstitute medications
- Perform mathematical calculations
- Prepare parenteral nutrient solutions and antineoplastic agents
- Prepare IV fluids and medications
- Repackage and label unit dose drugs

Medication Dispensing

- Certify the complete drug order/prescription
- Check the work of other technicians:
  - Check medication orders/prescriptions filled by other technicians
  - Check IV admixtures made by other technicians
  - Check order entries made by other technicians
- Deliver medications and controlled substances to patient care areas
- Fill and price outpatient prescriptions
- Fill orders for floor stock drugs
- Fill patient medication carts/cabinets
- Inspect and maintain emergency medication carts
- Inspect drug storage and patient care areas
- Provide drugs for medical emergency responses
- Receive oral requests from a nurse or oral orders/prescriptions from a physician (may be prohibited in some states)
- Review patient profiles for completeness of information (e.g., allergy history, patient age, height, and weight)
- Verify the completeness (e.g., drug name, strength, and directions) of a physician's order/prescription

Medication Inventory Management

- Audit controlled substances
- Control pharmacy purchases and inventory
- Initiate purchase orders
- Obtain drugs for decentralized pharmacists

Training

- Train other technicians

accurate and easier to access. Checks and balances (e.g., checks for drug interactions, patient allergies, and duplicate therapy) are built into computer systems, resulting in fewer errors. Automation of these checks and balances and other traditional functions allows pharmacists more time for activities that require their professional judgment and expertise. In turn, pharmacists are relying more than ever on technicians to operate and maintain these new systems.

Increasing Use of Outpatient Services

More and more, patients are cared for and treated as outpatients. This is a result of the increased need to contain the skyrocketing costs of health care. Patients who in the past would have been admitted to a hospital 2 or 3 days before surgery now are admitted on the day of the procedure and discharged earlier as well. Many hospitals have established outpatient surgery centers that admit patients for surgery and release them a few hours later. For many diagnostic tests, patients are no longer admitted to a hospital; they are seen as outpatients and allowed to go home shortly after the tests.

The practice of pharmacy is changing to adapt to this new environment. Some clinics and outpatient centers have pharmacists and pharmacies available on-site. In these settings, pharmacists have less time to gather patient information and provide pharmaceutical care.[22]

Summary

Pharmacy technicians now commonly review and fill medication orders or prescriptions that are later checked by a pharmacist. Technicians also do most of the IV admixture and sterile compounding. More and more of the computer-entry functions, such as patient billing and order entry, are also the responsibility of technicians. In some settings, technicians may check each other's work,[13,16] dispense medications from a pre-approved list,[18] or even administer medications.[19,20]

Given the changes occurring in the pharmacy profession, the roles of pharmacy technicians are expanding, and more is expected from technicians than in the past. Increasingly, technicians have become primarily responsible for the mechanical and routine aspects of pharmacy practice, allowing pharmacists to expand their practices.

Recommended Reading

American Society of Health-System Pharmacists. Model curriculum for pharmacy technician training. 2nd ed. Bethesda, MD; 2001. http://www.ashp.org/ technician/model_curriculum/ UserGuide.pdf (accessed 2003 Dec 2).

American Society of Health-System Pharmacists. Chronology of ASHP activities for pharmacy technicians. http://ashp.org/technician/ chronology.cfm?cfid=24092673&CFToken=32010507 (accessed 2003 Dec 2).

American Society of Hospital Pharmacists. ASHP statement on pharmaceutical care. Am J Hosp Pharm. 1993; 50:1720–3.

American Society of Hospital Pharmacists. ASHP accreditation standard for pharmacy technician training programs. http://ashp.org/technician/ FinalDraftAugust2002.pdf (accessed 2003 Dec 2).

American Society of Hospital Pharmacists. Technician training programs accreditation regulations and standards: ASHP regulations on accreditation of pharmacy technician training programs. http:// ashp.org/technician/techregs.pdf (accessed 2003 Dec 2).

Blake KM. How to achieve teamwork between pharmacists and technicians: a technician's perspective. Am J Hosp Pharm. 1992; 49:2133, 2137.

Knapp DA. Pharmacy practice in 2040. Am J Hosp Pharm. 1992; 49:2457–61.

McFarland HM. How to achieve teamwork between pharmacists and technicians: a pharmacist's perspective. Am J Hosp Pharm. 1992; 49:1665–6.

Smith JE. The national voluntary certification program for pharmacy technicians. Am J Health-Syst Pharm. 1995; 52:2026–9.

Whitney HAK Jr. Pharmacy's version of "The Wizard of Oz." Ann Pharmacother. 1992; 26:996–8.

References

1. Credentialing in pharmacy. Am J Health-Syst Pharm. 2001; 58:69–76.

2. White paper on pharmacy technicians: Recommendations of pharmacy practitioner organizations on the functions, training, and regulation of technicians. Am J Health-Syst Pharm. 1996; 53:1793–6.

3. Zellmer WA. Pharmacy technicians, part 1: national certification. Am J Health-Syst Pharm. 1995; 52:918. Editorial.

4. Landis NT. Certification now required for Texas pharmacy technicians. *Am J Health-Syst Pharm.* 2001; 58:204.

5. NAPB proposes national competence assessment of technicians. *Am J Health-Syst Pharm.* 2000; 57:1204.

6. American Society of Hospital Pharmacists. White paper on pharmacy technicians 2002: needed changes can no longer wait. *Am J Health-Syst Pharm.* 2003; 60:37–51.

7. Vandel JH. A board of pharmacy member's viewpoints on the technician issue. *Am J Hosp Pharm.* 1989; 46:545–7.

8. Schafermeyer KW. Overview of pharmacy in managed health care. In: A pharmacist's guide to principles and practices of managed care pharmacy. Alexandria, VA: Foundation for Managed Care Pharmacy; 1995:15–26.

9. American Society of Health-System Pharmacists. ASHP guidelines: minimum standard for pharmacies in hospitals. *Am J Health-Syst Pharm.* 1995; 52:2711–7.

10. Catania PN. Introduction to home health care. In: Home health care practice. 2nd ed. Palo Alto, CA: The Pocket Press; 1994:1–11.

11. American Society of Hospital Pharmacists. ASHP guidelines on the pharmacist's role in home care. *Am J Hosp Pharm.* 2000; 57:1252–7.

12. Henderson D, Johnson-Choong S, Wiles S. Pharmacy technician's role in an ambulatory care infusion clinic. *Am J Health-Syst Pharm.* 2000; 57:1664–5.

13. Ambrose PJ, Saya FG, Lovett LT et al. Evaluating the accuracy of technicians and pharmacists in checking unit dose medication cassettes. *Am J Health-Syst Pharm.* 2002; 59:1183–8.

14. Scott DM, Hospodka RJ. Pedersen CA et al. Pharmacist's assessment of technician use in Nebraska. *Am J Health-Syst Pharm.* 2000; 57:2206–10.

15. Ervin CKA, Skledar S, Hess MM et al. Data analyst technician: an innovative role for the pharmacy technician. *Am J Health Syst Pharm.* 2001; 58:1815–8.

16. Andersen SR, St Peter JV, Macres MG et al. Accuracy of technicians versus pharmacists in checking syringes prepared for a dialysis program. *Am J Health-Syst Pharm.* 1997; 54:1611–13.

17. Koch KE, Weeks A. Clinically oriented pharmacy technicians to augment clinical services. *Am J Health-Syst Pharm.* 1998; 55:1375–81.

18. Kalman MK, Witkowski DE, Ogawa GS. Increasing pharmacy productivity by expanding the role of pharmacy technicians. *Am J Hosp Pharm.* 1992; 49:84–9.

19. Scala SM, Schneider PJ, Smith GL Jr et al. Activity analysis of pharmacy directed drug administration technicians. *Am J Hosp Pharm.* 1986; 43:1702–6.

20. Fillmore AD, Schneider PJ, Bourret JA et al. Costs of training drug administration technicians. *Am J Hosp Pharm.* 1986; 43:1706–9.

21. Hepler CD, Strand LM. Opportunities and responsibilities in pharmaceutical care. *Am J Hosp Pharm.* 1990; 47:533–43.

22. American Society of Health-System Pharmacists. ASHP guidelines: minimum standard for pharmaceutical services in ambulatory care. http://www.ashp.com/bestpractices/PracticeSettings/Guide/264-272-%20Amb.%20care.pdf (accessed 2002 Sep 20).

Self-Assessment Questions

1. What is certification?
   a. the process of formally verifying and assessing professional or technical competence
   b. a voluntary process by which a nongovernmental agency or association grants recognition to an *individual* who has met certain predetermined qualifications specified by that agency or association
   c. the process of granting recognition or vouching for conformance with established criteria
   d. the process by which an agency of government grants permission to an individual to engage in a given occupation upon finding that the individual applicant has attained a minimal degree of competency

2. What is the process of granting recognition or vouching for conformance with established criteria called?
   a. accreditation
   b. certification
   c. licensure
   d. registration

3. Who is ultimately responsible for a pharmacy technician's activities and performance?
   a. the technician
   b. the patient's physician
   c. the technician with the most experience and seniority
   d. the supervising pharmacist

4. How can a pharmacy technician become certified?
   a. by submitting the proper application and documentation to the state board of pharmacy
   b. by working as a pharmacy technician for a number of years as specified by the state medical board
   c. by passing a national examination that evaluates the technician's knowledge and skills needed to perform the work of pharmacy technicians
   d. by passing a test offered by the National Association of Boards of Pharmacy that assesses the technician's knowledge of drug therapy and pharmacokinetics

5. Which of the following activities is a typical pharmacy technician duty?
   a. recommending an antibiotic to treat an ear infection in an infant to a physician
   b. filling a unit-dose cassette for a nursing home
   c. giving a nurse an order for an alternative medication to morphine in a patient who has had an allergic reaction to morphine in the past
   d. filling in for a pharmacist when she is on her lunch break

6. What does *pharmaceutical care* refer to?
   a. proper storage and handling of medication
   b. medication-related advertising that is directed to consumers from the drug manufacturers
   c. information provided to physicians and other health care professionals by pharmacists
   d. cooperation among a pharmacist, patient, and other health care professionals to best serve the patient's drug-related needs

7. A(n)_____ pharmacy practice setting is one where pharmacists care for patients in their own places of residence.
   a. home health care
   b. institutional
   c. acute care
   d. ambulatory

8. A_____ provides guidance in areas such as personnel orientation, training and evaluation, correct aseptic (sterile) technique, and administration of medications by personnel other than registered nurses.
   a. technician's manual
   b. policies and procedures manual
   c. pharmacy guidebook
   d. medication dispensing regulation

9. As a pharmacy technician, you may perform all *except* which of the following activities?
   a. entering orders into a computer or patient profile
   b. performing mathematical calculations
   c. checking the work of other technicians
   d. changing the dose of a prescribed medication on the basis of a patient's poor kidney function

10. A pharmacy technician job (or position) description_____.
    a. is the same as a pharmacist's, but the technician's work must be checked by the pharmacist
    b. is the same for each technician position within a practice setting
    c. outlines the expectations, functions, and tasks of a specific technician position
    d. formally verifies and assesses the competence of a pharmacy technician working in a specific technician position

Self-Assessment Answers

1. b. Certification is a voluntary process achieved by meeting established criteria. Letter a corresponds to credentialing; c is accreditation and is generally granted to the organization while certification is personal; and d is licensure.

2. a. Certification is associated with personal achievement of standard criteria, while accreditation is associated with organizational achievement. Licensure is a governmental recognition of the right to perform a specific occupation. Registration is a listing function.

3. d. While the physician may be ultimately responsible for a patient's care, the pharmacist is ultimately responsible for the actions of technicians working under his or her supervision.

4. c. Certification is offered by an independent organization and is not affiliated with either the State Boards of Pharmacy or the National Association of Boards of Pharmacy. Although working as a technician for a number of years might increase the likelihood of passing the certification exam, it is not sufficient to earn certification.

5. b. All the other answers are tasks that must be done by a pharmacist.

6. d. Medication storage and handling as well as both consumer and professional information may be parts of pharmaceutical care, but the more comprehensive definition of serving the patient's drug related needs is the correct answer.

7. a. Home health care pharmacists serve the patients in their own homes. Institutional and acute care pharmacists generally work in hospitals or long term care facilities. Ambulatory pharmacists generally see patients in an outpatient setting but do not serve patients directly in their homes.

8. b. Policies and procedures generally guide the technician in a number of training and performance areas. A technician manual is generally more related to job tasks and would not typically include information about evaluation, for example.

9. d. The other functions listed are acceptable for technicians to perform, but a pharmacist must do all dose adjustments.

10. c. Technicians would typically not have the same job description as pharmacists. A technician job description may be the same for each technician position within a practice setting, or it may vary based on job assignment and expected activities. Job descriptions express expectations but do not serve to assess competence.

Ambulatory Care Pharmacy Practice

RICHARD K. LEWIS

This chapter describes those characteristics of pharmacy practice that are unique to ambulatory care and the important role pharmacy technicians play in providing pharmacy services in this setting. Specifically, this chapter will offer a review of ambulatory care pharmacy history and current practices; compare and contrast different types of ambulatory care practices; and describe the activities performed by pharmacy technicians in this environment. It will also emphasize the importance of customer service and communication skills and discuss third-party payer programs, claims processing, and formularies as components of pharmacy workflow. Finally, a list of abbreviations for this chapter appears at the end of the chapter.

Many of the issues important to an ambulatory care setting are covered in other chapters. In particular, it may be useful to review the chapters on law, calculations, and interpreting medication orders.

Historical Overview and Current Practices

The majority of pharmacy practice takes place in an ambulatory care setting, and this setting has been the basis of the public's perception of pharmacy for hundreds of years. Over time, pharmacy practice in ambulatory care has changed significantly. Historically, the pharmacist (or apothecary) compounded medications in the corner drug store and often was consulted by patients to help treat their common ailments. In fact, prior to the enactment of the 1951 Durham–Humphrey Amendment to the Food, Drug and Cosmetic Act, there was no definition of prescription drugs, allowing pharmacists to dispense medications without a physician's order. Of course, now pharmacists can dispense prescription drugs only upon receipt of a valid prescription.

The mass production of pharmaceuticals by large drug companies began in the 1950s and resulted in several changes. The need for pharmacists to compound prescriptions decreased, and many community pharmacies became more focused on selling a large variety of retail items. As this trend continued, pharmacists spent less time talking to patients about

Learning Objectives

After completing this chapter, the technician should be able to

1. Discuss the history and current practices of pharmacy in ambulatory care.

2. List the similarities and differences among the variety of ambulatory care practice sites (chain, independent, clinic, managed care, and mail order).

3. Explain the importance of exceptional customer service and communication skills in the outpatient pharmacy environment.

4. Explain the typical prescription distribution process in an ambulatory care pharmacy.

5. Describe the role of the technician in ambulatory care pharmacy.

6. Describe the impact of third-party payment programs on prescription processing in ambulatory care.

their medications. In fact, in the 1960s, many professional pharmacy organizations encouraged pharmacists to refrain from discussing medication issues with patients, and many pharmacy schools taught students that such activity would interfere with the physician–patient relationship.

During the 1970s, some pharmacists began practicing "clinical pharmacy." Clinical pharmacists, who primarily practiced in hospitals, were monitoring specific drugs, rounding with the medical team, and filling an important role in hospital patient care. One of the reasons this practice occurred in the hospital was because of the pharmacists' ability to reduce costs. In addition, pharmacy organizations and pharmacy schools began encouraging patient–pharmacist interaction. During this time, pharmacists practicing in ambulatory care settings continued to focus on prescription dispensing, and there was an expansion in chain pharmacies. Unlike the hospital setting, there was little financial pressure to reduce unnecessary prescription use in the ambulatory care setting because most patients still paid cash for their prescriptions.

In the 1980s, the cost of health care became a significant public policy issue, and managed care began to grow. With managed care came restructuring of health care reimbursement and the movement to minimize the amount of time patients spend in hospitals. In ambulatory care, pharmacist–patient communication was emphasized, and the role of the pharmacy technician was expanded to include more prescription-filling activities.

In the 1990s, health care reform became a major item on political agendas. While "health care reform" was debated, little was accomplished on the legislative level. However, major payers forced market change by demanding lower costs for health care. With respect to pharmacy, there was a great deal of debate about the cost of pharmaceuticals. Attempts to manage the cost of pharmacy services and products resulted in the expansion of managed care and mail-order pharmacy operations and the advent of pharmacy benefit management firms (PBMs). One of the most significant changes during this period was the enactment of the Omnibus Budget Reconciliation Act of 1990 (OBRA 90), which required states to implement drug use review (DUR) programs within their Medicaid systems. A major component of DUR programs was the requirement that pharmacists review a patient's prescriptions for drug-related problems and, at least, offer counseling on prescription medications at the time of dispensing. Many states added the DUR/counseling requirement to their pharmacy practice acts to include all patients, not just Medicaid patients.

As health care progresses into the new millennium, interesting changes have taken place. The move to restrictive managed care plans, such as staff model health maintenance organizations (HMOs), has slowed and perhaps reversed. Concern over health care reform has been replaced by concern over patient safety, patient privacy via Health Insurance Portability and Accountability Act (HIPAA) regulations, and the potential for Medicare to cover prescription drugs for the elderly. However, the concern over controlling health care costs remains. Some mechanisms to control cost have changed. For instance, Medicare has implemented an Ambulatory Payment Classification System (APCS) to control outpatient costs. In the 90s, there was considerable discussion about including ambulatory care pharmacy in capitation plans (a set payment amount per patient per month regardless of the health and related expenses associated with the patient). Today, the focus has shifted to multitier copays for patients, giving them more responsibility for deciding on the need for expensive therapy.

Practice Sites in Ambulatory Care

Traditionally, the ambulatory care practice site has been the community pharmacy. However, in recent years, the number and type of ambulatory care practice sites have grown to include hospital-based clinic pharmacies (general and specialty), mail-order pharmacies, pharmacies in physician office buildings, and nondispensing practices, such as pharmacist-managed clinics, office practices, and PBMs. The roles and responsibilities of technicians in most of the dispensing operations are very similar.

Community Pharmacies

Community pharmacies are often stand-alone businesses that fill prescriptions and sell a variety of nonprescription products (e.g., cough and cold preparations, toiletries). Most community pharmacies employ pharmacists and technicians, and the pharmacists often counsel patients about proper use of their medications. There are two distinct types of community pharmacies: independent and chain.

Independent Community Pharmacies

Independent pharmacies are likely to be recognized as "corner drugstores." Their services vary, depending on the pharmacist, location, and patient population served. The owner of an independent pharmacy is most likely the pharmacist-in-charge. Many independent pharmacies specialize in such areas as durable medical equipment (DME) or medical supplies and compounding. Some independent pharmacies also serve nursing homes.

Chain Pharmacies

A corporate-owned group of pharmacies is generally recognized as a chain pharmacy. These pharmacies are usually large business entities with common policies and procedures. Pharmacists as well as technicians are employees of the corporation. Chain pharmacies often offer discount prescription-filling services, accept a large number of insurance plans, and offer the convenience of multiple locations. Some chains (as well as some independents) also offer cholesterol screening, flu shots, and blood pressure monitoring services.

Chain pharmacies may be further divided into (1) mass merchandisers with a large inventory and variety of products, (2) pharmacy chains located within a grocery store chain, and (3) apothecary shop chains focused primarily on pharmaceutical services, with little to no front-end merchandise.

Some pharmacies are considered "small chains" or "independent chains." They are often independent pharmacies that have grown to add new locations in a community. These small chains usually consist of three to seven pharmacies.

Clinic Pharmacies

Clinic pharmacies and pharmacies in physician office buildings usually offer the same scope of services as many community pharmacies but may have less focus on selling retail products other than medications. Because of the proximity of these pharmacies to the prescribers (i.e., physicians), the pharmacies generally have greater access to patient information.

Clinic pharmacies and physician office building pharmacies may differ in ownership and licensure. Clinic pharmacies associated with a hospital are likely to be owned by the hospital and operated under the direction of the hospital pharmacy department. Because of this relationship, the hospital-owned pharmacy may receive contract pricing from a buying group, through the manufacturer or through disproportionate share pricing (hospitals and clinics serving a disproportionate share of indigent patients are eligible to buy pharmaceuticals at government rates). In these instances, the pharmacies are not allowed to dispense prescriptions to nonhospital patients because their

pricing may give them an unfair advantage over community pharmacies. In other words, if a patient enters a hospital-owned pharmacy receiving contract prices with a prescription from the physician's office down the street, the pharmacy may not legally fill the prescription.

In the private physician office building, pharmacy services are more likely to be contracted with a local independent or chain pharmacy. In this case, the pharmacy operates just like any other community pharmacy. Clinics associated with a hospital may also hire an outside vendor to provide pharmacy services.

Specialty Clinic Pharmacies

Because of the specific needs of some specialty clinics, pharmacies occasionally will be located in these clinics. For example, oncology clinics often have their own pharmacies, which usually specialize in the preparation of chemotherapeutic agents for on-site administration.

Managed Care Pharmacies

Some managed care organizations own and operate physician office buildings or clinic practices and may also operate pharmacies in these buildings. These pharmacies operate much like community or other ambulatory care pharmacies but may carry only drugs on the organization's formulary and serve only the patients enrolled in the managed care plan.

Mail-Order Pharmacies

Mail-order pharmacies are mostly large-scale operations that mail maintenance medications (i.e., medications that patients take on a regular basis) to patients' homes. Mail-order pharmacies have become increasingly popular because they are convenient and are often thought to have lower prices. These pharmacies can process thousands of prescriptions per day. The role of the technician in these pharmacies is usually the same as in other ambulatory care sites, except the technician has no face-to-face patient contact. Instead, most communication with patients occurs over the telephone. Therefore, good telephone communication skills are essential.

Technician Responsibilities in Ambulatory Care

The role of pharmacy technicians in ambulatory care practice is essential to an efficient and effective operation. Generally, the technicians are responsible for maintaining and operating all aspects of the drug distribution process under the supervision of pharmacists. This includes receipt of the prescription order, computer order entry, claims processing, prescription filling and labeling, compounding, inventory maintenance, and other activities as directed by the pharmacist. The demands on the pharmacist to assess the patient and prescription for drug-related problems and to counsel the patient appropriately require technician support that is timely, complete, and accurate.

Customer Service and Communication Skills

Possibly the most important qualifications of those who serve the public are the abilities to provide good customer service and practice good communication skills. These abilities are especially necessary in the health care setting, where the patient is the customer. Patients are often not feeling well and have a low tolerance for inconvenience and perceived rudeness of employees. Technicians should always approach patients in a positive, polite, and caring manner. In addition to being a good business practice, a positive interaction with the technician helps prepare the patient for an open and productive interaction with the pharmacist. Technicians must also respect and be considerate of the patient's confidentiality and maintain a sense of privacy when discussing medications.

Technicians must be prepared to handle demanding patients appropriately. Sometimes demanding patients will create difficult situations, and the technician should work closely with the pharmacist to develop a game plan for handling such situations. For example, a patient may demand a quickly filled prescription or argue over the price of a copay. In such situations, the technician should always clarify the issue (perhaps it is a simple misunderstanding) and should never escalate an argument by speaking loudly or challenging the patient's knowledge. Part of the game plan should include when to refer the situation to a pharmacist.

The use of the telephone in a community pharmacy also requires proper communication skills. Physicians, patients, and other pharmacies may be calling, so the technician should identify him- or herself as the pharmacy technician. This may prevent the caller from taking the time to ask a lengthy question, only to be put on hold and then have to repeat the question to the pharmacist.

Third-Party Payment Programs

One of the most unusual and time-consuming activities in the ambulatory care pharmacy setting is dealing with third-party payment programs. Third-party programs are insurance or entitlement programs that reimburse the pharmacy for products delivered and services rendered. Although hundreds of third-party programs are administered by organizations ranging from large insurance companies to small employer- or union-sponsored employee benefit programs, there are only two major mechanisms for pharmacy reimbursement: fee-for-service and capitation.

Fee-for-service

In a fee-for-service system, either patients pay cash for the prescription and submit receipts to their insurance carrier or the pharmacy bills the insurance carrier directly each time an eligible product is dispensed or services rendered. The third party then reimburses the pharmacy. The amount charged and amount reimbursed depend on the cost and time involved. For patients without insurance, this is an "out-of-pocket" expense.

Capitation

Under a capitated payment program, a pharmacy receives a set amount of money for a defined group of patients, regardless of the number of prescriptions or amount of services received. The dollar amount is usually in terms of per patient (member) per month. For example, the third-party payer may agree to pay the pharmacy $2 per member per month. Therefore, if the program has 100 patients, the pharmacy receives $200 each month. Even if one of the patients does not use the pharmacy during one month, the pharmacy still receives the $2 for that patient. Likewise, if a patient receives multiple medications and uses the pharmacy 10 times per month, the pharmacy still receives only $2 for that patient. As noted earlier, the concept of capitation was popular in the 1990s, but rarely implemented. Today, very little capitation exists at the pharmacy level.

Eligibility Verification

Because of the variety of third-party programs, there are a variety of methods of ensuring eligibility. Most programs offer membership cards to their patients. These cards often carry basic information, such as name and identification number. However, the technician may have to collect additional information from the patient, such as date of birth and address. Most third-party programs are on-line through the pharmacy computer, which will notify the pharmacist or pharmacy technician if there is a problem with eligibility. Another situation to be aware of is that some third parties cover family members, but the membership card lists only the primary beneficiary.

Formularies

A formulary is a list of drugs approved by a third party for reimbursement. Formularies are developed to help control costs and improve the quality of the drug therapy patients receive (i.e., cost-effective therapy). However, formulary drugs will vary among third parties because of differences in contract prices and rebate agreements with the manufacturers, among other reasons. If a patient presents a prescription for a drug that is not on the formulary, the pharmacist should be alerted to the problem so that he or she can take appropriate action. One option would be for the patient to pay full price for the nonformulary drug.

CoPayments/Deductibles/Spend-Downs

Many third parties require the patient to pay a copayment, or deductible, each time a prescription is received. Third parties designate three basic copayment arrangements: (1) flat rate, (2) variable rate, and (3) straight percentage. A flat rate requires a specific copay regardless of the drug received and its cost. A variable-rate copay changes depending on the product being dispensed. In perhaps its simplest form, the variable-rate copay is higher for brand name products and lower for generics. Today, a popular version of the variable-rate copay is the multitier copay, which may be low for a generic, mid-level for a brand product on formulary, and high for a brand name off formulary. For instance, the copay structure may be $5, $10, and $25, respectively.

A straight percentage copay requires the patient to pay a percentage of the total cost of any medication. The amount paid by the patient would then increase as the cost of the prescription increased. For instance, if the copay is 10 percent, the patient pays $10 for a $100 prescription or $20 for a $200 prescription.

A spend-down (also known as a front-end deductible) differs from a copay or deductible in that it is assessed over a defined period of time and not on a per prescription basis. A spend-down requires a patient to spend a defined amount of out-of-pocket dollars on prescriptions within a year before the third party pays anything. For example, a patient may have a spend-down of $500 over a year. This patient will have to pay for $500 worth of prescription drugs first, and then the third party will pay for the remaining prescriptions during the rest of the year. The process would then start over the following year.

Prescription Processing and Workflow

The objective of this section is to highlight the unique components of prescription processing in the ambulatory care setting. The specific role of a technician in a pharmacy will vary depending on the preference of the pharmacist or the policies of the employer.

Prescription Reception

The patient will bring his or her prescription(s) to the prescription reception area (or "In Window") of the pharmacy. This is often the patient's first contact with the pharmacy, so good customer service is essential. Because it is the first contact, gathering accurate data about the patient and verifying that the prescription is complete is also important (see Chapter 9 for a list of items needed for a complete prescription). The typical data that should be collected about the patient include the following:

- Correct spelling of name
- Address and phone number
- Allergies
- Birth date
- Weight for children and infants
- Payment information
- Desire for generic substitution

If the patient is hesitant to provide this information, explain the purpose of collecting it (i.e., for insurance reimbursement, recall notices, dosage calculations).

If the patient has previously experienced an allergic reaction to a medication, the technician should document the reaction and alert the pharmacist. The technician's role is only to document the reaction. The assessment of the reaction and discussion with the patient should be left to the pharmacist. The pharmacist will need to evaluate the type of allergic reaction experienced by the patient, determine if it may be a potential problem with the patient's current prescription, and make recommendations as appropriate.

Many pharmacies accept a large number of insurance plans, and the technician should be familiar with the requirements of each plan or at least know where to find the information.

The laws and regulations regarding generic substitution vary from state to state, but usually the prescriber, patient, and pharmacist must agree before a generic product is dispensed in place of a brand name product. If the prescription is written generically (e.g., furosemide), then the generic can usually be dispensed.

However, if the prescription is written for the brand name product (e.g., Lasix) and marked "may substitute," the patient should be asked if he or she prefers the generic or brand name product. Because not all drugs are available as generics, the technician should be familiar with which generics are available. When unsure of availability, the technician should ask if the patient prefers the generic product if one is available. In certain cases, it is important to inform the patient that some insurance plans will not cover brand name products when a generic is available or that the insurance plan may require a higher copay for brand name products.

The last question that should be asked at the reception area is whether the patient plans to wait or return later for the prescription. From a customer service perspective, it is important to prioritize the prescription-filling process and efficiently adjust workflow as necessary to provide timely service and accommodate the customer's needs.

Prescription Computer Entry

After the prescription has been received, the next step is to enter it into the pharmacy computer system. There are hundreds of pharmacy software vendors, and some pharmacies develop their own software, so the details of the prescription entry process will differ between sites. However, the basic process of keying in the patient and prescription information and generating a label should be the same. Additionally, most insurance plans are on-line, which allows for virtually immediate responses to the pharmacy's insurance claims.

As the patient and prescription information is entered into the computer, the software or the on-line third party will verify the patient's eligibility for payment, as well as formulary and therapeutic problems. The technician should be prepared to handle payment problems; however, therapeutic problems should be referred to the pharmacist. When a problem does occur, the computer generates an alert message for the pharmacy. The following are some common error messages:

Refill Too Soon

This message deals specifically with refill prescriptions and the time period between filling prescriptions. Typically, third parties allow patients to receive a 30-day supply of medications. If the patient attempts to refill a prescription within a significantly shorter time period (e.g., 15 days after the last prescription), the prescription cannot be processed without prior approval from the third-party payer.

Missing/Invalid Patient ID

This or a similar message indicates that the patient who is entered into the pharmacy computer does not appear to be enrolled in the insurance program. On receiving this message, the technician should examine the patient information entered for mistakes. Perhaps the name was misspelled, identification number mistyped, or other required information left out. Because many insurance plans use a PBM to manage their pharmacy services, the prescription may need to be processed under the name of the PBM instead of the name of the third-party payer.

Drug–Drug or Drug–Allergy Interaction

Most pharmacy software will screen the patient profile for drug and allergy information. If interactions are detected, the program will alert the user. Some software will not only identify an interaction but also indicate the potential severity of the reaction. On receiving this message, the technician should alert the pharmacist to the problem.

Nonformulary/Not Covered

Many third-party payers have formularies. If a nonformulary drug is entered into the pharmacy computer, the message will indicate that the drug is not covered, and payment will not be made for that drug. On receiving this message, the technician should alert the pharmacist.

Patient Profile Maintenance

The patient profile is a list of the prescriptions received by a patient and all corresponding prescription information (original date, refill dates, prescribing physician). The patient profile assists the pharmacist in evaluating the appropriateness and efficacy of the patient's drug therapy. One use of the patient profile in ambulatory care that is unique in comparison with the inpatient environment is to assess patient compliance. For example, if a patient received a 30-day supply of medication but did not return to the pharmacy for a refill until 45 days later, the pharmacist will likely investigate the discrepancy to determine if a problem has occurred, if the patient is noncompliant, or if the prescribed therapy has been changed. The patient profile contains private and confidential information; therefore, this information should never be discussed with anyone other than the patient and the pharmacist.

Prescription Filling and Labeling

The actual filling and labeling of prescriptions is one of the most common pharmacy technician activities in ambulatory care. This process must be completed in a timely and accurate manner. Any mistakes in the process are not only dangerous but time-consuming and obstructive to the workflow. Pharmacy technicians should be careful to ensure that all prescriptions meet the "five rights": (1) the right drug, (2) in the right dose, (3) in the right dosage form, (4) with the right label, and (5) for the right patient. Any error discovered by the pharmacist will often be returned to the technician for correction.

Automation

The use of automated devices to fill and label prescriptions in ambulatory care is increasing and is likely to grow rapidly over the next several years. Such automation will increase the productivity of the pharmacy and the pharmacy technician and assist with inventory control. With automation comes an increase in the technician's responsibility for maintaining and filling automated devices; however, the final check still remains with the pharmacist. Technicians should strictly follow the policies, procedures, and standards developed within the pharmacy in filling automated devices. An error in filling the automated device could result in a large number of misfilled prescriptions if not caught by a pharmacist.

Compounding

One of the valuable services provided by an ambulatory care pharmacy is compounding prescriptions. The majority of compounding in this setting involves making suspensions for pediatric patients who need a smaller dose than what is available commercially or for patients who cannot swallow tablets or capsules. In addition, many combination topical products are prepared in ambulatory care settings. (Refer to Chapter 13, Nonsterile Compounding and Repackaging, for more detailed information on compounding.)

Most pharmacies keep a "recipe book" or "compounding log" that contains step-by-step guidance on how to prepare compounds that are routinely ordered. It serves as a reference on what ingredients to use, how to prepare the compound, and stability information (e.g., refrigeration requirements and expiration dates). The technician's role is to compound the prescription following the appropriate compounding instructions, document all necessary information, and label the product appropriately for the pharmacist to complete the final check.

Dispensing

The last step in the prescription-processing function is dispensing. Technicians can assist pharmacists in the dispensing process by making sure all the medications for a patient are ready to be dispensed and by collecting payment from the patient when appropriate.

A large and important component of the dispensing function is patient counseling. Many potential drug-related health problems and prescription errors could be prevented through effective communication between the patient and the pharmacist. A technician should always defer patient questions regarding the use and side effects of medications to the pharmacist.

Transferring Prescriptions

The laws regarding the transfer of prescriptions between pharmacies vary among states and among different classes of drugs. However, the pharmacist is always ultimately responsible for the information transferred. The transfer of a prescription to another pharmacy is usually initiated by a phone call from the pharmacy needing a transferred prescription. A technician may pull the original prescription from files or pull up the data on the computer, but the actual transfer of information is usually the responsibility of the pharmacist.

The same is true for prescriptions being transferred into the pharmacy. In this case, the process begins when a patient asks to transfer the prescription from another location. At that point, it is important for the technician to obtain as much information as possible from the patient about the prescription. At a minimum, the pharmacist needs the patient's name and the name of the pharmacy currently holding the prescription. If a patient brings in his or her old bottle, it may be useful to troubleshoot the labels. For example, if the label indicates that there are no refills, the physician will have to be called to authorize the refill.

Nonprescription Medications

Nonprescription medications, or over-the-counter (OTC) drugs, can be purchased without a prescription. Because of their availability to consumers and relatively low out-of-pocket expense, some third-party payers will not include OTCs on their formulary or will require that a provider have written a prescription for the OTC before covering it under the benefit. Some of the common OTC products available include drugs for cough and cold, antacids, laxatives, pain medications, topical preparations, antidiarrheal products, diabetic care products, weight control products, ophthalmic products (eye preparations), otic products (ear preparations), and nutritional supplements. In addition, a variety of home health care supplies, such as ostomy bags, crutches, and wheel chairs, are available.

In recent years, consumers have become increasingly interested in taking care of their health through self-education, exercise, and proper diet. In addition, more and more patients are choosing self-treatment for their acute illnesses (e.g., coughs, colds, heartburn). The increasing cost of health care, lack of medical insurance, inaccessibility of medical care, availability of more diverse and sophisticated self-care products, and increasing number of prescription drugs being switched to nonprescription status are some of the reasons patients are getting more involved in their own health care. These trends present tremendous opportunities for the pharmacy profession to give patients the guidance and information they need to use OTC products effectively.

Pharmacy technicians are usually the first to encounter patients when they approach the pharmacy; therefore, the technicians should familiarize themselves with the location of the OTCs and be able to direct patients to specific products. However, technicians must know when to answer a patient's question and when to refer the patient to the pharmacist. For example, if a patient asks a technician to help with returning a crutch the patient rented for a sprained ankle, the technician can usually take care of the patient. However, if the patient also asks if he or she can take aspirin for the pain, the technician should refer the patient to a pharmacist.

Referring Patients to a Pharmacist

Technicians should always refer patients to the pharmacist whenever clinical judgment is involved in answering a question. There are at least three specific reasons why technicians should always refer patients with drug (prescription or OTC) or health-related questions to a pharmacist: (1) drug–drug interactions, (2) drug–disease state interaction, and (3) need for physician referral.

Drug–Drug Interactions
The patient may be taking prescription or nonprescription drugs that may interact with OTC drugs. For example, drugs for use in heartburn and acid indigestion that were previously available only by prescription have recently entered the OTC market. Some of these drugs interact with prescription drugs, such as medica-

tions used for heart disease, blood pressure, seizure disorders, and so on. They may also interact with other OTC drugs. Therefore, these drugs may not be appropriate for all patients.

Drug–Disease State Interaction
Some OTC drugs may adversely affect the patient's existing disease state by making the condition worse or precipitating a disease that is in remission. Pharmacists are trained to know the effect of drugs on disease states and can make appropriate recommendations.

Need for Physician Referral
Often, patients may come to the pharmacy with seemingly simple problems that in reality are complex. For example, a patient may ask for an OTC drug recommendation for a headache. The technician may feel pressured to give a recommendation based on his or her own experience or what he or she heard a pharmacist recommend previously. However, the appropriate response is to refer the patient to a pharmacist. Pharmacists are trained to interview patients and determine if a patient's complaint is an indication of a more serious medical condition that requires further evaluation.

Another common question a technician may receive concerning nonprescription medications is whether insurance companies pay for OTC products. In general, many insurance companies do not pay for OTC products. But there are a few exceptions to the rule, so it is best to check the insurance plan before giving a patient a yes or no answer.

Summary
This chapter has provided an overview of ambulatory care pharmacy practice. As more and more health care is provided in the outpatient setting and as the complexity and breadth of OTC and prescription drugs continue to increase, the role of pharmacists in counseling and monitoring patients becomes increasingly critical to the safe and effective use of medications. The role of pharmacy technicians in maintaining an effective and efficient drug distribution process is critical to the success of ambulatory care pharmacies. Technicians must be knowledgeable and proficient in the use of automation and pharmacy computer systems and efficient in filling prescriptions. Technicians must also maintain a working knowledge of third-party payers and their prescription policies. Finally, technicians must provide excellent customer service through friendly and caring interactions with patients.

Recommended Reading

Rovers JP, Currie JD, Hagel HP eds. A practical guide to pharmaceutical care. Washington, DC: APhA; 1998.

Hagel HP, Rovers JP eds. Managing the patient-centered pharmacy. Washington, DC: APhA; 2002.

Cooke C, Wilson M. Managed care organizations, today and tomorrow. *Am Drug.* 1994; Nov: 67–74.

Abramowitz PW, Mansur JM. Moving toward the provision of comprehensive ambulatory care pharmaceutical services. *Am J Hosp Pharm.* 1987; 44:1155–63.

Fincham JE, Wertheimer AI eds. Pharmacy and the U.S. health care system. Binghamton, NY: Pharmaceuticals Products Press; 1991.

List of Abbreviations

APCS: Ambulatory Payment Classification System

DME: durable medical equipment

DUR: drug use review

HIPAA: Health Insurance Portability and Accountability Act

OBRA 90: Omnibus Budget Reconciliation Act of 1990

OTC: over-the-counter

PBM: pharmacy benefit management firms

Self-Assessment Questions

1. The Durham–Humphrey amendment:
   a. defined "prescription" drugs.
   b. required pharmacists to offer patients counseling on their medication.
   c. allowed pharmacists to dispense any drug without a prescription.
   d. defined rules regarding the privacy of patient information.

2. Typical data collected from the patient at the prescription take-in window does *not* include:
   a. weight for children and infants.
   b. allergies.
   c. hair color.
   d. phone number.

3. An important aspect of an ambulatory care pharmacy technician's job is:
   a. counseling patients about drug interactions.
   b. good customer service and communication skills.
   c. educating physicians about pharmacology.
   d. recommending specific nonprescription medications to patients.

4. If a patient is noted to have experienced an allergic reaction to a medication, the technician should:
   a. tell the patient the physician made a mistake and refuse to fill the prescription.
   b. assume the physician knew about the allergy and fill the prescription.
   c. ask the patient about the type of allergic reaction experienced and alert the pharmacist.
   d. recommend the patient call the physician before taking the medication.

5. If a prescription is written generically and is marked "may not substitute":
   a. a generic product can usually be dispensed.
   b. the specific brand name drug must be dispensed.
   c. send the patient back to the physician for clarification.
   d. charge a higher copay.

6. Which of the following questions or statements is the most important for the technician to ask of patients turning in prescriptions?
   a. "Will you be waiting for your prescriptions or returning at a later time?"
   b. "If you need to pick up any greeting cards while shopping today, they are half price."
   c. "You look really sick, I hope I don't catch your cold."
   d. "If your insurance information doesn't go through, you will have to pay cash."

7. Which of the following statements regarding pharmacy automation is false?
   a. Automation will assist with inventory control.
   b. Automation ensures error-free prescription filling.
   c. Technicians should strictly follow the policies, procedures, and standards developed within the pharmacy in filling automated devices.
   d. With the increase in automation comes an increase in the technician's responsibility for maintaining and filling such devices; however, the final check still remains with the pharmacist.

8. Which of the following is generally *not* included in the technician's responsibilities in ambulatory care practice?
   a. receipt of the prescription order.
   b. recommending therapeutic alternatives to the prescribing physician.
   c. prescription filling and labeling.
   d. inventory maintenance.

9. A formulary is:
   a. a list of drugs that are covered under a particular third-party plan.
   b. a recipe book for compounding prescriptions.
   c. a multitiered copayment plan.
   d. utilized by the pharmacist only and is outside of the scope of technician practice.

10. The patient profile:
    a. is strictly an inventory management tool.
    b. is maintained at the physician's office.
    c. is "off limits" to the pharmacy technician.
    d. has multiple purposes, including the storage of the patient's insurance information, potential drug interactions, allergy contraindications, and patient compliance.

Self-Assessment Answers

1. a. The 1951 Durham–Humphrey Amendment to the Food, Drug and Cosmetic Act gave a definition to "prescription" drugs and prohibited pharmacists from dispensing these drugs without a valid medication order. The OBRA 90 regulations required pharmacists to offer counseling to Medicaid patients. Many state practice acts quickly expanded the OBRA 90 guidelines to cover all patients.

2. c. The typical data that should be collected include correct spelling of name, address and phone number, allergies, birth date, weight for children and infants, payment information, and desire for generic substitution. Hair color would not likely be relevant information.

3. b. Good customer service and communication skills are essential in ambulatory care practice (for both the technician and the pharmacist). Some patients will not be feeling well and may be less tolerant of delays in receiving their prescriptions or perceived rudeness of employees. A friendly and caring interaction between the technician and the patient sets the stage for a productive patient interaction with the pharmacist.

4. c. Take each potential allergy seriously. Patients may believe minor side effects to be allergies, but leave that determination to the pharmacist. Never send the patient away, and never assume the physician is already aware.

5. a. If the prescription is written generically (e.g., furosemide), then the generic can usually be dispensed. However, if the prescription is written for the brand name product (e.g., Lasix) and marked "may substitute," the patient should be asked if he or she prefers the generic or brand name product.

6. a. The last question the patient should be asked at the reception area is if he or she plans to wait or return later for the prescription. From a customer service perspective, it is important to prioritize the prescription-filling process and efficiently adjust workflow as necessary to provide timely service and accommodate the customer's needs.

7. b. With the increase in automation comes an increase in the technician's responsibility for maintaining and filling such devices; however, the final check still remains with the pharmacist. Technicians should strictly follow the policies, procedures, and standards developed within the pharmacy in filling automated devices. An error in filling the automated device could result in a large number of misfilled prescriptions if not caught by a pharmacist.

8. b. Receiving the prescription from the patient, prescription filling/labeling, and inventory maintenance are all product workflow issues and well within the responsibilities of the technician. Recommending therapeutic alternatives to the physician is a patient care activity reserved for the pharmacist.

9. a. A formulary is a list of drugs approved by a third party for reimbursement. Formularies are developed to help control costs and improve the quality of the drug therapy patients receive (i.e., cost-effective therapy).

10. d. The patient profile is a list of the prescriptions received by a patient and all corresponding prescription information (i.e., original date, refill dates, prescribing physician). The patient profile assists the pharmacist in evaluating the appropriateness and efficacy of the patient's drug therapy. The patient profile is a tool for both the pharmacist and technician and is an essential part of the prescription-filling process.

Institutional Pharmacy Practice

3

STEVEN LUNDQUIST

Institutional settings are facilities, such as hospitals and nursing homes, where patients receive health care in a structured manner. Pharmacy plays an important role in institutional settings. The primary responsibility of the pharmacy department is to provide medications and services that help ensure safe and effective use of medications. However, the scope of responsibilities for pharmacy is ever changing and expanding to meet the challenges of rising health care costs, reduced health care resources, and advances in technology.

Institutional pharmacy practice centers around products and patient care services. Traditional product-focused services include procurement, storage, preparation, administration, and distribution of drugs and supplies to patients. Technicians are an integral part of the pharmacy team that provides these services. As the pharmacy profession continues to expand its realm of activities toward direct patient care, however, the responsibilities and opportunities for technicians also expand. This chapter provides a general overview of institutional pharmacy practice, discusses the current roles and responsibilities of pharmacy technicians, and identifies the potential impact of the changing health care environment on pharmacy technicians. Although this chapter concentrates on institutional pharmacy practice, it does not describe all aspects of that practice. Refer to "Recommended Reading" for further detail.

Historical Overview and Current Practices

Pharmacy services have existed in institutional settings in one form or another for many years. Pharmacy services 30 years ago usually consisted of a central pharmacy located in the basement of the hospital. These pharmacy services were often very limited in responsibilities and number of personnel. The focus was on medication products, including compounding, repackaging, and relabeling multidose supplies, to be used by nurses for patient care. Bulk supplies of medications were often kept on the nursing station as floor stock. When a patient needed a medication,

Learning Objectives

After completing this chapter, the technician should be able to

1. Describe the forces causing changes in health care practices in institutions.

2. Understand the differences between centralized and decentralized pharmacy services. Understand the roles and responsibilities of technicians in each of these different settings.

3. Understand and define the differences between product-focused and patient-focused services. Understand the roles and responsibilities of technicians in each of these different services.

4. Define pharmaceutical care and how it relates to the technician's new roles.

5. Explain how quality control and quality improvement are used in institutional pharmacy practice.

the nurse would obtain the medication from the floor stock, perform all calculations, and prepare the product. The nurse would also prepare all intravenous (IV) medications directly in the patient care area without the use of a laminar flow hood.

Fortunately, the practice of institutional pharmacy has made tremendous advances over the past 30 years. Pharmacy has moved from a profession focused primarily on medication preparation and distribution to one focused on providing services to help get the best outcome from the drug therapy. This evolution has occurred as a result of many internal and external forces. Two major forces are the impact of new technology and the enormous burden placed on health care by rising costs and diminishing resources.

Technology and Pharmacy

Technology has had an impact on our normal daily lives. We are able to obtain information and communicate faster and easier with the use of cellular phones, satellites, fax machines, and computer networks. Technology has helped industries improve the quality of the goods they produce and speed of production. These technological advances have certainly found their way into the health care system. Drug companies can now manufacture mass quantities of medications in a ready-to-use, unit-dose form (which will be discussed later in this chapter). This has made a significant impact on pharmacy by eliminating the burden of extemporaneous preparation of medications and the errors, waste, and cost associated with the process.

Another significant technological advance is automation. Automation technologies have replaced many of the manual tasks within pharmacy. Automation allows pharmacy technicians and pharmacists to devote more time and resources to patient-focused activities. Examples of automation in institutional practices are the Micromix® and Automix® machines and medication dispensing systems. The Micromix® and Automix® machines are used to prepare hyperalimentation solutions (see Chapter 18). Medication dispensing systems, as well as the use of robotics (e.g., Pyxis Medstation® and Baxter SureMed®), can be used in the pharmacy and in patient care areas to allow health care providers to obtain medications at the point of use. These systems can keep track of which medication was removed, who removed it, and to whom it was to be administered. A more detailed description and example of automation appears in Chapter 18.

Computers are commonly used to streamline the medication use process and reduce the chance of making an error. For example, some physicians now enter medication orders directly into an institution's computer system. On-line entry of medication orders eliminates the need to transcribe, manipulate, or re-enter medication orders, and it generates a typed label that is affixed to the final product. Physician order entry significantly reduces the number of steps in the medication use process and can reduce both interpretation and transcription errors and the time it takes to get medications to patients.

These are just a few examples of how technological advances reduce the time pharmacy personnel spend performing routine tasks, increase productivity, and improve the quality of pharmacy services. Although automation has replaced certain tasks performed by technicians, it has also created new opportunities. Technicians are often responsible for operating and maintaining these forms of automation. The time saved on traditional product-focused tasks can now be used to assist the pharmacist with patient-focused tasks. For example, technicians may be asked to obtain lab results for pharmacists to use when evaluating the appropriateness of certain drug regimens.[1] In addition, technicians are playing innovative roles relating to technology, such as data analysis of pharmacy-related patient care and financial information.[2]

Financial Implications

The financial burden on health care systems continues to have huge ramifications for patients and institutions. Health care costs have increased for many reasons. One reason may be that, in the past, Medicare and Medicaid legislation allowed institutions to receive full reimbursement for services determined to be necessary by the physician. This removed the incentive for institutions to control their costs and did not promote competition, which meant institutions were not stimulated to provide the best services at the lowest cost. Today, institutions and payers are trying to reduce costs and improve the quality of care by developing alternative practice settings, establishing reimbursement guidelines, and implementing changes to streamline patient care services. The diagnosis-related group (DRG) is an example of a system with reimbursement guidelines. In general terms, compensation is determined by the DRG assigned to a patient, regardless of how many health care resources are used to treat that patient.

Health maintenance organizations (HMOs) are an example of an alternative practice setting. Employers may use an HMO to provide health benefits for their employees. The HMO centralizes the delivery of care to improve efficiency and reduce waste and cost. The reimbursements HMOs receive from employers are capitated, which means HMOs receive a fixed amount of money for each employee enrolled in the plan, regardless of the care the patient receives. HMOs in turn pay health care providers an agreed-upon reimbursement based on the number of patients and types of diagnosis and treatments provided. Thus, it is in the best interests of HMOs and the health care institutions they partner with to provide cost-effective care. This is why HMOs are also focused on preventive care and wellness. Examples of other alternative practice settings include home health care, mail order prescription services, and managed care companies.

In addition, annual drug expenditures are now increasing in the double digits and were forecast to be 15.5 percent for hospitals and 18.5 percent for outpatient and ambulatory care in 2002. This increase is a result of many factors, including the use of newer,

more expensive drugs replacing older, less expensive drugs; the aging patient population; and increased marketing by direct-to-consumer advertising as well as to physicians and other health care providers.[3]

Organizational Structure of Institutions

Health care institutions are usually organized into several levels of management. Managers at the top of an organization are primarily involved in setting a direction and vision for the hospital. As you move down the organizational structure, the responsibilities become more defined and are targeted to meet the goals of the hospital. Each level of management is designed to allow a diverse range of activities to be performed in an organized manner. Without clear levels of responsibility and a chain of command, the activities of employees would be unorganized, inefficient, and unproductive. **Figure 3-1** is an example of a typical organizational structure.

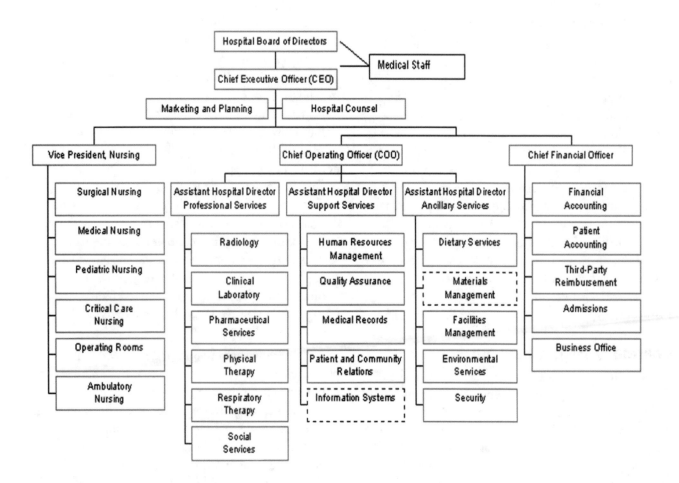

Figure 3-1. Example of a hospital organizational chart.
Source: Brown TR, ed. Handbook of institutional pharmacy practice. 3rd ed. Bethesda, MD: ASHP; 1992.

At the top of an organization is the chief executive officer (CEO), president, or hospital director. The CEO helps set a direction for the hospital by creating a vision and mission for the institution. The CEO reports to the hospital's board of directors and is responsible for ensuring that necessary budget, personnel, and operations are in place to help achieve the mission of the hospital. The medical staff and the second level of management report directly to the CEO.

Hospitals usually have a chief operating officer (COO), or vice president, representing a second level of management. The COO is responsible for the daily operations of the hospital. A chief financial officer (CFO) is also a second-level manager responsible for the financial management of the hospital. Another second level of management becoming more common is the vice president of patient care services. This manager is responsible for the patient-focused care departments, such as pharmacy, nursing, respiratory, and so on. The number of additional levels of management is a factor of the size and scope of services the health care institution provides.

The individual departments are routinely grouped by either patient care (e.g., nursing, pharmacy, radiology), ancillary (e.g., materials management, environmental services), or support (e.g., medical records information systems) services. Variations of this organizational structure are being used to improve quality of patient care, improve efficiency, and reduce cost. One example of a variation is the patient-focused care model (explained later in this chapter), in which managers are given responsibility for all employees and activities provided to specific patient types (i.e. surgery, pediatric, or medicine patients). The philosophy of this structure is for the employees to function as a team, with everyone having a role in providing patient care, regardless of discipline or the tasks performed.

Pharmacy Department Structure

The director or chief of pharmacy services is at the top of the pharmacy department hierarchy. The number and levels of management below the director of pharmacy depend on the department's size and scope of services. For example, a hospital affiliated with a university may need a manager to coordinate the residency program and another manager to coordinate pharmacy students, staff development, and all clinical

pharmacy services. However, pharmacy department structure is most often based on the types of operations the institution provides, such as centralized or decentralized pharmacy services.

Centralized Pharmacy Services

Centralized pharmacy services, as the name implies, handle pharmacy personnel, resources, and functions from a central location. Central pharmacies are often located in the basement of hospitals. A typical centralized pharmacy may contain an area for the preparation of IV medications (i.e., antibiotic piggybacks, large-volume parenterals with additives, total parenteral nutrition, chemotherapeutic agents), a medication cart filling area, an outpatient prescription counter, and a storage area for medications and supplies. Central pharmacy services are often used when resources (personnel, equipment, and space) are limited. The advantage of centralized services is that less staff is needed to control, store, inspect, prepare, and dispense medications for the entire institution.

The main disadvantages of offering only centralized pharmacy services are the lack of face-to-face interactions with patients and other health care providers and the time it takes to deliver medications. Many centralized pharmacies now have better access to patient care information through the use of computerized documentation. However, pharmacists in the central pharmacy still have difficulty accessing all patient information needed to make appropriate therapeutic assessments of medication orders, such as the patient's complete medical record. In addition, it may take a long time to deliver medication orders to all areas of the institution from a central location. Technology and automation, such as Pyxis® is an option that can shorten delivery time of medications to patient care areas. Another option for the pharmacy department is to offer decentralized pharmacy services, which are described in the next section.

The technician's responsibilities in a central pharmacy may involve preparing IVs, hyperalimentation, and chemotherapeutic agents; filling patient medication carts; delivering narcotics; restocking drugs for medication dispensing systems; extemporaneous compounding (i.e., products not available from a manufacturer); functions related to quality control and quality improvement; billing; and filling out miscellaneous paperwork.

Decentralized Pharmacy Services

Decentralized pharmacy services do not replace centralized pharmacy services but are used in conjunction with a central pharmacy. Decentralized pharmacy services are provided from within a patient care area. One common form of decentralized pharmacy is a pharmacy satellite, which is a designated area where drugs are stored, prepared, and dispensed for patients. Pharmacy satellites are often staffed by one or more pharmacists and technicians. The proximity of the pharmacy satellite to the patients and other health care providers gives the pharmacist more opportunities to interact with patients to obtain pertinent information, monitor and assess their response to drug therapy, and disseminate patient education materials. The pharmacist also has more opportunities to discuss the plan of care, answer drug information questions, and make appropriate drug therapy recommendations face to face with other health care providers.

The disadvantage of decentralized pharmacies is that they require additional resources. Additional resources include personnel to staff a decentralized satellite, equipment (e.g., laminar flow hood, computers, printers), references, and a second inventory of medications and supplies.

The technician's role in decentralized pharmacies varies from institution to institution. The technician's role in the satellite is a major factor in the ability of the pharmacist to provide pharmaceutical care. Some responsibilities of satellite technicians are maintaining appropriate inventory (e.g., medications and supplies), keeping the inventory free of expired medications, cleaning and maintaining laminar flow hoods, and preparing all unit-dose and IV medication orders in a timely fashion. Experienced technicians also may answer some questions from nurses and make judgments on when to refer a question to the pharmacist. Thus, some technicians are responsible for all aspects of running the satellite under the supervision of a pharmacist.

Use of Clinical Practitioners

Pharmacy departments may also be structured by nonproduct services. For example, services referred to as patient-focused care may require the use of clinical pharmacy skills. A clinical practitioner is a pharmacist who provides patient-focused care. Clinical practitioners are involved in all aspects of drug therapy to ensure appropriate, safe, and cost-effective care. Patient-focused care is accomplished by ensuring all patient-specific problems requiring drug therapy are being treated, the medication selected is appropriate for the indication, the dose ordered is correct, and the dosage form and administration technique meet the patient's needs. After the medication has been administered, clinical practitioners will monitor the effects of the medication through laboratory results (e.g., drug levels, culture and sensitivity results, or serum creatinine) as well as patient-specific parameters (e.g., heart rate, temperature, or respiration rate). Clinical practitioners also play a significant role in the education of patients and other health care providers regarding the use of medications. Clinical practitioners can spend more time directly with patients and in the patient care area than centralized pharmacists.

Product-Focused Services

Pharmacy services are changing and expanding. Pharmacy is still responsible, however, for the provision of medications directly to patients or other health care providers who care for patients. Fulfilling that responsibility efficiently requires that several processes, such as ordering, storing, preparing, delivering, administering, documenting, and monitoring, be integrated properly.

As an example, for a patient to receive one acetaminophen tablet, the following steps must occur. First, the drug has to be in the inventory, which means it was ordered from the manufacturer, received, inspected, stored, inventoried, and periodically reviewed to ensure that it has not expired. Next, the medication order must be received and processed by the pharmacy so the drug can be dispensed and delivered to the nursing station. Once at the nursing station, the drug is administered to the patient, and the dose is documented. In the past, compounding and repackaging was part of this process. However, the advent of the unit-dose drug distribution system eliminated this time-consuming process for most of the solid dosage forms dispensed.

Investigational drug services, if provided by the institution, represent another form of product-focused service in which the technician can play an important role. The technician may be involved in the record keeping, inventory control, preparation, and dispensing of investigational drugs. This is an important responsibility because the validity of the results and conclusions of every drug study depend on the accuracy of the dispensing records.

Unit-Dose System

Unit-dose drug distribution systems prepare medications in a single-unit package. In other words, the package contains a single dose that is ready to be administered to a patient. Understanding a unit-dose system is essential because technicians spend a significant part of their time obtaining, preparing, and labeling medications in a unit-dose form.

Unit-dose drug distribution systems allow a limited number of doses in a single unit of use (usually a 12- or 24-hour supply) to be dispensed in unit-dose medication carts or via automated floor stock systems. The advantages of using a unit-dose system are as follows:[4]

1. A reduction in the incidence of medication errors.

2. A decrease in the total cost of medication-related activities.

3. A more efficient use of pharmacy and nursing personnel, allowing for more direct patient-care involvement by pharmacists and nurses.

4. Improved overall drug control and drug use monitoring.

5. More accurate patient billings for drugs.

6. The elimination or minimization of drug credits.

7. Greater control by the pharmacist over pharmacy workload patterns and staff scheduling.

8. A reduction in the size of drug inventories located in patient-care areas.

9. Greater adaptability to computerized and automated procedures.

10. A reduction in the potential for drug waste.

Most medications are commercially available in unit-dose form, but pharmacy personnel still must package some medications as unit-dose units (see Chapter 13). IV medications are the best examples of those prepared in a unit-dose form by pharmacy personnel. Many IV medications are not stable in solution and must be mixed by a technician just prior to administration. (See Chapter 14.)

Patient-specific characteristics are often a reason to extemporaneously prepare medications in a unit-dose form. Pediatric patients, for example, require very small doses that may not be available from the manufacturer in a unit-dose form. Some doses required for pediatric patients (especially neonates) are so small that they cannot be measured accurately from commercially available products. The following scenario is an example of how a pediatric dose might be prepared in a unit-dose form:

> The doctor writes an IV 3-mg dose of clindamycin for a patient in the neonatal intensive care unit. Clindamycin is available in a concentration of 150 mg/ml vial. The final volume for a 3-mg dose at 150 mg/ml would be 0.02 mls. Because this volume is too small to measure accurately, the technician will have to prepare a dilution. An appropriate dilution would be a 1:25 dilution, which would result in a final concentration of 6 mg/ml. The final volume for a 3-mg dose of the new concentration would be 0.5 ml (see Chapter 5). The technician can now, under the supervision of a pharmacist, measure, label, and dispense this medication.

Solid dosage forms also may need to be diluted. A technician may need to crush tablets; add a filler ingredient, such as lactose; measure each dose using a calibrated balance; and then fold each powdered dose using a paper (referred to as powder paper) into single unit-dose packages.

Patient-Focused Services

Approximately 30 years ago pharmacists began to provide patient-focused services, called clinical pharmacy services, in addition to product services. These clinical services included pharmacokinetic dosing services, drug information services, and nutritional support services. The profession realized that to achieve optimal outcomes and improve patient satisfaction, pharmacy had to be accountable for the patient's medication-related needs.

Clinical services were eventually incorporated into the model of pharmaceutical care. Pharmaceutical care is defined as "the responsible provision of drug therapy to achieve definite outcomes intended to improve a patient's quality of life."[5] The pharmacist becomes an advocate for the patient. Not only are all medication therapy decisions made for the patient's benefit, but the patient has input into the decision-making process.

This approach also incorporates new roles for the technician. For example, institutions are now reporting the use of technicians to record laboratory results in the pharmacist's patient database.[1] At one institution, one of the pharmacy satellites uses the technician to record the serum creatinine level for patients receiving certain medications. The pharmacist uses the serum creatinine value to assess kidney function and make appropriate recommendations for dosing the medications. Technicians also obtain other laboratory test results for the pharmacist, such as cultures, sensitivities, and electrolytes (e.g., potassium and sodium). Technicians can screen medication orders for nonformulary and restricted medications and notify the pharmacist when there is a need to take action on those orders. Technicians can also review and collect missing information for a patient's database, such as allergies, height, and weight.

The ultimate goals of pharmaceutical care are to improve patient outcomes, enhance quality of care, heighten patient satisfaction, and decrease costs. Because of the fierce competition for health care dollars, quality care at the lowest cost may be the key to an institution's financial survival. W. Edwards Deming is known for his work in quality improvement techniques and philosophies. Deming often used the chain reaction shown in **Figure 3-2** to illustrate the effects of quality improvement.[6]

Quality Control and Quality Improvement Programs

Whether the pharmacy department is providing product- or patient-focused services, these services must be provided in a manner that guarantees a high level of quality. Quality and the prevention of adverse events is a popular topic not only for pharmacy but for any organization providing a product or service.[7] Medication safety continues to be in the public spotlight, and many accrediting agencies, including the Joint Commission on Accreditation of Healthcare Organizations (JCAHO), have made it a key agenda for institutional practices.

Quality itself is difficult to describe because the term has a positive connotation but denotes nothing measurable. Quality may be identified when a product or service meets predetermined standards, such as accreditation or certification. Quality may also be defined by what customers perceive. The pharmacy's customers may be patients, nurses, other pharmacists, or even accrediting agencies like JCAHO. Two methods or concepts can help to ensure quality: quality control and quality improvement. Each is important and has a specific role in pharmacy.

Quality Control

Quality control is a process of checks and balances (or procedures) followed during the manufacturing of a product or provision of a service to ensure that the end products or services meet or exceed specified standards (e.g., zero errors, zero problems). The start of any quality control program requires complete written procedures and training for all staff involved in that procedure. Checks and balances usually occur at critical points in the process. For example, a quality control system for the preparation of Cefazolin 1-gm IVPB may start with the technician pulling the Cefazolin vial from stock and checking to make sure it is the right drug and strength. Next, the technician will calculate the correct volume to withdraw, draw up the correct volume of drug, inject it into the bag, and check for any particulate matter or leaks. Finally, the technician will check the label for accurate and complete information (i.e., correct patient's name, drug, dose, route, diluent). Quality control is necessary to prevent defective products from reaching the patient and is especially desirable when IV products are being prepared. An error or defect in an IV medication may cause significant morbidity and even death.

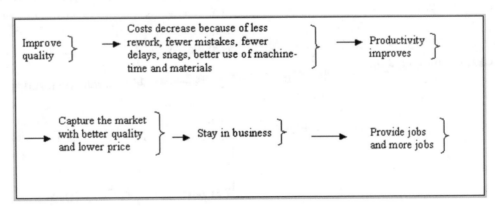

Figure 3-2. The Deming Chain Reaction.

Reprinted from *Out of the Crisis* by W. Edwards Deming by permission of MIT and the W. Edwards Deming Institute.

Published by MIT, Center for Advanced Educational Services, Cambridge, MA 02139. Copyright 1986 by the W. Edwards Deming Institute.

A disadvantage of quality control is the time and resources it adds to the process. Although quality control identifies and prevents errors or defects, the underlying cause is not always identified or corrected. As a result, the underlying problem still exists, and defects will continue. Quality improvement, an alternative method, reduces the problems and improves the product or service.

Quality Improvement

Quality improvement, also referred to as continuous quality improvement (CQI), is a scientific and systematic process involving monitoring, evaluating, and identifying problems and developing and measuring the impact of the improvement strategies. CQI concentrates on problems within a system, not on people. It requires that decisions be based on facts (data), not on a hunch or opinion. Various tools have been used to identify problems, assist in the data collection, and analyze the data. The use of these tools requires an understanding of when, how, and why they are used. For example, brainstorming is an excellent method of generating ideas and breaking down barriers between individuals or departments, because everyone in the group is given an opportunity to express an opinion. Another tool is a workflow diagram, which is a visual display of a given procedure. Everyone should participate in creating a workflow diagram, because each individual may have a unique role in the process not known to others in the CQI group. A workflow diagram ensures that everyone has the same understanding of the process. An example of a tool involving statistics is a run chart, which tracks patterns and trends over a period of time. The temperature of a medication refrigerator, for example, can be plotted each day on a run chart, allowing immediate action before medications are affected if the temperature becomes too high or low.

CQI requires everyone's participation. All employees are encouraged to offer ideas in the CQI cycle. An example of a CQI program used by many health care institutions is the FOCUSPDCA® cycle, which was developed by a health care organization, Hospital Corporation of America (HCA). FOCUSPDCA® is an acronym that can be broken into two sections: FOCUS and PDCA. FOCUS stands for

- Find a process to improve
- Organize a team
- Clarify the current process
- Understand the sources of the problem and the process variation

- Select the improvement or change

PDCA, which is continuous cycle, stands for

- Plan the improvement
- Do the improvement
- Check the results
- Act, or do, to hold the gain

Many accrediting agencies, such as JCAHO and the Centers for Medicare and Medicaid Services (CMS), require quality control and quality improvement programs. The technician can be a valuable resource in preparing surveys or inspections by these agencies. For example, the technician may be responsible for ensuring that refrigerator logs are completed, medication units are inspected, and IV hoods are inspected on a routine basis and the inspections documented. The technician may also assist in the database management for other pharmacy quality improvement services, such as adverse drug reaction (ADR) reports, medication occurrence reports, and drug use evaluations.

The Future

The trend is for hospitals to become more involved in critically ill and intensive care patients. In critical care settings, the technicians are already valuable assets because they can accurately prepare emergency IV drips. Automation and technology continue to change trends in health care. The role of technicians is already integral to automation. The growing use of automation, such as automated dispensing machines, will increase opportunity for technicians.

The role of the pharmacy technician has changed and will continue to change as health care systems change. The pharmacy technician must continue to be flexible, adaptable, and knowledgeable about new technologies and services. Thus, the technician is encouraged to attend any educational sessions or inservices on new skills, automation, and technology. The technician should volunteer and participate in any available programs, such as CQI or data collection for upcoming JCAHO inspections. Following these guidelines, the technician can stay one step ahead of change.

Recommended Reading

Brown TR. Handbook of institutional pharmacy practice. 3rd ed. Bethesda, MD: American Society of Hospital Pharmacists; 1992.

References

1. Hudkins JE, Crane VS. Role of pharmacy technicians in hospital formulary maintenance. *J Pharm Technol.* 1988; 4(Jul/Aug):144–56.

2. Ervin KC, Skledar S, Hess MM et al. Data analyst technician: An innovative role for the pharmacy technician. *Am J Health-System Pharm.* 2001; 58:1815–8.

3. Shah ND, Vermeulen LC, Santell JP et al. Projecting future drug expenditures—2002. *Am J Health-System Pharm.* 2002; 59:131–42.

4. American Society of Health-System Pharmacists. Practice standards of ASHP 1995–1996. Bethesda, MD: ASHP, 1995; p.11.

5. Hepler CD, Strand LM. Opportunities and responsibilities in pharmaceutical care. *Am J Hosp Pharm.* 1990; 47:533–43.

6. Walton M. The Deming management method. New York: Putnam Publishing Co; 1986, p. 25.

7. Bates DW, Laird N, Peterson LA et al. Incidence of adverse drug events and potential adverse drug events. Implications for prevention. ADE Prevention Study Group. *JAMA.* 1995; 274:29–34.

Self-Assessment Questions

1. Which of the following have had a role in rising health care costs?
   a. Medicare
   b. Medicaid
   c. JCAHO
   d. a and b
   e. none of the above

2. Which of the following are forms of technology used by pharmacy technicians in an institutional pharmacy?
   a. Micromix®, Automix®
   b. Pyxis®, SureMed®
   c. computers
   d. all of the above
   e. none of the above

3. Which of the following health care settings have been developed to reduce cost or increase patient satisfaction?
   a. managed care companies
   b. home health care companies
   c. mail order prescription companies
   d. health maintenance organizations
   e. all of the above

4. Which of the following statements regarding shrinking health care dollars is false?
   a. Technicians now have less responsibility.
   b. Hospitals are now looking for the most cost-effective means of providing services.
   c. Alternative practice settings, such as HMOs, are more common.
   d. The use of automation to streamline services is increasing.

5. Which of the following are advantages to a centralized pharmacy?
   a. easy to control medications
   b. reduces inventory compared with a decentralized pharmacy
   c. reduces the number of personnel required to operate a pharmacy
   d. all of the above

6. Which of the following are advantages of a decentralized pharmacy?
   a. Pharmacy services are closer to the patient.
   b. Fewer resources are required.
   c. The technician can assist the pharmacist in providing pharmaceutical care.
   d. a and c
   e. all of the above

7. Indicate which functions the technician can perform from a decentralized pharmacy.
   a. prepare doses in a unit-dose form
   b. perform pharmacokinetic calculations for gentamicin dosing regimen
   c. collect patient laboratory results for the pharmacist
   d. screen questions in the satellite
   e. a, c, and d
   f. a and d

8. Which of the following statements regarding pharmaceutical care is false?
   a. Pharmaceutical care is the responsible provision of drug therapy to achieve definite outcomes intended to improve a patient's quality of life.
   b. Pharmaceutical care affects only the activities of the pharmacist.
   c. Pharmaceutical care allows the patients to have input into decisions regarding their drug therapy.
   d. none of the above

9. In which of the following activities can a technician assist in the provision of pharmaceutical care?
   a. obtaining laboratory results
   b. counseling a patient
   c. screening orders for nonformulary/restricted drugs
   d. pharmacokinetic dosing of a medication
   e. a and c

10. Which of the following are disadvantages of a centralized pharmacy?
    a. lack of face-to-face interaction with other health care providers
    b. difficulty accessing information kept in the patient's medical chart
    c. increased time to deliver medications
    d. a and b
    e. all of the above

11. Which of the following best defines a unit-dose system?
    a. All medications are kept on the nursing station in bulk quantities.
    b. All medications are packaged in a single dose that is ready to be administered to a patient.
    c. A unit-dose system increases the number of errors compared with a system where bulk supplies of medications are dispensed.
    d. none of the above

12. Which of the following statements is true regarding unit-dose ready-to-use systems?
    a. increase waste
    b. increase errors
    c. increase cost
    d. all of the above
    e. none of the above

13. Which of the following statements regarding pharmacy directors is false?
    a. Pharmacy directors are typically at the top of the pharmacy department hierarchy.
    b. Pharmacy directors are responsible for all the activities of the department.
    c. Pharmacy directors often report to one of the hospital administrators (COO or one of the vice presidents).
    d. Pharmacy directors can operate all activities independent of other departments or managers.

14. Which of the following statements regarding organizational structures is (are) false?
    a. A typical organizational structure will have a CEO at the top of the hierarchy.
    b. All health care institutions have the same organizational structure.
    c. Organizational structures are important to maintain clear levels of responsibility and chain of command.
    d. none of the above
    e. all of the above

15. Which of the following is a true statement regarding unit-dose systems?
    a. Unit-dose systems are helpful in preparing medications for specialty patients, such as pediatric patients.
    b. Unit-dose systems increase the chance of errors.
    c. Unit-dose systems increase workload for nurses.
    d. Unit-dose systems decrease the level of drug control.

16. Which of the following statements regarding quality is false?
    a. Quality control is a process of checks and balances.
    b. Quality may be defined by what customers perceive.
    c. Because quality is something that cannot be directly measured, it is more important to

focus on the quantity of products made.
    d. none of the above

17. Which of the following is (are) false about quality improvement?
    a. Quality improvement falls under the total responsibility of the pharmacy director.
    b. Quality improvement is an important part of preparing for a JCAHO survey.
    c. Quality improvement concentrates on problems within a system, rather than on individuals.
    d. all of the above

18. Which of the following statements on technology is (are) false?
    a. Technology will continue to be used to help improve the efficiency of pharmacy services.
    b. Technology in pharmacy has provided new opportunities for pharmacy technicians.
    c. Technology and automation continue to interfere with pharmacy in the provision of patient-focused pharmaceutical care.
    d. a and c
    e. All of the above are true.

19. Which of the following regarding quality control is (are) false?
    a. Quality control is a method used only after a medication has been prepared.
    b. Quality control is a process of checks and balances.
    c. The checks and balances often occur at critical points in the process.
    d. Although quality control prevents errors or defects from occurring, the underlying cause may not be identified or corrected.
    e. none of the above

20. Which of the following statements about CQI is (are) false?
    a. CQI focuses on people problems.
    b. CQI is a scientific/systematic approach to quality.
    c. CQI allows decisions to be made on the basis of objective data alone.
    d. b and c
    e. a and b

21. Which of the following statements is (are) true?
    a. Computers have frequently been used with success by pharmacy departments; however, physicians using computers for medication

order entry have increased errors and added several steps to the medication use process.

b. Physician order entry can decrease the number of steps in the system and reduce the potential for errors.

c. Physician order entry will eliminate the role of pharmacists in the review of appropriate medication therapy.

d. all of the above

22. Which of the following statements is (are) false?

a. The CEO of the hospital is the individual to whom the board of directors reports.

b. CFO stands for Chief Financial Officer, and the CFO is responsible for the financial management of the hospital.

c. COO stands for Chief Operating Officer, and the COO is responsible for the daily operation of the hospital.

d. The CEO helps set a direction for the hospital by creating a vision and mission for the institution.

e. b and c

23. Which of the following statements is (are) true about a pharmacy satellite?

a. A pharmacy satellite is a decentralized form of pharmacy services.

b. Pharmacy services from a satellite pharmacy are performed in or near the patient care area.

c. Pharmacy satellites are located in the central pharmacy.

d. Pharmacy satellites eliminate the need for pharmacy technicians.

e. a and b.

f. a, b, and d

24. Which of the following are strategies to cut the costs of a health care institution?

a. Cut personnel.

b. Reduce the length of time that patients spend in the hospital.

c. Shift patient care to the ambulatory care setting.

d. Improve efficiency of existing services.

e. all of the above

25. Which of the following statements about quality control is (are) false?

a. Quality control builds checks and balances throughout the process.

b. Training is important for a quality control program.

c. Written policies and procedures are not needed if you have a quality control program.

d. Quality control is extremely useful for IV products because of the potential for morbidity and mortality.

e. all of the above

Self-Assessment Answers

1. d. Medicare and Medicaid have contributed to rising health care costs.
2. d. Micromix®, Automix®, Pyxis®, SureMed®, and computers are all examples of technology used by technicians in pharmacies.
3. e. All have been developed to reduce health care cost and increase patient satisfaction.
4. a. Technicians are being used for more activities. Technicians are now responsible for many activities formerly reserved for pharmacists (e.g., managing investigational drug programs, using automated technology).
5. d. All are advantages to a centralized pharmacy. A centralized pharmacy allows for efficient control, storage, inspection, preparation, and dispensing of medications with fewer personnel.
6. d. A decentralized pharmacy allows pharmacy services to be closer to the patients and expands the role of the pharmacy technician, but increases the need for resources (i.e., equipment, references, inventory, etc.).
7. e. The technician can perform many tasks from a decentralized pharmacy, including, but not limited to, preparing unit-dose products, collecting laboratory results, and screening questions for the pharmacist. The application of pharmacokinetics is a clinical skill that pharmacists are trained to provide.
8. b. Technicians participate in the provision of pharmaceutical care by gathering patient-specific laboratory results that are used to assess drug therapy.
9. e. Obtaining laboratory results and screening orders for nonformulary/restricted drugs are activities the technician can perform to assist the pharmacist in the provision of pharmaceutical care.
10. e. All are disadvantages of a centralized pharmacy. These disadvantages are based primarily on the location of the pharmacy.
11. b. A unit-dose system prepares each dose in ready-to-use form. To review the advantages of a unit-dose system, please refer to the "Unit-Dose System" section of this chapter.
12. e. None of the above is true about unit-dose systems. Please refer to the "Unit-Dose System" section of this chapter.
13. d. Pharmacy directors must collaborate with many departments to provide the best services for patients.
14. b. Many organizational structures may exist, depending on the size, the type of institution (e.g., teaching vs. community), and other factors.
15. a. Unit-dose systems are particularly valuable in specialty practices, such as pediatrics.
16. c. Quality should always be more important than quantity.
17. a. Quality improvement requires the participation of all individuals involved, not just a few.
18. c. Technology may change the focus of pharmacy's responsibilities, but these changes offer new opportunities and responsibilities.
19. a. Quality control consists of checks and balances built in throughout the process.
20. a. CQI looks at the entire system. CQI is based on the principle that most problems are system related, not people related.
21. b. Although computers cannot eliminate errors, they have reduced errors related to transcription and manipulation of orders. In addition, computer order entry reduces the number of steps in a medication use process.
22. a. CEO stands for Chief Executive Officer. The CEO is at the top of the organizational structure but reports to the board of directors.
23. e. A pharmacy satellite is a decentralized form of pharmacy services and is located on or near the patient care area. The pharmacy technician has many opportunities to work in a pharmacy satellite. Please refer to the "Decentralized Pharmacy Services" section of this chapter for a more detailed description of the technician's role in the pharmacy satellite.
24. e. All are examples of methods for cutting costs. All these strategies may affect the technician. These strategies offer opportunities for the technician to obtain new responsibility and knowledge about pharmacy services.
25. c. Written procedures are very important in quality control. Without written procedures, the potential for deviating from the production process may introduce errors and defects into the product.

Home Care Pharmacy Practice

KAREN E. BERTCH

Home health care is the provision of health care services in the patient's home, rather than an institutional setting or provider's office.[1] Home care pharmacy is part of home health care practice. The majority of pharmaceuticals in noninstitutional settings are provided through the community pharmacy system. The role of home care pharmacy is to provide intravenous (IV) medications and high-technology services in the home. Much of the material covered in Chapter 14, Aseptic Technique, Sterile Compounding, and Intravenous Admixture Systems, complements this chapter. Technicians planning to practice in a home care setting should review both chapters thoroughly.

Historical Overview and Current Practices

Patients first began receiving infusion therapy in the home, rather than in an institutional setting, in the late 1970s. The driving force for sending patients home was twofold: keeping patients in the hospital to receive long-term intravenous antibiotic therapy or parenteral nutrition was becoming too expensive, and it was a hardship for patients and their families to "live" in the hospital for the duration of their treatment. These long-term patients often required minimal intensive medical care other than the care associated with their infusion therapy. The search for alternatives to hospitalization led to the development of programs to treat long-term infusion patients at home, and the home infusion industry was born. In the past 20 years, home care, and in particular home infusion, has become one of the fastest growing segments of health care. Currently, approximately $5 billion per year is spent on home infusion services in the United States.[2]

Home infusion has grown so rapidly for several reasons. First, a number of studies have shown that administration of long-term IV therapy in the home is safe and effective, as well as less expensive, which helped physicians and insurance companies overcome any fear or reluctance they may have had in sending their patients to home health care agencies. In addition, the explosion of technology has supported the movement of patients to the home care setting. New developments have brought infusion pumps that are portable, small, easily programmable for a wide range of therapies, and, in some cases, disposable. These new infusion pumps have made it easier to teach nonprofessionals, such as patients and their families, to administer complicated therapies at home. Although consumers have demanded home care, citing improved quality of life, ability to return to work, and greater independence, the strongest impetus for home health care came from the dramatic changes in our health care system. Escalating health care costs forced hospitals to decrease the length of time patients spent in the hospital. As a result, patients are discharged earlier in the course of treatment and often need additional care when they get home. The need for more intensive medical care and support in the home provided opportunities for the home health care industry to grow. Finally, treating patients at home has the advantage, in some cases, of helping them to avoid the development of new infections in the hospital, such as hospital-acquired pneumonia.

Home infusion services are provided by a number of organizations, including hospitals, community pharmacies, home health nursing companies, integrated health care systems, and independent home infusion companies. After the tremendous expansion of home health care organizations, we are now seeing a consolidation, with mergers of companies and shifting of dominance among the providers of home infusion services.

Summary of Home Care Practice

Purpose and Goals of Home Infusion Therapy
The purpose of home care pharmacy practice is to provide high-technology therapy, which is usually provided in an institutional setting, at home. The intentions of these services are summarized in **Table 4-1**. Overall, the major goal is to provide safe and effective infusion therapy in the home. However, this therapy must also be cost-effective.

The Home Care Process
A patient may enter the home care process a number of ways. Usually a physician will recommend that a patient complete therapy at home. In some instances, the patient and the patient's family advocate home therapy, or the patient's insurance company may dictate where therapy will be provided. Sometimes an individual called a case manager will mediate the location of the therapy. The case manager may work for the insurance company, the hospital, or the home care

company. The case manager works to manage the cost of medical care for the patient and may be very influential in steering a patient to home care. The hospital may also initiate the process as it tries to control its costs by reducing patients' length of stay.

Once the decision has been made to send a patient home, a social worker or a discharge planner contacts the home care agency and initiates the process. In many hospitals, the discharge planner is a registered nurse with home care experience, and will begin preparing the patient for home therapy.

An intake coordinator at the home care company receives the patient referral. This person is responsible for retrieving the patient's demographic information (address, phone number, etc.), diagnosis, requested home care therapy, pertinent medical data, and insurance information. Home care personnel must keep the information provided on the patient in the strictest confidentiality, especially in light of the new regulations in the Health Insurance Portability and Accountability Act (HIPAA). The intake coordinator is often a nurse, or may be a technician specially trained for the job.

When all the necessary data have been obtained, the home care team decides whether to accept or refuse the referral. This determination is based on the ability and willingness of the patient or the caregivers to perform the tasks required to administer therapy at home. Other factors used to decide if a referral is acceptable include the appropriateness and feasibility of the therapeutic plan and the assurance that home care therapy will not place too much of a financial burden on the patient or the home infusion company.

Once the patient is accepted, the home care team begins providing services, which include determining the necessary medical supplies (e.g., tubing, dressing, needles, and syringes); selecting an appropriate infusion device (e.g., gravity system, pump) depending on the

TABLE 4-1. GOALS OF HOME CARE
■ Allow patients to leave the hospital earlier
■ Allow patients to receive therapy without being hospitalized
■ Allow patients to return to work or normal activities sooner
■ Allow patients to recuperate in the comfort of the home environment
■ Decrease health care costs
■ Provide safe and effective therapy and care
■ Achieve a smooth, nonstressful transition of therapy between the hospital and the patient's home

patient's therapy; preparing the drug for the infusion device in a sterile environment; assembling the appropriate patient educational materials and home care paperwork; and negotiating charges with the insurer. When all materials and supplies are ready, a delivery is made to the patient's home. The pharmacy technician may be involved in gathering supplies, educational material, and paperwork and in arranging delivery. The technician is always involved in preparing the drugs.

A registered nurse trained in home infusion makes the initial patient visit. Once the patient has been informed of his or her rights and responsibilities as a home care patient, the nurse begins to teach the patient about the supplies and drugs and how to care for the catheter so the patient can eventually administer the medications. If a patient cannot administer the medications, a caregiver learns how to do it, or, on rare occasions, a nurse will administer the medications. Several nursing visits are often required to ensure that the patient can perform medication administration and other procedures properly.

The initial referral process usually extends from 24 to 48 hours; occasionally, it must be performed in just a few hours. Empathy is essential in this process. Many times the idea of home infusion of medications overwhelms the patients and their caregivers. What is routine for the home care professional is often very foreign to the patient. Therefore, crucial members of the team (home care nurse, pharmacist) must be available (usually by pager) to the patient 24 hours a day, 7 days a week.

After the initial visit, the home care team develops a care plan for the patient. The care plan includes how the home care team will monitor the patient's therapy and watch for complications of therapy, as well as signs that the therapy is effective. Home care team members visit or contact the patients on a regular basis to assess their status, inventory their supplies, and make interventions when necessary. Generally, supplies and drugs are prepared and delivered weekly. This schedule may vary, however, depending on the stability of the medications or solutions and the laboratory work that is being conducted on the patient. The home care team maintains records of the patient's home care course. These records become the patient's home care chart and include documentation of all communications concerning the patient, physician orders and prescriptions, records of drugs and supplies sent to the patient, and laboratory results. The goal of the home care process is for the patient to experience a successful course of therapy without any adverse events. Once home care therapy is completed, the patient is discharged from the home care service.

The Home Care Team and Specific Roles

The members of the home care team are listed in **Table 4-2**. The primary team members are actively involved in the care of the majority of home infusion patients. Secondary members are involved only when a particular patient requires their services.

Physician

The physician is the leader of the team and ultimately responsible for the care of the patient. The physician provides the direction of care. Any major changes in therapy require the physician's approval. To ensure that the physician remains in charge of the patient's care, the physician reviews and signs the Certificate of Medical Necessity and Plan of Treatment. Physician drug orders (prescriptions) are usually given to the pharmacist over the phone, as in the community pharmacy setting. Written and signed physician orders received via facsimile machine, however, are becoming more common. Rules and regulations regarding prescriptions may be specific to each state, especially for narcotics. The technician should be aware of the regulations of the state in which the home care pharmacy is located. In the home care environment, the

TABLE 4-2. MEMBERS OF THE HOME HEALTH CARE TEAM

Primary Members

- Physician
- Registered nurse with infusion skills
- Registered pharmacist
- Pharmacy technician
- Reimbursement specialist
- Delivery representative
- Patient service representative
- Patient and caregiver

Secondary Members

- Registered dietitian
- Respiratory therapist
- Social worker
- Physical therapist
- Occupational therapist
- Certified nursing assistant (CNA)

physician does not see the patient daily or even weekly. The physician often relies on the nurse or pharmacist to evaluate and report the patient's clinical condition.

Nurse and Pharmacist

The infusion nurse and pharmacist are key members of the team. They work together to coordinate patient supplies, develop a plan of care, monitor and document the patient's status, communicate with the physician, coordinate physician orders, and make appropriate interventions. The nurse and pharmacist not only select the infusion device but also should be proficient in programming and troubleshooting the devices. Both disciplines are intensely involved in assessing and educating home care patients and work jointly to perform the organization's clinical quality assurance activities, such as measuring and documenting catheter infections, rehospitalizations, adverse events (including adverse drug reactions), and outcomes of the plan of care. Together, the nurse and pharmacist are responsible for communicating and coordinating all patient care activities.

Nurse

The nurse is the primary educator of the patient, responsible for teaching all aspects of home care therapy. When visiting the patient, the nurse assesses the patient's physical status, the patient's adherence to treatment plan, the condition of the catheter, and the psychosocial issues the patient may be facing. Maintenance of all intravenous catheters is the sole responsibility of the nurse. Home care infusion nurses are skilled in placement of peripheral catheters, and many are skilled in the insertion of peripheral long-term catheters or the peripherally inserted central venous catheter (PICC), discussed later in this chapter. Nurses also schedule and perform all blood work that is ordered.

Pharmacist

The pharmacist is solely responsible for the proper acquisition, compounding, dispensing, and storage of drugs. The pharmacist is also an educator, responsible for instructing the patient and the nurse on the drugs being administered. The pharmacist regularly assesses the home care patient with a focus on monitoring the laboratory data, the patient's symptoms, and the patient's compliance with drug therapy. Important additional clinical pharmacy roles are pharmacokinetic dosing of vancomycin and aminoglycosides, providing nutritional support services, and having an input in selection of the most appropriate drug for the patient.

The pharmacist is the drug information source for all other team members.

Pharmacy Technician

Pharmacy technicians support the pharmacist by performing the majority of the technical pharmacy functions. These functions consist of generating medication labels; compounding, preparing, and labeling medications; and maintaining the compounding room and drug storage areas. The technician is the coordinator of the IV room, working with the pharmacist to arrange the mixing schedule, ordering and maintaining drug and mixing supplies, and performing quality assurance on compounding activities. Other functions the technician may be responsible for are managing the warehouse and inventory of nondrug supplies, keeping track of accounts receivable, picking and packaging supplies for shipment to patients, and arranging for delivery of supplies to patients. In smaller companies, the pharmacy technician may wear many of these hats. In larger companies, separate individuals (who may be pharmacy technicians) perform each of these functions. For example, some technicians may be experienced drivers and only make patient deliveries.

Reimbursement Specialist

Although not active in direct patient care, the reimbursement specialist is a key to the economic viability of the company. The reimbursement department is the interface among the insurer, the home infusion company, and the patient. The primary responsibility of this department is to coordinate all the billing and collection for services provided. To fulfill this responsibility, reimbursement specialists brief staff regarding the services and drugs that are paid for by the insurers, negotiate the price of services with insurers, and brief the insurers regarding the status of the patient and the therapeutic plan. The timeliness of this function is crucial to the financial survival of the organization. The reimbursement specialist is also well versed in public aid and government reimbursement programs, such as Medicaid and Medicare.

Patient Service Representative

Many companies employ a patient service representative. The representative is responsible for controlling the patient's inventory of supplies and screening for problems. This person's job is to contact the patient or caregiver weekly or on a routine basis, depending on the anticipated delivery schedule. Often this individual helps coordinate pickup of supplies and equipment when the patient's therapy is completed. Occasionally a pharmacy technician may be responsible for this job.

Patient and Caregiver

Not to be forgotten as team members are the patient and the caregivers. In home care, much of the burden falls on their shoulders. They must be involved in the decision-making and the development of the care plan. The patient's right to be involved is clearly stated in the rights and responsibilities document that is presented on the initial visit. This document outlines how the patient and caregivers are included in the management of the patient at home.

Types of Home Care Therapies

Antibiotic Therapy

The administration of antibiotic therapy is the leading home infusion service, comprising 40 to 70 percent of the current home infusion business.[3,4] Four classes of antibiotics constitute more than 80 percent of home infusion antibiotic therapy (see **Table 4-3**).[4] Because antibiotics are discussed in Chapter 12, this discussion focuses on the use of these drugs in home infusion.

Cephalosporins, such as ceftriaxone, cefazolin, cefotetan, and cefoperazone, comprise 33 percent of IV antibiotic courses in the home.[4] Cephalosporins are very easy to use in home care because they have a low incidence of adverse reactions[4] and require minimal monitoring. Ceftriaxone is often prescribed because it can be given once daily, which decreases the costs of supplies and requires less work for the patient or caregiver. Most cephalosporins are stable for 10 days after admixture, so they are ideal for weekly deliveries. The only exceptions are cefotetan and cefoperazone, which are stable for 4 and 5 days, respectively. Moreover, many of the cephalosporins can be administered as an IV push, which is a convenience for the patient because of the short administration time.

TABLE 4-3. MOST COMMON ANTIBIOTICS USED IN HOME CARE

- Cephalosporins
- Penicillins
- Vancomycin
- Therapy for AIDS-related infections:

Ganciclovir	Foscarnet
Acyclovir	Amphotericin B
Pentamidine	

Penicillins comprise 23 percent of IV antibiotic courses in the home.[4] The top four drugs in this class are ampicillin/sulbactam (Unasyn®), ticarcillin/clavulanate (Timentin®), nafcillin or oxacillin, and penicillin G. Penicillins are more difficult to use in the home because they need to be given so frequently (every 4 to 6 hours). These types of dosing regimens are difficult for some patients to adhere to because of the time they take out of their day. Portable pumps, called ambulatory pumps, that can automatically give intermittent doses throughout the day are often required for penicillin therapy. Stability is another problem with this class. Ampicillin has short stability and must be mixed in the home prior to infusion. The availability of the ADD-Vantage®, Add-a-vial®, and Add-Ease® systems (see Chapter 14) has made mixing in the home much easier and safer. Most of the other penicillins have just 7 days of stability. Pushing penicillins to their stability limit is of concern because they may break down as they expire, and the breakdown products are associated with an increased risk of allergic reactions. The most common adverse effect in this class is allergic reaction, such as rash. Penicillins are also very irritating to veins, frequently causing phlebitis (redness and inflammation of the vein). It is highly recommended that patients receiving penicillins at home have a central catheter.

Vancomycin is the third most frequently prescribed drug in home care, accounting for 21 percent of the orders.[4] Vancomycin should be infused at a rate of no greater than 1 gm over 60 minutes to prevent Red Man Syndrome (discussed in Chapter 12). This can be accomplished by using a pump or infusion control device or by placing vancomycin in larger amounts of fluid (e.g., 150 to 250 mls). The pharmacist, using pharmacokinetics and the results of vancomycin blood levels, may do individualized patient dosing of vancomycin. Vancomycin is irritating to the veins and in the home setting is best given through a central catheter. If a peripheral catheter is used, vancomycin should be placed in 150 to 250 mls of solution to avoid vein irritation.

Additional antibiotics that are becoming more frequently used in the home care setting include azithromycin, doxycycline, and the fluoroquinolones. Azithromycin, doxycycline, and many of the newer fluoroquinolones can be given once daily via IV dosing, thus making them convenient for patients receiving therapy at home.[5]

Most available IV antibiotics can be used in the

home environment. However, relatively few infectious diseases require long-term infusion therapy. Five of the more common infectious diseases seen in home care patients are listed in **Table 4-4**.

Osteomyelitis

Osteomyelitis is an infection that occurs when bacteria invade bone. Bacteria can enter bones via the blood (e.g., in patients with bacteria in the blood); via nearby tissues, such as muscle and skin (e.g., when infections of the skin pass to adjacent bone); or via the external environment (e.g., because of a penetrating wound or a fracture where the bone breaks through the skin). The most common bacteria causing osteomyelitis is *Staphylococcus aureus*. This is a gram-positive organism that is commonly found on skin. Osteomyelitis caused by other types of bacteria, such as gram negatives and anaerobes, is becoming more common.

The main symptoms of osteomyelitis are fever and pain and tenderness near the affected bone(s). The diagnosis is usually based on X rays and a blood value called erythrocyte sedimentation rate (ESR). The ESR is abnormally high in patients with osteomyelitis. The antibiotic chosen to treat the infection is based on bone cultures when available or on the organism most likely to cause osteomyelitis. Treatment usually depends on how the patient got the infection. The duration of therapy is usually 4 to 6 weeks, but it may be longer. Patients' symptoms and ESR are monitored. With treatment of the infection, the ESR should return to normal.

Septic Arthritis

Septic arthritis is an infection of the tissue that lines the joints, which is called the *synovium*. The synovium has an extensive blood supply that allows bacteria in blood to enter the joint space easily. People with trauma to a joint, who have artificial joints, or who have had arthroscopy are more susceptible to this infection. Patients with diabetes, arthritis, or cancer are also at higher risk for septic arthritis. Therapy consists of surgical drainage of pus from the joint followed by 2 to 3 weeks of IV antibiotic therapy. Antibiotics are chosen on the basis of cultures of the drainage. If the causative bacterium is *Staphylococcus*,

TABLE 4-4. COMMON INFECTIOUS DISEASES IN HOME CARE PATIENTS	
■ Osteomyelitis	■ Septic arthritis
■ Cellulitis	■ Endocarditis
■ AIDS-related infections	

treatment is recommended for 4 weeks. For other bacteria, the duration of treatment depends on the specific organism. Therapy could range from 4 to 6 weeks.

Septic arthritis in patients with artificial joints is an extremely painful and costly experience. These patients often require surgical removal of the joint, followed by 6 weeks of IV antibiotic therapy, and then replacement of the joint with a new artificial joint.

Cellulitis

Cellulitis is an acute inflammatory infection of the skin that often extends deep into the subcutaneous tissue (tissue under the skin). Cellulitis is often secondary to events such as puncture wounds, ulcers, bites, and illicit drug injections. *Streptococcus* and *Staphylococcus* bacteria found on the skin are the most common causes of cellulitis. Usually cellulitis can be treated with 14 days of oral antibiotics. However, serious infections, such as diabetic foot ulcers and human or animal bites, may require IV therapy. Intravenous therapy duration for these infections may be anywhere from 4 to 6 weeks, or until 3 days after the acute inflammation disappears.

Endocarditis

Endocarditis is an infection of the heart valves or heart tissue. Patients who get endocarditis usually have an underlying heart defect, such as congenital heart disease (born with heart defect), rheumatic heart disease (result of an infection), an artificial heart valve, or a history of illicit drug abuse. Endocarditis can be difficult to diagnose because the symptoms, such as fevers, night sweats, fatigue, weakness, and malaise, can be caused by several different medical conditions. The diagnosis of endocarditis is based on blood cultures and ultrasound images of the heart. Endocarditis is treated with 4 weeks of IV antibiotics. Antibiotics are chosen on the basis of the organism identified in the blood cultures. Depending on the causative bacteria, combination therapy with two drugs may be required for the first 2 weeks of the 4-week course.

Infections in Acquired Immunodeficiency Syndrome Patients

Patients with acquired immunodeficiency syndrome (AIDS) often contract a number of different infections. The virus that causes AIDS, the human immunodeficiency virus (HIV), suppresses the patients' immune systems and makes them more susceptible to infections. *Pneumocystis carinii* pneumonia (PCP) is the most common opportunistic infection in AIDS patients. The symptoms of PCP are a dry cough and labored or difficult breathing. Therapy begins with 3 weeks of IV pentamidine or trimethoprim/sulfamethoxazole. Chronic maintenance therapy with oral antibiotics usually follows. Both pentamidine and trimethoprim/sulfamethoxazole have the potential for serious toxicity in AIDS patients. Pentamidine can cause severe hypotension if infused too fast, and it can also cause acute and severe drops in blood glucose because of a direct toxic effect on the pancreas. In the home setting, pentamidine should be placed in a pump to control the infusion rate. Many home care protocols require the immediate availability of normal saline infusion and a syringe of 50 percent dextrose so these side effects may be treated. Trimethoprim/sulfamethoxazole can cause a high number of allergic reactions in patients with AIDS. AIDS patients have a particularly greater risk for rash from this drug.

Fungal Infections

Infections with fungi, such as *Candida albicans, Histoplasmosis,* and *Coccidiomycosis,* are also common in patients without a competent immune system. Amphotericin B is the primary treatment for these infections. Patients may need to receive amphotericin B infusions for 1 to 2 months. Many patients experience fever, chills, and shakes from amphotericin infusions. This reaction often requires premedication with oral acetaminophen and diphenydramine. Some patients have such severe reactions that IV meperidine and hydrocortisone are given. The home care infusion pharmacy usually supplies these premedications. Infusions of amphotericin should always be given with an infusion pump. Normal saline, commonly used to flush the catheter before and after infusion of medication, is incompatible with amphotericin B—mixing the two results in precipitate. Therefore, the pharmacy compounds dextrose 5 percent syringes for flushing the catheter when amphotericin is used in the home. Lipid-based amphotericin B formulations are also available and are usually reserved for patients who cannot tolerate plain amphotericin B or who have compromised renal function. Three lipid-based amphotericin B products are currently available. Technicians should become familiar with these products because each requires a slightly different method of preparation owing to the lipid emulsion component. In some cases, because of short stability, the patient may have to admix these formulations in the home. AIDS patients require maintenance therapy following their treatment courses of IV antifungal agents, which is often accomplished with the oral antifungal agent fluconazole.

Immunosuppressed patients are susceptible to *Mycobacterium avium intracellulare* (MAI), part of the tuberculosis family. This infection is very difficult to treat, often requiring a patient to take up to five different medications concurrently. Therapy options include the oral agents clarithromycin, ethambutol, rifabutin or rifampin, ciprofloxacin, and clofazine. Amikacin is the only IV agent for treating MAI. The duration of therapy is indefinite. However, most patients cannot remain on amikacin for more than several months because of side effects.

Viral Infections

Cytomegalovirus is a common viral infection in AIDS patients. The infection manifests itself primarily as retinitis (infection of the retina or back portion of the eye), with blurred vision, or enteritis (infection of the intestines), with diarrhea. The infection is treated with 3 weeks of IV ganciclovir or 2 weeks of foscarnet followed by daily maintenance therapy. Ganciclovir almost always causes bone marrow toxicity in AIDS patients. Filgrastim (Neupogen®) therapy is often added to offset the bone marrow toxicity. Foscarnet can cause kidney damage if the patient does not drink plenty of fluids or if the drug is infused too fast. To help prevent kidney damage, foscarnet is compounded in 500 to 1,000 ml of fluid and infused with a pump, or 500 to 1,000 ml of normal saline is given prior to each infusion.

Provision of antimicrobial therapy for patients with AIDS was a mainstay of many home infusion programs 10 years ago. The advent of highly active antiretroviral therapy, however, has brought about marked declines in the number of these patients with cytomegalovirus or serious fungal infections. Many patients with HIV are now managed as chronic disease-state patients. As such, they may rarely develop complex infections, and a major shift to the treatment of these infections with oral rather than IV medications has occurred. The technician should still be aware of the IV medications used in these patients, because on occasion a patient may still require parenteral therapy.

Parenteral Nutrition

Patients with Crohn's disease (inflammatory disease of the small and large intestines) and bowel loss or dysfunction are the major recipients of parenteral nutrition. Malnutrition associated with cancer and AIDS is another indication for parenteral nutrition. Patients who absorb some nutrients from the food they eat, but not enough to completely sustain them, may require supplementation with parenteral nutrition. These patients require smaller volumes of parenteral nutrition and may not need daily infusions.

Patients receiving parenteral nutrition often require other IV medications. Many of these medications are not compatible with parenteral nutrition, which creates a difficult situation to manage in the home. The patient must learn to stop and start the parenteral nutrition and adequately flush the catheter to administer other medications. One solution is for these patients to have a central catheter with at least two separate lumens. Another solution is for the parenteral nutrition to be cycled to infuse over 12 to 14 hours at night instead of continuously over 24 hours.

Common parenteral nutrition 3-in-1 solutions (containing lipids) are stable for 9 days, and bags without lipids are stable for 14 days. Extended stability may be achieved with 3-in-1 solutions by using a dual-chamber bag in which the lipids are housed separately above the dextrose and amino acids. The patient "activates" the bag just before infusing it. A number of ingredients in parenteral nutrition, however, are stable for only 24 hours. These drugs are called *patient additives* and must be injected into the bag prior to infusion by the patient or caregiver. Examples of drugs that the patient must add are insulin, heparin, vitamins, and H_2-receptor antagonists (e.g., cimetidine, ranitidine). Drugs a patient needs to add should be supplied in vials rather than ampoule whenever possible. It is also advisable to limit the medications a patient must add to a parenteral nutrition bag to those that are absolutely indicated. This limitation is not only for sterility reasons but also for the sake of compliance and patient stress. The more medications are added, the greater the complexity of the solution and the greater the chance for incompatibility or contamination.

Parenteral nutrition patients require intensive monitoring, which usually includes weekly laboratory tests [chemistry and complete blood count (CBC)], glucose and fluid status monitoring, and patient weight monitoring. Monitoring progress toward the therapeutic goals of increasing the patient's weight and improving his or her nutritional status, as well as screening for complications such as liver toxicity and bone breakdown, is a continual process. Before a week's supply of solution is mixed, the pharmacist must review these parameters, as well as others. If these values are abnormal, the pharmacist must make recommendations to the physician, followed by appropriate changes in the parenteral nutrition formula (e.g., electrolyte content; volume; or

amount of glucose, lipid, or protein in the solution). The pharmacist may do this in consultation with a dietician. To avoid making parenteral nutrition bags that cannot be used, the technician should coordinate mixing of a patient's parenteral nutrition to follow scheduled laboratory blood draws and pharmacist and nursing assessments and visits. Changes to parenteral nutrition formulas are common, especially in the first few months of therapy. Patients on long-term parenteral nutrition tend to stabilize after several months and require less monitoring.

Chemotherapy

Most chemotherapy is given in a clinic setting, but a number of chemotherapy agents have been given in the home environment. Chemotherapy regimens reserved for home are those requiring prolonged infusion, usually greater than 24 hours. The agents that tend to be used in this manner are 5-fluorouracil, cyclophosphamide, adriamycin, vincristine, vinblastine, and paclitaxel.

5-Fluorouracil is the most common agent administered in the home care environment. Continuous infusions of 5-fluorouracil are used in treatment protocols for gastrointestinal (stomach, intestine, colon) and liver cancers. A central line is highly recommended for patients receiving chemotherapy at home to avoid the risk of extravasation (leaking of chemotherapy agents into the skin, resulting in severe skin damage). Side effects, primarily bone marrow toxicity and stomatitis (sores in the mouth), are frequent with this class of drugs. Many patients require the addition of filgrastim therapy to counteract the chemotherapy-induced drop in white blood cells. Other supportive therapies, such as IV fluids and antiemetic medications (e.g., $5-HT_3$-receptor antagonists such as ondansetron), are often administered to patients receiving chemotherapy.

Some oncology clinics and offices have home infusion pharmacies mix chemotherapy for their patients. The chemotherapy is usually compounded for IV push or short IV infusion in the clinic or office. When the home infusion company assumes this role, the home care team does not routinely monitor the patients.

Pain Management

The term *pain management* identifies infusion therapy for patients with chronic pain and pain associated with terminal illnesses. Intravenous medications are used when oral, rectal, or transdermal alternatives are not effective. Ninety percent of home care narcotic orders are for morphine.[4] When morphine is not acceptable, other drugs used for pain control are hydromorphone, meperidine, fentanyl, or fentanyl with bupivacaine. Usually one bag or cassette with enough narcotic to last the patient a week is dispensed at a time. The morphine solution is usually provided in concentrations of 5 to 50 milligrams per milliter (mg per ml).

In the home environment, narcotics can be given intravenously, subcutaneously, intrathecally, or epidurally. When the patient has an IV catheter, pain management is given via this route. The subcutaneous route is often used in patients without IV access. Intrathecal and epidural routes are saved for those patients who cannot achieve adequate pain control with IV therapy. Infusion of narcotics is accomplished using patient-controlled analgesia (PCA) pumps (see Chapter 14 for a complete description). Patients receiving PCA therapy will often receive a continuous basal infusion with or without patient-activated bolus doses. Attainment of adequate pain control, such that the patient has a decent quality of life, is the goal of the home care team. Team members assess the patient's pain on a continual basis.

Enteral Nutrition Therapy

Some home infusion pharmacies may also provide enteral nutrition therapy. Enteral nutrition is the administration of specialized formulas, high in required nutrients, through the stomach or part of the small intestine (jejunum) to meet a patient's nutritional needs. Patients who can eat will drink the enteral formula. Patients who cannot eat (e.g., are comatose) but have a working stomach or small intestine receive the formula through tubes placed either through their nose down into their stomach or surgically to their stomach or jejunum. Home infusion companies become involved when enteral nutrition is being administered continuously via a feeding tube, with or without a pump. When this technology is used, the expertise of the home health care team is often required. Patients who can drink their enteral formulas can usually get their therapy much cheaper through a community pharmacy system and do not require home care services. Monitoring of enteral nutrition patients includes monitoring their nutritional status and detecting drug-nutrition interactions.

Biological Response Modifiers

The biological response modifiers include filgrastim (Neupogen®), a long-acting colony stimulating factor called pegfilgrastim (Neulasta®), erythropoietin (Epogen®, Procrit®), a long-acting erythropoietin called darbepoetin alfa (Aranesp®), interferons, and growth hormone. These agents are called *high-technology drugs* because they are produced through genetic engineering. They are fairly easy to administer through conventional subcutaneous and IV routes.

Filgrastim is used for treatment of chemotherapy- and AIDS-induced neutropenia (low white cell count). Erythropoietin is used to treat anemia. Interferons have roles in the treatment of multiple sclerosis, chronic hepatitis, cancer, and certain rare diseases. Growth hormone is used in children less than 14 years old who are short in stature because of a deficiency in the hormone. All these agents are proteins that should not be shaken and require refrigeration for stability.

Other Therapies

Numerous other therapies are becoming more common in the home health care setting. In some cases, patients with congestive heart failure, women with premature labor, patients with the genetic disorder alpha-1 antitrypsin deficiency, and patients with simple dehydration are being treated at home with drugs that were previously infused in institutional settings. Additional parenteral medications that have been marketed in the past 2 to 3 years,[6] which the technician may see used more in the home health care setting, include the following:

- Alemtuzumab (Campath®), a monoclonal antibody for chronic lymphocytic leukemia
- Anakira (Kineret®), an interleukin-1 inhibitor for rheumatoid arthritis
- Caspofungin (Cancidas®), an antifungal for aspergillosis
- Ertapenem (Invanz®), a carbapenem antibiotic
- Moxifloxacin (Avelox®), a fluoroquinolone for a variety of infections
- Nesiritide (Natrecor®), a naturetic hormone for congestive heart failure
- Pantoprazole (Protonix® IV), a proton pump inhibitor for gastroesophageal reflux disease
- Treprostinil sodium (Remodulin®), a direct pulmonary and systemic arterial vasodilator
- Voriconazole (Vfend®), an antifungal agent for invasive aspergillosis and other serious fungal infections
- Zoledronic acid (Zometa®), a bisphosphonate for malignant hypercalcemia

Compounding in the Home Care Setting

Pharmacy technicians, under the supervision of pharmacists, are responsible for the correct preparation of sterile products. The pharmacy technician must become familiar with appropriate procedures to ensure that pharmacy-prepared sterile products are of high quality.

Clean Rooms

A clean room is an enclosed space, containing one or more clean zones, where the concentration of airborne particles is controlled. Most home infusion companies have either a clean room or sterile compounding area. The major difference between the two is the designated specifications for control of potential particulate and microbial contamination. In a clean room, the whole room environment is controlled for microorganisms within designated specifications. In a sterile compounding area, the sterile product preparation space only needs to be functionally separate from nonsterile product preparation and constructed to minimize particulate and microbial contamination. Although a clean room would seem to be the best option, new technology and products allow companies to prepare products safely in sterile compounding areas. A few state boards of pharmacy have mandated the use of clean rooms, but generally the home infusion company decides which type of space to use.

Clean rooms minimize the accumulation of particulates and microbial growth by using smooth, seamless, nonporous, and nonshedding building materials; temperature and relative humidity controls; and air filtration devices.[7] These rooms, coupled with policies that prohibit shedding materials (e.g., cardboard boxes) and porous and nonsterile materials from entering the room and require personnel to be properly trained and dressed in sterile garments, establish the cleanest compounding environment possible.

Clean rooms are classified on the basis of the number of particles in the room. A room with no more than 1 particle of 0.5 micron size per cubic foot of space is a Class 1 clean room. A room with no more than 100,000 particles of 0.5 micron size per cubic foot of space is a Class 100,000 clean room. At a minimum, clean rooms must be certified by a qualified contractor every 6 months or whenever the room is relocated.

Sterile compounding areas do not require formal certification.[7] The number of particles per cubic foot of space in a sterile compounding area can increase the chances of contaminating a product during preparation. When products are prepared in a sterile compounding area, however, different techniques and approaches to preparing sterile products are employed to reduce the risk of contamination.

Most infusion providers look to voluntary practice standards for guidance on quality assurance. Two professional pharmacy organizations have provided guidelines to help pharmacy personnel ensure that

TABLE 4-5. STERILE PRODUCT RISK LEVELS

Risk Level	Storage Conditions* Room Temperature	Refrigerator	Freezer	Products	Quality Assurance Level
1	Completely administered within 28 hrs	≤ 7 days	≤ 30 days	Unpreserved sterile products for one patient; batch-prepared products with preservatives; closed-system aseptic transfer of pharmaceutical obtained from licensed manufacturer into sterile final container	least
2	Storage and administration exceeds 28 hrs	> 7 days	> 30 days	Batch-prepared products without preservatives; closed-system aseptic transfer of combined multiple sterile ingredients obtained from licensed manufacturer in a sterile reservoir before subdivision into multiple units	more
3	N/A	N/A	N/A	Compounded from nonsterile ingredients or compounded with nonsterile components, containers, or equipment; use of open-system transfer or open reservoir for sterile or nonsterile combined multiple ingredients before terminal sterilization or subdivision into multiple units	most

*Storage Conditions: Room Temperature (15 to 30°C), refrigerator (2 to 8°C), freezer (−20 to −10°C); N/A = not applicable.

Adapted from: ASHP guidelines on quality assurance for pharmacy-prepared sterile products. *Am J Health-Syst Pharm.* 2000; 57:1150–69.

pharmacy-prepared IV admixtures are of high quality. The American Society of Health-System Pharmacists (ASHP) published the "ASHP Guidelines on Quality Assurance for Pharmacy-Prepared Sterile Products."[8] The United States Pharmacopeial (USP) Convention issued an informational chapter (chapter 797) on "Sterile drug products for home use."[9] This chapter was recently revised and renamed "Pharmaceutical compounding— sterile preparations." The revised USP chapter focuses on the practices of personnel who compound sterile formulations for patients' use rather than the site in which sterile formulations are used. In the ASHP guidelines, sterile products are grouped into three levels of risk to the patient. These categories depend on how much time elapses between when the drug is compounded and when it is administered—in other words, the expiration dating—as well as the use of nonsterile ingredients. These levels increase from least (level 1) to greatest (level 3) potential risk and have different quality assurance recommendations for product integrity and patient safety[8] (see **Table 4-5**).

The rationale behind the risk-level approach is that the greater the chance of contamination or the greater the risk of microbial growth in the product, the more careful providers should be to safeguard the sterility of the IV admixture. For example, a parenteral nutrition solution prepared by gravity transfer from manufacturers' bottles or bags, refrigerated for 7 days or fewer before administration, and given to a patient over a period not exceeding 24 hours is a relatively low-risk product in level 1. The highest risk of contamination would entail batch preparation of parenteral nutrition solutions with investigational L-glutamine prepared from nonsterile powdered glutamine in an open reservoir. Most products prepared for use by home care patients fall into risk level 2 because they are stored for more than 7 days.

Methods to assess an individual's aseptic techniques and environmental monitoring programs are two ways of identifying potential sources of contamination. Once a source is identified, steps can be taken to improve the environment. Pharmacy technicians can play a major role in preserving clean environments by maintaining them properly. Chapter 14 reviews the principles relating to sterile compounding and maintaining clean environments.

High-Technology Systems

The home infusion therapy industry's needs for technology to improve the patient's quality of life and save the infusion companies money have resulted in a number of products that allow medications to be delivered to patients at home. In most cases, the device chosen by the home care provider dictates the type of bag the medication or solution will be dispensed in and, to a greater extent, the type of supplies (e.g., tubing, needles) the technician will have to assemble for the patient. Technicians should become familiar with the infusion products and supplies the home infusion company uses to care for its patient population.

Five types of infusion systems are available for patients to use at home: (1) minibag infusion via gravity system, (2) syringe infusion via syringe device, (3) syringe infusion via IV push method, (4) rate-restricted IV administration set systems, and (5) ambulatory electronic infusion pumps. Home care providers select the most appropriate infusion device on the basis of several factors, the most important being the patient's needs (see **Table 4-6**). In addition to the patient's needs, cost and reimbursement are important factors that home care providers consider when selecting a system.[10,11] A range of issues to consider when selecting an infusion system are listed in

TABLE 4-6. PATIENT NEEDS ASSESSMENT FOR SELECTING INFUSION SYSTEMS

■ Age	■ Diagnosis
■ Clinical condition	■ Manual dexterity
■ Ambulatory status	■ Working status
■ Number of therapies	■ Training ability for self-administration
■ Language interpreters	■ Caregiver presence in the home
■ Nursing support requirements	
■ Travel time from home infusion provider	

Adapted from: Saladow J. Ambulatory systems for IV antibiotic therapy: making sense of the options. *Infusion.* 1995; April:17–29.

TABLE 4-7. ISSUES ASSOCIATED WITH INFUSION SYSTEM SELECTION

■ Product design	■ Product efficacy
■ Product reliability	■ Product availability
■ Product compatibility and stability	
■ Ease of staff training	■ Ease of patient/caregiver training
■ Nursing interaction time	■ Pharmacy handling time
■ Pharmacy filling time	
■ Ability of device to minimize complications	
■ Ability of device to minimize waste	
■ Storage space needed at provider's facility	
■ Storage space needed in patient's home	
■ Manufacturer and/or distributor support	
■ Ease of product disposal	■ Downtime and repair cost
■ Inventory costs	

Adapted from: Saladow J. Ambulatory systems for i.v. antibiotic therapy: making sense of the options. *Infusion.* 1995; April:17–29.

Table 4-7. All these factors have an impact on the cost-effectiveness and appropriate selection of infusion devices. Unfortunately, the industry has yet to quantify and analyze this impact. Selection is also complicated by the vast array of products that are marketed as the most economical method for therapy delivery.

Minibag Infusion via Gravity System

The minibag infusion via gravity system can be one of the most cost-effective methods to deliver medications. In fact, it is the standard IV administration set used for hospitalized patients in the United States. However, this system may be more expensive in the home care setting than in the institutional setting because of the cost associated with nurses teaching patients and caregivers and troubleshooting problems.[10] Other limitations of the system are the expectation that patients or caregivers will manually connect the bag to the infusion tubing and set and maintain the infusion rate; the increased risk for touch contamination; and the problems the cumbersome IV pole (on which the bag hangs) causes patients who are ambulatory or trying to work.

The AddVantage®, Add-Ease®, and Add-a-Vial® systems are special types of minibags used for drugs with short stability. With these systems, the patient or caregiver activates the vial just before administration so that the drug mixes with the diluent in the minibag. This is more expensive than the minibag system mentioned above because of the specially designed minibags these systems use and the special drug vials used with the AddVantage® system. All these systems have the same limitations as the traditional minibag system. See Chapter 14 for a more detailed description of special types of minibags.

Syringe Infusion System

The syringe infusion system is very cost-effective. Syringes are also easier to prepare and store than the containers used with other systems. The limitation of the syringe systems is the small volume of fluid that can be stored in one syringe, resulting in the preparation of concentrated dilutions. The potential for increased time spent educating patients and caregivers, for malfunctions of the electrical devices used to push the solution from the syringe, and restrictions on ambulatory or working patients are other concerns associated with syringe infusion systems.[10] Syringe infusion systems include the Baxa MicroFuse® Dual Rate Infuser (marketed in partnership with Abbott Laboratories), Baxa MicroFuse® Extended Rate Infuser, Baxa MicroFuse® Rapid Rate Syringe Infuser, Baxter Auto Syringe® AS50 Infusion Pump, Baxter InfusO.R.™ Syringe Pump, B. Braun Medical Perfusor™ basic and compact S, Excelsior ESP Infusion System, and Medfusion 2001 and 2010 models.[12] These devices are commonly used to administer IV antibiotics to home care patients. The Repro-Med Systems, Inc., Freedom 60™ syringe system is unique in that it uses a mechanical rather than electronic syringe driver along with a series of proprietary infusion sets that control the medication rate.

Rate-Restricted IV Administration Systems

Rate-restricted IV administration sets are used with proprietary fluid reservoirs that are designed specifically for use in the home care setting. The tubing used with these systems is designed to infuse the solution at a set rate. The only way to change the rate of infusion is to change the tubing. Three general types of proprietary fluid reservoirs can be used in this system: (1) the elastomeric balloon system, (2) the mechanical system, and (3) the electronic controlled pressure system.

Elastomeric Balloons

Elastomeric balloon systems were first used to deliver antibiotics and chemotherapy agents to patients outside the hospital setting. Infusion Systems developed the first device of this type, now called the Baxter Intermate® Elastomeric Infusion System. As the home care industry grew, so did the number of elastomeric balloon infusion systems. These reservoirs consist of multiple layers of elastomeric (i.e., stretchy, elastic-like) membranes within a hard or soft shell. When the device is filled with diluent and drug, the elastomeric material expands like a balloon filling up with air. When tubing is attached to the device and the patient's catheter, the elastic balloon forces the solution through the tubing and into the patient. The tubing controls the rate of the infusion, which can range from 0.5 to 200 ml/hour.[10] These devices do not have alarms or safety features, so they may not be suitable for medications that require a critical infusion rate (e.g., dobutamine) or that cause tissue damage if extravasation occurs.[11] The advantages of elastomeric balloons are that they are small and lightweight, thus convenient for use in ambulatory or working patients, and they are easy to use, which makes patient training simple.

The elastomeric balloon systems that are available besides Baxter's Intermate® Elastomeric Infusion System include Alaris Medical Systems ReadyMED®, I-Flow Homepump Eclipse®, and the Metrix Company Medflo II™.[12] Baxter Healthcare's Infusor™ System and I-Flow's Homepump® C Series Continuous Infusion System are designed specifically for administering chemotherapy and other long-term continuous infusions.[12] Elastomeric balloon reservoirs can be filled with syringes manually, via an automated filling pump, or by using a pump designed specifically for filling the elastomeric system. It is important that the technician or pharmacist prime the tubing to remove air before sending the elastomeric balloon device to a patient. Manipulation of these devices may take the pharmacy technician more time than other systems because of the need to add diluent and drug. Automated filling pumps can reduce the preparation time.

Mechanical Systems

Several mechanical systems that rely on positive pressure similar to elastomeric balloons have been developed. The I-Flow SideKick® infusion system was introduced in 1992. It consists of a round pump housing that unscrews and opens in two halves, a round disposable plastic bag that holds either 50 ml or 100 ml of fluid, and an IV flow control set. Once the two halves are screwed together, a spring-loaded pressure plate in the upper half of the pump housing applies positive pressure to the lower half containing the diluent and drug. As the clamp on the attached IV set is opened, the positive pressure forces fluid out of the bag at a rate controlled by the tubing. Infusion sets are available as disposable, preattached, or as a separate set that is detached from the disposable bag and reused for future doses. The reusable set lowers the overall cost per dose.[10] I-Flow also developed two additional devices similar in design and concept, the Paragon® and Paragon Elite®. The Paragon® is like the SideKick® except that it holds 110 ml of fluid and its spring mechanism is designed for more accurate delivery and slower infusion rates. It was designed to give longer-term continuous infusions, such as chemotherapy. The Paragon Elite® has the additional feature of a built-in battery, which can provide a series of alarm conditions. All these devices are manually filled with a syringe or a pharmacy-automated filling pump.

Electronic Controlled Pressure Systems

In early 1994, an electronic controlled pressure device, the Maxx®100 by Medication Delivery Devices, was introduced. Baxter Healthcare eventually acquired it. This system consists of a rectangular housing and a series of disposable reservoir bags with preattached IV flow control sets.[10] Detachable IV sets may be reused for multiple doses, reducing the cost per dose. A proprietary plastic bag is placed inside the device housing on top of a bladder, which expands with air and applies pressure to the bag when the device is closed and turned on. The IV tubing controls the drug administration rate once the clamp on it is opened. It differs from the previously discussed rate-restricted systems in that it provides controlled pressure pumping via an electronic system rather than by positive pressure. It also has audible and visible alarms. The Maxx®250 infusion system, a 250-ml version of the Maxx®100 system, was recently released. Proprietary minibags prefilled with diluent may be used in this device.

A unique rate-restricted IV administration system is the Eureka™ infusion pump by Universal Medical Technologies, Inc. The delivery rate of the IV solution is determined by the selection of the IV administration set, which is designed to deliver solution at a controlled flow rate. The pumping mechanism on this device is a controlled positive pressure displacement. It maintains a constant pressure on an IV solution container to evacuate all of its solution. The Eureka™ infusion pump will accommodate standard solution containers plus the reconstituted drug solution.[12]

Rate-restricted IV administration systems offer significant advantages in the delivery of antibiotics and other medications to home care patients. Unfortunately, many of them still require addition of diluent to the reservoirs. When more are available with prefilled diluents, these systems will be more convenient, reduce pharmacy admixture time, increase flexibility of use, and be more cost-effective.

Ambulatory Electronic Infusion Pumps

A number of ambulatory electronic infusion pumps are designed to deliver therapies to home care patients. Many of these devices integrate infusion and computer technologies. Some are designed to administer a single therapy, such as parenteral nutrition, while others can accommodate multiple types of therapies used in the home.[10,11] Today, more than 30 ambulatory electronic infusion devices are available.

Ambulatory electronic infusion pumps are small, are lightweight, and can be worn by the patient during infusions. They offer a wide range of infusion rate settings and volumes that are controlled by the electronic components of the individual device. Moreover, these pumps can infuse out of standard IV containers or proprietary reservoirs. Selection of an ambulatory device depends on patient-, therapy-, and infusion service-related factors. **Table 4-8** reviews these factors. The device selected for a patient on home infusion therapy may ultimately determine how the patient views the home care experience.[13,14]

TABLE 4-8. FACTORS INFLUENCING SELECTION OF AMBULATORY INFUSION DEVICE[13,14]		
Patient-Related	**Therapy-Related**	**Infusion Service-Related**
■ Age	■ Number of drugs	■ Distance from home care office
■ IV access	■ Drug stability and compatibility	■ Reimbursement issues
■ Ambulatory status	■ Duration of infusion	■ Nursing support requirements
■ Level or presence of caregiver assistance	■ Dosing schedule or pattern	
	■ Volume of infusate	
■ Environment	■ Patient-controlled dose needs	
■ Language interpreters	■ Accuracy of small volume delivery	
	■ Life of battery	

Ambulatory infusion devices are typically divided into two broad categories: therapy-specific and multiple-therapy devices.[15] Therapy-specific devices are designed to provide single therapies, such as pain management or total parenteral nutrition (TPN). Operation of these devices is fairly straightforward and can be done by clinicians or patients. Common therapy-specific devices include the Abbott Provider® 6000, Abbott Pain Manager II for PCA, McKinley Medical WalkMed® pumps, and some of the SIMS Deltec CADD® infusion pumps. Other therapy-specific devices are found in **Table 4-9**. The CADD® pumps are some of the most widely used ambulatory infusion devices in the United States. Most of these devices are therapy-specific and relatively simple to program.[12,14] The CADD-TPN®, CADD-Legacy™ PCA, and CADD-Legacy™ Plus are designed specifically for TPN infusions, pain medications, and antibiotics, respectively. The CADD-TPN® has two proprietary sets that connect to standard TPN containers, one containing a 0.22 micron filter for non-lipid-containing TPN

solutions and one containing a 1.2 micron filter for lipid-containing solutions. The CADD-Legacy™ PCA and CADD-Legacy™ Plus devices use proprietary 50-ml or 100-ml cassettes with attached tubing that contain the diluent or drug. These devices are manually filled using a luer-lock syringe. Other IV containers can be used with these two devices by attaching a bypass spike adaptor with tubing. Filling the cassettes or containers requires the technician to remove air from them because the pumps do not contain air-eliminating filters.

The growth of the product offerings in ambulatory electronic infusion devices took hold in the mid-1990s with the introduction and acceptance of the multiple-therapy devices. Multiple-therapy devices allow providers to carry a single device that may be used for patients with different therapies. Inventory can be consolidated, capital equipment costs can be overcome more quickly, and clinical staff training is simplified. These devices can infuse continuously or intermittently and may be used to infuse TPN solutions, antibiotics, antineoplastic agents, and pain medications. Most are

TABLE 4-9. THERAPY-SPECIFIC AMBULATORY INFUSION DEVICES[12,15]

Device	Manufacturer	Primary Therapy
Provider® 6000	Abbott Laboratories, Inc.	Continuous and intermittent infusions, patient-controlled analgesia
Pain Manager II	Abbott Laboratories, Inc.	Patient-controlled analgesia
6060 Epidural™ PCA*	Baxter Healthcare Corporation	Epidural PCA
Epic™	McKinley Medical	Epidural pain management
WalkMed® IC	McKinley Medical	Chemotherapy, antibiotics
WalkMed® 350	McKinley Medical	Low-dose continuous infusions
WalkMed® PCA	McKinley Medical	Patient-controlled analgesia
WalkMed® Plus	McKinley Medical	Continuous only, intermittent infusions, PCA, PCA + intermittent infusion
MiniMed 407 C	MiniMed	Microinfusions (terbutaline)
MiniMed 508	MiniMed	Insulin
CADD-Prizm® PCS	SIMS Deltec Inc.	PCA, continuous infusions
CADD-TPN®*	SIMS Deltec Inc.	Parenteral nutrition, continuous infusions
CADD-Legacy™ 1	SIMS Deltec Inc.	Continuous infusions
CADD-Legacy™ Plus	SIMS Deltec Inc.	Continuous and intermittent infusions
CADD-Legacy™ PCA	SIMS Deltec Inc.	Patient-controlled analgesia
CADD-Micro	SIMS Deltec Inc.	Microinfusions (insulin, terbutaline)
30 Pump	Sorenson Medical	Chemotherapy, inotropes, etc.
200 Pump	Sorenson Medical	Antibiotics
PCA Pump	Sorenson Medical	Patient-controlled analgesia
PCEA Pump	Sorenson Medical	Epidural patient-controlled analgesia

* PCA = patient-controlled analgesia; TPN = total parenteral nutrition.

single-channel, allowing infusion of only one medication at a time. Others are multiple-channel, capable of infusing up to four different drugs at different rates.[13,15] In addition, newer devices offer telemedicine capabilities whereby information can be transmitted over standard telephone lines via the use of modems from the patient's home to the health care provider's office. Providers can change infusion rates, correct alarm conditions, track patient compliance, and view or print infusion status reports without making a home visit. **Table 4-10** lists the multiple-therapy devices.

New ambulatory infusion devices continue to be developed. Disposable devices that infuse large volumes of fluid using disposable batteries are on the horizon. Home infusion providers must keep up with the latest infusion device technology so they can provide the high quality of care that patients and third-party payers expect. Pharmacy technicians must become familiar with the different ambulatory infusion devices available. This knowledge will allow technicians to choose the appropriate supplies when preparing products and sending the supplies patients need to use the devices.

Automated Compounding Devices

Automated compounding devices are based on peristaltic pump principles similar to infusion pumps. Peristaltic pumps control rate by squeezing tubing. Patient-specific parenteral nutrition formulations and the benefits of providing 24-hour, single-container TPN and hydration bags have driven the need for automated compounding devices. The need is especially prevalent in home care practice because the patient usually gets a 1- to 2-week supply of TPN or fluids. Automated compounding devices are also used to prepare complex multicomponent sterile products, such as nutrition formulations and cardioplegia solutions, as well as batch preparations of other solutions.

TABLE 4-10. MULTIPLE THERAPY AND MULTIPLE CHANNEL AMBULATORY INFUSION DEVICES[12,15]

Device	Manufacturer	Therapies Delivered
AIM Plus™†¨	Abbott Laboratories	Antibiotics, chemotherapy, continuous infusions, PCA*, TPN*
Gemstar®†¨	Abbott Laboratories	Continuous and intermittent infusions, pain management, TPN; variable, weight-dosed, and mL/hr*
6060 Homerun™†¨	Baxter Healthcare Corporation	Antibiotics, chemotherapy, continuous infusions, PCA, TPN
2000 Plus™†¨	Curlin Medical	Continuous and intermittent infusions, PCA with IV*, epidural or subcutaneous delivery, TPN with ramping, variable with 24 specified doses
Panomat® 3 mL* (C-3,T-3, V-3)†	Disetronic Medical Systems	Continuous, intermittent, or circadian infusions with demand or automatic dosing, subcutaneous or IV microinfusion, intrathecal pain control
Panomat® 5 mL (C-5,T-5, P-5,V-5)†	Disetronic Medical Systems	Continuous, intermittent, or circadian infusions with demand or automatic dosing, subcutaneous or IV microinfusion, intrathecal pain control
Panomat® 10 mL (C-10,T-10, P-10,V-10)†	Disetronic Medical Systems	Continuous, intermittent, or circadian infusions with demand or automatic dosing, subcutaneous or IV microinfusion, intrathecal pain control
Verifuse® Plus†	I-Flow Corporation	Antibiotics, chemotherapy, continuous infusions, PCA, TPN
I-Flow VIP†	I-Flow Corporation	Antibiotics, chemotherapy, continuous infusions, PCA, TPN
Vivus™ 4000†‡¨	I-Flow Corporation	Antibiotics, chemotherapy, continuous infusions, PCA, TPN
EZ Pump§	SIGMA International	Antibiotics, chemotherapy, circadian infusions, continuous infusions, microinfusions, PCA
CADD-Prizm® VIP†¨	Sims Deltec, Inc.	Antibiotics, chemotherapy, continuous and intermittent infusions, PCA, TPN

* PCA = patient-controlled analgesia; TPN = total parenteral nutrition; mL/hr = milliliters per hour; IV = intravenous; mL = milliliters.

† Denotes devices with telecommunications capabilities.

‡ Can infuse four medications, either continuously or sequentially.

§ Can infuse up to two medications with the addition of pump modules.

Automated compounding systems currently marketed include Nutrimix Macro® (Abbott Laboratories), Nutrimix Micro® (Abbott Laboratories), MicroMacro 12® (Baxa), Exacta-Mix® (Baxa), Automix® 3+3, Automix® 3+3/AS, Micromix® (Baxter Healthcare Corporation), and Hyper-Former® (B. Braun Medical). The advantages of these devices over manual compounding are increased efficiency and accuracy, automatic calculations (software-driven systems), potential reduction in labor, reduction in materials, and demonstrated cost-effectiveness.[16,17] The disadvantages of a completely automated system are the potential for equipment malfunction and power outages. Automated compounding devices are available with proprietary tubing that attaches to the device. Proprietary or other manufacturers' containers are then connected to the tubing. The device operator must remove air from the filled container before sending it to the patient. Removing air avoids setting off device alarms and eliminates other problems.

Special considerations are needed when using automated compounding devices. Home infusion companies use a compounding sequence or manufacturing practice that minimizes the potential for gross (large) or subtle (slight) incompatibilities, especially when mixing total nutrient admixtures (TNAs). It is essential that technicians recognize the importance of these sequences and practices, because technicians often play a major role in, or are completely responsible for, following the sequence. The order of mixing of components as well as their final concentrations is important for TPN solution stability. Many manufacturers of automated compounding devices have predetermined additive sequences available for use by operators of these devices.[18] Since many pharmacies are using automated compounding devices, ASHP has developed guidelines to outline the key issues that should be considered to incorporate this type of technology into pharmacy operations safely and cost-effectively.[19] The development of dual-chamber bags in which the lipid is in the upper portion of the bag while the other TPN components are in the lower portion also may improve the safety of TNA formulations. These bags extend stability (up to 30 days). The patient or caregiver activates the bag by removing a white strip and gray bar just prior to infusing. These bags can be filled using an automated compounding device. To ensure stability throughout the administration period, the patient adds some medications, such as multivitamins and insulin, just prior to infusion.

Labeling and Expiration Dating

Labeling in home care practice is similar to labeling in institutions. However, home care has some unique requirements. The product is considered an outpatient prescription, so it must meet state board of pharmacy requirements (see Chapter 9). The label should be written so that lay people (people who are not medically trained, such as patients and caregivers) can interpret and understand the directions.

The information required by law for a home care product label includes the patient's name, prescription number, prescribing physician, and date (see **Figure 4-1**). The patient's address is optional; however, an address may simplify delivery procedures. Directions for use should state the rate and frequency of administration and any special handling or storage requirements. The name and amount of drug contained in one dose and the appropriate volume for that amount are listed. Then, the name and volume of admixture solution equivalent to one dose of drug is indicated. The actual expiration date established for the product is noted. The individual(s) who prepared and checked the admixture must initial the label. Finally, auxiliary labeling should include federal transfer labeling, and, as an option, specific precautionary labels or storage instruction labels may be applied to the product. The bottle or bag sequence may be listed as well to help track the number of doses ordered or the total number of doses administered.[8]

Expiration dating has important implications in home care practice because it may dictate whether the pharmacy can prepare batches, reduce waste, and decrease the frequency of deliveries to the patient. Expiration dates for admixtures are based on stability and sterility data.[8,9] Most home care pharmacists have references that list expiration dates for products or their components. The most common reference is the *Handbook on Injectable Drugs*, but many pharmacists keep files containing published research articles on stability. *Extended Stability for Parenteral Drugs* is a relatively new reference that contains stability information on the most commonly used medications in alternate site infusion practice. Technicians need to be aware of expiration dates on products they use to make sterile admixtures. When a product expiration date is a particular month, it can be used through the last day of that month.

A product can quickly change or deteriorate as a result of changes in pH, temperature, and drug structure that may cause solubility problems; drug adsorp-

```
┌──────────────────────────────────────────────────────────────┐
│          Facility/Pharmacy Name, Address, Telephone Number⁽⁷⁾   │
│  Rx: 1234567⁽¹⁾                          Date: 2/11/04⁽¹⁾        │
│  Patient:      Jane A. Doe⁽²⁾            Physician: J.R. Smith⁽¹⁾ │
│                110 S. Elm St.            No refills⁽¹⁾           │
│                Anywhere, MD⁽²⁾           Bag: # 1 of 5⁽⁸⁾        │
│                                                                │
│  Nafcillin 24gm/250ml SWFI⁽⁴⁾                                  │
│  Cadd Prizm Pump to infuse Nafcillin 2 GM⁽⁴⁾ IV every 4 hours   │
│  via intermittent infusion for 10 days. Change bag every 48    │
│  hours. Keep bag refrigerated and warm to room temperature     │
│  prior to infusion.⁽³⁾                                          │
│                                                                │
│  Pump Settings ⁽³⁾: Res Vol = 250ml; Dose = 20ml⁽⁴⁾; Dose       │
│  Infusion Time = 1 hour                                        │
│  Cycle = 4 hours; KVO = 0.2ml/hour                             │
│              ***Bag will last 48 hours****                     │
│  Use before 12N 2/24/04⁽⁵⁾                                     │
│  Prepared by: AP⁽⁶⁾                    Checked by: TK⁽⁶⁾        │
└──────────────────────────────────────────────────────────────┘
```

Figure 4-1. Sample home care label.

KEY: Required Labeling

1 - Prescription number, date, and prescribing physician—These are typically required by state boards of pharmacy. Used by dispensing pharmacist to verify original order.

2 - Patient name and address—The patient's name should be printed as part of the label.

3 - Directions to the patient for use of the medication—These should be easy to understand. They should include rate and frequency of administration. Any special handling or storage requirements should be stated.

4 - Name and volume of admixture solution—The amount of admixture solution per dose should be stated. In the case of a container housing more than one dose, the volume listed should be equivalent to the total volume in the container.

5 - Beyond-use date—The date is usually the actual beyond-use date established for the product.

6 - Initials of persons who prepare and check IV admixture—State boards of pharmacy often require that this information appear on the label. In addition, this information is helpful when questions arise about product preparation.

7 - Name, address, and telephone number of the compounding facility/pharmacy—This information provides an easy mechanism for the patient to contact the dispensing pharmacy when questions arise.

8 - Optional labeling—The bottle or bag sequence number can help to track the doses ordered and/or doses administered.

Adapted from: Kuban PJ. Labeling sterile preparations. In: Compounding sterile preparations, 2nd ed. Bethesda, MD: ASHP; 2005:102.

tion to, and absorption within, product containers; and chemical degradation due to hydrolysis, oxidation, reduction, or exposure to light. The method of delivery—either the system or technique—and environment of drug administration can also affect stability.[8,9] Home care practice demands that the pharmacist assign a maximum expiration date that is still within appropriate stability limits. A common problem is the use of drugs with limited stability at room temperature. For drugs to be given via an ambulatory infusion device, at least 24-hour stability at room temperature or warmer is required.[13] For drugs that have limited room temperature stability, the patient or caregiver may be taught how to prepare the drug immediately before administration. Although a product may be stable for an extended period, its sterility and potential for bacterial growth must also be considered in assigning an expiration date. Sterile products not intended for prompt use should be stored at no higher than 4°C to inhibit microbial growth, unless room temperature storage is warranted.[9]

Packaging and Transport

Temperature control during transportation of sterile products to a patient's home is critical. Appropriate packaging must be used to keep the temperature near the midpoint of the product's specified range.[9] Technicians should be familiar with the pharmacy's procedures for packaging products so they can abide by them. Most admixtures are placed in a zip-lock bag to prevent a problem if leakage occurs. Hazardous substances should be double bagged to protect the shipper, patient, and caregiver if leakage occurs. These individuals should be trained to deal with a spill in case it occurs. Certain product containers, such as prefilled syringes, should be packaged in hard plastic or cardboard tubes or within bubble packs to prevent movement during transit. Refrigerated items should be transported in coolers, and postdelivery temperature checks should be made to ensure that an adequate temperature was maintained. Delivery personnel should be familiar with the shipping requirements for each package. In some cases, technicians may make deliveries, so they must understand the delivery requirements.

Supplies for the Home Care Patient

Technicians should become familiar with the supplies used by home care patients so the technicians can communicate about supply issues with the patient and other health care professionals. Familiarity entails being aware of the various venous access devices (catheters that reside in the patient's vein through which medication or solution flows) as well as specific supplies that the patient or caregiver uses to set up an infusion, such as tubing and needles.

Venous Access Devices

Peripheral access (infusing drugs through a needle placed in the veins of an arm) is one of the most common ways patients receive infusions in the hospital, but it does not always work well in the home care environment. Peripheral access is better for short courses of therapy than long courses of therapy. Peripheral veins often collapse or rupture, so a new vein must be used, and, in some cases, no usable peripheral veins are available. To avoid this scenario, other types of venous access devices are used for patients who need long-term access. A number of extended venous access devices that can be used for weeks to months, even years have been developed for patients who require repeated venipuncture (the puncture of a vein for any therapeutic purpose) or who have suboptimal peripheral venous access due to advanced age, obesity, or previous irritating drug therapy. These devices are classified as tunneled central venous catheters, subcutaneous vascular access ports, or peripherally inserted central venous catheters (PICC).[13] A general understanding of the venous access devices commonly used is important for technicians. This knowledge helps technicians select patient supplies more accurately and efficiently.

Two commonly used tunneled central venous catheters are the Broviac and Hickman catheters. These catheters were introduced in the 1970s and are made of barium-impregnated silicone rubber (Silastic®). They facilitate long-term vascular access with minimal complications. These catheters are surgically inserted into a central venous site, such as the subclavian vein, and passed through the vein until the tip of the catheter stops at the entrance of the heart's right atrium. After insertion, the catheter is tunneled subcutaneously for a short distance to establish a barrier between the skin exit site and vascular entrance site. An external dressing or bandage is applied to the site. Available tunneled models are distinguished by the catheter material (silicone or polyurethane), number of lumens (single, double, or triple), catheter diameter (French size 3 = pediatric to 12.5 or 13.0 = double or triple lumen), lumen diameter (0.2 to 2.0 mm), and type of catheter tip.[13,20,21] Manufacturers of these catheters include Arrow International, Inc., Bard Access Systems, Inc., Cook Critical Care, and Quinton. The lumens (access ports on the catheters) are separate within the catheter, so incompatible solutions can be administered at the same time. To prevent the formation of blood clots when the catheter is not in use, a heparin solution of 100 units/ml should be locked into each lumen at least daily. Another type of tunneled catheter, the Groshung® catheter, is unique in that it has a pressure-sensitive, distal-tip slit valve (a valve at the end of the catheter with a slit in the rubber). Infusing or withdrawing fluid causes pressure that opens the valve. When the valve is closed, blood cannot flow back into the catheter. This eliminates the need for heparin locking and also decreases the risk of air embolism. These catheters are flushed with 5 to 10 ml of saline after each use and weekly when the catheter is not in use. Infections are the most common complications of tunneled venous access devices. Other complications include catheter occlusion (clogging), dislodgement (moving out of the vein), incorrect catheter positioning, and venous thrombosis (blood clots).

The subcutaneous vascular access port consists of a small-volume reservoir with a self-sealing septum that is connected to a central venous catheter. This system is placed subcutaneously (under the skin) by a surgeon, usually in the chest wall, and is hardly noticeable. A dressing or bandage is unnecessary. The device is accessed by inserting a specially designed, noncoring needle, called a Huber needle, through the skin and port septum.[13] Single- and double-lumen devices are available. Products on the market include Port-a-Cath®, Infusaport®, Mediport®, and Davol®. These devices are suitable for intermittent or prolonged continuous infusions. Between infusions, the port is flushed and locked with heparin 100 units/ml, 5 ml at monthly intervals. Complications are similar to those of tunneled catheters and include infections, occlusion, and thromboses. Needle dislodgement from the septum may occur, as may pocket (the opening under the skin where the device resides) infections.

The use of PICCs has continued to increase because of their unique features. PICCs can be inserted at the hospital bedside or at home by specially trained nurses. They are inserted through a vein in the arm, threaded through other veins in the arm, and end up with the tip resting in the superior vena cava.[13,21] PICCs can remain in place for weeks to months. An X ray is used to confirm placement before infusing solutions that are very hypertonic, such as TPN. PICC lines, also known as *long-arm* or *long-line* catheters, are made of silicone (Silastic®) or flexible polyurethane and are available in single- and multilumen designs. They require daily flushing with heparin and dressing changes. Complications include phlebitis at the insertion site or along the vein, infection, cellulitis, occlusion, catheter tip migration, and thrombosis.[13,21,22]

Peripheral catheters are available in a number of gauges and lengths, commonly from 18- to 24-gauge and three quarters to one inch in length. These catheters are desirable for short-term therapies. Most home care providers' protocols call for changing peripheral catheters every 72 hours.

Midline catheters are peripheral catheters but have the advantage of being 6 inches long and able to remain in place on average 7 to 10 days or even up to months. For this reason, they are appropriate for longer term therapy, such as the treatment of endocarditis with IV antibiotics. Midline catheters are usually placed in one of the large veins of the upper arm, the basilic or cephalic veins. Because of this, midline catheters are particularly ideal for infusing caustic drugs, unlike other peripheral catheters. A Landmark® catheter is a common type in home care.

Other Supplies

Patients on home infusion therapy require a number of other supplies. Many home care providers have standard supplies that are sent to most patients, whether they have a peripheral or central venous catheter. In general, these supplies include alcohol pads, injection caps (caps that go onto the end of the catheters), nonsterile gloves, a sharps container, medical waste bags, and tubing. Additional supplies depend on the type of venous access and therapy, the physician, or account specifications. For drugs or fluids requiring filtration, an appropriate filter should be included. If a patient has a peripheral line, an IV start kit will be needed, whereas a CVC (central venous catheter) kit is required for midline or central lines. These kits are self-contained packets of supplies required to insert IV lines or change the dressing at the line insertion site. Several catheters should be available in the home for patients with peripheral lines so that the nurse has one when the catheter is scheduled to be changed. The only centrally placed catheters that are inserted in the home are PICC lines. Other central venous access devices are placed in the hospital, outpatient clinic, or surgical setting.

For patients requiring an ambulatory infusion device, the appropriate tubing should be sent. Thus, keeping a record of which device a patient is using is important. Batteries are required for devices that are battery-operated. Patients receiving their therapy via minibag or using a nonambulatory infusion device may need an IV pole. IV poles are available in portable, collapsible designs or the standard, rugged type seen in hospitals. Pitch-It, by SCI, a line of disposable IV poles designed specifically for home infusion therapy patients, is also available.

Heparin is supplied in different concentrations depending on the type of venous access device. Generally, heparin 10 units/ml is used for peripheral catheters, while 100 units/ml is used for central venous catheters. The concentration of heparin used may also differ in neonatal, pediatric, and adult patients. Many home infusion companies or institutions have specific protocols that are followed for heparin flushes. Technicians should be familiar with these protocols so the appropriate flushing materials accompany the patient's supply order. If flush materials are sent in vial form or if drugs will need to be drawn from vials, the appropriate syringe(s) and needles should be included.

Patients on a needleless system should receive the proper materials, including injection caps, vial adaptors, syringes, and syringe cannulas. Interlink®, CLAVE®, and Smartsite™ are some of needleless system products currently available.[22] Home care personnel should determine the appropriate supply use on the basis of anticipated delivery frequency and send supplies accordingly. In many cases, patients are taught to take inventory of their supplies and review the inventory with the appropriate personnel each time a delivery is anticipated. This minimizes over- or undersupply and helps to reduce costs.

Infection Control and Safety

All patients in the home care setting should be treated as if they are potentially infectious. Thus, home care personnel must follow "universal precautions." Nurses should wear sterile gloves when manipulating catheters to maintain their integrity and nonsterile gloves when drawing blood to protect themselves. Delivery personnel should also wear nonsterile gloves or rugged work gloves when picking up medical waste and unused supplies to prevent needlestick injuries or contact with contaminated spills.

Patients or their caregivers are taught to use appropriate sterile technique when preparing their medications or fluids and when manipulating the catheter. Occasionally, a break in technique may occur that could lead to a catheter infection or sepsis. In many cases, these infections can be treated with IV antibiotics, but some cases require removal of the catheter.

Collection and Disposal of Medical Waste

Most state boards of pharmacy prohibit reuse of repackaged or compounded items, including sterile products. Thus, products returned from the home environment are not recycled. Supplies returned by patients to the home infusion company should be dealt with as described by the company's disposal policies and procedures.

In the 1980s, improper disposal of medical waste was a national issue. Since then, disposal methods and recycling of waste have become more regulated. All home care patients and their caregivers should be taught to dispose of hazardous and nonhazardous wastes properly.[9] Needles and other sharp materials should be placed in a hard plastic or cardboard sharps container to prevent injury. An isolated area in the home should be identified for storage of medical waste. A schedule for waste removal should be developed and agreed on by the patient and the home care provider. If patients notice that their sharps container will be full before their next scheduled delivery, they should contact their home care provider as soon as possible. Some home infusion companies offer patients the use of a mail-back medical disposal process whereby medical waste is sent in commercially available containers via the U.S. Postal Service to regulated collectors.

Conclusion

Home infusion pharmacy offers a unique and challenging opportunity for the pharmacy technician. The role of the home care pharmacy technician involves substantial responsibility, and the technician's role in the maintenance of the mixing room, inventory control, and product preparation continues to expand. Home care technicians have an opportunity to learn skills not found in other types of practice sites, such as dealing with specialized technologies, infusion supplies, and venous access systems. Often, there is opportunity for patient contact as well. Home infusion pharmacy is a growing field that depends on skilled pharmacy technicians to help the team provide pharmaceutical care to its patients.

References

1. Anon. Home health care. *Ann Int Med.* 1986; 105:454–460.

2. American Society of Hospital Pharmacists. Increase in market for home infusion products and services predicted. *Am J Hosp Pharm.* 1990; 47:958.

3. Anon. Report provides profile of home infusion services patients. *Am J Hosp Pharm.* 1993; 50:846–9.

4. Kliethermes MA. Adverse drug reactions in home care: report of five-year data collection. Paper presented at HomeCare 95 Meeting of ASHP. Boston, MA, August 1995.

5. Tice AD, Nolet BR. Update on outpatient parenteral antimicrobial therapy. *Home Health Care Consultant.* 2001; 8(12):22–29.

6. Nowobilski-Vasilios A. New drugs and biologicals. *Infusion.* 2002; July/August:32–42.

7. Kaplan LK. How clean is clean enough? *Infusion.* 1995; August:11–8.

8. American Society of Health-System Pharmacists. ASHP guidelines on quality assurance for pharmacy-prepared sterile products. *Am J Health-Syst Pharm.* 2000; 57:1150–69.

9. Sterile drug products for home use. In: United States Pharmacopeia, 24th rev./national formulary. 19th ed. Rockville, MD: United States Pharmacopeial Convention; 1999:2130–43.

10. Saladow J. Ambulatory systems for i.v. antibiotic therapy: making sense of the options. *Infusion.* 1995; April:17–29.

11. Kwan JW. High-technology i.v. infusion devices. *Am J Hosp Pharm.* 1991; 48(Suppl. 1):S36–51.

12. Saladow J. Infusion device technologies: consolidation and change. *Infusion.* 2000; June:9–42.

13. Finley RS. Drug-delivery systems: infusion and access devices. *Highlights on Antineoplastic Drugs.* 1995; 13:15–20,23–9.

14. Bowles C, McKinnon BT. Selecting infusion devices. *Am J Hosp Pharm.* 1993; 50:228–30.

15. Saladow J. Ambulatory electronic infusion systems. Making sense of the options. *Infusion* 1995; July:9–21.

16. Dickson LB, Somani SM, Herrmann G, Abramowitz PW. Automated compounder for adding ingredients to parenteral nutrient base solutions. *Am J Hosp Pharm.* 1993; 50:678–82.

17. Seidel AM, Woller TW, Somani S, Abramowitz PW. Effect of computer software on time required to prepare parenteral nutrient solutions. *Am J Hosp Pharm.* 1991; 48:270–5.

18. Driscoll DF. Total nutrient admixtures: theory and practice. *Nutr Clin Pract.* 1995; 10:114–9.

19. American Society of Health-System Pharmacists. ASHP guidelines on the safe use of automated compounding devices for the preparation of parenteral nutrition admixtures. *Am J Health-Syst Pharm.* 2000; 57:1342–8.

20. Viall CD. Your complete guide to central venous catheters. *Nursing 90.* 1990; 20:34–41.

21. Masoorii S, Angeles T. PICC lines: the latest home care challenge. *RN.* 1990; 44–51.

22. Moureau N. Vascular access with a focus on safety. *Infusion.* 1991; October:16–35.

Self-Assessment Questions

Case 1

Tom is a 54-year-old with a 10-year history of diabetes. Tom stepped on a tack while working in the garage. He did not notice the tack in his shoe until he took off his shoes and socks that evening. The tack had cut his right foot behind the big toe and caused it to bleed. He cleaned the wound. Three weeks later, Tom began experiencing severe pain and tenderness in his right foot. He went to his doctor, who noted a swollen and red right foot with a 2 cm wide and 4 cm deep ulcer behind the big toe. The patient was hospitalized for surgery to drain the wound. Cultures of bone were obtained during surgery. A diagnosis of osteomyelitis of the right foot with *Staphylococcus aureus* was made.

Tom supports a family of six. Three of his children are in college. Because of recent layoffs at his place of employment, he is concerned about his illness causing him to lose time at work. He is also concerned about the financial drain this illness will cause his family because his HMO requires him to pay 20 percent of all health care expenditures.

1. Tom's diagnosis is often treated in the home health care environment.
   a. True
   b. False

2. Which of the following would be home care goals for this patient?
   a. Allow the patient to leave the hospital earlier.
   b. Allow the patient to return to work sooner.
   c. Decrease the health care costs associated with his therapy.
   d. all of the above.

Tom's physician started nafcillin 2 gms IV every 6 hours to treat his infection and gave orders to arrange home care services for him. Tom is very nervous about going home. He is not sure he will be able to do what the nurses have been doing for him in the hospital. Although he knows going home will be less costly, he is still concerned about how much this is going to cost.

3. Which of the following hospital employees coordinates Tom's transfer into the home care system?
   a. pharmacy technician
   b. reimbursement specialist
   c. discharge planner
   d. intake coordinator

4. The most appropriate team member with whom Tom should discuss the cost of therapy is the
   a. pharmacy technician.
   b. reimbursement specialist.
   c. home care nurse.
   d. home care pharmacist.

5. The pharmacist and nurse decide to use an ambulatory pump to administer Tom's nafcillin so he can return to work. The temporary technician is complaining about mixing the nafcillin for the pump because it is so much harder than minibags. The home health care technician explains to the temporary technician that the pump is used because
   a. the company will make more money.
   b. the ambulatory pump will automatically infuse the drug every 6 hours, allowing the patient the time to work.
   c. nafcillin is more stable in ambulatory pumps.
   d. None of the above.

6. Which team member would be the most appropriate to teach Tom how to use the system chosen to administer his medication?
   a. home care nurse
   b. physician
   c. pharmacy technician
   d. delivery personnel

The day has come for Tom to go home. Besides the prescription, orders are written for a PICC catheter to be inserted at home and for a CBC and erythrocyte sedimentation rate to be done weekly.

7. Which home care team member is responsible for giving the above orders?
   a. home care nurse
   b. home care pharmacist
   c. physician
   d. discharge planner

8. Which team member will insert the PICC catheter?
   a. nurse
   b. physician
   c. pharmacist
   d. none of the above

9. The pharmacy technician needs to order enough nafcillin to provide Tom with the appropriate

course of therapy. The technician notes that Tom's diagnosis is osteomyelitis. Based on this, how long will his therapy last?
a. 5 days
b. 4 to 6 weeks
c. 1 week
d. 3 months

10. The technician is entering the orders for Tom into the computer system at the technician's organization. He or she comes to the CBC and erythrocyte sedimentation rate orders and recognizes these as
a. orders nursing will need to schedule blood draws
b. orders the pharmacist will need to set up a monitoring plan
c. orders that will require the patient to have blood draw supplies in the home
d. all of the above

Tom has now received 5 weeks of therapy without complications. At the weekly patient rounds, the nurse reports Tom's right foot looks great. There is no more swelling or redness, and the ulcer has completely healed.

11. The patient service representative tells the technician that the patient needs seven more cassettes of nafcillin. She is a little concerned because Tom has not been feeling "quite right" the last few days. He thinks he may have prickly heat because he has red bumps all over his chest. The technician should take what action?
a. Tell the pharmacist about the patient service representative's concerns and wait to make the nafcillin until the pharmacist has evaluated the situation.
b. Mix 7 days worth of nafcillin, because a rash is a common reaction to nafcillin.
c. Arrange to return the nafcillin to the drug supplier because you will not be using it any more.
d. all of the above

Case 2
Ken is a 35-year-old who was diagnosed with AIDS 2 years ago. He was recently started on ganciclovir for CMV retinitis. Over the past 6 months, Ken has lost 60 pounds, and now he feels very weak. Ken

and his physician have decided to treat his malnutrition with parenteral nutrition.

12. Parenteral nutrition is used to treat malnutrition associated with AIDS.
a. True
b. False

13. Parenteral nutrition is a very complicated therapy and needs to be administered in an institutional setting. Ken will have to be admitted to a hospital or long-term care facility.
a. True
b. False

14. Ken would like to continue his job as an accountant and wishes to start his parenteral nutrition at home. His physician and insurance case manager approve this plan because home care therapy
a. allows patients to receive therapy without being hospitalized.
b. allows patients to return to work or normal activities sooner.
c. decreases health care costs.
d. all of the above

15. The pharmacist recommends the following formula for Ken:

Dextrose 50%	1,000 ml
Amino Acids 10%	1,000 ml
Lipids 20%	500 ml
Multiple Electrolyte vial	40 ml
Sodium Phosphate	30 mMol
Trace Metals	5 ml
Multivitamins	10 ml

The technician is preparing to compound Ken's parenteral nutrition solutions. Which of the following will the technician *not* add to the solution?

a.	Lipids 20%	500 ml
b.	Trace Metals	5 ml
c.	Sodium Phosphate	30 mMol
d.	Multivitamins	10 ml

After 2 weeks on parenteral nutrition, it becomes clear that Ken is not tolerating the high dextrose load. His physician orders Regular Human Insulin. The stress of Ken's disease causes stomach pain, and his physician orders ranitidine, an H_2-receptor antagonist, 100 mg IV daily, to be added to his parenteral nutrition.

16. Ranitidine and insulin are incompatible with his TPN formula and therefore cannot be given when

the TPN is infusing.
a. True
b. False

17. The nurse plans to draw Ken's weekly labs and change his central line dressings on Tuesdays. The technician should plan to mix his TPN on which day?
a. Monday
b. Tuesday
c. Wednesday
d. Sunday

18. Ken is planning to take a 2-week vacation to Hawaii. Is this possible, given his TPN therapy?
a. Yes, but he would not be able to infuse his TPN during the 2 weeks.
b. Absolutely not, it would be too dangerous. He cannot go on vacation while receiving this therapy.
c. A 9-day supply could be sent with him, but because of limited stability, the remainder would have to be shipped.
d. none of the above

19. The pharmacist tells you that the electrolytes on Ken's most recent labs are all normal, but his liver enzymes are elevated. The pharmacist reviews potential reasons as to why Ken's liver enzymes are abnormal. The pharmacist tells the technician to
a. go ahead and mix his TPN because the electrolytes are good.
b. hold the mix of TPN because the elevated liver enzymes may be TPN-induced and result in a change in formula.
c. hold the mix because the elevated liver enzymes are due to the ganciclovir.
d. none of the above

20. As the technician is preparing Ken's ganciclovir, he or she makes a mental note to check on how much stock is in the refrigerator for a drug that is often given to patients on ganciclovir, just in case Ken may need it. Which drug would the technician check for?
a. filgrastim (Neupogen)
b. insulin
c. ranitidine
d. none of the above

21. Which of the following groups was responsible for establishing three levels of risk to patients who are receiving a sterile product?
a. American Society of Health-System Pharmacists
b. Food and Drug Administration
c. United States Pharmacopeial Convention
d. National Institutes of Health

22. A pharmacy technician is preparing a 1-week supply of TPN for a patient at home, using an automated compounding device. Investigational L-glutamine is being added at the end of the mixing process. Which risk level of compounding describes this situation?
a. risk level 1
b. risk level 2
c. risk level 3
d. no risk level

23. What is/are the disadvantage(s) of minibags?
a. the need for an IV pole
b. increased risk for touch contamination
c. requirement for more nursing interaction
d. all of the above

24. Advantages to delivering medications via syringe infusion include which of the following?
a. Syringes are easy to batch fill.
b. Syringes require less storage space.
c. The drugs stored in syringes are stable for longer.
d. a and b

25. Which of the following systems is considered an elastomeric balloon device?
a. SideKick®
b. Homepump Eclipse®
c. Paragon®
d. Maxx®100

26. Which of the following rate-restricted systems provides controlled pressure pumping via an electronic system rather than by positive pressure?
a. ReadyMED®
b. Paragon Elite®
c. Maxx®100
d. SideKick®

27. Which of the following manufacturers offers a therapy-specific device designed specifically for infusion of TPN, pain medication, antibiotics, and insulin?
a. Baxter Healthcare Corporation
b. SIMS Deltec, Inc.
c. MiniMed
d. Abbott Laboratories, Inc.

28. A patient will be receiving TPN and pain management at home through a home infusion therapy provider. The patient is very debilitated and his wife does not feel very comfortable with programming an infusion pump. Which of the following devices would be most suitable for use in this patient?
    a. 6060 Homerun™
    b. CADD-Prizm® VIP
    c. VIVUS™ 4000
    d. Provider 6000®

29. Required labeling information for a product going to a home care patient includes which of the following?
    a. patient name, address, prescribing physician
    b. prescription number, date, prescribing physician
    c. precautionary labels, patient name, date of dispensing
    d. bag sequence, patient address, federal transfer label

30. Selecting an appropriate expiration date for sterile products used in home care practice is important because it dictates
    a. whether the product can be prepared in batches.
    b. how much of the product will be wasted.
    c. the frequency of deliveries to the patient.
    d. all of the above

31. Which of the following statements is true regarding expiration dating for sterile products used in the home care setting?
    a. A 24-hour stability at room temperature is required for drugs to be given via an ambulatory infusion device.
    b. Changes in pH and drug structure do not affect extended stability for sterile products.
    c. Sterile products not intended for prompt use should be stored at no more than 25°C to inhibit microbial growth.
    d. Physical degradation due to hydrolysis, oxidation, and reduction can cause a product to deteriorate.

32. Tunneled central venous catheter models are distinguished from each other by which of the following features?
    a. surgery versus bedside placement
    b. likelihood that it will become occluded
    c. flushing protocol
    d. number of lumens

33. Which of the following is true about peripherally inserted central venous catheters (PICCs)?
    a. They are also called midlines.
    b. They do not require flushing with heparin.
    c. They may be inserted in the hospital or at home.
    d. Their complication rate is less than any other catheter.

Self-Assessment Answers

1. a. Osteomyelitis is one of the most common diseases seen in the home care environment, primarily because it requires long-term IV antibiotic therapy.

2. d. All the goals listed are primary goals of home care and are personal goals for the patient as well.

3. c. The discharge planner or a social worker coordinates the discharge of a patient to home care from the hospital.

4. b. The reimbursement specialist is the most knowledgeable about the cost of home care therapy and insurance coverage.

5. b. Ambulatory infusion pumps can be used to automatically infuse doses throughout the day. They are ideal for patients who may have a problem adhering to an infusion schedule that requires frequent dosing. In addition, ambulatory infusion pumps are convenient for patients who may require ambulation during their therapy.

6. a. The nurse is the primary educator of the patient at home.

7. c. Only the physician can give orders that alter the therapeutic plan.

8. a. The home care nurse has primary responsibility for IV catheters. Many home care nurses are trained in the insertion and maintenance of PICC catheters.

9. b. Osteomyelitis is usually treated for 4 to 6 weeks.

10. d. The nurse is responsible for scheduling and drawing blood for laboratory tests on the patient. The pharmacist is responsible for evaluating laboratory results as part of the patient assessment and monitoring function. The home care company is usually the source for all the patient's medical supplies.

11. a. A rash developing well into therapy with nafcillin is a common occurrence in the home care environment. However, it is best to find out how the rest of the home care team wants to deal with the rash before mixing or returning the nafcillin. That way the nafcillin will not be wasted.

12. a. Parenteral nutrition may be used to treat malnutrition associated with AIDS. AIDS patients, because of chronic diarrhea, often cannot absorb enough nutrients from the food they eat to sustain adequate nutrition.

13. b. This may have been the thought 35 years ago; however, long-term infusion therapy such as parenteral nutrition has been shown to be safe, effective, and less costly in the home care environment.

14. d. All three goals listed are part of the seven goals of home care therapy.

15. d. Multivitamins are the only components of Ken's formula that have limited stability (24 hours) and must be added by the patient in the home prior to infusion. The remaining ingredients—lipids, electrolytes, sodium phosphate, and trace metals—are stable in solution for 9 days.

16. b. The home care pharmacy staff will most likely be preparing a 7-day supply of TPN for the patient. Both these drugs are compatible with Ken's TPN but have short-term stability of 48 hours or less. Therefore, they should be added by the patient prior to infusion.

17. c. Wednesday would be the optimal day to mix because lab results would be available that day and the nurse would have made a patient assessment for any problem or complications on Tuesday. Any changes in the formula could be made then before mixing a 7-day supply of TPN.

18. c. Ken could take up to nine bags (9-day supply) or more with him, depending on how long his TPN formula is stable. Other arrangements would have to be made for the remainder of his therapy. Often a home infusion company will ship the medication overnight to the vacation spot.

19. b. Because elevated liver enzymes are a long-term complication of parenteral nutrition, the TPN order may be changed to avoid further complications. It is best to wait until a decision has been made regarding the composition of the TPN, rather than to mix the wrong TPN and waste material, time, and money.

20. a. Ganciclovir commonly causes bone marrow toxicity and resulting neutropenia (low white blood cell count) in AIDS patients. Filgrastim is frequently used as therapy for this side effect.

21. a. The American Society of Health-System Pharmacists (ASHP) published the "ASHP

Guidelines on Quality Assurance for Pharmacy-Prepared Sterile Products." The United States Pharmacopeial Convention issued an informational chapter on "Sterile Drug Products for Home Use." In the ASHP guideline, sterile products are grouped into three levels of risk to the patient. These categories depend on how much time elapses between when the drug is compounded and when it is administered, in other words, the expiration dating. These levels increase from least (level 1) to greatest (level 3) potential risk and have different quality assurance recommendations for product integrity and patient safety.

22. c. The rationale behind the risk-level approach is that the greater the chance of contamination or the greater the risk of microbial growth in the product, the more careful providers should be to safeguard the sterility of the IV admixture. The product being prepared by the pharmacy technician falls into risk level 3 because of the preparation of investigational L-glutamine from a powder (a nonsterile component) in an open reservoir. Indeed, the TPN solutions are being prepared using an automated compounder, which alone renders them risk level 2. Because of the L-glutamine, however, risk level 2 is superceded by risk level 3.

23. d. From an acquisition standpoint, minibags are considered one of the most cost-effective methods to deliver medications. Their limitations in home care practice include the need for an IV pole; patient or caregiver needs to manually set and maintain the infusion rate; patient or caregiver needs to connect the set and the bag in the home, increasing the risk of touch contamination; and the need for more nursing interaction with the patient than other systems. Use of minibags for drugs that are given frequently can pose a problem for patients who are ambulatory or working because of the cumbersome IV pole.

24. d. A revived interest has surged in the delivery of medications via syringe infusion because of attempts to reduce cost. As drug

containers, syringes are the least expensive. In addition, syringes are easy to batch fill and require less storage space.

25. b. Elastomeric balloon systems besides Baxter's Intermate® Elastomeric Infusion System are Alaris Medical Systems ReadyMED®, I-Flow Homepump Eclipse®, and the Metrix Company Medflo II™. Baxter Healthcare's Infusor™ System and I-Flow's Homepump® C Series Continuous Infusion System are designed specifically for administering chemotherapy and other long-term continuous infusions.

26. c. In early 1994, an electronic controlled pressure device, the Maxx®100 by Medication Delivery Devices, was introduced. However, Baxter Healthcare eventually acquired this device. This system consists of a rectangular housing and a series of disposable reservoir bags with preattached IV flow control sets. A proprietary plastic bag is placed inside the device housing on top of a bladder that expands with air and applies pressure to the bag when the device is closed and turned on. The IV tubing controls the drug administration rate once the clamp on it is opened. The Maxx®100 differs from other rate-restricted systems in that it provides controlled pressure pumping via an electronic system rather than by positive pressure.

27. b. Therapy-specific devices are designed to provide single therapies, such as pain management or TPN. Operation of these devices is fairly straightforward and can be readily done by clinicians and patients. Common therapy-specific devices include the Abbott Provider® product and the SIMS Deltec CADD® infusion pumps. The CADD® pumps are some of the most widely used ambulatory infusion devices in the United States. Most of these devices are therapy-specific and relatively simple to program. The CADD-TPN®, CADD-Legacy™ PCA, CADD-Legacy™ Plus, and CADD-Micro are designed specifically for infusion of TPN, pain medications, antibiotics, and insulin, respectively.

28. c. The VIVUS™ 4000 pump will allow infusion of up to four medications simultaneously, which would be ideal for this patient receiving

Self-Assessment Answers

two therapies. In addition, it offers telecommunications capabilities that would be pertinent in this case because of the inability of caregivers to operate the device. The home care provider can program it over the phone via a modem. The other devices cannot infuse two medications through the same device.

29. b. Required labeling information includes prescription number, date, and prescribing physician, usually required by state boards of pharmacy and useful to the dispensing pharmacy to verify an original order. The patient's name is mandatory but the address is optional; however, an address may simplify delivery procedures. Directions for use should be simple and easy to understand. The name and amount of drug contained in one dose and the appropriate volume for that amount is listed. Then, the name and volume of admixture solution equivalent to one dose of drug is indicated. The actual expiration date established for the product is noted. The individual who prepared and checked the admixture must initial the label. Finally, auxiliary labeling should include federal transfer labeling, and, as an option, specific precautionary labels or storage instruction labels can be applied to the product. The bottle or bag sequence may be listed as well to help track the specific number of doses ordered or the total number of doses administered.

30. d. Expiration dating has important implications in home care practice because it may mean the ability to do batch preparation in the pharmacy, a reduction in waste, and less frequent deliveries to the patient.

31. a. Expiration dates for admixtures must be based on stability and sterility considerations. Physical and chemical breakdowns are possible. Changes in pH, temperature, and drug structure may cause solubility problems. Chemical degradation due to hydrolysis, oxidation, reduction, or photolysis can quickly cause a product to deteriorate. Home care practice demands that the pharmacist assign a maximum expiration date that is still within appropriate stability limits. A common problem is the use of drugs with limited room temperature stability. For drugs to be given via an ambulatory infusion device, at least 24-hour stability at room temperature or warmer is required. For drugs that have limited room temperature stability, the patient or caregiver may be taught how to prepare the drug immediately before administration. Although a product may be stable for an extended period, its sterility must also be a factor in assigning an expiration date. The potential for bacterial growth must be considered. Sterile products not intended for prompt use should be stored at no more than 4°C to inhibit microbial growth, unless room temperature storage is warranted.

32. d. Available tunneled central venous catheter models are distinguished by the catheter material (silicone or polyurethane), number of lumens (single, double, or triple), catheter diameter (French size 3 = pediatric to 12.5 or 13.0 = double or triple lumen), lumen diameter (0.2 to 2.0 mm), and type of catheter tip.

33. c. The use of PICCs is continuing to increase because of their unique features. PICCs can be inserted at the bedside or at home by specially trained nurses. These lines may remain in place for weeks to months. PICC lines, also known as *long-arm* or *long-line* catheters, are made of silicone (Silastic®) or flexible polyurethane and are available in single- and multilumen designs. They require daily flushing with heparin and dressing changes. Complications include phlebitis at the insertion site or along the vein, infection, cellulitis, occlusion, catheter tip migration, and thrombosis.

Pharmacy Calculations

GERALD A. STORM, REBECCA S. KENTZEL

GERALD A. STORM, REBECCA S. KENTZEL

5

Learning Objectives

After completing this chapter, the technician should be able to

1. Calculate conversions between different numbering and measuring systems.

2. Calculate medication doses from various medication dilutions.

3. Calculate and define osmolarity, isotonicity, body surface area, and flow rates.

4. Calculate and define arithmetic mean, median, and standard deviation.

Most calculations pharmacy technicians and pharmacists use involve basic math; however, basic math is easily forgotten when it is not used routinely. This chapter reviews the fundamentals of calculations and how those calculations are applied in pharmacy.

Review of Basic Mathematics

Numerals
A numeral is a word or a sign, or a group of words or signs, that expresses a number.

Kinds of Numerals

Arabic
    Examples: 0, 1, 2, 3, 4, 5, 6, 7, 8, 9

Roman
    In pharmacy practice, Roman numerals are used only to denote quantities on prescriptions.

ss or $\overline{ss}$ = 1/2	L or l = 50
I or i = 1	C or c = 100
V or v = 5	D or d = 500
X or x = 10	M or m = 1000

It is important to note that when a smaller Roman numeral (e.g., "I") is placed before a larger Roman numeral (e.g., "V"), the smaller Roman numeral is subtracted from the larger Roman numeral. Conversely, when a smaller Roman numeral is placed after a larger one, the smaller one is added to the larger.

Example 1: I = 1 and V = 5; therefore, IV = 4 because 5 – 1 = 4.

Example 2: I = 1 and V = 5; therefore, VI = 6 because 5 + 1 = 6

Problem Set #1
Convert the following Roman numerals to Arabic numerals:

a. ii = 2   b. DCV = 605   c. xx = 20

d. iii = 3   e. vii = 7   f. iv = 4

Numbers

A number is a total quantity or amount that is made of one or more numerals.

Kinds of Numbers

Whole Numbers

    Examples: 10, 220, 5, 19

Fractions

    Fractions are parts of whole numbers.

    Examples: 1/4, 2/7, 11/13, 3/8

    Always try to express a fraction in its simplest form.

    Examples: 2/4 = 1/2; 10/12 = 5/6; 8/12 = 2/3

    The whole number above the fraction line is called the numerator, and the whole number below the fraction line is called the denominator.

Mixed Numbers

These numbers contain both whole numbers and fractions.

    Examples: 1 1/2, 13 3/4, 20 7/8, 2 1/2

Decimal Numbers

Decimal numbers are actually another means of writing fractions and mixed numbers.

    Examples: 1/2 = 0.5, 1 3/4 = 1.75

    Note that you can identify decimal numbers by the period appearing somewhere in the number. The period in a decimal number is called the decimal point.

    The following two points about zeros in decimal numbers are VERY important:

1. Do NOT write a whole number in decimal form.

    In other words, when writing a whole number, avoid writing a period followed by a zero (e.g., 5.0). Why? Because periods are sometimes hard to see, and errors may result from misreading the number. For example, the period in 1.0 may be overlooked, and the number could appear to be 10 instead, causing a 10-fold dosing error, which could kill someone.

2. On the contrary, when writing a fraction in its decimal form, always write a zero before the period.

    Why? Once again, periods are sometimes difficult to see, and .5 may be misread as 5.

However, if the period in 0.5 were illegible, the zero would alert the reader that a period is supposed to be there.

Working with Fractions and Decimals

Please note that this section is meant to be only a basic overview. A practicing pharmacy technician should already possess these fundamental skills. The problems and examples in this section should serve as building blocks for all calculations reviewed later in this chapter. If you do not know how to do these basic functions, you need to seek further assistance.

Review of Basic Mathematical Functions Involving Fractions

When adding, subtracting, multiplying, or dividing fractions, you must convert all fractions to a common denominator. Also, when working with fractions, be sure that you express your answer as the smallest reduced fraction (i.e., if your answer is 6/8, reduce it to 3/4).

Addition

Use the following steps to add 3/4 + 7/8 + 1/4.

1. Convert all fractions to common denominators.

    3/4 × 2/2 = 6/8

    1/4 × 2/2 = 2/8

2. Add the fractions.

    6/8 + 7/8 + 2/8 = 15/8

3. Reduce to the smallest fraction.

    15/8 = 1 7/8

Subtraction

Use the following steps to subtract 7/8 – 1/4.

1. Convert the fractions to common denominators.

    1/4 × 2/2 = 2/8

2. Subtract the fractions.

    7/8 – 2/8 = 5/8

Multiplication

Use the following steps to multiply 1/6 × 2/3.

    When multiplying and dividing fractions, you do NOT have to convert to common denominators.

1. Multiply the numerators: 1 × 2 = 2

2. Multiply the denominators: 6 × 3 = 18

3. Express your answer as a fraction: 2/18

4. Be sure to reduce your fraction: 2/18 = 1/9

Division

Use the following steps to divide 1/2 by 1/4.

Once again, you do NOT have to convert to common denominators.

To divide two fractions, the first fraction must be multiplied by the inverse (or reciprocal) of the second fraction:

$1/2 \div 1/4$ is the same as $1/2 \times 4/1$

1. Multiply the fractions.

$1/2 \times 4/1 = 4/2$

2. Reduce to lowest fraction.

$4/2 = 2$

Review of Basic Mathematical Functions Involving Decimals

As with fractions, when adding, subtracting, multiplying, or dividing decimals, all units (or terms) must be alike.

Addition

Remember to line up decimal points when adding or subtracting decimal numbers.

Add the following: $0.1 + 124.7$

Add the terms by lining up the decimal points:

```
   0.1
+ 124.7
 124.8
```

Subtraction

Subtract the following: $2100 - 20.5$

Subtract the terms by lining up the decimal points:

```
2100.0
- 20.5
2079.5
```

Multiplication

When multiplying decimal numbers, the number of decimal places in the product must equal the total number of decimal places in the numbers multiplied, as shown below.

Multiply the following: 0.6×24

In this example, there is a total of one digit to the right of the decimal point in the numbers being multiplied, so the answer will have one digit to the right of the decimal point.

Answer: $0.6 \times 24 = 14.4$

Division

The dividend is the number to be divided, and the divisor is the number by which the dividend is divided. When dividing decimal numbers, move the divisor's decimal point to the right to form a whole number. Remember to move the dividend's decimal point the same number of places to the right. When using long division, place the decimal point in the answer immediately above the dividend's decimal point.

Divide the following: $60.75 \div 4.5$

Move the decimal points: $607.5 \div 45$

Answer: $607.5 \div 45 = 13.5$

Converting Fractions to Decimal Numbers

To convert a fraction to a decimal, simply divide the numerator by the denominator.

For example, $1/2$ = one divided by two = 0.5

Converting Mixed Numbers to Decimal Numbers

This process involves the following two steps:

1. Write the mixed number as a fraction.

   Method: Multiply the whole number and the denominator of the fraction. Add the product (result) to the numerator of the fraction, keeping the same denominator.

   Example: $2\ 3/4$ = two times four plus three over four = $11/4$

2. Divide the numerator by the denominator.

   Example: $11/4$ = eleven divided by four = 2.75

An alternate method involves the following three steps:

1. Separate the whole number and the fraction.

   Example: $2\ 3/4$ = 2 and $3/4$

2. Convert the fraction to its decimal counterpart.

   Example: $3/4$ = three divided by four = 0.75

3. Add the whole number to the decimal fraction.

   Example: 2 plus $0.75 = 2.75$

Converting Decimal Numbers to Mixed Numbers or Fractions

To convert decimal numbers to mixed numbers or fractions, follow these three steps:

1. Write the decimal number over one, dividing it by one. (Remember that dividing any number by one does not change the number.)

Example: 3.5 = 3.5/1

2. Move the decimal point in the numerator as many places to the right as necessary to form a whole number. Then move the decimal point in the denominator the same number of places.

   Example: Because there is only one digit following the decimal point in 3.5, move the decimal point one place to the right in both the numerator and the denominator: 3.5/1 = 35/10.

Remember that the number will remain the same as long as you do exactly the same things to the numerator and the denominator. You also have to remember that the decimal point of a whole number always follows the last digit.

3: Simplify the fraction.

Example: 35/10 = 7/2 = 3 1/2

Problem Set #2

Convert the following fractions to decimal numbers:

a. 1/2	b. 3/4	c. 1	d. 2/5
e. 1/3	f. 5/8	g. 50/100	h. 12/48
i. 11/2	j. 2 2/3	k. 5 1/4	l. 3 4/5

Convert the following decimal numbers to fractions or mixed numbers:

m. 0.25	n. 0.4	o. 0.75	p. 0.35
q. 2.5	r. 1.6	s. 3.25	t. 0.33

Percentages

Percentage means "by the hundred" or "in a hundred." Percents (%) are just fractions, but fractions with a set denominator. The denominator is always one hundred (100).

   Example: "50%" means "50 in a hundred" or "50/100" or "1/2"

Converting Percentages to Fractions

Write the number preceding the percent sign over 100 and simplify the resulting fraction.

   Example: 25% = 25/100 = 1/4

Converting Fractions to Percentages

Convert the fraction to one in which the denominator is a hundred. This is easiest when the fraction is in the form of a decimal. Follow these four steps:

1. Write the fraction in its decimal form.

   Example: 3/4 = three divided by four = 0.75

2. Write the decimal over one.

   Example: 0.75/1

3. To obtain 100 as the denominator, move the decimal point two places to the right. To avoid changing the number, move the decimal point two places to the right in the numerator as well.

   Example: 0.75/1 = 75/100

4. Because you already know that "out of a hundred" or "divided by a hundred" is the same as percent, you can write 75/100 as 75%.

Concentration Expressed as a Percentage

Percent weight-in-weight (w/w) is the grams of a drug in 100 grams of the product.

Percent weight-in-volume (w/v) is the grams of a drug in 100 ml of the product.

Percent volume-in-volume (v/v) is the milliliters of drug in 100 ml of the product.

   The above concentration percentages will be discussed in further detail a little later in this chapter.

Problem Set #3

Convert the following percentages to fractions (remember to simplify the fractions):

a. 23%	b. 67%	c. 12.5%	d. 50%
e. 66.7%	f. 75%	g. 66%	h. 40%
i. 100%	j. 15%		

Convert the following fractions to percentages:

k. 1/2	l. 1/4	m. 2/5	n. 6/25
o. 4/100	p. 0.5	q. 0.35	r. 0.44
s. 0.57	t. 0.99		

Units of Measure

Metric System

The metric system is based on the decimal system, in which everything is measured in multiples or fractions of 10. The appendix lists the conversion charts reviewed on the following pages.

Standard Measures

The standard measure for length is the meter; the standard measure for weight is the gram; and the standard measure for volume is the liter.

Prefixes

The prefixes below are used to describe multiples or

fractions of the standard measures for length, weight, and volume.

Latin Prefixes

micro- (mc): 1/1,000,000 = 0.000001

milli- (m): 1/1000 = 0.001

centi- (c): 1/100 = 0.01

deci- (d): 1/10 = 0.1

Note that Latin prefixes denote fractions.

Greek Prefixes

deca- (da): 10

hecto- (h): 100

kilo- (k): 1000

mega- (M): 1,000,000

Note that Greek prefixes denote multiples.

Prefixes with Standard Measures

Length

The standard measure is the meter (m).

1 kilometer (km) = 1000 meters (m)

0.001 kilometer (km) = 1 meter (m)

1 millimeter (mm) = 0.001 meter (m)

1000 millimeters (mm) = 1 meter (m)

1 centimeter (cm) = 0.01 meter (m)

100 centimeters (cm) = 1 meter (m)

Volume

The standard measure is the liter (L).

1 milliliter (ml) = 0.001 liter (L)

1000 milliliters (ml) = 1 liter (L)

1 microliter (mcl) = 0.000001 liter (L)

1,000,000 microliters (mcl) = 1 liter (L)

1 deciliter (dl) = 0.1 liter (L)

10 deciliters (dl) = 1 liter (L)

Weight

The standard measure is the gram (g).

1 kilogram (kg) = 1000 grams (g)

0.001 kilogram (kg) = 1 gram (g)

1 milligram (mg) = 0.001 gram (g)

1000 milligrams (mg) = 1 gram (g)

1 microgram (mcg) = 0.000001 gram (g)

1,000,000 micrograms (mcg) = 1 gram (g)

Apothecary System

The apothecary system was developed after the Avoir-dupois system (see below) to enable fine weighing of medications. Today, the apothecary system is used only for a few medications, such as aspirin, acetaminophen, and phenobarbital.

Weight

The standard measure for weight is the grain (gr).

Pound	Ounces	Drams	Scruples	Grains
1 =	12 =	96 =	288 =	5760
	1 =	8 =	24 =	480
		1 =	3 =	60
			1 =	20

Volume

The standard measure for volume is the minim (m.).

Gallons	Pints	Fluid ounces	Fluid drams	Minims
1 =	8 =	128 =	1024 =	61,440
	1 =	16 =	128 =	7,680
		1 =	8 =	480
			1 =	60

Avoirdupois System

This system is used mainly in measuring the bulk medications encountered in manufacturing. Be sure to note that the pounds-to-ounces equivalent is different in the apothecary and avoirdupois systems. The avoirdupois system is most commonly used to measure weight, and the apothecary system is most commonly used to measure volume. Be sure also to note the difference in symbols used for the two systems. In addition, note that a fluid ounce, which measures volume, is often mistakenly shortened to an "ounce," which is actually a measure of weight. Because ounces measure weight, pay close attention to the measure you are working with and convert accordingly.

Weight

The standard measure for weight is the grain (gr).

Pound (lb)	Ounces (oz)	Grains (gr)
1 =	16 =	7000
	1 =	437.5

Household System

The household system is the most commonly used system of measuring liquids in outpatient settings. The measuring equipment usually consists of commonly used home utensils (e.g., teaspoons, tablespoons).

1 teaspoonful (tsp) = 5 ml

1 dessertspoonful = 10 ml

1 tablespoonful (TBS) = 15 ml = 0.5 fluid ounces (fl oz)

1 wineglassful = 60 ml = 2 fl oz

1 teacupful = 120 ml = 4 fl oz

1 glassful/cupful = 240 ml = 8 fl oz

3 tsp = 1 TBS

2 TBS = 1 fl oz

8 fl oz = 1 cup

2 cups = 1 pint (pt)

2 pt = 1 quart (qt)

4 qt = 1 gallon (gal)

The term *drop* is commonly used; however, caution should be exercised when working with this measure, especially with potent medications. The volume of a drop depends not only on the nature of the liquid but also on the size, shape, and position of the dropper. To accurately measure small amounts of liquid, use a 1-ml syringe (with milliliter markings) instead of a dropper. Eye drops are an exception to this rule; they are packaged in a manner to deliver a correctly sized droplet.

Problem Set #4

Fill in the blanks:

a. 1 liter (L) = __1000__ ml

b. 1000 g = __1__ kg

c. 1 g = __1000__ mg

d. 1000 mcg = __1__ mg

e. 1 TBS = __3__ tsp

f. 1 TBS = __15__ ml

g. 240 ml = __1__ cupfuls

h. 1 cup = __240__ ml

i. 15 ml = __1__ TBS

j. 1 tsp = __5__ ml

k. 240 ml = __16__ TBS

l. 1 pt = __480__ ml

m. 1 fl oz = __2__ TBS

n. 1 qt = __2__ pt

Equivalencies Among Systems

The apothecary, avoirdupois, and household systems lack a close relationship among their units. For this reason, the preferred system of measuring is the metric system. The table of weights and measures below gives the approximate equivalencies used in practice.

Length Measures

1 meter (m) = 39.37 (39.4) inches (in)

1 inch (in) = 2.54 centimeters (cm)

Volume Measures

1 milliliter (ml) = 16.23 minims

1 fluid ounce (fl oz) = 29.57 (30) milliliters (ml)

1 liter (L) = 33.8 fluid ounces (fl oz)

1 pint (pt) = 473.167 (480) milliliters (ml)

1 gallon (gal) = 3785.332 (3785) milliliters (ml)

Weight Measures

1 kilogram (kg) = 2.2 pounds (lb)

1 pound (avoir) (lb) = 453.59 (454) grams (g)

1 ounce (avoir) (oz) = 28.35 (28) grams (g)

1 ounce (apoth) (oz) = 31.1 (31) grams (g)

1 gram (g) = 15.432 (15) grains (gr)

1 grain (gr) = 65 milligrams (mg)

1 ounce (avoir) (oz) = 437.5 grains (gr)

1 ounce (apoth) = 480 grains (gr)

Temperature Conversion

Temperature is always measured in the number of degrees centigrade (°C), also known as degrees Celsius, or the number of degrees Fahrenheit (°F). The following equation shows the relationship between degrees centigrade and degrees Fahrenheit: [9(°C)] = [5(°F)] – 160°

Example: Convert 110°F to °C.

[9(°C)] = [5(110°F)] – 160°

°C   = (550 – 160)/9

°C   = 43.3°

Example: Convert 15°C to °F

[9(15°C)] = [5(°F)] – 160°

(135 + 160)/5 = °F

59°   = °F

Conversion Among Systems

To find out how many kilograms are in 44 lbs, follow these three steps:

1. Write down the statement of equivalency between the two units of measure, making sure that the unit corresponding with the unknown in the

question is on the right.

2.2 lbs = 1 kg

2. Write down the problem with the unknown underneath the equivalency.

Equivalency: 2.2 lbs = 1 kg

Problem: 44 lbs = ? kg

3: Cross multiply and divide.

1 times 44 divided by 2.2 = [(1 × 44) / 2.2] = 20 kg

Determining Body Surface Area

The Square Meter Surface Area (Body Surface Area, or BSA) is a measurement that is used instead of kilograms to estimate the amount of medication a patient should receive. BSA takes into account the patient's weight and height. BSA is always expressed in meters squared (m^2) and is frequently used to dose chemotherapy agents. When using the equation below, units of weight (W) should be kilograms (kg) and height (H) should be centimeters. The following equation is used to determine BSA:

$$BSA = (W^{0.5378}) \times (H^{0.3964}) \times (0.024265)$$

Now, using the formula, follow these three steps to calculate the BSA of a patient who weighs 150 pounds and is 5 feet 8 inches tall.

1. Convert weight to kilograms.

$$\frac{150 \text{ lb}}{2.2 \text{ lb/kg}} = 68.2 \text{ kg}$$

2. Convert height to centimeters.

5 feet × 12 inches/foot = 60 inches

+ 8 inches = 68 inches

68 inches × 2.54 cm/inch = 172.7 cm

3. Insert the converted numbers into the formula.

$BSA = (W^{0.5378}) \times (H^{0.3964}) \times 0.024265$

$BSA = (68.2^{0.5378}) \times (172.7^{0.3964}) \times 0.024265$

$BSA = (9.69) \times (7.71) \times 0.024265$

$BSA = 1.81 m^2$

Problem Set #5

Convert or solve the following:

a.   30 ml = __1__ fluid ounces

b.   500 mg = __0.5__ g

c.   3 teaspoons = __0.5__ fluid ounces

d.   20 ml = __4__ teaspoons

e.   3.5 kg = _____ g

f.   0.25 mg = _____ g

g.   1500 ml = _____ L

h.   48 pints = _____ gallons

i.   6 gr = _____ mg

j.   120 lb = _____ kg

k.   3 fluid ounces = _____ ml

l.   72 kg = _____ pounds

m.   946 ml = _____ pints

n.   800 g = _____ lb

o.   3 tsp = _____ milliliters

p.   2 TBS = _____ fluid ounces

q.   2 TBS = _____ ml

r.   2.5 cups = _____ fl oz

s.   0.5 gr = _____ mg

t.   0.5 L = _____ ml

u.   325 mg = _____ gr

v.   2 fl oz = _____ TBS

w.   60 ml = _____ fl oz

x.   144 lb = _____ kg

y.   1 fl oz = _____ tsp

z.   4 tsp = _____ ml

aa.   83°F = _____ °C

bb.   –8°F = _____ °C

cc.   5°C = _____ °F

dd.   32°C = _____ °F

ee.   What is the BSA of a patient who weighs 210 pounds and is 5 feet 1 inch tall?

Ratio and Proportion

A ratio states a relationship between two quantities.

Example: 5 g of dextrose in 100 ml of water (this solution is often abbreviated "D5W").

A proportion is two equal ratios.

Example: 5 g of dextrose in 100 ml of a D5W solution equals 50 g of dextrose in 1000 ml of a D5W solution; or

$$\frac{5 \text{ g}}{100 \text{ ml}} = \frac{50 \text{ g}}{1000 \text{ ml}}$$

A proportion consists of two unit (or term) types (e.g., kilograms and liters, or milligrams and milliliters). If you know three of the four terms, you can calculate the fourth term.

Problem Solving by the Ratio and Proportion Method

The ratio and proportion method is an accurate and simple way to solve some problems. To use this method, you should learn how to arrange the terms correctly, and you must know how to multiply and divide.

There is more than one way to write a proportion. The most common is the following:

$$\frac{\text{Term \#1}}{\text{Term \#2}} = \frac{\text{Term \#3}}{\text{Term \#4}}$$

This expression is read Term #1 is to Term #2 as Term #3 is to Term #4.

By cross multiplying, the proportion can now be written as:

(Term #1) × (Term #4) = (Term #2) × (Term #3)

Example 1: How many grams of dextrose are in 10 ml of a solution containing 50 g of dextrose in 100 ml of water (D50W)?

1. Determine which is the known ratio and which is the unknown ratio. In this example, the known ratio is "50 g of dextrose in 100 ml of solution." The unknown ratio is "X g of dextrose in 10 ml of solution."

2. Write the unknown ratio (Terms #1 and #2) on the left side of the proportion. Be sure the unknown term is on the top.

$$\frac{X \text{ g}}{10 \text{ ml}} = \frac{\text{Term \#3}}{\text{Term \#4}}$$

3. Write the known ratio (Terms #3 and #4) on the right side of the proportion. The units of both ratios must be the same—the units in the numerators and the units in the denominators must match. In this case, that means grams in the numerator and milliliters in the denominator. If units of the numerators or the denominators differ, then you must convert them to the same units.

$$\frac{X \text{ g}}{10 \text{ ml}} = \frac{50 \text{ g}}{100 \text{ ml}}$$

4. Cross multiply.

X g × 100 ml = 50 g × 10 ml

5. Divide each side of the equation by the known number on the left side of the equation. This will leave only the unknown value on the left side of the equation:

$$X \text{ g} = \frac{50 \text{ g} \times 10 \text{ ml}}{100 \text{ ml}}$$

6. Simplify the right side of the equation to solve for X grams:

Answer: X g = 5 g

Example 2: You need to prepare a 500-mg chloramphenicol dose in a syringe. The concentration of chloramphenicol solution is 250 mg/ml. How many milliliters should you draw up into the syringe?

1. Determine the known and unknown ratios.

Known: $\dfrac{1 \text{ ml}}{250 \text{ mg}}$

Unknown: $\dfrac{X \text{ ml}}{500 \text{ mg}}$

2. Write the proportion.

$$\frac{X \text{ ml}}{500 \text{ mg}} = \frac{1 \text{ ml}}{250 \text{ mg}}$$

3. Cross multiply.

X ml × 250 mg = 1 ml × 500 mg

4. Divide.

$$X \text{ ml} = \frac{1 \text{ ml} \times 500 \text{ mg}}{250 \text{ mg}}$$

5. Simplify.

X ml = 2 ml

Answer: Draw up 2 ml in the syringe to prepare a 500-mg dose of chloramphenicol.

Problem Set #6

a. How many milligrams of magnesium sulfate are in 10 ml of a 100 mg/ml magnesium sulfate solution?

b. A potassium chloride (KCl) solution has a concentration of 2 mEq/ml.

   1. How many milliliters contain 22 mEq?

   2. How many milliequivalents (mEq) in 15 ml?

c. Ampicillin is reconstituted to 250 mg/ml. How many milliliters are needed for a 1-g dose?

Concentration and Dilution

Terminology

- 5% dextrose in water is the same as D5W.

- 0.9% sodium chloride (NaCl) is the same as normal saline (NS).

- Half-normal saline is half the strength of normal saline (0.9% NaCl), or 0.45% NaCl. This may also be referred to as 0.5 NS or 1/2 NS.

Concentration Expressed as a Percentage

The concentration of one substance in another may be expressed as a percentage or a ratio strength.

As stated earlier in this chapter, concentrations expressed as percentages are determined using one of the following formulas:

1. Percent weight-in-weight (w/w) is the grams of a drug in 100 grams of the product.

2. Percent weight-in-volume (w/v) is the grams of a drug in 100 ml of the product.

3. Percent volume-in-volume (v/v) is the milliliters of drug in 100 ml of the product.

Example 1:

0.9% sodium chloride (w/v) = 0.9 g of sodium chloride in 100 ml of solution.

Example 2:

5% dextrose in water (w/v) = 5 g of dextrose in 100 ml of solution.

Example 3:

How many grams of dextrose are in 1 L of D5W?

Use the ratio and proportion method to solve this problem:

Known ratio: D5W means $\dfrac{5 \text{ g}}{100 \text{ ml}}$

Unknown ratio: $\dfrac{X \text{ g}}{1\text{L}}$

1. Write the proportion:

$$\frac{X \text{ g}}{1 \text{ L}} = \frac{5g}{100 \text{ ml}}$$

2. Are you ready to cross multiply? No. Remember, you must first convert the denominator of either term so that both are the same. Because you know that 1 L = 1000 ml, you can convert the unlike terms as follows:

$$\frac{X \text{ g}}{1000 \text{ ml}} = \frac{5g}{100 \text{ ml}}$$

3. Now that the units are both placed in the same order and the units across from each other are the same, you can cross multiply.

$$X \text{g} \times 100 \text{ ml} = 5 \text{ g} \times 1000 \text{ ml}$$

4. Divide:

$$X \text{g} = \frac{5g \times 1000 \text{ ml}}{100 \text{ ml}}$$

5. Simplify:

$$X \text{g} = 50 \text{ g}$$

Answer: There are 50 g of dextrose in 1 L of D5W.

Before you attempt problem sets #7 and #8, here are a few suggestions for solving concentration and dilution problems:

1. First calculate the number of grams in 100 ml of solution. That is your "known" side of the ratio.

2. Then calculate the number of grams in the volume requested in the problem by setting up a ratio.

3. Check to make sure your units are in the same order in the ratio.

4. Make sure the units that are across from each other in the ratio are the same.

5. After you have arrived at the answer, convert your answer to the requested units.

Problem Set #7

a. In 100 ml of a D5W/0.45% NaCl solution:

1. How many grams of NaCl are there?

2. How many grams of dextrose are there?

b. How many grams of dextrose are in 1 L of a 10% dextrose solution?

c. How many grams of NaCl are in 1 L of 1/2 NS?

d. How many milligrams of neomycin are in 50 ml of a 1% neomycin solution?

e. How many grams of amino acids are in 250 ml of a 10% amino acid solution?

Problem Set #8

a. An order calls for 5 million units (MU) of aqueous penicillin. How many milliliters are needed if the concentration is 500,000 units/ml?

b. How many milliliters are needed for a 15-MU aqueous penicillin dose if the concentration of the solution is 1 MU/ml?

c. Pediatric chloramphenicol comes in a 100 mg/ml

concentration. How many milligrams are present in 5 ml of the solution?

d. How many milliliters of a 250 mg/ml chloramphenicol solution are needed for a 4-g dose?

e. Oxacillin comes in a 500 mg/1.5 ml solution. How many milliliters will be required for a 1.5-g dose?

f. How many grams of ampicillin are in 6 ml of a 500 mg/1.5 ml solution?

g. How many milliliters contain 3 g of cephalothin if the concentration of the solution is 1 g/4.5 ml?

h. Use these concentrations to solve the following 20 problems:

Hydrocortisone 250 mg/2 ml

Tetracycline 250 mg/5 ml

Potassium chloride (KCl) 2 mEq/ml

Amoxicillin suspension 250 mg/5 ml

Mannitol 12.5 g/50 ml

Heparin 10,000 units/ml

Heparin 1000 units/ml

1. 10 mEq KCl = _____ml
2. 125 mg amoxicillin = _____ml
3. 750 mg hydrocortisone = _____ml
4. 1 g tetracycline = _____ml
5. 25 g mannitol = _____ml
6. 20,000 units heparin = _____ml OR _____ml
7. 35 mEq KCl = _____ml
8. 6000 units heparin = _____ml OR _____ml
9. 40 mEq KCl = _____ml
10. 600 mg hydrocortisone = _____ml
11. _____mg hydrocortisone = 4 ml
12. _____mg tetracycline = 15 ml
13. _____mEq KCl = 15 ml
14. _____g mannitol = 75 ml
15. _____units or _____units heparin = 2 ml
16. _____mEq KCl = 7 ml
17. _____g tetracycline = 12.5 ml
18. _____units or _____units heparin = 10 ml
19. _____mEq KCl = 45 ml
20. _____mg amoxicillin = 10 ml

i. How many grams of magnesium sulfate are in 2 ml of a 50% magnesium sulfate solution?

j. How many grams of dextrose are in 750 ml of a D10W solution?

k. How many milliliters of a D5W solution contain 7.5 grams of dextrose?

l. How many grams of NaCl are in 100 ml of a NS solution?

m. How many grams of NaCl are in 100 ml of a 1/2 NS solution?

n. How many grams of NaCl are in 100 ml of a 1/4 NS solution?

o. How many grams of NaCl are in 1 L of a 0.45% NaCl solution?

p. How many grams of NaCl are in 1 L of a 0.225% NaCl solution?

q. How many grams of dextrose are in 100 ml of a D5W/0.45% NaCl solution?

r. How many milliliters of a 70% dextrose solution are needed to equal 100 g of dextrose?

s. How many milliliters of a 50% dextrose solution are needed for a 10-g dextrose dose?

t. How many grams of dextrose are in a 50 ml NS solution?

Concentration Expressed as a Ratio Strength

Concentration of weak solutions is frequently expressed as ratio strength.

> Example: Epinephrine is available in three concentrations: 1:1000 (read one to one thousand); 1:10,000; and 1:200.
>
> A concentration of 1:1000 means there is 1 g of epinephrine in 1000 ml of solution.

What does a 1:200 concentration of epinephrine mean?

> It means there is 1 g of epinephrine in 200 ml of solution.

What does a 1:10,000 concentration of epinephrine mean?

> It means there is 1 g of epinephrine in 10,000 ml of solution.

Now you can use this definition of ratio strength to set up the ratios needed to solve problems.

Problem Set #9

a. How many grams of potassium permanganate should be used in preparing 500 ml of a 1:2500 solution?

b. How many milligrams of mercury bichloride are needed to make 200 ml of a 1:500 solution?

c. How many milligrams of atropine sulfate are needed to compound the following prescription?

R̸

Atropine sulfate   1:200

Dist. water qs ad   30 ml

d. How many milliliters of a 1:100 solution of epinephrine will contain 300 mg of epinephrine?

e. How much cocaine is needed to compound the following prescription?

R̸

Cocaine   1:100

Mineral oil qs ad   15 ml

f. How much zinc sulfate and boric acid are needed to compound the following prescription?

R̸

Zinc sulfate 1%

Boric acid 2:100

Distilled water qs ad 50 ml

Note: "qs ad" means "sufficient quantity to make."

Dilutions Made from Stock Solutions

Stock solutions are concentrated solutions used to prepare various dilutions. To prepare a solution of a desired concentration, you must calculate the quantity of stock solution that must be mixed with diluent to prepare the final product.

Calculating Dilutions

Example 1: You have a 10% NaCl stock solution available. You need to prepare 200 ml of a 0.5% NaCl solution. How many milliliters of the stock solution do you need to make this preparation? How much more water do you need to add to produce the final product?

1. How many grams of NaCl are in the requested final product?

$$\frac{X \text{ g NaCl}}{200 \text{ ml soln}} = \frac{0.5 \text{ g NaCl}}{100 \text{ ml soln}}$$

Therefore, 200 ml of 0.5% NaCl solution contains 1 g of NaCl.

2. How many milliliters of the stock solution will contain the amount calculated in step 1 (1 g)?

Remember, 10% means the solution contains 10 g/100 ml.

$$\frac{X \text{ ml}}{1 \text{ g}} = \frac{100 \text{ ml}}{10 \text{ g}}$$

$$X \text{ ml} = 10 \text{ ml}$$

The first part of the answer is 10 ml of stock solution.

3. How much water will you need to finish preparing your solution?

Keep in mind the following formula:

(final volume) – (stock solution volume) = (volume of water)

Therefore, for our problem,

200 ml – 10 ml = 190 ml of water

The second part of the answer is 190 ml of water.

Example 2: You have to prepare 500 ml of a 0.45% NaCl solution from a 10% NaCl stock solution. How much stock solution and water do you need?

1. How many grams of NaCl are in the requested volume? In other words, 500 ml of a 0.45% NaCl solution contains how much NaCl?

$$\frac{X \text{ g NaCl}}{500 \text{ ml}} = \frac{0.45 \text{ g}}{100 \text{ ml}}$$

$$X \text{ g} \times 100 \text{ ml} = 0.45 \text{ g} \times 500 \text{ ml}$$

$$X \text{ g} = \frac{0.45 \text{ g} \times 500 \text{ ml}}{100 \text{ ml}}$$

$$X \text{ g} = 2.25 \text{ g}$$

2. How many milliliters of stock solution will contain the amount in step 1 (2.25 g)?

$$X \text{ ml} \times 10 \text{ g} = 2.25 \text{ g} \times 100 \text{ ml}$$

$$X \text{ ml} \times 100 \text{ g} = 2.25 \text{ g} \times 100 \text{ ml}$$

$$X \text{ ml} = \frac{2.25 \text{ g} \times 100 \text{ ml}}{10 \text{ g}}$$

$$X \text{ ml} = 22.5 \text{ ml}$$

You will need 22.5 ml of stock solution.

3. How much water will you need?

(Final volume) – (stock solution volume) = volume of water

500 ml – 22.5 ml = 477.5 ml water

Answer: You will need 22.5 ml of stock solution and 477.5 ml of water to make the final product.

Problem Set #10

a. You need to prepare 1000 ml of a 1% neomycin solution for a bladder irrigation. You have only a 10% neomycin stock solution available in the pharmacy.

1. How many milliliters of the stock solution do you need to make this preparation?

2. How many milliliters of sterile water do you need to add to complete the product?

b. Sorbitol is available in a 70% stock solution. You need to prepare 140 ml of a 30% solution.

1. How many milliliters of the stock solution are needed to formulate this order?

2. How much sterile water still needs to be added to complete this product?

c. You need to make 1 L of dextrose solution containing 35% dextrose.

1. How many milliliters of the D70W do you use?

2. How much sterile water for injection still has to be added?

d. You have a 10% amino acid solution. You need to make 500 ml of a 6% amino acid solution.

1. How many milliliters of the stock solution are needed to prepare this solution?

2. How many milliliters of sterile water for injection need to be added?

e. You receive the following prescription:

℞

Boric acid 300 mg

Dist. water qs ad   15 ml

1. How many milliliters of a 5% boric acid solution are needed to prepare this prescription?

2. How many milliliters of distilled water do you need to add?

f. You need to prepare 180 ml of a 1:200 solution of potassium permanganate ($KMnO_4$). A 5% stock solution of $KMnO_4$ is available.

1. How much stock solution is needed?

2. How much water is needed?

g. How many milliliters of a 1:400 stock solution should be used to make 4 L of a 1:2000 solution?

h. You receive the following prescription:

℞

Atropine sulfate   0.05%

Dist. water qs ad   10 ml

You have a 1:50 stock solution of atropine sulfate available.

1. How many milliliters of stock solution are needed?

2. How many milliliters of water are needed to compound this prescription?

Dosage and Flow Rate Calculations

Dosage Calculations

Basic Principles

1. Always look for what is being asked:

- Number of doses
- Total amount of drug
- Size of a dose

If you are given any two of the above, you can solve for the third.

2. Number of doses, total amount of drug, and size of dose are related in the following way:

$$\text{Number of doses} = \frac{\text{Total amount of drug}}{\text{Size of dose}}$$

This proportion can also be rearranged in the following two ways:

Total amount of drug = (number of doses) × (size of dose)

OR

$$\text{Size of dose} = \frac{\text{Total amount of drug}}{\text{Number of doses}}$$

Calculating Number of Doses

Problem Set #11

a. How many 10 mg doses are in 1 g?

b. How many 5 ml doses can be made out of 2 fl oz?

Calculating Total Amount of Drug

Problem Set #12

a. How many milliliters of ampicillin do you have to dispense if the patient needs to take 2 teaspoonfuls four times a day for 7 days?

Note: First, calculate the total number of doses the patient needs to receive; then, multiply this number by the dose.

b. How many milligrams of theophylline does a patient receive per day if the prescription indicates 300 mg tid?

c. How many fluid ounces of antacid do you have to dispense if the patient is to receive 1 TBS with meals and at bedtime for 5 days?

Calculating Dose Size

Problem Set #13

a. If a patient is to receive a total of 160 mg of propranolol each day, and the patient takes one dose every 6 hours, how many milligrams are in each dose?

b. If a daily diphenhydramine dose of 300 mg is divided into six equal doses, how much do you have to dispense for every dose?

Calculating the Correct Dose

Dosage calculations can be based on weight, body surface area, or age.

Calculating Dose Based on Weight

Dose (in mg) = [Dose per unit of weight (in mg/kg)] × [Weight of patient (in kg)]

Dose/day (in mg/day) = [Dose/kg per day (in mg/kg per day)] × [Weight of patient (in kg)]

To find the size of each dose, divide the total dose per day by the number of doses per day as illustrated in the following formula:

$$\text{Size of Dose} = \frac{\text{Total amount of drug}}{\text{Number of doses}}$$

Problem Set #14

a. A patient who weighs 50 kg receives 400 mg of acyclovir q8h. The recommended dose is 5 mg/kg every 8 hours.

1. Calculate the recommended dose for this patient.

2. Is the dose this patient is receiving greater than, less than, or equal to the recommended dose?

b. The test dose of amphotericin is 0.1 mg/kg. What dose should be prepared for a patient weighing 220 lbs? (Remember, terms must be in the same units before beginning calculations.)

c. A 20-kg child receives erythromycin 25 mg q6h. The stated dosage range is 30 to 100 mg/kg per day divided into four doses.

1. What is the dosage range (in mg/day) this child should receive?

2. Is the dose this child is being given within the dosage range you have just calculated?

Calculating Dose Based on Body Surface Area

As noted previously in this chapter, BSA is expressed as meters squared (m^2).

Problem Set #15

a. An adult with a BSA of 1.5 m^2 receives acyclovir. The dose is 750 mg/m^2 per day given in three equal doses.

1. Calculate the daily dose for this patient.

2. Calculate the size of each dose for this patient.

Note: These problems are done exactly like the weight problems; however, you should substitute meters squared everywhere kilograms appeared before.

Calculating Dose Based on Age

The following is an example of information that might be found on the label of an over-the-counter children's medication:

St. Joseph's Cough Syrup for Children

Pediatric Antitussive Syrup

Active ingredient: Dextromethorphan hydrobromide 7.5 mg per 5 ml

Indications: For relief of coughing associated with colds and flu for up to 8 hours

Actions: Antitussive

Warnings: Should not be administered to children for persistent or chronic cough such as occurs with asthma or emphysema, or when cough is accompanied by excessive secretions (except under physician's advice)

How supplied: Cherry-flavored syrup in plastic bottles of 2 and 4 fl oz

Dosage: (see table below)

Age	Weight	Dosage
Under 2 yr	below 27 lb	As directed by physician
2 to under 6 yr	27 to 45 lb	1 tsp every 6 to 8 h (not to exceed 4 tsp daily)

Age	Weight	Dosage
6 to under 12 yr	46 to 83 lb	2 tsp every 6 to 8 h (not to exceed 8 tsp daily)
12 yr and older	84 lb and greater	4 tsp every 6 to 8 h (not to exceed 16 tsp daily)

Problem Set #16

a. Based on the preceding dosing table:

1. What is the dose of St. Joseph's for a 5-year-old child?

2. What should you dispense for a 12-year-old child weighing 30 kg?

b. The usual dose of ampicillin is 100 mg/kg per day. The prescription for a 38-kg child is written as 1 g q6h.

1. Is this dose acceptable?

2. If not, what should it be?

c. Propranolol is given as 0.5 mg/kg per day, divided every 6 h.

1. What should a 10-kg child receive per day?

2. What is the size of every dose?

d. Aminophylline is given at a rate of 0.6 mg/kg per hr.

1. What daily dose will a 50-kg patient receive?

2. If an oral dose is given every 12 h, what will it be?

IV Flow Rate Calculations

Using flow rates, you can calculate the volume of fluid or the amount of drug a patient will be receiving over a certain period of time. Prefilled IV bags are available in a number of volumes, including: 50, 100, 250, 500, and 1000 ml.

Calculating Volume of Fluid

Daily volume of fluid (in ml/day) =
[Flow rate (in ml/h)] × [24 h/day]

Problem Set #17

a. D5W is running at 40 ml/hr.

1. How many milliliters of D5W does the patient receive per day?

2. Which size D5W container will you dispense?

b. D5W/NS is prescribed to run at 100 ml/h.

1. How much IV fluid is needed in 24 h?

2. How will you dispense this volume?

c. A patient has two IVs running: D5W/0.5NS at 10 ml/h and a hyperalimentation solution at 70 ml/h. How much fluid is the patient receiving per day from these IVs?

Calculating Amount of Drug

Problem Set #18

a. An order is written as follows: 1 g of aminophylline in 1 L D5W/0.225% NaCl to run at 50 ml/h. How much aminophylline is the patient receiving per day?

b. The dose of aminophylline in a child is 1 mg/kg per hour.

1. If the child weighs 40 kg, at what rate should the IV in question "a" be running?

2. What should the daily dose be?

c. You add 2 g of aminophylline to 1 L of D5W. If this solution is to run at 10 ml/h, how much drug will the patient receive per day?

d. If the dose of aminophylline should be 0.6 mg/kg per hour and the patient weighs 40 kg, at what rate should the IV in question "c" be running?

Calculation of IV Flow (Drip) Rates

Calculation of IV flow (drip) rates is necessary to ensure that patients are getting the amount of medication the physician ordered. For example, if an order is written as 25,000 units of heparin in 250 ml D5W to infuse at 1000 units/h, what is the correct rate of infusion (in ml/h)?

$$\text{Concentration of IV} = \frac{\text{Total amount of drug}}{\text{Total volume}}$$

$$\text{Concentration of IV} = \frac{25,000 \text{ units heparin}}{250 \text{ ml D5W}}$$

$$\text{Concentration of IV} = 100 \text{ units/ml of D5W}$$

Now that you have calculated the concentration per milliliter, you can determine exactly what the rate should be by using the following formula:

$$\text{IV Rate} = \frac{\text{Dose desired}}{\text{Concentration of IV}}$$

$$\text{IV Rate} = \frac{(1,000 \text{ units/h})}{(100 \text{ units/ml})}$$

$$\text{IV Rate} = 10 \text{ ml/h}$$

Problem Set #19

a. An order is written for 2 g of lidocaine in 250 ml of D5W to infuse at 120 mg/h. What is the correct rate of infusion (in ml/h)?

b. An order is written for 25,000 units of heparin in 250 ml of D5W. The doctor writes to infuse 17 ml/h. How many units of heparin will the patient receive in a 12-hour period?

Moles, Equivalents, Osmolarity, Isotonicity, and pH

Moles and Equivalents

A mole is one way of expressing an amount of a chemical substance or a drug.

> Examples: A mole of NaCl (sodium chloride) weighs 58.45 g.
>
> A mole of KCl (potassium chloride) weighs 74.55 g.
>
> An equivalent usually expresses the amount of each part (or element) of a chemical substance or a drug.
>
> Examples: One mole of NaCl contains one equivalent of Na+ (which weighs 23 g).
>
> One mole of NaCl also contains one equivalent of Cl- (which weighs 35.45 g).
>
> Remember, 1 equivalent (Eq) = 1000 milliequivalents (mEq).

Numbers to Remember

If you forget these numbers, these equivalents can be found on the labels of the large-volume sodium and dextrose solutions.

a. 0.9% NaCl contains 0.9 g NaCl in every 100 ml of solution,
   or
   0.9% NaCl contains 9 g NaCl in every liter of solution.

b. 0.9% NaCl contains 15.4 mEq Na+ in every 100 ml of solution,
   or
   0.9% NaCl contains 154 mEq Na+ in every liter of solution.

c. 0.45% NaCl (1/2 NS) contains 0.45 g NaCl in every 100 ml of solution, or 7.7 mEq of Na+ in every 100 ml of solution,
   or
   0.45% NaCl contains 4.5 g NaCl in every liter of solution, or 77 mEq of Na+ in every liter of solution.

d. The table below summarizes some of the data.

	grams of NaCl/100 ml	grams of NaCl/liter	milliequivalents of Na+/liter
0.9% NaCl (NS)	0.9	9	154
0.45% NaCl (1/2 NS)	0.45	4.5	77
0.225% NaCl (1/4 NS)	0.225	2.25	38.5

Problem Set #20

a. You need to make 1 L of NS. You have 1 L of SWI (Sterile Water for Injection) and a vial of NaCl (4 mEq/ml). How will you prepare this solution?

b. An order calls for D10W/0.45% NaCl to run at 40 ml/h. You have 1 L of D10W and a vial of NaCl (4 mEq/ml) available. How would you prepare this bottle?

c. How would you prepare 500 ml of a D10W/ 0.225% NaCl solution if you have SWI, NaCl (4 mEq/ml), and a 50% dextrose solution available?

d. You have D10W and a vial of NaCl (4 mEq/ml). How would you prepare 250 ml of a D10W/NS solution?

Osmolarity and Isotonicity

Osmolarity expresses the number of particles (osmols) in a certain volume of fluid.

> Remember, 1 osmol (Osm) = 1000 milliosmols (mOsm).
>
> The osmolarity of human plasma is about 280 to 300 mOsm/L.
>
> The osmolarity of NS is about 300 mOsm/L, and the osmolarity of D5W is about 280 mOsm/L.
>
> Solutions of the same osmolarity are called isotonic.

> Example: NS and plasma are isotonic.
>
> If parenteral fluids are administered that are not isotonic, the result could be irritation of veins and swelling or shrinking of red blood cells.
>
> Solutions having osmolarities higher than that of plasma are known as hypertonic solutions.
>
> Examples: Hyperalimentation solutions and D5W/ NS are hypertonic.
>
> Solutions having osmolarities lower than that of plasma are called hypotonic solutions.
>
> Example: 1/2 NS is hypotonic.

pH

pH refers to the acidity or basicity of a solution.

The pH scale ranges from 1 to 14.

pH = 7 is neutral

pH < 7 is acidic

pH > 7 is basic

Normal human plasma has a pH of approximately 7.4.

Parenteral solutions with pHs different from that of normal human plasma can be very irritating to tissue when injected. Examples are phenytoin and diazepam. Ophthalmologic preparations are buffered to maintain a pH as close to 7.4 as possible.

Some drugs are not stable at a certain pH. One example is ampicillin, which is not very stable in acidic solutions. D5W solutions are slightly acidic, whereas NS solutions are more neutral. Therefore, ampicillin injection is dispensed in NS rather than D5W.

Statistics

The arithmetic mean is a value that is calculated by dividing the sum of a set of numbers by the total number of number sets. This value is also referred to as an *average*. The following formula is used to determine the average:

$$M = \frac{\sum X}{N}$$

where $\sum$ = sum

M = mean (average)

X = one value in set of data

N = number of values X in data set

Now, using the formula, follow these two steps to calculate the arithmetic mean age of five pharmacists whose ages are 25, 28, 33, 47, and 54 years.

1. Find the sum of all ages.

2. Divide the sum by total number of pharmacists:

$$\frac{25 + 28 + 33 + 47 + 54}{5} = \frac{187}{5} = 37.4 \text{ years}$$

The median is a value in an ordered set of values below and above which there are an equal number of values. When an even number of measurements are arranged according to size, the median is defined as the mean of the values of the two measurements that are nearest to the middle.

Example 1: Determine the median temperature for a medication refrigerator whose temperature reading was 37°F, 39°F, 40°F, 44°F, and 38°F on 5 consecutive days.

1. Arrange the temperature readings according to size, smallest to largest.

   37° 38° 39° 40° 44°

2. The median is 39°.

Example 2: Determine the median temperature for a medication refrigerator whose temperature reading was 45°F, 40°F, 43°F, 39°F, 46°F, and 40°F on 6 consecutive days.

1. Arrange the temperature readings according to size, smallest to largest.

   39° 40° 40° 43° 45° 46°

2. The median is $\frac{40 + 43}{2} = \frac{83}{2} = 41.5$

Standard deviation is a statistic that tells you how tightly clustered the data points are around the mean in a set of data. Standard deviation can be calculated by using the following formula:

$$\Omega = \sqrt{\sum(X-M)^2 \times 1/(N-1)}$$

Where Ω = standard deviation

X = one value in set of data

M = the mean of all values X in your set of data

N = the number of values X in your set of data

Graphically, when the individual values are bunched around the mean in a set of data, the bell-shaped curve is steep. Conversely, when the individual values are widely spread around the mean in a set of data, the bell-shaped curve is flat (see **Figure 5-1**).

One standard deviation away from the mean in either direction on the X axis accounts for about 68% of the individual values in the data set. Two standard deviations away from the mean in either direction on the X axis accounts for about 95% of the individual values in the data set. Three standard deviations away from the mean in either direction on the X axis accounts for about 99% of the individual values in the

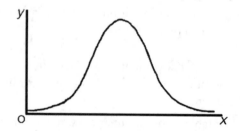

Figure 5-1. Bell Curve

data set. If the curve were flatter and more spread out, the standard deviation would be larger to account for 68% of the individual values in the data set. The standard deviation can help you explain data and evaluate various studies.

Example: Using the following steps, calculate the standard deviation for body weight of normal males according to the table below:

Normal Males	Body Weight (pounds)
1	154
2	175
3	162
4	213
5	191
6	187
7	158
8	202
9	185
10	230

1. Calculate the mean (average) of all body weights by adding all body weights and dividing by the total number of normal males.

$$\overline{X} = \frac{\sum X}{N}$$

$\sum X$ = 154 + 175 + 162 + 213 + 191 + 187 + 158 + 202 + 185 + 230 = 1,857 pounds

N = 10

$$\overline{X} = \frac{1,857 \text{ pounds}}{10} = 185.7 \text{ pounds}$$

2. For each of the individual male body weights, subtract the mean (average) body weight from the individual male body weights, then multiply that value by itself (also known as determining the square).

$(154 - 185.7)^2 =$	1004.89
$(175 - 185.7)^2 =$	114.49
$(162 - 185.7)^2 =$	561.69
$(213 - 185.7)^2 =$	745.29
$(191 - 185.7)^2 =$	28.09
$(187 - 185.7)^2 =$	1.69
$(158 - 185.7)^2 =$	767.29
$(202 - 185.7)^2 =$	265.69
$(185 - 185.7)^2 =$	0.49
$(230 - 185.7)^2 =$	1962.49

3. Sum up all the squared values.

1004.89 + 114.49 + 561.69 + 745.29 + 28.09 + 1.69 + 767.29 + 265.69 + .49 + 1962.49 = 5452.1

4. Multiply the sum of all the squared values by 1/(N-1) and take the square root of the resulting value to obtain the standard deviation for male body weights.

$(5452.1) \times (1/(N-1)) =$

$(5452.1) \times (1/(10-1)) = 605.79$

$\sqrt{605.79} = 24.61$

Ideal Body Weight (IBW)

You need to know a patient's IBW to determine the estimated creatinine clearance of an individual patient. The estimated creatinine clearance is needed to determine the appropriate dose of renally excreted medications, such as tobramycin. The following formula is used for calculating the IBW for a male:

IBW male (kg) = 50 + $\dfrac{(2.3 \times \text{height in inches})}{5 \text{ feet}}$

The following formula is used for calculating the IBW for a female:

IBW female (kg) = 45.5 + $\dfrac{(2.3 \times \text{height in inches})}{5 \text{ feet}}$

Example: Calculate the IBW for a male who is 6 feet 2 inches tall.

1. Convert the height to inches.

6 feet x 12 inches/foot = 72 inches + 2 inches = 74 inches

2. Using the formula for calculating the IBW for a male, multiply 2.3 times 74 inches.

2.3 × 74 = 170.2

3. Divide 170.2 by 5 feet.

170.2 inches/5 feet = 34.04

4. Add 50 to 34.04 to obtain the ideal body weight.

50 + 34.04 = 84.04 kg

Practice Calculations 1

1. What does $\overline{ss}$ mean?_____

2. Write II as an Arabic numeral:_____

3. Write 2/5 as a decimal fraction:_____

4. The fraction form of 0.1 is:_____

5. Express 25% as a fraction:_____

6. Write 0.88 as a percentage:_____

7. Express 1/4 as a percentage:_____

8. The fraction form of 0.4 is:_____

9. Express xiv in Arabic numerals:_____

10. Write 1 1/2 in decimal form:_____

11. The standard metric system measure for weight is the:_____

12. The standard metric system measure for length is the:_____

13. The standard metric system measure for volume is the:_____

14. 1 km = _____ m

15. 1 L = _____ ml

16. 1 kg = _____ g

17. 1 g = _____ mg

18. 1 mg = _____ g

19. 0.01 g = _____ mg

20. 1 ml = _____ L

21. 1 tsp = _____ TBS

22. 1 cup = _____ ml

23. 1 TBS = _____ fl oz

24. 15 ml = _____ TBS

25. 1 cup = _____ fl oz

26. 1000 ml = _____ L

27. 2 kg = _____ g

28. 1 gal = _____ qt

29. 1 pt = _____ cups

30. 1 mm = _____ m

31. 1 tsp = _____ ml

32. 5 gr = _____ g

33. 3 cups = _____ ml

34. 70 kg = _____ lb

35. 45 ml = _____ fl oz

36. 80 mg = _____ gr

37. 250 mg = _____ g

38. 3 TBS = _____ tsp

39. 2 fl oz = _____ TBS

40. 3 qt = _____ pt

41. 120 ml = _____ cups

42. 10 ml = _____ tsp

43. 45 ml = _____ TBS

44. 50 mg = _____ mg

45. 2 gal = _____ qt

46. 0.5 pt = _____ ml

47. 20 kg = _____ lb

48. 750 mg = _____ g

49. 25 ml = _____ tsp

50. 6 tsp = _____ TBS

Practice Calculations 2

1. 6% (w/w) = _____

   10% (w/v) = _____

   0.5% (v/v) = _____

2. A patient needs a 300-mg dose of amikacin. How many milliliters do you need to draw from a vial containing 100 mg/2 ml of amikacin?

3. A suspension of naladixic acid contains 250 mg/5 ml. The syringe contains 15 ml. What is the dose (in milligrams) contained in the syringe?

4. How many milligrams of neomycin are in 200 ml of a 1% neomycin solution?

5. 1/2 NS = _____ g NaCl / _____ ml solution

6. How many grams of pumpkin are in 300 ml of a 30% pumpkin juice suspension?

7. Express 4% hydrocortisone cream as a ratio. (Remember that solids, such as creams, are usually expressed as weight-in-weight.)

8. You have a solution labeled D10W/NS.

   a) How many grams of NaCl are in 50 ml of this solution?

   b) How many milliliters of this solution contain 50 g dextrose?

9. A syringe is labeled "inamrinone 5 mg/ml, 20 ml." How many milligrams of inamrinone are in the syringe?

10. Boric acid 2:100 is written on a prescription. This is the same as _____ boric acid in _____ solution.

11. How much epinephrine do you need to prepare 20 ml of a 1:400 epinephrine solution?

12. Calculate the amounts of boric acid and zinc sulfate to fill the following prescription:

    R

    Zinc sulfate   0.5%

    Boric acid   1:50

Distilled water qs. ad   100 ml

13. Use the following concentrations to solve the problems:

Gentamicin   80 mg/ml

Magnesium sulfate 50%

Atropine 1:200

a) 120 mg gentamicin = _____ ml

b) 100 mg atropine = _____ ml

c) _____ g magnesium sulfate = 150 ml

Practice Calculations 3

1. You need to prepare 1 L of 0.25% acetic acid irrigation solution. The stock concentration of acetic acid is 25%.

   a. How many milliliters of stock solution do you need to use?

   b. How many milliliters of sterile water do you need to add?

2. A drug order requires 500 ml of a 2% neomycin solution.

   a. How much neomycin concentrate (1 g/2 ml) do you need to fill the order?

   b. How many milliliters of sterile water must you add to the concentrate before dispensing the drug?

3. a. Calculate the amount of atropine stock solution (concentration 0.5%) needed to compound the following prescription:

   ℞

   Atropine sulfate   1:1500

   Sterile water qs ad 300 ml

   b. How much sterile water do you have to add to complete the order?

4. How many tablets do you have to dispense for the following prescription?

   ℞

   Obecalp ii tablets tid for 10 days

5. How many 2 tsp doses can a patient take from a bottle containing 3 fl oz?

6. A patient is receiving a total daily dose of 2 g of acyclovir. How many milligrams of acyclovir is he receiving per dose if he takes the drug five times a day?

7. The recommended dose of erythromycin to treat an ear infection is 50 mg/kg per day given q6h. Answer the following questions regarding this drug:

   a. If a child weighs 20 kg, how much erythromycin should he receive per day?

   b. How much drug will he receive per dose?

8. The dose of prednisone for replacement therapy is 2 mg/m² per dose. The drug is administered twice daily. What is the daily prednisone dose for a 1.5-m² person?

9. An aminophylline drip is running at 1 mg/kg per hour in a 10-kg child. How much aminophylline is the child receiving per day?

10. A child with an opiate overdose needs naloxone. The recommended starting dose is 0.1 mg/kg. The doctor writes for 0.3 mg naloxone stat. Answer the following questions on the basis of the child's weight of 26.4 lbs.:

    a. What is the child's weight in kg?

    b. On the basis of the answer to "a," does 0.3 mg sound like a reasonable dose?

11. An IV fluid containing NS is running at 80 ml/h.

    a. How much fluid is the patient receiving per day?

    b. How many 1-L bags will be needed per day?

12. A patient has two IVs running: an aminophylline drip at 20 ml/h and saline at 30 ml/h. How much fluid is the patient receiving per day from the IVs?

13. a. You prepare a solution by adding 2 g of Bronkospaz to 1 L of NS. What is the concentration of Bronkospaz?

    b. If the solution of Bronkospaz you made in "a" runs at 30 ml/h, how much Bronkospaz is the patient receiving per day?

    c. If a 60-kg patient should receive 1 mg/kg per hour, will the dose in "b" be appropriate?

Answers to Problem Sets

Problem Set #1:

a. 2	b. 605	c. 20	d. 3
e. 7	f. 4	g. 9	h. 15
i. 11	j. 1030	k. 14	l. 16

Problem Set #2:

a. 0.5	b. 0.75	c. 1	d. 0.4

e. 667/1000   f. 0.625   g. 0.5   h. 0.25   n. 1.76 lb

i. 5.5   j. 2.67   k. 5.25   l. 3.8   o. 15 ml

m. 1/4   n. 2/5   o. 3/4   p. 7/20   p. 1 fl oz

q. 2 1/2   r. 1 3/5   s. 3 1/4   t. 1/3   q. 30 ml

r. 20 fl oz

Problem Set #3:

a. 23/100   b. 67/100   c. 1/8   d. 1/2   s. 32.5 mg

e. 66.7/100   f. 3/4   g. 33/50   h. 2/5   t. 500 ml

i. 1   j. 3/20   k. 50%   l. 25%   u. 5 gr

m. 40%   n. 24%   o. 4%   p. 50%   v. 4 TBS

q. 35%   r. 44%   s. 57%   t. 99%   w. 2 fl oz

x. 65.5 kg

Problem Set #4:

a. 1000 ml

b. 1 kg

c. 1000 mg

d. 1 mg

e. 3 tsp

f. 15 ml

g. 1 cup

h. 240 ml

i. 1 TBS

j. 5 ml

k. 16 TBS

l. 480 ml

m. 2 TBS

n. 2 pt

y. 6 tsp

z. 20 ml

aa. 28.3°C

bb. –22.2°C

cc. 41°F

dd. 89.6°F

ee. 2.1 m^2

Problem Set #6:

a. 1000 mg

b. 1. 11 ml

   2. 30 mEq

c. 4 ml

Problem Set #7:

a. 1. 0.45 g

   2. 5 g

b. 100 g

c. 4.5 g

d. 500 mg

e. 25 g

Problem Set #8:

a. 10 ml

b. 15 ml

c. 500 mg

d. 16 ml

e. 4.5 ml

f. 2 g

g. 13.5 ml

h. 1. 5 ml

Problem Set #5:

a. 1 fl oz

b. 0.5 g

c. 0.5 fl oz

d. 4 tsp

e. 3500 g

f. 0.00025 g

g. 1.5 L

h. 6 gal

i. 390 mg

j. 54.5 kg

k. 90 ml

l. 158.4 lb

m. 1.97 pt

1. 5 ml

2. 2.5 ml

3. 6 ml

4. 20 ml

5. 100 ml

6. a. 2 ml of heparin 10,000 units/ml or

   b. 20 ml of heparin 1000 units/ml

7. 17.5 ml

8. a. 0.6 ml of heparin 10,000 units/ml or

   b. 6 ml of heparin 1000 units/ml

9. 20 ml

10. 4.8 ml

11. 500 mg

12. 750 mg

13. 30 mEq

14. 18.75 g

15. 20,000 units or 2000 units

16. 14 mEq

17. 0.625 g

18. 100,000 units or 10,000 units

19. 90 mEq

20. 500 mg

i. 1 g

j. 75 g

k. 150 ml

l. 0.9 g

m. 0.45 g

n. 0.225 g

o. 4.5 g

p. 2.25 g

q. 5 g

r. 142.9 ml

s. 20 ml

t. 0

Problem Set #9:

a. 0.2 g

b. 400 mg

c. 150 mg

d. 30 ml

e. 150 mg

f. 500 mg of zinc sulfate and 1 g of boric acid

Problem Set #10:

a. 1. 100 ml of stock solution

   2. 900 ml of water

b. 1. 60 ml of stock solution

   2. 80 ml of water

c. 1. 500 ml of D70W

   2. 500 ml of sterile water

d. 1. 300 ml of stock solution

   2. 200 ml of sterile water

e. 1. 6 ml of 5% boric acid

   2. 9 ml of distilled water

f. 1. 18 ml of stock solution

   2. 162 ml of water

g. 800 ml of stock solution

h. 1. 0.25 ml of stock solution

   2. 9.75 ml of water

Problem Set #11:

a. 100 doses

b. 12 doses

Problem Set #12:

a. 280 ml of ampicillin

b. 900 mg of theophylline

c. 10 fl oz

Problem Set #13:

a. 40 mg of propranolol

b. 50 mg for every dose

Problem Set #14:

a. 1. 250 mg q8h

   2. greater than the recommended dose

b. 10 mg

c. 1. 600–2000 mg/day

   2. no

Problem Set #15:

a. 1. 1125 mg

   2. 375 mg

Problem Set #16:

a. 1. 1 tsp every 6 to 8 h not to exceed 4 tsp daily

2. 2 tsp every 6 to 8 h not to exceed 8 tsp daily
   (Defer to weight when there is a difference
   between the weight-based dose and the age-based
   dose, since weight is a more accurate basis for
   dosing medications in general.)

b. 1. no (Depending on your facility's rounding
   conventions, this dose may be considered
   correct.)

   2. 3800 mg/day

c. 1. 5 mg/day

   2. 1.25 mg per dose

d. 1. 720 mg

   2. 360 mg every 12 hours

Problem Set #17:

a. 1. 960 ml

   2. 1000 ml

b. 1. 2400 ml

   2. 3000 ml, three 1-L bags

c. 1920 ml of fluid

Problem Set #18:

a. 1.2 g

b. 1. 40 ml/h

   2. 960 mg/day

c. 480 mg/day

d. 12 ml/hr

Problem Set #19:

a. 15 ml/h

b. 20,400 units

Problem Set #20:

a. Add 38.5 ml NaCl to 1 L SWFI

b. Add 19.25 ml NaCl to 1 L D10W

c. 4.81 ml NaCl plus 100 ml D50W; qs with SWFI to
   500 ml

d. 9.625 ml NaCl; qs with D10W to 250 ml

Answers to Practice Calculations 1

1. 1/2
2. 2
3. 0.4
4. 1/10
5. 1/4
6. 88%
7. 25%
8. 2/5
9. 14
10. 1.5
11. gram
12. meter
13. liter
14. 1000
15. 1000
16. 1000
17. 1000
18. 0.001
19. 10
20. 0.001
21. 1/3
22. 240
23. 0.5
24. 1
25. 8
26. 1
27. 2000
28. 4
29. 2
30. 0.001
31. 5
32. 0.325
33. 720
34. 154
35. 1.5
36. 1.23
37. 0.25
38. 9
39. 4
40. 6
41. 0.5
42. 2
43. 3
44. 0.05
45. 8

46. 240

47. 44

48. 0.75

49. 5

50. 2

Answers to Practice Calculations 2

1. 6 g/100 g

    10 g/100 ml

    0.5 ml/100 ml

2. 6 ml

3. 750 mg

4. 2000 mg

5. 0.45 g/100 ml

6. 90 g

7. 4 g/100 g

8. a. 0.45 g

    b. 500 ml

9. 100 mg

10. 2 g in 100 ml

11. 0.05 g or 50 mg

12. 0.5 g zinc sulfate and 2 g boric acid

13. a. 1.5 ml

    b. 20 ml

    c. 75 g

Answers to Practice Calculations 3

1. a. 2.5 g acetic acid = 10 ml stock solution

    b. 990 ml sterile water

2. a. 10 g neomycin = 20 ml stock solution

    b. 480 ml sterile water

3. a. 0.2 g atropine sulfate = 40 ml stock solution

    b. 260 ml sterile water

4. 60 tablets

5. 9 doses

6. 400 mg per dose

7. a. 1000 mg per day

    b. 250 mg per dose

8. 6 mg per day

9. 240 mg per day

10. a. 12 kg

    b. No, the calculated dose is 1.2 mg.

11. a. 1920 ml per day

    b. 2 1-L bags per day

12. 1200 ml per day

13. a. 2000 mg/1000 ml or 2 mg/ml or
    2 g/1000 ml or 2 g/L or 2:1000

    b. 1440 mg/day

    c. Yes, dose is appropriate.

APPENDIX

Table 1

micro-(mc):	1/1,000,000	= 0.000001
milli-(m):	1/1000	= 0.001
centi-(c):	1/100	= 0.01
deci-(d):	1/10	= 0.1

Table 2

deca-(da) :	10
hecto-(h):	100
kilo-(k):	1000
mega-(M):	1,000,000

Table 3

1 kilometer (km)	= 1000 meters (m)
0.001 kilometer (km)	= 1 meter (m)
1 millimeter (mm)	= 0.001 meter (m)
1000 millimeters (mm)	= 1 meter (m)
1 centimeter (cm)	= 0.01 meter (m)
100 centimeters (cm)	= 1 meter (m)

Table 4

1 milliliter (ml)	= 0.001 liter (L)
1000 milliliters (ml)	= 1 liter (L)
1 microliter (mcl)	= 0.000001 liter (L)
1,000,000 microliters (mcl)	= 1 liter (L)
1 deciliter (dl)	= 0.1 liter (L)
10 deciliters (dl)	= 1 liter (L)

Table 5

1 kilogram (kg)	= 1000 grams (g)
0.001 kilogram (kg)	= 1 gram (g)
1 milligram (mg)	= 0.001 gram (g)
1000 milligrams (mg)	= 1 gram (g)
1 microgram (mcg)	= 0.000001 gram (g)
1,000,000 micrograms (mcg)	= 1 gram (g)

Table 6

Pound	Ounces	Drams	Scruples	Grains
1 =	12 =	96 =	288 =	5760
	1 =	8 =	24 =	480
		1 =	3 =	60
			1 =	20

Table 7

Gallon	Pints	Fluid ounces	Fluid drams	Minims
1 =	8 =	128 =	1024 =	61,440
	1 =	16 =	128 =	7,680
		1 =	8 =	480
			1 =	60

Table 8

Pound (lb)	Ounces (oz)	Grains (gr)
1 =	16 =	7000
	1 =	437.5

Table 9

1 meter (m)	=	39.37 (39.4) inches (in)
1 inch (in)	=	2.54 centimeters (cm)
1 micron (mc)	=	0.000001 meter (m)

Table 10

1 milliliter (ml)	= 16.23 minims (m.)
1 fluid ounce (fl oz)	= 29.57 (30) milliliters (ml)
1 liter (L)	= 33.8 fluid ounces (fl oz)
1 pint (pt)	= 473.167 (480) milliliters (ml)
1 gallon (gal)	= 3785.332 (3785) milliliters (ml)

Table 11

1 kilogram (kg)	= 2.2 pounds (lb)
1 pound avoir (lb)	= 453.59 (454) grams (g)
1 ounce avoir (oz)	= 28.35 (28) grams (g)
1 ounce apoth (oz)	= 31.1 (31) grams (g)
1 gram (g)	= 15.432 (15) grains (gr)

1 grain (gr)	= 65 milligrams (mg)		
1 ounce (avoir) (oz)	= 437.5 grains (gr)		
1 ounce (apoth)	= 480 grains (gr)		

Table 12

	grams of NaCl/100ml	grams of NaCl/liter	milliequiva-lents of Na+/liter
0.9% NaCl (NS)	0.9	9	154.5
0.45% NaCl (1/2 NS)	0.45	4.5	77
0.225% NaCl (1/4 NS)	0.225	2.25	38.5

Footnotes

This chapter was adapted with permission from the Johns Hopkins Hospital Technician Training Course 1991: 106–38.

Pharmacy Law

PHILIP R. TORF

To work as a pharmacy technician is a privilege, not a right. This privilege can be lost when the pharmacy technician violates the law or ethical standards. Therefore, the pharmacy technician is responsible for knowing the laws and ethical standards that govern his or her professional conduct.

Federal and state laws regulate the practice of pharmacy, and the pharmacy technician must comply with them. Federal law is the same throughout the country, whereas individual state laws affect only the persons, actions, and items within that state. This chapter will consider only federal laws. Pharmacy technicians must become familiar with their own state laws for a more complete understanding of pharmacy law.

Introduction

Congress has enacted laws as both statutes and acts. The Food, Drug, and Cosmetic Act (FDCA), the Controlled Substance Act, and the Poison Prevention Packaging Act are the most commonly referenced laws in regulating the practice of pharmacy. These acts have been amended numerous times to add, delete, or modify portions of the original acts.

Administrative agencies, such as the Food and Drug Administration (FDA), create rules that have the effect of law. The rules, enacted by the United States Department of Justice, the Drug Enforcement Administration (DEA), and the FDA, are found in the Code of Federal Regulation (CFR). Volume 21 of the CFR regulates foods and drugs. Its sections address everything from food additives to investigational drugs to controlled substances.

Following the laws and rules that govern an industry such as pharmacy is called regulatory compliance. Violation of laws can lead to prosecution in a court of law; violation of a rule can lead to discipline within an administrative agency. This chapter will focus on the aspects of pharmacy regulatory compliance that are relevant to the pharmacy technician.

In addition to the need for regulatory compliance, pharmacy technicians should be aware of pharmacy malpractice. Technicians should understand their personal responsibility to each patient. A pharmacy

6

Learning Objectives

After completing this chapter, the technician should be able to

1. Define "legend drug."

2. Explain what is meant by a drug being "safe and effective."

3. Distinguish between compounding and manufacturing.

4. Identify the components of the prescription label.

5. Identify the components of over-the-counter drug labels.

6. Explain the Poison Prevention Packaging Act as it relates to pharmacy.

7. Distinguish between "expiration date" and "beyond-use" date.

8. Name the five classes of controlled substances.

9. Distinguish between brand and generic drugs.

10. Explain how to use DEA Order Form 222.

technician dispensing an incorrect drug that results in catastrophic personal injury to a patient could well find him- or herself in the middle of a law suit for negligently filling the prescription. Negligence will not be discussed in detail here because this chapter's focus is on regulatory compliance. Besides, knowing more about malpractice per se will not make one a better technician. Rather, filling each prescription correctly and following the regulatory requirements will likely prevent involvement in civil, criminal, or administrative litigation.

Most federal laws pertaining to pharmacy practice are directed toward retail pharmacy, but they do apply to hospital and long-term care pharmacy settings with some variations. For example, over-the-counter products are required to have certain information on their labels. Floor stock, common in long-term care and hospital pharmacies, is generally not sold to the general public, but it still must meet the requirements for over-the-counter drug labeling. Therefore, it would be wrong to send a bottle of Tylenol®, for example, to a nursing station within a health care facility without proper over-the-counter labeling.

This chapter will primarily examine the federal Controlled Substance Law, the FDCA, the Poison Prevention Packaging Act, and the Omnibus Budget Reconciliation Act, but it will also review the common law.

Federal Food, Drug, and Cosmetic Act

The foundation of pharmacy law is the FDCA. Originally enacted in the 1900s as the Pure Food and Drug Act, it has been amended numerous times to address many issues, such as safety and efficacy. The original Pure Food and Drug Act and later amendments were enacted to protect people from fraudulent claims about drugs, contaminated and mislabeled drugs,[1] drugs that were unsafe or ineffective,[2] and drugs that were dangerous without a physician's guidance.[3] In 1962, the FDCA was amended to ensure more safety and efficacy.[4]

The FDCA is so vast in its applications that hundreds of books have been written about it. This chapter will discuss the important parts of the FDCA as they pertain to the practice of pharmacy.

Legend Drugs

A drug is any chemical that causes a response in the body. Some drugs are regulated by the government and others are not. Caffeine and codeine, for example, are both drugs but are not subject to the same government control. Some drugs are sold only pursuant to a prescription, whereas others are available over the counter. Drugs that require prescriptions have either of the following on their label: "Federal Law prohibits dispensing without prescription" or "Rx." These drugs are considered *legend drugs*. Legend drugs can be dispensed only pursuant to a prescription from a licensed practitioner. The authority to prescribe varies from state to state. Some states allow mid-level practitioners, such as physician assistants and nurse practitioners, to prescribe legend drugs. A state's licensing board will give details as to a state's laws regarding the dispensing of legend drugs. The technician cannot assume that any items in the pharmacy that do not have a legend may be unconditionally sold. This subject will be discussed more fully later in this chapter.

Safe and Effective

The FDCA has been amended to require that all drugs be safe and effective, regardless of their status as a legend or over-the-counter (OTC) drug. For a legend drug to be safe and effective, the manufacturer of the drug must have filed with the FDA evidence of the safety and efficacy of the drug in both human and animal studies and must monitor the drug (post-marketing surveillance) after its approval to assure the FDA that the drug is safe. This monitoring involves the receipt and evaluation of adverse drug reaction reports as well as other documentation that may be relevant to maintaining the status of a drug's safety and efficacy.

The fact that a drug has been approved by the FDA should give the technician confidence that it is safe and effective. However, based on post-marketing surveillance, the FDA may reverse the safety and efficacy of a drug. Older drugs may be pulled off the market if no studies have been performed to establish that they are safe and effective. Furthermore, because of litigation, many drugs that were approved by the FDA have been withdrawn either by the manufacturer or by the FDA because they were demonstrated not to be as safe and effective as originally claimed. The pharmacy technician, as a member of the health care team, has a responsibility to report adverse drug reactions to the manufacturer as well as to the FDA.

Compounding and Manufacturing

A pharmaceutical manufacturer transforms a chemical into a final dosage form (such as extended- and sustained-release capsules or tablets, suspensions, elixirs and solutions, creams, ointments and gels). This final dosage form can be sold to pharmacies or prescribers and can be marketed and advertised for uses approved by the FDA. A drug must be proven safe and effective to be manufactured or sold. In contrast, no such proof is needed for compounded pharmaceutical products when they are made in a pharmacy pursuant to a prescription.

The United States Supreme Court has defined compounding as "A process by which a pharmacist or doctor combines, mixes, or alters ingredients to create a medication tailored to an individual patient's needs." Prescriptions are frequently written for a combination of drugs that need to be compounded in the pharmacy. These may include parenteral products, ophthalmics, and dermatologicals and can take the form of sterile IV solutions, capsules, suppositories, elixirs, suspensions, creams, and ointments. The preparation of these compounded drugs in a pharmacy is not considered manufacturing if it is done pursuant to a prescription that is intended for an individual patient's use. The FDA does not require proof that the final compounded product will be safe or effective. It is important to know that a pharmacy cannot sell the final compounded product to another pharmacy or physician. Doing so would constitute manufacturing and hence require proof of the safety and efficacy of the product to the FDA.

Vitamins and Nutritionals

Vitamins and nutritionals have carved out an exception from the new drug approval process and have escaped the requirement of being effective because of recent amendments to the FDCA. Whereas some vitamins have proven to be clinically useful, other vitamins have received acceptance by the public and perhaps are effective in helping to maintain a healthy body or even improving its state of well-being. So long as the manufacturers of these vitamins and nutritionals do not make clinical claims or market them for specific diseases, the FDA allows these chemicals to be sold without a prescription, whether or not they have been proven safe and effective.

The basis for classifying a chemical as either a drug or nutritional is beyond the scope of this chapter. A pharmacy technician will not make a decision as to whether an item in the pharmacy requires a prescrip-

tion. The most important thing a technician can do is to be certain that a prescription has been issued whenever a legend drug is being dispensed.

Prescription Labeling

All drugs must be properly labeled. The information required to be on the label depends on whether the drug is dispensed pursuant to a prescription, sold over-the-counter without a prescription, or sold to the pharmacy by a manufacturer. The patient's location (i.e., long-term care, general public, or hospital) may also have an impact on what is required on the label.

The FDCA requires that all (retail) prescription labels have the following information: name and address of pharmacy, prescription number, date of prescription filling or refilling, name of prescriber, name of patient, directions for use, and cautionary statement (as indicated on the prescription). "Medication orders" in long-term care facilities and hospitals are different from "retail" prescriptions, so the labels do not require the same information. Labels on medicines in long-term care facilities or hospitals may not include quantity dispensed, cautionary statements, original filling date, prescriber's name, or even the name and address of the pharmacy. Most states have rules for what must appear on prescription or medication order labels. Therefore, the technician should review the state's rules regarding labeling.

Over-the-Counter Drugs

If a pharmacy sells an OTC product to the public not pursuant to a prescription, that container must be labeled as if the pharmacy were a manufacturer. This requirement is waived if the pharmacy dispenses the OTC drug pursuant to a prescription and labels it as a prescription.

The FDCA requires the following information to be on all OTC labels:

- name of product;
- name of manufacturer,
- distributor or packer;
- quantity;
- established name of all active ingredients and the quantity of other ingredients, whether active or not;
- name of any habit-forming drug contained in the preparation;
- directions for use;
- cautionary statements;

- purpose for which drug is intended;
- normal dose for each intended use; and
- dosages for persons of different age groups and physical conditions.

Repackaging of an OTC product by a pharmacy requires compliance with this federal labeling law. For example, if a patient walks into a pharmacy to purchase a bottle of milk of magnesia off the shelf, the manufacturer of that product should have labeled it with all the information listed above. If the same customer were to go to the pharmacy counter and request some milk of magnesia and the pharmacy technician were to repackage a quantity of the milk of magnesia from a stock bottle for that customer, the technician would be required to label the package exactly as the manufacturer had.

Contrast this situation with a customer who comes to the pharmacy with a prescription for milk of magnesia. Pursuant to a prescription, the product need only be labeled with the following information by the pharmacy: *See handout in email*

- pharmacy's name and address,
- patient's name,
- prescriber's name, and
- directions for use.

A prescription label can be affixed to an OTC drug container only if there is a valid prescription. Affixing a prescription label to an OTC drug, or even to a legend drug, without a valid prescription would be misbranding and a violation of federal law.

All legend drugs must contain the following information on their packaging when sold to a pharmacy:

- manufacturer, packer, or distributor's name and address;
- ingredient information;
- generic and proprietary names;
- weight measure of drug (e.g., 500 mg);
- size of package (e.g., 480 ml);
- dosage information or a reference to the package insert for dosage information;
- expiration date; and
- lot number.

The drug's indication, pharmacological action, adverse reactions, contraindications, and pregnancy category also may be included. This information is usually found on the package insert. The insert or leaflet, which is generally the same information found in the *Physicians' Desk Reference®* (PDR), can be given to the patient. In addition to the package insert, some drugs must have patient package inserts (PPIs) provided to the patient at each dispensing. There is state case law that holds that this PPI be provided to both retail and hospital patients.

Poison Prevention Packaging Act

The Poison Prevention Packaging Act was enacted to reduce the number of poisonings in children from drugs and chemicals. It has been remarkably successful. The law requires that all prescriptions and most OTC drugs be dispensed in containers with child-resistant closures, unless the drug or container falls under one of the many exceptions. These child-resistant prescription containers cannot be reused for refills. This law usually applies to retail settings. It does not apply to dispensing prescriptions to inpatients in long-term care facilities or hospitals, but it does apply to prescriptions dispensed to those patients upon discharge. Therefore, prescriptions for a patient who is being discharged from an institution to return home must be dispensed in a container with a child-resistant closure.

Some drugs, such as nitroglycerin, oral contraceptives, and other drugs packaged for patient use by the manufacturer, do not require the child-resistant container. **Table 6-1** provides a partial list of chemicals that do not have to be packaged in child-resistant containers. The complete list can be found in the CFR.[5] A list of drugs that require safety closures and exceptions to the list are also available from the U.S. Consumer Product Safety Commission's website: **http://www.cpsc.gov/CPSCPUB/PUBS/384.pdf**.

Because many patients do not have children at home or may have a disease that impairs their ability to open child-resistant containers, the patient, caregiver, or physician can request that the prescription be dispensed in a non-child-resistant container. Federal law does not require a written request to have the prescription dispensed in a non-child-resistant container; however, physicians must make this request on a patient-by-patient basis and not in the form of a blanket request for all or a group of patients.

TABLE 6-1

1. Sublingual dosage forms of nitroglycerin.

2. Sublingual and chewable forms of isosorbide dinitrate in dosage strengths of 10 milligrams or less.

3. Erythromycin ethylsuccinate granules for oral suspension andoral suspensions in packages containing not more than 8 grams of the equivalent of erythromycin.

4. Cyclically administered oral contraceptives in manufacturers' mnemonic (memory-aid) dispenser packages that rely solely upon the activity of one or more progestogen or estrogen substances.

5. Anhydrous cholestyramine in powder form.

6. All unit dose forms of potassium supplements, including individually-wrapped effervescent tablets, unit dose vials of liquid potassium, and powdered potassium in unit-dose packets, containing not more than 50 milliequivalents of potassium per unit dose.

7. Sodium fluoride drug preparations including liquid and tablet forms, containing not more than 110 milligrams of sodium fluoride (the equivalent of 50 mg of elemental fluoride) per package or not more than a concentration of 0.5 percent elemental fluoride on a weight-to-volume basis for liquids or a weight-to-weight basis for non-liquids and containing no other substances.

8. Betamethasone tablets packaged in manufacturers' dispenser packages, containing no more than 12.6 milligrams betamethasone.

9. Pancrelipase preparations in tablet, capsule, or powder form and containing no other substances subject to this Sec. 1700.14(a)(10).

10. Prednisone in tablet form, when dispensed in packages containing no more than 105 mg. of the drug, and containing no other substances.

11. Mebendazole in tablet form in packages containing not more than 600 mg. of the drug, and containing no other substance.

12. Methylprednisolone in tablet form in packages containing not more than 84 mg of the drug and containing no other substance.

13. Colestipol in powder form in packages containing not more than 5 grams of the drug and containing no other substance.

14. Erythromycin ethylsuccinate tablets in packages containing no more than the equivalent of 16 grams erythromycin.

15. Conjugated Estrogens Tablets, U.S.P., when dispensed in mnemonic packages containing not more than 32.0 mg of the drug and containing no other substances.

16. Norethindrone Acetate Tablets, U.S.P., when dispensed in mnemonic packages containing not more than 50 mg of the drug and containing no other substances.

17. Medroxyprogesterone acetate tablets.

18. Sacrosidase (sucrase) preparations in a solution of glycerol and water.

19. Hormone Replacement Therapy Products that rely solely upon the activity of one or more progestogen or estrogen substances.

20. Certain iron-containing drugs, i.e., animal feeds used as vehicles for the administration of drugs, and (ii) those preparations in which iron is present solely as a colorant.

21. Effervescent tablets or granules containing acetaminophen, provided the dry tablet or granules contain less than 15 percent acetaminophen, the tablet or granules have an oral LD-50 of 5 grams or greater per kilogram of body weight, and the tablet or granules contain no other substance.

22. (ii) Unflavored acetaminophen-containing preparations in powder form (other than those intended for pediatric use) that are packaged in unit doses providing not more than 13 grains of acetaminophen per unit dose and that contain no other substance.

23. Diphenhydramine. Preparations for human use in a dosage form intended for oral administration and containing more than the equivalent of 66 mg diphenhydramine base in a single package.

24. Ibuprofen. Ibuprofen preparations for human use in a dosage form intended for oral administration and containing one gram (1,000 mg) or more of ibuprofen in a single package.

25. Loperamide. Preparations for human use in a dosage form intended for oral administration and containing more than 0.045 mg of loperamide in a single package (i.e., retail unit).

26. Lidocaine. Products containing more than 5.0 mg of lidocaine in a single package (i.e., retail unit).

27. Dibucaine. Products containing more than 0.5 mg of dibucaine in a single package (i.e., retail unit).

28. Naproxen. Naproxen preparations for human use and containing the equivalent of 250 mg or more of naproxen in a single retail package.

29. Ketoprofen. Ketoprofen preparations for human use and containing more than 50 mg of ketoprofen in a single retail package.

30. Fluoride. Household substances containing more than the equivalent of 50 milligrams of elemental fluoride per package.

31. Minoxidil. Minoxidil preparations for human use and containing more than 14 mg of minoxidil in a single retail package. Any applicator packaged with the minoxidil preparation and which it is reasonable to expect may be used to replace the original closure.

Code of Federal Regulation

The CFR is a compilation of the rules that have been created by various federal administrative agencies, including the FDA and the Department of Justice. These rules are an important reference source for pharmacy-related laws. "Food and Drugs" is the title of chapter 21 of the CFR. Some states require that pharmacies have chapter 21 of the CFR as part their reference library. Chapter 16 of the CFR contains information about the Poison Prevention Packaging requirements. The CFR has the effect of law, and everyone who practices pharmacy should become familiar with it.

Expiration Dating

The pharmacy technician will notice that on every stock bottle of medication, the manufacturer has indicated an expiration date, after which the medication should not be used. This expiration date is based on stability studies performed by the manufacturer for that drug in that type of sealed container. Once the container is opened, the manufacturer's expiration date is no longer valid because the contents have been exposed to moisture, light, and air.

The expiration date is critical when a pharmacy technician repackages medication from stock containers into packaging for distribution to patients or nursing staff. Although each state has its own guidelines for the expiration date of a repackaged medication, these guidelines almost certainly rely on current United States Pharmacopeia (USP) standards. It is up to the pharmacy technician to check the law in his or her state.

Generally speaking, the expiration date of a repackaged medication from a sealed medication stock bottle will be 25 percent of the expiration date of the sealed bottle or 1 year from the date of packaging, whichever is less. This general rule is based on the repackager's use of class A packaging material. Class A packaging material is considered the standard for preventing light, moisture, and air permeation and often requires a heat-sealing machine to ensure uniform closure of the container.

Consider some examples of expiration dating for repackaged pharmaceuticals. If a sealed container has an expiration date of 1 year and the contents of that container are repackaged with Class A materials, the expiration date of the repackaged drug would be 3 months, which is 25 percent of 1 year. If the expiration date is 2 years and the medication is repackaged, the expiration date of the repackaged drug would be 6 months. If the expiration date of the sealed container is 10 years, then the expiration date of the repackaged product would be 1 year.

Beyond-Use Dating

Beyond-use dating is the date beyond which a drug should no longer be used by a patient. This date is different from the expiration date of repackaged drugs or of the manufacturer's stock container, but it can never exceed either expiration date. For example, amoxicillin suspension in an unreconstituted form may have an expiration date of 1 year. However, once the amoxicillin has been reconstituted, the product stability usually cannot be guaranteed beyond 14 days. The date of the 14th day would be the beyond-use date. The same holds true for many parenteral drugs, whose expiration date far exceeds the beyond-use date once the medication has been prepared for administration to a patient. The technician must know the beyond-use date for every medication that is compounded, reconstituted, and otherwise modified from its original packaging for immediate patient administration. The pharmacy technician should look to the manufacturer's guidelines and the pharmacy's policies for determining the beyond-use date for individual medications.

Federal Controlled Substance Law

The Federal Controlled Substance Act was enacted to protect the public by controlling the flow of dangerous drugs into the community. The United States Department of Justice Drug Enforcement Agency (DEA) takes responsibility for vigilance over the distribution of these drugs in research, institutions, and the community. This agency plays an important role in creating the rules that govern the practice of pharmacy.[6]

Drugs that are watched by the DEA are called controlled substances. Controlled substances are divided into five categories, or Schedules. Schedule I drugs are substances with a high abuse potential and no legitimate medical purpose. Schedule II drugs are those with high abuse potential and a recognized medical purpose. Schedules III, IV, and V drugs have a legitimate medical purpose but less abuse potential. For all practical purposes, Schedules III, IV, and V drugs are treated alike from a regulatory perspective.

To order a prescription for a controlled substance, a prescriber must be registered with the Department of Justice and be issued a DEA registration number. Similarly, to dispense a controlled substance, a pharmacy, too, must have a DEA registration number.

Calculation of Valid DEA Numbers

A valid DEA number consists of two letters and seven numbers, for example, BB 1 1 9 7 9 6 7. If the holder of the DEA number is a registrant, such as a physician or pharmacy, the first letter is an "A" or "B." If the holder of the DEA number is a mid-level practitioner, such as a qualified nurse practitioner, the first letter is an "M." The second letter is related to the registrant's name. In the case of a physician, it is the first letter of the physician's last name.

The seven numbers also are used to determine a legitimate DEA number. The odd group consisting of the 1st, 3rd, and 5th numbers in the sequence and the even group consisting of the 2nd, 4th, and 6th numbers are added in the following manner so that the sum relates to the 7th number. The following example should make it clear:

BB 1 1 9 7 9 6 7

Odd Group— 1 + 9 + 9 = 19

Even Group— 1 + 7 + 6 = 14

Sum of odd (19) and 2x even group (14 x 2)= 19 + 28 = 47

The last digit of this odd/even group sum is the same as the last digit of the DEA number.

Schedules of Controlled Substances

Schedule II. Some examples of single-entity Schedule II narcotics include morphine, codeine, hydrocodone, and opium. Other Schedule II narcotic substances and their common name-brand products are hydromorphone (Dilaudid®), methadone (Dolophine®), meperidine (Demerol®), oxycodone (Percodan®), and fentanyl (Sublimaze®). Some examples of Schedule II stimulants include amphetamine (Dexedrine®, Adderall®), methamphetamine (Desoxyn®), and methylphenidate (Ritalin®). Other Schedule II substances are cocaine, amobarbital, glutethimide, pentobarbital, and secobarbital.

Schedule III. Some examples of Schedule III narcotics include products containing less than 15 milligrams of hydrocodone per dosage unit (Vicodin®, Lorcet®, Tussionex®), and products containing not more than 90 milligrams of codeine per dosage unit (codeine with acetaminophen, aspirin, or ibuprofen). Other Schedule III substances include anabolic steroids; benzphetamine (Didrex®); phendimetrazine; and any compound, mixture, preparation, or suppository dosage form containing amobarbital, secobarbital, pentobarbital, dronabinol (Marinol®), or ketamine.

Schedule IV. The substances in this schedule have an abuse potential less than those in Schedule III and more than those in Schedule V. Some examples of Schedule IV narcotics include propoxyphene (Darvon®), butorphanol (Stadol®), and pentazocine (Talwin-NX®). The following benzodiazepine substances are also found in Schedule IV: alprazolam (Xanax®), clonazepam (Klonopin®), clorazepate (Tranxene®), diazepam (Valium®), flurazepam (Dalmane®), halazepam (Paxipam®), lorazepam (Ativan®), midazolam (Versed®), oxazepam (Serax®), prazepam (Verstran®), temazepam (Restoril®), triazolam (Halcion®), and quazepam (Doral®). Other Schedule IV substances include barbital, phenobarbital, chloral hydrate, ethchlorvynol (Placidyl®), chlordiazepoxide (Librium®), ethinamate, meprobamate, paraldehyde, methohexital, phentermine, diethylpropion, pemoline (Cylert®), mazindol (Sanorex®), and sibutramine (Meridia®).

Schedule V. The substances in this schedule have an abuse potential less than those in Schedule IV and consist primarily of preparations containing limited quantities of certain narcotic and stimulant drugs, generally for antitussive, antidiarrheal, or analgesic purposes. Some examples are cough preparations containing not more than 200 milligrams of codeine per 100 milliliters or per 100 grams (e.g., Robitussin AC®, Phenergan with Codeine®) and buprenorphine (Buprenex®).

List I & II Chemicals. In addition to Schedules I–V controlled substances, the DEA has designated List I and List II chemicals. These chemicals can be used in the synthesis of other chemicals that are controlled substances. The pharmacy must account for List I and List II chemicals. Three common List I chemicals are ephedrine, phenylpropanolamine (PPA), and pseudoephedrine. A state may require that the use of these chemicals in compounding be reported to the DEA.

States also will place certain drugs into a Schedule. Occasionally, a conflict will arise when a state and the federal government do not agree on which schedule a drug should be. If such a conflict arises, the stricter scheduling will apply.

Ordering Controlled Substances

Schedule I and II Substances

Schedule I and II controlled substances are ordered

with a DEA Form-222 (Official Order Form). The Official Order Form is required for each distribution, purchase, or transfer of a Schedule II controlled substance from one DEA registrant to another, such as from wholesaler to pharmacy, pharmacy to pharmacy, or pharmacy to physician. These federal forms are used only when purchasing, distributing, or transferring drugs that are federally Schedule I or II.

Completing the Official 222 Order Form. Anyone can enter information on the 222 form. The person filling out the form must fill in the number of packages, the size of the package(s), and the name of the item(s). It is also a good idea to enter the National Drug Code (NDC) of the item being ordered. However, *each Official 222 Order Form can be signed and dated only by the person on the pharmacy registration application* or a person who has been given a power of attorney to sign the order form (see "Power of attorney").

The 222 is a triplicate form. The top page and middle pages go to the supplier of the drugs, who sends the middle page to the DEA, and the last page stays with the purchaser. When the items are received, the pharmacist must document on the purchaser's copy (copy 3) the number of packages received and the date received. These forms must be maintained separately from the purchaser's (pharmacy's) other business records. The pharmacy can attach its copy to a copy of the supplier's invoice for that order.

The CFR requires that the Official Order Form be "complete, legible, and properly prepared, with no signs of alteration, erasure or change of any description." A supplier may refuse to accept an order if any of these conditions is not met. However, DEA has acknowledged that a supplier may accept some minor changes or alterations. For example, suppliers may correct Official Order Forms that have minor errors, such as in inconsequential information or an incorrect date unintentionally annotated by the purchaser. If the supplier refuses to fill an order, the supplier must return the Official Order Form (copies 1 and 2) to the purchaser with a statement explaining why the order was refused.

DEA policy does not prohibit the substitution of identical products differing in packaging size from those initially ordered, provided the actual quantity received does not exceed the amount initially ordered. For example, if a pharmacy orders 500 secobarbital capsules, the distributor may ship either one bottle of 500 capsules or five bottles of 100 capsules.

Power of attorney to sign an Official Order Form. Any registrant (e.g., pharmacy, physician) may authorize one or more individuals, including technicians, to obtain and execute Official Order Forms by granting a power of attorney to each individual. *The power of attorney must be signed by the same person who signed the most recent application for registration or renewal registration, as well as the individual being authorized to obtain and execute Official Order Forms.*

The power of attorney may be revoked at any time by the person who granted it. It should be filed in the pharmacy along with the completed Official Order Forms and be readily retrievable (see **Figure 6-1** for a sample power of attorney form). The power of attorney is not submitted to DEA.

Lost or stolen order forms. When the pharmacist fails to receive an expected shipment of controlled substances, he or she should first contact the supplier to determine whether the original DEA Form-222 was received. If the original order form has been lost or stolen, the pharmacist must complete a second order form so the supplier can fill the original order. The pharmacist must also prepare a statement that includes the first order form's serial number and date, verify that the drugs ordered were never received, attach a copy of the statement to the second order form that is sent to the supplier, and keep a copy of the statement with copy 3 from the first and second order forms. Upon discovery of the loss or theft of unused order forms, a pharmacy must immediately report the loss to the nearest DEA Diversion Field Office and provide the serial numbers of each lost or stolen order form. If an entire book or multiple books of order forms are lost or stolen and the serial numbers of the missing forms cannot be identified, the pharmacist must report the approximate date of issuance (in lieu of the serial numbers) to DEA. If an unused order form reported stolen or lost is later recovered or found, the pharmacy must immediately notify the nearest DEA Diversion Field Office.

Schedule III–V Substances
The DEA registrant (pharmacy) must record on a receipt (i.e., invoice or packing slip) on which record the date the drugs were received is recorded and confirm that the order is accurate. These receipts must be readily retrievable for inspection by DEA.

Prescribing Authority
Physicians (M.D. and D.O.), dentists (D.D.S.), podiatrists (D.P.M.), and veterinarians (D.V.M.)

POWER OF ATTORNEY FOR DEA ORDER FORMS

_____ (Name of registrant)

_____ (Address of registrant)

_____ (DEA registration number)

I,_____(name of person granting power), the under-signed, who is authorized to sign the current application for registration of the above-named registrant under the Controlled Substances Act or Controlled Substances Import and Export Act, have made, consti-tuted, and appointed, and by these present, do make, constitute, and appoint _____ (name of attorney-in-fact), my true and lawful attorney for me in my name, place, and stead, to execute applications for books of official order forms and to sign such order forms in requisition for Schedule I and II controlled substances, in accordance with Section 308 of the Controlled Substances Act (21 U.S.C. 828) and part 1305 of Title 21 of the Code of Federal Regulations. I hereby ratify and confirm all that said attorney shall lawfully do or cause to be done by virtue hereof.

(Signature of person granting power)

I, _____, (name of attorney-in-fact), hereby affirm that I am the person named herein as attorney-in-fact and that the signature affixed hereto is my signature.

Witnesses:

1._____

2._____

Signed and dated on the _____ day of _____in the year_____ at_____.

NOTICE OF REVOCATION OF POWER OF ATTORNEY

The foregoing power of attorney is hereby revoked by the undersigned, who is authorized to sign the current application for registration of the above-named registrant under the Controlled Substances Act or the Controlled Substances Import and Export Act. Written notice of this revocation has been given to the attorney-in-fact _____ this same day.

(Signature of person revoking power)

Witnesses:

1._____

2._____

Signed and dated on the _____ day of _____, in the year _____at _____.

Figure 6-1.

generally can prescribe any drug in the course of their practice for legitimate medical conditions. DEA has provided examples of mid-level practitioners who could have the authority to prescribe medications, including midwives, homeopathic physicians, nursing homes, advance nurse practitioners, physician assistants, and optometrists. Mid-level prescribing authority is determined on a state-by-state basis. Therefore, the technician must know the laws in his or her state that specify which professionals have prescribing authority.

Brands, Generics, and Branded Generics

The terms *generic* and *brand name* are used daily in pharmacy practice. The brand name is usually a trademark name owned by a drug manufacturer. The generic name identifies the chemical. A patent gives its owner the right to exclude others from making that drug. Once the patent expires, any company is free to manufacture the drug or a generic version of the original drug. The original patent-holder of the drug retains the right to exclude others from using the original trade name.

Once the manufacturer loses the patent rights and other companies manufacture the drug and receive FDA approval for the generic drug, generally, the generic drug can be dispensed in place of the brand. For example, Motrin® (ibuprofen) was patented and owned by Upjohn. No other company was allowed to manufacture ibuprofen until the patent expired. Today, numerous companies make ibuprofen. If these companies obtain approval from the FDA, their generic version of Motrin® can be sold. Some states require additional data before allowing a "substitution" of a federally approved generic for a brand name. Generally speaking, if a prescription is written for ibuprofen, any federally approved ibuprofen can be dispensed. Substituting generics requires knowledge of proper prescription labeling. Generic substitution should not be confused with therapeutic substitution or pharmaceutical alternatives, which are a subject for advanced clinical discussions with the prescriber.

If a generic drug is dispensed, the prescription label cannot state that the brand name was dispensed even though it is the pharmaceutical equivalent. That is misbranding. Some generic manufacturers have successfully created "branded generics," such as Roxicet® and Endocet®. These two are each a combination of the same two generics. Neither drug has patent protection on the drug itself, but both have trademark protection on the names. Therefore, to dispense Roxicet® and label it Endocet® would be misbranding.

The Omnibus Budget Reconciliation Act of 1990

The Omnibus Budget Reconciliation Act of 1990 (OBRA) required states that use federal funding to create programs to improve the quality of pharmaceutical care and save money by educating patients on the proper use of drugs. The program required pharmacists to obtain certain information from the patient, including personal identifying information, disease state, and medication allergies, that would be important for determining proper drug therapy. This federal program targeted only Medicaid and Medicare patients, but most states expanded it to include all patients.

Whereas most states require the pharmacist to provide the counseling, the pharmacy technician's role in this program is important in obtaining information from the patient. The extent of the technician's involvement in gathering information from the patient will be related directly to the technician's ability to communicate effectively with patients and his or her knowledge of disease and pharmaceutical terminology.

Privacy Laws

All patients have a right to privacy. Privacy laws are found in federal law, state law, and the common law. Violating privacy rights can have serious consequences for the technician, pharmacist, and pharmacy. The privacy laws are complicated and will not be addressed completely in this chapter. However, a general rule is that no patient information can be given to any person other than the patient or patient's legal representative. The person or company that pays for the patient's medication is not necessarily a legal representative. Information is not to be given to an insurance company, spouse, child, relative, or caregiver unless there is an express authorization by the patient to do so. If a request is made by telephone, it is unwise to release the information because the pharmacist or technician cannot verify the caller's identity. Some government agencies have a statutory right to obtain information. A gray area exists as to when a parent can ask for medical information about a child. Does a 16-year-old girl using oral contraceptives have a right to keep that information from her parents? Because law varies from state to state, the technician should check with the compliance officer in his or her state to find the applicable law.

The Health Insurance Portability and Accountability Act of 1996

The Health Insurance Portability and Accountability

Act of 1996 (HIPAA) has strengthened patient privacy rights. Although this was not the only purpose of the law, the pharmacy's role in maintaining confidentiality also has increased. Patient records must be guarded from disclosure to unauthorized individuals and companies. Pharmacy employees are forbidden to discuss a patient's medical history except for purposes relevant to the patient's care. All written information concerning a patient must be discarded in such a manner as to protect the patient's identity. Using shredders or professional document disposal services is now common pharmacy practice. Pharmacy technicians should discuss information regarding a patient's therapy in such a way that unauthorized persons will not overhear the discussions. Technicians should also be aware that using overhead paging systems to announce a patient's name could undermine a patient's privacy. Most facilities that employ pharmacy technicians will have policies and procedures in place to address the requirements of HIPAA.

Malpractice

Negligence is part of the law that is based on tradition (common law) rather than on written laws created by the government. Malpractice is negligence by professionals, such as physicians, pharmacists, and lawyers, that injures someone. The exact requirements to prove negligence and the compensation for the injury are governed by state law, not by federal law. Recently, however, the U.S. House of Representatives passed legislation that may affect all malpractice litigation. Therefore, although malpractice litigation is currently a state matter, technicians should stay alert to pending federal legislation that may have an impact on it.

Basically, to prove malpractice the injured party must prove that the professional breached a duty of care owed to the patient and that breach of duty caused the injury. If so proven, the professional will be ordered to pay the injured party. Usually there is sufficient insurance to protect the professional insofar as covering the cost of the determined compensations.

State licensing agencies may discipline the professional whose negligence was found to have caused injury. The administrative agency may determine that the professional's conduct fell below the standard of care for the profession and may impose a penalty ranging from a reprimand to a revocation of a professional license. Some states have enacted laws that mandate the reporting of drug-dispensing errors to state agencies.

The pharmacy technician who is negligent in dispensing a prescription is as liable for personal injury and as likely to be the subject of litigation and administrative proceedings as the negligent pharmacist would be. It is very important for the technician to seek advice from the pharmacist whenever doubt arises about a prescription. Errors in clinical judgment rarely result in liability; however, errors in filling a prescription will certainly result in liability. Whether negligent conduct ends up in a courtroom usually depends on the extent of the injury. The greater the injury, the greater the likelihood of litigation.

State Law and Federal Law

While the pharmacologic action of a drug is the same from state to state, the law is not. Each state has its own laws about pharmacist-to-technician staffing ratios, long-term care standards, parenteral product record keeping, labeling, and numerous of other aspects of pharmacy practice. Some of these laws are in conflict with federal law. In many cases, no federal law exists. Also, the law is constantly changing. For example, 20 years ago fax machines were uncommon and no federal law covered their use. As fax machines became common and faxing prescriptions became routine, new regulations were established. Because the laws are changing and are different from state to state, the technician must become familiar with the laws of the state in which he or she is licensed. If help is needed to clarify or interpret a law or to unravel a discrepancy between state and federal law, the technician should consult a member of the state board of pharmacy or the state agency responsible for issuing the licenses. And just as pharmacy record keeping is a vital component of pharmacy practice, it is a good idea to document each conversation with a consultant, including the name of the consultant, the date of the consultation, the questions raised, and the responses provided. Should a technician's conduct be called into question, such documentation would be evidence of his or her effort to perform professional duties with diligence and to maintain regulatory compliance.

Ethics

The philosophy of ethics can be discussed for hours. Consider the following definitions.

Society's Definition

ethics. The study of standards of and moral judgment; moral philosophy. The system or code of morals of a particular philosopher, religion, group, profession, etc.

—*Webster's Dictionary of the English Language Unabridged*

The Medical Profession's Definition

ethics [G. *ethikos* etherial arising from custom, fr *ethos*, custom]. The science of morality. In relation to medical practice, the principles of correct professional conduct with regard to the rights and duties of the physician himself, his patients, and his fellow practitioners.

—Stedman's Medical Dictionary, 22nd Edition

code of ethics. A set of rules established for the guidance of the medical practitioner in his professional conduct.

—Stedman's Medical Dictionary, 22nd Edition

The Legal Profession's Definition

ethics. "What is generally called the 'ethics' of the profession is but consensus of expert opinion as to necessity of profession standards."

—Black's Law Dictionary, Revised 4th Edition

legal ethics. Usages and customs among members of the legal professional, involving their moral and professional duties toward one another, toward clients, and toward the courts; that branch of moral science which treats of the duties which a member of the legal profession owes to the public, to the court, to his brethren and to his client.

—Black's Law Dictionary, Revised 4th Edition

The Pharmacy Profession's Definition

ethics. Ethics and law are related in that both share the social purpose of encouraging "right" conduct. Law attempts to achieve its purpose through the sovereign power of government while the ethics, in particular the ethics of a profession, attempts to achieve its purpose without the intervention of government.

—Remington's Pharmaceutical Science, 14th Edition

Summary of Definitions

As you have read, different sources define ethics differently. Medical ethics are different from legal and pharmacy ethics. But they are all related to how a professional is to behave within society. Ethics begin as goals for standards of conduct created by an association for a specific group. For example, pharmacists created ethical standards for pharmacists. Boards of pharmacy determine whether a pharmacist's conduct has been ethical and whether and how to discipline the pharmacist. If the boards of pharmacy fail to adequately police the unethical conduct of pharmacists that is dangerous to society, then the government will create laws to police pharmacy practice.

Law enforcement agencies will discipline pharmacists for violations of pharmacy statutes but not for ethical violations. Boards of pharmacy enforce pharmacy ethics violations. A technician who violates a statute can expect law enforcement action. A technician who violates an ethical standard can expect board of pharmacy action.

The American Pharmacists Association's Code of Ethics appears on page 109. Although the Code is not a law, it should be followed to avoid disciplinary actions by a board of pharmacy.

Conclusion

Pharmacy is an ancient and modern profession holding one of highest places with society's trust. A pharmacy technician becomes part of this heritage and agrees to conduct him- or herself accordingly. The government, society, and a technician's peers expect professional conduct and compliance with the law. If a technician does not know the law, he or she should check with the board of pharmacy or DEA; the answers are free.

Recommended Reading

Strauss S, Ph.D., R.Ph. Strauss's federal drug laws. 5th ed. Lancaster, PA: Technomic Publishing Co., Inc.; 2000.

References

1. Code of Federal Regulation, 21 CFR 1300 et seq.

2. Food Drug and Cosmetic Act, 21 USC 301 et seq.

3. Poison Prevention Packaging Act, 15 USC 1471.

4. Omnibus Budget Reconciliation Act, 42 USC 201.

5. Dietary Supplement Health and Education Act, 21 USC 321.

6. *Tommy G. Thompson, Secretary of Health and Human Services, et al., Petitioners v. Western States Medical Center et al.*, 122 S. Ct. 1497; 2002.

7. Department of Justice. Pharmacist's manual. http://www.deadiversion.usdoj.gov/pubs/manuals/pharm2/index.htm (accessed 4/5/04).

PREAMBLE

Pharmacists are health professionals who assist individuals in making the best use of medications. This Code, prepared and supported by pharmacists, is intended to state publicly the principles that form the fundamental basis of the roles and responsibilities of pharmacists. These principles, based on moral obligations and virtues, are established to guide pharmacists in relationships with patients, health professionals, and society.

I. A pharmacist respects the covenantal relationship between the patient and pharmacist.

Considering the patient–pharmacist relationship as a covenant means that a pharmacist has moral obligations in response to the gift of trust received from society. In return for this gift, a pharmacist promises to help individuals achieve optimum benefit from their medications, to be committed to their welfare, and to maintain their trust.

II. A pharmacist promotes the good of every patient in a caring, compassionate, and confidential manner.

A pharmacist places concern for the well-being of the patient at the center of professional practice. In doing so, a pharmacist considers needs stated by the patient as well as those defined by health science. A pharmacist is dedicated to protecting the dignity of the patient. With a caring attitude and a compassionate spirit, a pharmacist focuses on serving the patient in a private and confidential manner.

III. A pharmacist respects the autonomy and dignity of each patient.

A pharmacist promotes the right of self-determination and recognizes individual self-worth by encouraging patients to participate in decisions about their health. A pharmacist communicates with patients in terms that are understandable. In all cases, a pharmacist respects personal and cultural differences among patients.

IV. A pharmacist acts with honesty and integrity in professional relationships.

A pharmacist has a duty to tell the truth and to act with conviction of conscience. A pharmacist avoids discriminatory practices, behavior or work conditions that impair professional judgment, and actions that compromise dedication to the best interests of patients.

V. A pharmacist maintains professional competence.

A pharmacist has a duty to maintain knowledge and abilities as new medications, devices, and technologies become available and as health information advances.

VI. A pharmacist respects the values and abilities of colleagues and other health professionals.

When appropriate, a pharmacist asks for the consultation of colleagues or other health professionals or refers the patient. A pharmacist acknowledges that colleagues and other health professionals may differ in the beliefs and values they apply to the care of the patient.

VII. A pharmacist serves individual, community, and societal needs.

The primary obligation of a pharmacist is to individual patients. However, the obligations of a pharmacist may at times extend beyond the individual to the community and society. In these situations, the pharmacist recognizes the responsibilities that accompany these obligations and acts accordingly.

VIII. A pharmacist seeks justice in the distribution of health resources.

When health resources are allocated, a pharmacist is fair and equitable, balancing the needs of patients and society.

adopted by the membership of the American Pharmacists Association October 27, 1994.

Footnotes

[1] 1906, Pure Food and Drug Act. Prohibited placing misbranded or adulterated drugs into interstate commerce.

[2] 1938, Food Drug and Cosmetic Act (which amended and renamed the Pure Food and Drug Act). Required drugs to be safe, and required manufacturers to get governmental approval before drugs could be sold.

[3] 1951, Durham–Humphrey Amendments. Two classes of drugs were created: legend and over-the-counter. "Legend" drugs could only be dispensed pursuant to a prescription. Established labeling requirements.

[4] 1962, Kefauver–Harris Amendments. Required drugs to be safe and effective.

[5] 17 CFR 1700.14.

[6] 21 CFR 1300-1306.

1. What is meant by a legend drug?
   a. a drug that is famous.
   b. a drug that is part of folklore.
   c. an herbal drug.
   d. a drug that requires a prescription to have a prescription label.
   e. a drug that can be dispensed only pursuant to a valid prescription.

2. What is a safe and effective drug?
   a. a medication that prevents pregnancy.
   b. a medication approved for getting high.
   c. a drug that has no side effects.
   d. a drug that has been approved by the FDA for sale in the United States on the basis of information provided by the manufacturer.

3. What is compounding?
   a. a process by which a pharmacist or doctor combines, mixes, or alters ingredients to create a medication tailored to an individual patient's needs.
   b. a process by which a pharmacist or doctor combines, mixes, or alters ingredients to create a medication tailored to an individual patient's needs that has been approved by the FDA.
   c. a process by which a pharmacist or doctor combines, mixes, or alters ingredients to create a medication tailored for sale to another pharmacy or physician.
   d. a type of interest used by financial institutions.

4. According to federal law, which of the following does *not* need be on a prescription label?
   a. the pharmacy's name.
   b. the prescriber's name.
   c. the patient's name.
   d. the name of the drug.
   e. All the above need to be on the prescription label.

5. Which of the following needs to be on a label of a container for an over-the-counter drug?
   a. place of manufacture.
   b. expiration date.
   c. quantity or size of container.
   d. established name of all active ingredients.
   e. all the above.

6. All of the following prescription drugs must be dispensed in a child-resistant container *except*:
   a. nitroglycerin tablets.
   b. controlled substances.
   c. Celebrex.
   d. methotrexate.
   e. iron-containing vitamins.

7. The beyond-use date is the date on which a pharmacy can no longer dispense a medication.
   a. True
   b. False

8. Which of the following Schedules of Controlled Substance drugs have the highest abuse potential and an accepted medical use?
   a. Schedule I Controlled Substances.
   b. Schedule II Controlled Substances.
   c. Schedule III Controlled Substances.
   d. Schedule IV Controlled Substances.
   e. List I Chemicals.

9. Which of the following statements is most correct?
   a. The patent holder of a brand name drug can exclude everyone in the world from manufacturing the same drug.
   b. Brand name drugs are always better than generic drugs.
   c. According to the FDA, generic drugs must look like their brand name counterparts.
   d. The brand name only of a drug can be used on a prescription label even though it is not dispensed.

10. Who has the authority to sign a DEA Form 222 when ordering Schedule II controlled substances?
    a. only a pharmacist.
    b. only the owner of the pharmacy.
    c. only the person who signed the application for pharmacy registration with DEA.
    d. only the person who has the power of attorney to sign the 222 Form.
    e. c and d.

Self-Assessment Answers

1. e. A drug is considered "legend" if it has the statement on its label "Caution: Federal Law Prohibits Dispensing Without a Prescription." Therefore, the drug cannot be dispensed without a prescription from an authorized prescriber.

2. d. For any drug to be sold in this country, it must be proven to the FDA that it is safe and effective for a specific disease or disorder.

3. a. The United States Supreme Court, in *Tommy G. Thompson, Secretary of Health and Human Services, et al., Petitioners, v. Western States Medical Center et al.*, 122 S. Ct. 1497, (2002), stated that this is how compounding is defined.

4. d. The name of the drug does not need to be included on the prescription label; it can be affixed to the dispensed medication.

5. e. The FDCA requires OTC labels include name of product; name of manufacturer; distributor or packer; quantity; established name of all active ingredients and quantity of other ingredients, whether active or not; name of any habit forming drug contained in the preparation; directions for use; cautionary statements; purpose for which drug is intended; normal dose for each intended use; and dosages for persons of different age groups and physical conditions.

6. a. Some drugs such as nitroglycerin, oral contraceptives, and other drugs packaged for patient use by the manufacturer, do not require the child-resistant container.

7. b. The beyond-use date is the date that a medication should no longer be used by the patient.

8. b. Schedule I drugs have no accepted use. Schedules II–V all have accepted medical uses and have decreasing abuse potential as you move through the list from II–V. List I chemicals do not have significant abuse potential, but are ingredients in manufacturing drugs with higher abuse potential.

9. a. Holding a patent on a drug means nobody else can produce that drug for the life of the patent. Generic drugs may be pharmaceutically equivalent to brand name drugs but may look very different. Only the actual name of the product dispensed may be used on the label. To use the brand name on the label when a generic product is dispensed is a violation called misbranding.

10. e. The person who signed the application for the pharmacy's registration with the DEA has the authority to sign DEA Form 222. He or she may delegate that authority to another by issuing a power of attorney. You do not have to be a pharmacist to sign a DEA Form 222 as long as you have a valid power of attorney from the registrant.

Medication Dosage Forms and Routes of Administration

MICHELE F. SHEPHERD

When most people think of taking a medication, they think of swallowing a tablet or capsule. Although this is the most common way people take medications, other forms of administration are used to introduce medications into the body by routes other than the mouth. Solutions, suspensions, suppositories, and sprays may be used to deliver medications into body areas such as the ear, nose, eye, rectum, or bloodstream.

This chapter describes many medication dosage forms and routes of administration. The chapter is not intended to be all inclusive, but rather to serve as an introduction to some commonly used and not-so-commonly used dosage forms and administration routes.

Medication Dosage Forms

Liquid Medication Dosage Forms

Liquid medication dosage forms deliver medication in a fluid medium. The fluid serves as a carrier, or delivery system, for the medication and is referred to as the *vehicle*. Common vehicles are water, alcohol, and mineral oil. The medication may be dissolved in the vehicle or may be present as very fine solid particles suspended, or floating, in the vehicle. Liquid dosage forms may pour as freely as water or have the thick consistency of syrup. They may be intended for oral consumption or for use in, or on, other parts of the body.

Liquid medication dosage forms have some advantages over other medication dosage forms (see **Table 7-1**):

- Oral liquid dosage forms usually are faster acting than solid dosage forms. Medications are absorbed into the bloodstream in a dissolved state. The medication in a liquid dosage form is already dissolved or is present in small particles, so it can be absorbed readily. In contrast, tablets must dissolve before they can be absorbed, so it takes more time for the medication to be absorbed.

- For patients who have difficulty swallowing, oral liquid medications may be easier to take than an oral solid dosage form.

- Liquid doses have more flexibility than some other dosage forms because liquid medications are usually dispensed in bulk containers rather than distinct dosage units. For example, a liquid medication

7

Learning Objectives

After completing the chapter, the technician should be able to

Medication Dosage Forms

1. List three advantages of liquid medication dosage forms over other dosage forms.
2. List three disadvantages of solid medication dosage forms.
3. Outline characteristics of solutions, emulsions, and suspensions.
4. Describe two situations in which an ointment may be preferred over a cream.
5. Explain the differences among various solid dosage forms, such as tablets, capsules, lozenges, powders, and granules.

Routes of Administration

6. List six routes of administration by which drugs may enter or be applied to the body.
7. Identify special considerations for each route of administration.
8. List five parenteral routes of administration.
9. Explain the difference between the topical and transdermal routes.
10. Distinguish between the sublingual and buccal routes.

TABLE 7-1. ADVANTAGES AND DISADVANTAGES OF LIQUID DOSAGE FORMS

Advantages

- Usually faster acting than solid dosage forms
- May be easier to take than an oral solid dosage form
- Has more flexibility in dosage than some other dosage forms
- May be more practical to administer than solid dosage forms

Disadvantages

- May have a shorter time to expiration than other dosage forms
- May have an unpleasant taste or sensation on the tongue
- May not be convenient to take because it may spill, require careful measurement, or have special storage or handling requirements

may contain 500 milligrams (mg) of a drug in 10 milliliters (mL) of liquid. The same medication is also available in 500 mg tablets. To take a 600 mg dose of the liquid medication, a patient would simply need to measure out 12 mL of liquid. However, to take a 600 mg dose of the tablet, the patient would need to take 1.2 tablets, which would be difficult.

- Liquid medications may be used where solid dosage forms are not practical to administer. For example, medications that need to be placed directly into the ear or eye may be administered more practically as a liquid than as a solid.

Liquid dosage forms also have some disadvantages:

- Often, liquid dosage forms have a shorter time to expiration than other dosage forms.

- Most drugs have an unpleasant taste as the drug dissolves or is chewed into small particles. Drug particles are already present in oral liquid medications and come in contact with the taste and sensory receptors of the tongue. People often find the taste or sensation of these drug particles objectionable. Sweeteners and flavoring agents are necessary to make these liquid medications more palatable. Tablets, on the other hand, are often coated and are swallowed quickly to avoid contact with the taste receptors.

- Patients do not always find liquid medications convenient to take because they may be spilled, require careful measuring before administration, or have special storage or handling requirements, such as refrigeration or shaking before use.

Liquid medication dosage forms are categorized on

the basis of several characteristics: the type of liquid medium (e.g., water or alcohol) in which the medication is delivered, whether the medication is dissolved or suspended as particles in the liquid, and the intended use of the medication. Other characteristics are explained in the following paragraphs. **Table 7-2** gives examples of liquid dosage forms.

Solutions

Solutions are evenly distributed, homogeneous mixtures of dissolved medication in a liquid vehicle. Molecules of a solid, liquid, or gaseous medication are equally distributed among the molecules of the liquid vehicle. Because the medication is already dissolved in

TABLE 7-2. EXAMPLES OF LIQUID MEDICATION DOSAGE FORMS

Solutions

- Aqueous (water) solutions

  Douches
  Irrigations
  Enemas
  Gargles
  Washes
  Sprays

- Viscous (thick) aqueous solutions
  Syrups
  Jellies
  Mucilages

- Nonaqueous solutions
  Hydroalcoholic
    Elixirs
    Spirits

  Alcoholic
    Collodions
    Spirits

  Glycerites

  Miscellaneous
    Inhalants
    Liniments

Emulsions

- Oil-in-water
- Water-in-oil

Suspensions

- Lotions
- Magmas and milks
- Gels

Extractives

- Tinctures
- Fluidextracts
- Extracts

the solution, the upper gastrointestinal tract, skin, or other site of administration absorbs it more quickly than other medication dosage forms.

Solutions may be subdivided on the basis of the characteristics of the vehicle:

- *Aqueous* and *viscous aqueous* solutions use purified water as the vehicle. Aqueous solutions may be ingested orally, applied topically, or injected into the bloodstream. Viscous aqueous solutions are sticky, thick, sweet solutions that are either liquid or semisolid.

- *Nonaqueous* solutions are those that use solvents, or dissolving liquids, in addition to or instead of water. Commonly used nonaqueous solvents include alcohol (ethyl alcohol or ethanol), glycerin, and propylene glycol. A *glycerite,* which uses glycerin as a solvent, vehicle, or both, is an example of a nonaqueous solution.
  Hydroalcoholic solutions are nonaqueous solutions that contain a mixture of alcohol and water. *Alcoholic* solutions are nonaqueous solutions that contain alcohol but no water.

- *Inhalants* and *liniments* do not fit neatly into any category and are classified as miscellaneous solutions.

Aqueous solutions. *Douches* are aqueous solutions that are directed into a body cavity or against a part of the body to clean or disinfect. Douches are used to remove debris from the eyes or to cleanse the nose, throat, or vagina. Examples of commercially available vaginal douche products are Massengill® (SK-Beecham) and Summer's Eve® (Fleet).

Irrigating solutions are used to wash or cleanse part of the body, such as the eyes, urinary bladder, open wounds, or abraded skin. These solutions often contain medications, such as antibiotics or other antimicrobial agents. Irrigating solutions may be used in surgical procedures to clear the surgical field of blood and surgical debris. Although similar to douches, irrigating solutions usually are used in larger volumes and over larger areas of the body for a more general cleansing than douches.

Enemas are solutions that are introduced into the rectum to empty the bowel or to treat diseases of the lower gastrointestinal tract. Enemas such as Fleet enemas (Fleet®) are often given to relieve serious constipation or to cleanse the bowel before surgery.

Gargles are solutions that treat conditions of the throat. The gargle is held in the throat as the patient gurgles air through the solution. Although gargles are admitted into the mouth, they should not be swallowed. A familiar commercial gargle is Cepacol® antiseptic mouthwash/gargle (J.B. Williams).

A *wash* is a solution used to cleanse or bathe a body part, such as the eyes or mouth. A *mouthwash* is a solution used to deodorize, refresh, or disinfect the mouth, primarily for cosmetic reasons. Although many people use mouthwashes as gargles, the two are technically in different classes of solutions: Gargles are used to treat throat conditions, such as a sore throat, whereas mouthwashes are used to freshen the mouth. Like gargles, mouthwashes should not be swallowed. Common mouthwashes include Plax® (Pfizer) and Listerine® (GlaxoWellcome).

Sprays are solutions that are delivered as a mist to the area to be treated. Some sprays target the mucous membranes of the nose and throat; other sprays are intended for use on the skin. Nasal decongestants (e.g., Afrin 12-Hour Original® [Schering-Plough Healthcare] and Neo-Synephrine 12-Hour® [Bayer Corp.]) and antiseptic throat solutions (e.g., Cheracol Sore Throat® [Roberts]) are spray formulations for the nose and throat, respectively.

Viscous aqueous solutions. A *syrup* is a concentrated mixture of sugar and purified water. The high sugar content distinguishes syrups from other types of solutions. Syrups may or may not contain medication or added flavoring agents. Syrups without a medication, but with a flavoring agent, are called nonmedicated or flavored syrups. Flavored syrups often are used as vehicles for unpleasant-tasting medications; the result is a medicated syrup. The amount of sugar present in syrups predisposes them to bacterial contamination, so they often contain a preservative.

The advantage of a syrup is its ability to disguise the bad taste of medications. Because syrups are thicker than aqueous solutions, only a portion of the medication dissolved in the syrup comes in contact with the taste buds. The remainder of the medication is held above the tongue by the thick syrup so it is not tasted as it is swallowed. The sweet taste of syrups help conceal the taste of the medicine, which is why syrups are commonly used for pediatric medications.

The thick character of syrups also has a soothing effect on irritated tissues of the throat, so syrups are often used for cough formulations. Robitussin® (Whitehall-Robins) and Triaminic® (Novartis) are two examples of well-known cough and cold syrups.

Jellies are semisolid solutions that contain a high proportion of water. Jellies are used as lubricants for surgical gloves and rectal thermometers. K-Y Jelly® (Johnson & Johnson) is an example of a commonly used biological lubricant. It may be used to aid in the insertion of rectal thermometers or other diagnostic probes into orifices, as a sexual lubricant, or to reduce surface friction during ultrasound procedures. Jellies are also used as vehicles for vaginal contraceptive agents.

Mucilages are thick, viscous, adhesive liquids. They are solutions of water containing the sticky, pulpy components of vegetable matter. Mucilages are useful dosage forms that prevent insoluble solid medication particles from settling to the bottom of liquids. Bulk-producing laxative/psyllium products, such as Metamucil® (Proctor & Gamble), form a mucilage when the powder is added to water or juice.

Hydroalcoholic solutions. Hydroalcoholic solutions are nonaqueous and differ from aqueous solutions in that they contain alcohol as well as water. Elixirs and spirits are examples of hydroalcoholic solutions.

Elixirs are clear, sweet, flavored water-and-alcohol mixtures intended for oral ingestion. The alcohol content in elixirs varies greatly depending on the ability of the other ingredients in the elixir to dissolve in water. Many drugs do not dissolve easily in pure water but do so in a water-and-alcohol mixture. Some elixirs may have as little as 3 percent alcohol, whereas others may contain almost 25 percent alcohol. The advantage of an elixir, its alcohol content, may also be a disadvantage or a contraindication in patients who should not or cannot ingest alcohol. In addition, alcohol can have undesired interactions with other medications the patients may be taking. Pediatric, elderly, and alcoholic patients should be made aware of the alcohol content of elixirs, because these patients may be especially sensitive to even a small amount of alcohol. Phenobarbital elixir and digoxin pediatric elixir are two widely prescribed medicated elixirs.

Aromatic and licorice elixirs are used as flavoring agents. An aromatic elixir is an unmedicated elixir commonly used as a vehicle for other medications. *Simple elixir*, which contains orange, lemon, coriander, or anise oils in syrup, water, and alcohol, is one example.

Spirits, or essences, are alcoholic or hydroalcoholic solutions that contain volatile, or easily evaporated, substances. Because the volatile substances dissolve more readily in alcohol, spirits can contain a greater concentration of these materials than water. Perhaps the most familiar spirits administered internally are the alcoholic beverages brandy (spiritus vini vitis) and whiskey (spiritus frumenti). Other spirits may be inhaled (e.g., aromatic ammonia spirits, popularly known as smelling salts), while still others, such as peppermint spirits, are used as flavoring agents.

Alcoholic solutions. Alcoholic solutions are nonaqueous solutions that contain alcohol but no water.

A *collodion* is a liquid preparation of pyroxylin (found in cotton fibers) dissolved in ethyl ether and ethanol. After application to the skin, the ether and ethanol evaporate and leave a pyroxylin film. Collodions that contain medication are useful in the treatment of corns and warts (e.g., Compound W® [Whitehall]). Unmedicated collodions, such as liquid adhesive bandages (e.g., New-Skin® [Medtech]) and skin protectants (e.g., BlisterGard® [Medtech]), may be applied to the skin for protection or to seal small wounds.

Glycerite solutions. *Glycerites* are nonaqueous solutions of medication dissolved in glycerin, a sweet oily fluid made from fats and oils. Glycerin can be used alone as a vehicle or in combination with water, alcohol, or both. Because glycerin easily mixes with water and alcohol, it can be used as a solvent for medications that do not dissolve in either alone. After a medication is dissolved in glycerin, the medication/glycerin mixture can then be added to a water or alcohol vehicle. Most glycerite solutions are very viscous, some to the point of being jelly-like. Glycerites are not commonly used today.

Miscellaneous solutions. *Inhalants* are fine powders or solutions of drugs delivered as a mist through the mouth into the respiratory tract. Many drugs used to treat asthma are formulated as inhalants. The over-the-counter product Primatene Mist® (Whitehall Robins) and the prescription drug Proventil® (Schering) are two examples.

A *liniment* is a medication dosage form that is applied to the skin with friction and rubbing. Liniments may be solutions, emulsions, or suspensions. Some liniments contain agents that produce a mild irritation or reddening of the skin. This irritation produces a counterirritation, or mild inflammation, of the skin that relieves inflammation of deeper structures, such as muscles. Ben-Gay Original Ointment® (Pfizer) is a liniment widely used to relieve minor aches and pains of muscles.

Emulsions

Emulsions are mixtures of two liquids that normally do not mix. In an emulsion, one liquid is broken into small particles evenly scattered throughout the other. The liquid present in small particles is referred to as the internal phase; the other liquid is called the external, or continuous, phase. To keep the two liquids from separating, an emulsifying agent is added to the formulation. The emulsifying agent prevents the small particles of the internal phase from fusing together and eventually separating from the external phase to form two distinct layers. Oil-and-vinegar salad dressing is a common household emulsion that is formed by shaking the two liquids together. Because no emulsifying agent is added, the oil and vinegar separate within seconds after shaking and the emulsion is broken.

In most emulsions, the two liquids are oil and water. An *oil-in-water* (O/W) emulsion consists of small oil globules dispersed throughout water; a *water-in-oil* (W/O) emulsion is the reverse—water droplets are distributed throughout the oil. Most emulsions intended for oral use are of the O/W type; those to be applied to the skin may be of either type.

Oil-in-water emulsions. The O/W emulsions are desirable for oral use for several reasons. Unpalatable oily medications are broken into small particles and dispersed throughout a sweetened, flavored aqueous vehicle. These small particles are then carried past the taste buds and swallowed without the patient tasting the oily medication. The small particle size increases medication absorption from the stomach and small intestine into the bloodstream. Mineral oil and castor oil are available as emulsions that make them taste better.

Water-in-oil emulsions. W/O emulsions are often used on unbroken skin. They spread more evenly than O/W emulsions because the natural oils on the skin readily mix with the external oil phase of the emulsion. They also soften the skin better because they retain moisture and are not washed off readily with water. However, they have a heavy, greasy feel and may stain clothing. O/W emulsions may be more desirable in some cases because they are water washable and do not stain clothing. They feel lighter and nongreasy and are particularly advantageous when the emulsion is to be applied to a hairy part of the body, such as the scalp.

The choice of O/W or W/O emulsion for preparations applied to the skin depends on several factors. Medications that are irritating to the skin are better tolerated if they are applied as small particles present in the internal phase. The external phase keeps them from directly contacting and irritating the skin. Therefore, medications that dissolve more readily in oil are applied to the skin as O/W emulsions, in which the oil is the internal phase, whereas those that dissolve in water are applied as W/O emulsions, in which the water is the internal phase.

Some emulsions may also be injected into the bloodstream. Intravenous fat emulsion (Intralipid® [Clintec] and Liposyn II® [Abbott]) is an example of an O/W emulsion that is infused into the bloodstream through a vein. O/W and W/O emulsions are compared in **Table 7-3**.

Suspensions

Suspensions are mixtures of fine particles of an undissolved solid distributed through a gas, liquid, or solid. Most suspensions are solids dispersed in liquids. The difference between a solution and a suspension is that in a solution the particles are dissolved, whereas in a suspension they are not. Suspensions are useful for administering a large amount of solid medication that would be inconvenient to take as a tablet or capsule. The fine particles dissolve more quickly in the stomach or small intestine and thus are absorbed into the bloodstream more quickly than the medication of a solid tablet or capsule. Usually, suspensions need to be shaken before use to redistribute particles that may

TABLE 7-3. COMPARISON OF O/W AND W/O EMULSIONS

Oil-in-Water (O/W)

Advantages

- Improves taste of oral medications
- Better absorption of oral medications into the bloodstream
- Light, nongreasy feel
- Water washable (may also be a disadvantage)

Disadvantages

- May easily wash off with water, or if patient sweats
- Does not spread easily on the skin

Water-in-Oil (W/O)

Advantages

- Spreads evenly on skin
- Softens skin
- Not easily washed off (may also be a disadvantage)

Disadvantages

- May stain clothing
- Heavy, greasy feel

have settled to the bottom or risen to the top of the container during storage.

Most suspensions are intended for oral use, but some may be administered by other routes, such as the rectal, otic, ophthalmic, or parenteral routes. Orally administered suspensions usually use water as the vehicle; some given by parenteral routes, such as the intramuscular route, use an oil as the vehicle.

Lotions are suspensions intended for external application. They contain finely powdered medications, and they cool, soothe, dry, or protect the skin. Lotions are usually applied without rubbing and work easily into large areas of the skin without leaving a greasy or oily feeling. Calamine lotion (Caladryl® [Parke-Davis]) is a common example of a protective lotion.

Magmas and *milks* are thick, viscous suspensions of undissolved drugs in water. Milk of magnesia may be the most familiar example of a magma. Magmas and milks are usually intended for oral administration and should be shaken well before each use.

Gels are similar to magmas and milks except that the suspended particle size in gels is smaller. Gels, too, are often intended for oral administration. Many commercially available antacids are gels.

Extractives

Extractives are concentrated preparations of active components obtained from plant or animal tissue. The crude drug is extracted, or withdrawn, from the dried plant or animal tissue by soaking it in a solvent. The solvent is then evaporated, leaving the active component behind. Tinctures, fluidextracts, and extracts are examples of formulations prepared in this manner. They differ only in their potency.

Tinctures are alcoholic or hydroalcoholic solutions whose potency is adjusted so that each milliliter of tincture contains the equivalent of 100 mg of crude drug. Iodine tincture and paregoric tincture are common examples.

Fluidextracts are more potent than tinctures; each milliliter of fluidextract contains the equivalent of 1,000 mg of crude drug. Cascara sagrada fluidextract and senna fluidextract are extracts that, in the past, were commonly used to clear the bowels.

Extracts are prepared in the same manner as tinctures and fluidextracts but are two to six times as potent as the crude drug. Vanilla, almond, and peppermint extracts, commonly used in cooking and baking, are examples of extracts.

Solid Medication Dosage Forms

Medications are commonly formulated in a solid form. Examples of solid medication dosage forms include tablets, capsules, suppositories, and lozenges. Solid medication dosage forms are used to deliver medications orally, rectally, or vaginally. Like some liquid medication dosage forms, some solid medication dosage forms may be used by more than one route. For example, tablets are used for oral medications, but they may also be used to deliver medications into the vagina. Suppositories are usually given rectally (e.g., glycerin rectal suppositories) but may also be used to deliver medications into the vagina (e.g., Monistat 3® [Advanced Care Products] vaginal suppositories) or, very rarely, into the urethra (e.g., MUSE® [Vivus] urethral suppositories). **Table 7-4** summarizes the solid medication dosage forms that are discussed in this chapter.

Solid medication dosage forms have several advantages over other dosage forms (see **Table 7-5**):

- They often have longer shelf lives and are easier to package, store, and transport.

- Patients receive accurate medication doses

TABLE 7-4. EXAMPLES OF SOLID MEDICATION DOSAGE FORMS

Tablets
- Sublingual
- Buccal
- Effervescent
- Chewable
- Vaginal

Capsules

Lozenges

Extended-Release

Miscellaneous
- Powders
- Granules
- Aerosols
- Ointments
  Oleaginous
  Anhydrous
  Emulsion; O/W, W/O
  Water soluble
- Creams
  O/W
  W/O

TABLE 7-5. ADVANTAGES AND DISADVANTAGES OF SOLID DOSAGE FORMS

Advantages

- May have longer shelf life than liquid dosage forms
- May be easier to package, store, and transport than liquid dosage forms
- Are formulated in distinct units so patients receive accurate medication dosage
- May be formulated in sustained-release dosage forms
- May be more convenient to self-administer than liquid dosage forms
- May have little or no taste

Disadvantages

- May be too large too swallow
- Cannot be used orally for unconscious patients
- Must be dissolved before they are absorbed into the bloodstream, which can delay the time before the drug can begin to act

---

because solid medications are formulated in distinct units.

- Techniques have been developed to create dosage forms of solid medications in which the medication is released from the solid over a long period of time; these are sustained-release dosage forms. Patients therefore need not take the medication as often as they would a non-sustained-release or immediate-release form.

- Patients find solid dosage forms more convenient to self-administer.

- Often, the oral solid medication dosage forms have little or no taste.

Oral solid dosage forms also have disadvantages:

- Some oral solid dosage forms are large enough to present a problem for patients unable to swallow larger tablets or capsules.

- Unconscious patients are not able to take oral solid medications. This is especially a problem if the desired medication is not available in a form that can be administered by another route.

- Solid dosage forms must be dissolved—in the stomach or rectum, for instance—before they are absorbed into the bloodstream. Thus, there is a time delay before the drug can begin to act. Delay is not desirable for such situations as a heart attack or severe asthma episode, in which immediate drug action is necessary.

Tablets

Tablets are compacted solid medication dosage forms; they may be further classified on the basis of their method of manufacture. *Molded tablets* are made from wet materials placed in molds. *Compressed tablets* are formed by die punch compression of powdered, crystalline, or granular substances.

Other ingredients that have no medicinal activity may be included in a compressed tablet. These inactive, or inert, ingredients (e.g., binders, lubricants, diluents, colorants) are necessary for the manufacturing process or to make the tablet more effective (e.g., disintegrators).

- Binders help keep the compressed tablet from crumbling and hold it together.

- Diluents are fillers that are added to the active medication to make the tablet a practical size.

- Lubricants ease removal of the tablet from the die.

- Colorants add color to the product.

- Disintegrators are included to help the tablet dissolve in the stomach, small intestine, or elsewhere in the body.

Compressed tablets may have a sugar, film, or enteric coating on the outside. Sugar coating or film coating may be used to mask noxious-tasting or -smelling drugs, to add color to the tablet, or to protect the drug from exposure to the air and humidity. A film coating coats the tablet with a hard shell to make it more durable and easier to swallow.

Enteric-coated oral tablets have a coating that protects the tablet from stomach acid and protects the lining of the gastrointestinal tract from irritation by the drug. Enteric-coating is also used in making sustained-release tablets.

Tablets may be described by a number of other terms as well. *Sublingual* and *buccal* tablets are useful solid dosage forms that are absorbed directly into the bloodstream through the lining under the tongue or of the cheek. Medications that are destroyed by stomach acid or are poorly absorbed into the bloodstream may be formulated as sublingual or buccal tablets.

Effervescent tablets contain ingredients that bubble and release the active drug when placed in a liquid. Their advantage is that they disintegrate and dissolve before administration so the drug can be absorbed quickly. Alka-Seltzer Effervescent Tablets® (Bayer) are an example.

Chewable tablets are those that do not need to be swallowed whole and may or should be chewed. They are pleasantly flavored and are especially useful for pediatric medications (e.g., chewable baby aspirin). Some adult tablets are also chewable. Antacid tablets (e.g., Rolaids Tablets® [Pfizer Inc.] and Tums® [SmithKline Beecham Consumer]) may be chewed before swallowing.

Vaginal tablets are inserted into the vagina. The tablet dissolves and the medication is absorbed through the vaginal mucous lining. Gyne-Lotrimin 3® (Schering-Plough) vaginal tablets is one example.

Capsules

Capsules are solid medication dosage forms in which the drug, with or without inactive or inert ingredients, is contained within a gelatin shell. Gelatin shells are made of protein derived from animals.

Hard gelatin capsules are two-piece oblong casings filled with powdered ingredients. Most often, they are intended for oral use and are swallowed whole. However, in some instances the capsule may be or should be opened and the powdered ingredients sprinkled on food or in water before administration (e.g., Depakote Sprinkle® [Abbott] and Topamax Sprinkle® [Ortho-McNeil] capsules). Other capsules contain powders that should be inhaled through the mouth into the lungs where the drug takes effect. These capsules are inserted into a mechanical device that punctures the capsule and releases the powder. Patients then inhale the powder through the mouthpiece on the mechanical device. Ventolin Rotacaps® (Glaxo Wellcome), a medication to treat asthma, is administered in this fashion.

Soft gelatin capsules have ingredients added to the gelatin to give it soft, squeezable, elastic consistency. The two halves of the capsule are sealed shut and, unlike hard gelatin capsules, cannot be opened. Soft gelatin capsules may be round, elliptical, or oblong in shape and filled with liquid, pasty, or powdered medications. Vitamin A and vitamin D preparations are often available in a soft gelatin capsule. Colace® (Roberts), a stool softener, is also a soft gelatin capsule.

Lozenges

Lozenges, also known as *troches* or *pastilles*, are hard disk-shaped solid medication dosage forms that contain medication in a sugar base. Lozenges are used to deliver antiseptic, local anesthetic, antibiotic, analgesic, antitussive, astringent, or decongestant drugs to the mouth or throat. The lozenge is held in the mouth and sucked. As it dissolves, the lozenge releases the medica-tion. Sucrets Sore Throat® (SK-Beecham) and Cepacol Throat® (J.B. Williams) lozenges contain local anesthetic, antiseptic, and other ingredients useful for treating minor sore throats. Mycelex® (Bayer) troches and Mycostatin Pastilles® (Bristol-Myers Oncology) contain a fungicide and are used to treat oral fungal infections.

Extended-Release Dosage Forms

In some instances, having a medication dosage form that slowly and consistently releases the drug over an extended period of time—instead of all at once—is desirable. These medication dosage forms are called extended-release, sustained-release, long-acting, or controlled-release. Although the exact meanings of these terms differ in some respects, each of these terms implies a gradual release of medication over a longer period than standard dosage forms. **Table 7-6** lists common abbreviations for extended release. Oral tablets and capsules are the most common dosage forms that are formulated as extended release. Other dosage forms, such as implants and some intramuscular injections, that are also extended release, will be discussed later.

Extended-release dosage forms offer several advantages:

- They deliver medication in a slow, controlled, and consistent manner so the patient is absorbing the same amount of medication throughout a given time period.

- The risk of drug side effects is reduced because the medication is delivered over an extended period.

- Patients may need to take the medication less frequently, perhaps only once or twice a day.

TABLE 7-6. COMMON ABBREVIATIONS FOR EXTENDED-RELEASE

CD	Controlled-diffusion
CR	Controlled-release, continuous-release
CRT	Controlled-release tablet
LA	Long-acting
SA	Sustained-action
SR	Sustained-release, slow-release
TD	Time delay
TR	Time-release
XL	Extra-long
XR	Extended-release

- Patients are more likely to take their medications properly if they have to take them less often and are less likely to experience side effects.

- The daily medication cost to patients may be decreased. Although extended-release products may be more expensive on a per-dose basis, the total daily cost may be less because the patient may need to take fewer doses per day.

Several technologies are available to give medication dosage forms extended-release properties. Many small beads of medication in varying sizes may have varying thicknesses of a coating material. These beads are then put in a hard gelatin capsule. In the stomach, the gelatin capsule quickly dissolves and releases the small beads, which then dissolve and release medication at varying rates over a period of time. The cold product Contac 12-Hour Capsules® (SmithKline Beecham Consumer) is formulated in this manner.

Other extended-release products use a slowly eroding matrix. In this case, a portion of the medication is treated and made into special granules. These granules are then combined with an untreated portion of the medication granules and made into a tablet or capsule. The untreated drug granules immediately release the drug in the stomach, while the treated ones slowly erode to provide the prolonged effect. Slow-K® (Summit) potassium tablets are such a product.

Some extended-release products are formulated in two or more layers. One layer dissolves immediately while the remaining layers dissolve more slowly and release the drug gradually.

Other products, such as Procanbid Extended-Release Tablets® (Monarch), embed the drug in an inert plastic or wax matrix core covered by a controlled-release layer. The drug is then released into the body as it slowly leaches from the matrix. The matrix does not dissolve and is passed through the gastrointestinal tract and excreted in the feces.

A very sophisticated extended-release system uses an osmotic pump to deliver medication over time. This system uses the principle of osmosis, which states that fluids tend to flow from areas with a low concentration of a substance to areas with a high concentration. The pump system is composed of a special membrane surrounding a core of medication. As fluid in the stomach passes through the membrane, the drug core inside swells and forces medication out of a small hole drilled in the membrane. Procardia XL® (Pfizer) is one product that uses an osmotic pump system.

Miscellaneous Dosage Forms

A number of medication dosage forms do not fit neatly into a specific category. They may be either unique in and of themselves or a combination of medication dosage forms.

Powders

Powders, as a medication dosage form, can be used externally or internally. External powders, or dusting powders, are finely ground mixtures of dry drugs and inactive ingredients that are sprinkled or dusted on the area to be medicated. An example is Mycostatin® (Westwood Squibb) powder, which is often used to treat fungal infections of the skin. Internal powders are dissolved in a liquid prior to ingestion. Many potassium products are available as powders to be dissolved in water or juice. Some powders, such as powdered toothpaste, are mixed with water and used in the wetted state.

Powders are packaged in bulk containers or, when the amount delivered must be accurate, in powder papers. Powder papers are folded paper envelopes that contain enough powder for one dose or application. BC Powder® and Arthritis Strength BC Powder® (Block) are analgesics packaged in powder papers.

Granules

When powders are wetted, allowed to dry, and ground into coarse pieces, the resulting medication dosage form is called a granule.

Granules differ from powders in that the particle size is larger and usually more stable. Many antibiotics are formulated as granules. The pharmacist or technician adds water to form a solution or suspension at the time of dispensing. Senokot Granules® (Purdue Frederick), a common laxative, for example, is added to water before administration.

Aerosols

Aerosols are suspensions of very fine liquid or solid particles distributed in a gas and packaged under pressure. Medication is released from the container in a spray (e.g., Bactine First Aid Antiseptic Anesthetic® [Bayer Consumer]), foam (e.g., ProctoFoam-HC® [Schwarz Pharma]), or solid (e.g., Tinactin® [Schering-Plough]). Aerosols are conveniently packaged and easy to use.

Aerosols may be used to deliver medications to internal and external sites. Aerosols inhaled internally, such as Proventil® (Schering) and Ventolin® (GlaxoSmithKline), are used to treat such conditions as asthma. The aerosol delivers the drug directly to the lungs, where it begins acting immediately. The drug does not first have to be dissolved in the stomach and absorbed into the bloodstream as it would if it were formulated as a tablet or capsule. External aerosols, such as Tinactin® (Schering-Plough) and Bactine First Aide Antiseptic Anesthetic® (Bayer Consumer) sprays, may be applied topically (externally) for skin conditions. An external aerosol can deliver medication to a hard-to-reach area of the skin and can be applied to inflamed or irritated skin without causing further irritation.

Ointments

Ointments are semisolid medication dosage forms intended to be applied to the skin or mucous membranes. They are used to lubricate and soften or as a base (a vehicle that contains a drug) for drug delivery. Not all ointments contain a drug. Ointments are categorized on the basis of their characteristics. The primary types are oleaginous, anhydrous, emulsion, and water soluble.

Oleaginous, or *hydrocarbon, bases* are emollients that soothe the skin or mucous membrane. They are occlusive and protect the skin or mucous membrane from the air. They are hydrophobic (repel water), and therefore do not wash off with water, and they feel greasy to the touch. Oleaginous bases are used primarily for their lubricating effect because they do not allow moisture to escape from the skin, do not dry out, and remain on the skin for a long time. Vaseline® (Cheesebrough Ponds) petroleum jelly is an example of an oleaginous base.

Anhydrous, or *absorption, bases* contain no water and are similar to oleaginous bases, but instead of repelling water, they absorb it. They also soften skin, but not to the same degree as the oleaginous bases. Anhydrous bases are used to absorb an aqueous, or water-based, drug into an ointment base. They do not contain water as part of their formula, but as they absorb water, a W/O emulsion is formed. Anhydrous lanolin and cold cream are widely used anhydrous bases.

Emulsion bases may be W/O or O/W. The W/O types are emollient, occlusive, and greasy. They contain water, and some may be able to absorb additional water. Lanolin, mentioned above as an anhydrous base, and cold cream are considered to be W/O emulsions when water is added to them.

Emulsion bases of the O/W type, or water-washable bases, are quite different. They are nongreasy and readily wash off with water. They are nonocclusive and may be diluted, or thinned, with the addition of water. In certain skin conditions, O/W emulsion bases are used to absorb watery discharge or to help the skin absorb certain medications. Hydrophilic ointment is an O/W ointment base.

Water-soluble bases are nongreasy, nonocclusive, and water-washable. They do not contain any fats and usually do not contain any water. Nonaqueous or solid medications are added to this type of ointment base. Polyethylene glycol ointment is one such base.

Ointment bases are chosen primarily on the basis of the characteristics described above. A W/O emulsion base may be used if a liquid medication is to be added to the ointment. Some medications may be more stable or more readily absorbed by the skin when delivered in a particular type of ointment base. The softening or drying characteristics of the ointment base may also influence the choice of a base. For instance, a nongreasy ointment base may be chosen if the ointment is to be applied to the face, because a greasy base may leave an unpleasant feeling.

Creams

Creams are semisolid O/W or W/O emulsions that may or may not contain medication. They are easily worked into the skin and feel lighter than ointments. They, too, serve to soften the skin. Creams may be preferred over ointments because they are easier to spread, have a cooling effect on the skin, and, in the case of O/W creams, are easier to wash off with water. Many drug products are available as either creams or ointments to cater to the preferences of patients and physicians. Creams are also widely used in many cosmetic products.

Routes of Administration

Drugs can be administered by several different routes (see Table 7-7). Although the oral route is most common, it may not always be the most convenient or practical. Drugs may be administered via any body orifice, through the skin, or into an artificially made opening.

Oral

Medications taken by the oral route are introduced into the body through the mouth. The oral route is abbreviated *PO*, which is from the Latin *per os* (by mouth). Tablets, capsules, solutions, suspensions, and emulsions are some of the medication dosage forms that may be taken orally.

TABLE 7-7. ROUTES OF MEDICATION ADMINISTRATION

Oral (through the mouth)
- *buccal* (inside the cheek)
- *sublingual* (under the tongue)

Enteral (by way of the intestine)

Parenteral (bypassing the gastrointestinal tract)
- *intraarterial* (IA—into an artery)
- *intraarticular* (into a joint)
- *intracardiac* (into the heart muscle)
- *intradermal* (ID—into the top layers of the skin)
- *intramuscular* (IM—into a muscle)
- *intraperitoneal* (into the peritoneal, or abdominal, cavity)
- *intrapleural* (into the pleura, the sac surrounding the lungs)
- *intrathecal* (into the space around the spinal cord)
- *intravenous* (IV—into a vein)
- *intraventricular* (into the ventricles, or cavities, of the brain)
- *intravesicular* (into the urinary bladder)
- *intravitreous* (into the eye)
- *subcutaneous* (SC, subQ, SQ—immediately under the skin)

Inhalation (drawn through the mouth into the lungs)

Nasal (into the nose)

Ophthalmic (into the eye)

Otic (into the ear)

Percutaneous (through the skin)

Rectal (through the anus into the rectum)

Topical (applied to skin or mucous membranes)

Transdermal (across the skin)

Vaginal (into the vagina)

The oral route has many advantages. It is safe and convenient, and medications taken orally are generally less expensive than those administered by other routes. Oral dosage forms may be modified to deliver drugs in an extended-release fashion.

The oral route, however, does have disadvantages. It cannot be used to administer medications to unconscious patients or those who have trouble swallowing. In addition, because an oral medication must be dissolved in the gastrointestinal tract before entering the bloodstream, there is a lag time between ingestion and the time the drug begins to act. This time lag is a problem if an immediate action is desired. Food, other drugs, and acid or lack of acid in the stomach may interfere with the dissolution or absorption of the drug.

There may be times when a patient cannot swallow a medication (e.g., the patient is mechanically ventilated with an endotracheal tube in the throat). In these situations, medications may be given enterally, bypassing the patient's mouth and entering the body by way of the intestine. Usually, liquid medication is poured down a tube inserted through the nose, throat, or even abdomen and enters the patient's stomach or small intestine. Although these tubes are usually inserted for other reasons, they may offer alternatives to the oral route.

Sublingual and Buccal

The terms *sublingual* (under the tongue) and *buccal* (inside the cheek) refer not only to types of tablets but also to routes of oral medication administration.

To administer a drug sublingually, a *sublingual* tablet is placed under the tongue, where the medication dissolves and is absorbed into the bloodstream through the underlining of the tongue. Hydergine® (Sandoz) and nitroglycerin sublingual tablets are administered under the tongue. Sublingual tablets are used when a rapid drug effect is desired, such as in the treatment of chest pain or migraine headache.

Buccal tablets are placed inside the pouch of the cheek, where the medication dissolves and is absorbed through the cheek lining into the bloodstream over time. Nitrogard® (Forest) controlled-release buccal tablets are administered to prevent and treat episodes of chest pain. Although not formulated as a tablet, nicotine gum (Nicorette® [GlaxoSmithKline Consumer]) uses the buccal route to deliver nicotine into the bloodstream of people who are trying to quit cigarette smoking.

Parenteral

Parenteral routes of administration are those that bypass the gastrointestinal tract. Medications administered parenterally are most commonly introduced into the body intravenously, intramuscularly, or subcutaneously. They may be injected over a short period of time (seconds to minutes) with a needle and syringe or infused into the body at a constant rate over hours or days. Drugs that are given parenterally are most commonly formulated as solutions (e.g., potassium chloride, dextrose, many antibiotics, regular insulin), and less often as suspensions (e.g., Sus-Phrine® [Forest Pharmaceuticals], penicillin G benzathine) and emulsions (e.g., intravenous fat emulsion).

Parenterally administered drugs are given when patients are unable to take oral medications, when faster drug action is desired, or when a drug is not available in a form that can be administered by another route. A disadvantage of parenteral routes is that they are often invasive—that is, a needle penetrates the skin to enter into veins, arteries, and other areas of the body. This penetration may be painful for the patient and could introduce bacteria or other contaminants into the body, resulting in infection or inflammation.

Intravenous (IV) medications are introduced into the body through a needle placed directly in a vein. These drugs are usually given as solutions, which must be sterile and free of particulate matter. Drugs given by the IV route are immediately available to act in the body. Because they act quickly, care must be taken giving IV medications. If too high a dose is given or if the patient experiences an adverse reaction, quick action may be needed to reverse the drug's effects.

IV drugs may be given as a *bolus* or by *continuous infusion*. A bolus drug dose is injected into the body over a relatively short period of time—seconds to minutes. The term *IV push* also refers to this administration technique; the drug is pushed into the body by means of a syringe. Lidocaine, a drug used to treat abnormal heart rhythms, may be given as a bolus. In contrast, some medications may be infused into veins over hours to days using a constant infusion or drip, which provides a constant supply of drug to the body. Bolus doses and continuous infusions are often used together. For example, after lidocaine is given as an IV push, a lidocaine drip is often started to maintain a certain level of lidocaine in the blood.

Intramuscular (IM) administration involves direct injection of medication into a large muscle mass, such as the upper arm, thigh, or buttock. The drug is then absorbed from the muscle tissue into the bloodstream. IM drugs may be given as solutions or suspensions. Drugs given by the IM route act more quickly than orally administered drugs but not as quickly as IV drugs. Some drugs may be formulated in extended-release forms that slowly release drug from the muscle tissue into the bloodstream over hours, days, or even months. Some types of penicillin are formulated in this manner. Disadvantages to the IM route are that it is difficult to reverse the drug's effects once the injection has been given, the injection is painful to receive and may cause bruising, and drug absorption from the muscle into the bloodstream may be erratic and incomplete.

Solutions or suspensions injected *subcutaneously* (SC, subQ, SQ), sometimes referred to as *hypodermic*

injections, are deposited in the tissue immediately under the skin. Drugs given by the SC route are absorbed to a lesser extent and act slower than those given by the IV or IM routes. Patients can easily be taught to self-administer SC injections. Many diabetic patients, for example, give themselves daily SC injections of insulin.

A limitation of both the SC and IM routes is the volume of drug that can be injected under the skin or into the muscle. It may be undesirable to use the SC route in patients with frail skin or the IM route in patients with decreased muscle mass or bleeding problems.

Caution must be exercised when interpreting abbreviations that refer to the route of medication administration. The abbreviation *IV* usually refers to the intravenous route, but it could also refer to the *intravitreous* (into the eye) or *intraventricular* (into the brain) routes, or it could be interpreted as the Roman numeral four. Like extended-release abbreviations, abbreviations for drug administration routes must be interpreted carefully in the context of each medication order.

The IV, IM, and SC routes are the most commonly used parenteral routes. However, drugs can be injected into almost any body space. Several other parenteral medication dosage routes are used for specialized purposes or to limit drug delivery to the immediate area of the injection. These routes include intradermal, intraarterial, intraarticular, intracardiac, intraperitoneal, intrapleural, intraventricular, intravesicular, intravitreous, and intrathecal.

The *intradermal* (ID) route involves injecting a drug into the top layers of the skin. ID injections are not injected as deep as SC injections. The ID route is used to administer drugs for skin testing to see if patients are allergic to drugs or other substances, such as dust, pet dander, or pollen. This route can also be used to administer diagnostic skin tests to check if patients have been exposed to certain microorganisms, such as those that cause mumps or tuberculosis.

Intraarterial (IA) injections involve administering an agent directly into arteries. These injections have the advantage of delivering drugs, such as cancer chemotherapy agents, directly to the desired location and thus may decrease some of the side effects caused when the drug acts in other parts of the body. This more direct route involves greater risk than the IV route and may be more toxic if the drug was not originally intended for arterial administration.

The *intraarticular* route involves injecting a drug into a joint, such as a knee or elbow. These drugs act to treat diseases in the joint. For example, steroid drugs are injected intraarticularly to treat the inflammation caused by arthritis.

The *intracardiac* route, injection directly into the heart muscle, is used in life-threatening emergencies. This route is not often used, because it entails the risk of rupturing the heart.

Intraperitoneal injections are given into the peritoneal, or abdominal, cavity. This route is used to administer antibiotics to treat infections in the peritoneal cavity. One method of dialysis, peritoneal dialysis, uses the intraperitoneal route to remove waste products from the blood of patients with kidney failure.

Intrapleural describes the injection of drugs into the sac surrounding the lungs, or the pleura. Drugs are injected intrapleurally to stimulate inflammation and scarring of the pleural tissues so that excessive fluid can no longer accumulate in the pleural sac.

The *intraventricular* route is used to administer drugs into the ventricles, or cavities, of the brain to treat infections or cancerous tumors of brain. Caution must be used when interpreting an order for the intraventricular route, because the heart also has ventricles.

The *intravesicular* route delivers drugs directly into the urinary bladder. This route is used to treat bladder infections or bladder cancer.

Intravitreous administration is direct injection into the eye. Many drugs do not enter the eye from the bloodstream, and often the only way to deliver medications inside the eye is to inject them intravitreously. Antibiotics to treat sight-threatening eye infections are administered intravitreously.

Intrathecal is the route by which drugs are injected into the space around the spinal cord. This route may be used to deliver agents that treat infections or cancerous tumors of the central nervous system.

An *implant* is a medication pump or device inserted semipermanently or permanently into the body. Medication is released from the implant and delivered in a controlled fashion. Implants are often used to treat chronic (long-term) conditions or diseases. Some diabetic patients have a small pump implanted in their bodies that delivers insulin. Certain types of cancers may be treated with chemotherapeutic agents delivered into the arteries that enter the cancerous organ. A small pump filled with the drug is implanted into the body and infuses the chemotherapy drug into the artery. A form of contraception, Norplant® (Wyeth-Ayerst), has been developed in which an implant inserted under the skin of a woman's arm slowly releases birth control medication for up to 5 years.

Topical

The topical route refers to the application of medications to the surface of the skin or mucous membranes. Medications administered topically include antibiotics, antiseptics, astringents, emollients, and corticosteroids. Topical medication dosage forms include creams, ointments, lotions, sprays, and aerosols. In most cases, the skin or mucous membrane acts as a barrier to prevent the medication from entering the bloodstream. As a result, drugs used for treating diseases of the skin and mucous membranes can be applied in higher concentrations than drugs administered internally.

Some ointments and creams (e.g., topical corticosteroid ointments) are formulated to deliver a drug into the skin to treat a condition of the deeper skin layers. Sometimes creams or ointments may be designed so that the drug diffuses through the skin into the bloodstream. The drug is then available to the whole body. This is called systemic absorption. Nitroglycerin ointment used to treat chest pain is an example.

In some cases, systemic absorption is not desired and may result in unwanted side effects. For example, when topical corticosteroids are absorbed systemically over prolonged periods of time, the patient may develop cataracts or glaucoma. Topical medications are more likely to penetrate into the bloodstream when the skin is not intact (e.g., when it is inflamed or burned).

Other Routes of Administration

Transdermal

The *transdermal*, or *percutaneous*, route of medication administration delivers drugs across, or through, the skin. The topical route is used for medications not intended to enter the body and bloodstream, but the transdermal route is meant to deliver medications to the bloodstream and, consequently, the rest of the body. Medications are continuously absorbed into the bloodstream when the transdermal route is used. Transdermal medications are applied to the skin, released from a vehicle, and absorbed into the bloodstream. Adhesive patches, similar to plastic bandages, that contain drugs in a small reservoir are commonly used to deliver medications transdermally. Patches are convenient to use. Depending on the patch, they may be applied to the skin from once a day to once a week.

Transdermal patches are formulated in one of two ways. One type of patch is formulated so the patch itself controls the rate of delivery of drug to the skin. A special membrane in the patch is in contact with the skin. The membrane controls the amount of drug delivered from a drug reservoir in the patch, through the membrane and skin, and into the bloodstream. The second type of transdermal patch is designed so that the skin controls the rate of drug delivery. The drug moves from an area of high concentration (the drug reservoir) into an area of low concentration (the skin and bloodstream). The disadvantage of this type of patch is that the release of drug is less controlled, and a large amount of drug could suddenly be released from the patch into the blood.

Medications available in a patch formulation include a narcotic analgesic (Duragesic® [Janssen]), female hormones (Estraderm® [Ciba-Geigy]), and drugs to treat high blood pressure (Catapres-TTS® [Boehringer Ingelheim]), chronic chest pain (Transderm-Nitro® [Summit] and others), and motion sickness (Transderm Scop® [Hope Pharmaceuticals]) and to help patients quit smoking (Nicotrol® [Pharmacia] and others).

Ointments are sometimes used to deliver drugs percutaneously. Nitroglycerin ointment for chronic chest pain was often used in the past. Its use has been widely replaced by nitroglycerin transdermal patches, although the ointment may still be used to transition, or wean, patients from continuous nitroglycerin IV infusions to oral nitroglycerin medications.

Rectal

Drugs delivered by the rectal route are inserted through the anus into the rectum. Rectally administered drugs may be formulated as solids (suppositories), liquids or suspensions (enemas), and aerosol foams. Once the drug reaches the rectum, its activity may be limited to the lower gastrointestinal tract, or the drug may be absorbed into the bloodstream and delivered to its site of action elsewhere in the body. The rectal route is often used for children and patients who are unable to take oral medications.

Vaginal

Drugs may also be inserted into the vagina. Drugs delivered by the vaginal route may be in the form of a vaginal suppository (e.g., Monistat-7® [Advanced Care Products] vaginal suppositories), tablet (e.g., nystatin vaginal tablets), cream (e.g., Terazol 3® [Ortho-McNeil]), ointment (Vagistat-1® [Bristol-Myers Squibb]), gel (e.g., Ortho-Gynol Contraceptive® [Advanced Care]), or solution (e.g., Massengill Douche® [SK-Beecham]). A contraceptive ring, Nuva Ring® (Organon), is one of the newer vaginal drug delivery forms.

The drug's activity may be limited to the vagina—as it is when vaginal medications are used to treat vaginal infections—or the drug may be absorbed into the bloodstream and delivered to another part of the body where the drug takes effect. Prostaglandin suppositories used for premenstrual syndrome are an example of a drug administered vaginally to produce effects in other parts of the body (systemic effects).

Otic

The otic route is used to deliver drugs into the ear canal. Otic drugs may be formulated as solutions or suspensions. Local conditions of the ear, such as ear infections or excessive earwax, may be treated with otically administered drugs.

Ophthalmic

Drugs given via the ophthalmic route are administered into the eye. Ophthalmic medications are formulated as solutions, suspensions, gels, or ointments. Special medicated inserts (e.g., Ocusert Pilo® [Alza]) placed in the pouch of the lower eyelid can also be used to deliver medications to the eye. The ophthalmic route is advantageous in that conditions of the eye, such as glaucoma and infections of the conjunctiva, may be treated without administering the drug systemically. As a result, medication can reach the intended site without exposing the patient to unnecessary side effects in other parts of the body.

Nasal

Drugs are administered into the nostrils by the nasal route. Solutions may be nasally administered as sprays or drops. This route enables conditions of the nose, such as nasal congestion or allergic rhinitis, to be treated without administering the drug systemically. Often, drugs given nasally act more quickly than if they were administered by a route, such as the mouth or vein, that introduces medication into the whole body. In other instances, drugs may be administered nasally to treat conditions not involving the nose (e.g., Stadol NS® [Mead Johnson] nasal spray for the relief of migraine headaches or Nicotrol NS® [Pharmacia] as an aid in smoking cessation).

Inhalation

Drugs may be inhaled through the mouth into the lungs. This route is used when a rapid drug effect is desired to treat lung conditions. The inhalation route is most often used to deliver medications for the treatment of asthma. Examples, such as the over-the-counter product Primatene Mist® and the prescription drug Proventil, have previously been discussed. Nicotrol® (Pharmacia) inhalers are used to aid in smoking cessation.

Dosage Form versus Route of Administration

A particular medication dosage form often implies a specific administration route; and a particular route often implies a specific dosage form. For instance, the tablet dosage form is most often administered orally, although it is also used to administer drugs intravaginally. When the rectal route is used, the suppository is the dosage form commonly considered. However, suppositories are not the only dosage form used for the rectal route, because many medications are formulated as rectal foams or enemas. Occasionally, a dosage form intended for use via one route may be delivered through another route when other options or routes are impractical or infeasible. For example, oral morphine tablets may be administered rectally to terminally ill cancer patients who are unable to swallow and do not have intravenous access. Finally, as discussed previously, one term may be used to describe both a route and a dosage form: for example, the terms *sublingual* and *buccal*.

Many drugs are available in a number of dosage forms and may be delivered via a number of administration routes. In some instances, a condition may be treated using two or more routes. For example, meningitis, an infection of the brain, may be treated with antibiotics administered intravenously and intraventricularly. Glaucoma, a condition of the eye, may be treated locally with ophthalmic drops or systemically with oral capsules. Physicians and pharmacists select the most appropriate dosage form and route on the basis of the patient's condition, the need for immediate drug action, or the availability of a drug in a particular dosage form or administration route.

Additional References

Ansel HC. Pharmaceutical dosage forms and drug delivery systems. 7th ed. Baltimore: Lippincott Williams & Wilkins; 1999.

Gennaro AR, ed. Remington: the science and practice of pharmacy. 20th ed. Baltimore: Lippincott Williams & Wilkins; 2000.

Self-Assessment Questions

1. Which of the following are common vehicles for liquid medication forms?
   a. water, isopropyl alcohol, glycerin, propylene glycol
   b. water, glycerin, propylene glycol, ethyl alcohol
   c. water, glycerite, propylene glycol, ethyl alcohol
   d. water, isopropyl alcohol, glycerin, ethanol

2. For which of the following situations would a liquid medication dosage form be a better choice than a solid one?
   a. A patient has just had throat surgery and cannot easily swallow.
   b. A patient is very sensitive to unpleasant tastes and refuses to take "bad-tasting" medicine.
   c. A traveling salesman needs to take a medication on a regular basis.
   d. A patient must take a medication that must be dosed very precisely.

3. The IV route of administration may be advantageous over the oral route for what reason?
   a. There is less chance of bacterial contamination of the bloodstream.
   b. The drug effects are easily reversed if too high a dose is given.
   c. The drug is absorbed from muscle tissue into the bloodstream, which may provide an extended-release effect.
   d. The drug is available to immediately act in the body.

4. Medication administered by the IV route usually means that the medication is injected directly into
   a. a ventricle of the heart
   b. an eye
   c. a vein
   d. a ventricle of the brain

5. A parenteral route of medication administration is one that bypasses
   a. the gastrointestinal tract
   b. the heart and circulatory system
   c. the kidneys
   d. the skin barrier

6. Injection of a drug into a joint, such as the knee or elbow, is known as the _____ route of medication administration.
   a. intraarterial
   b. intrapleural
   c. intraarticular
   d. intrarthritic

7. Advantages of liquid oral dosage forms include all of the following EXCEPT:
   a. Oral liquid dosage forms usually are faster acting than solid dosage forms.
   b. Oral liquid dosage forms may be easier to take for a patient who has difficulty swallowing than an oral solid dosage form.
   c. Oral liquid dosage forms may be used where solid dosage forms are not practical to administer.
   d. Oral liquid dosage forms often have a shorter expiration time than other dosage forms.

8. A tincture is an alcoholic or hydroalcoholic extractive solution whose potency is adjusted so that each milliliter contains the equivalent potency of _____ of crude drug.
   a. 100 mg
   b. 1,000 gm
   c. 10 mg
   d. 100 gm

9. Which of the following statements about W/O emulsions is false?
   a. W/O emulsions are often used on unbroken skin.
   b. W/O emulsions spread more evenly than O/W emulsions because the natural oils on the skin readily mix with the external phase.
   c. W/O emulsions soften the skin better than O/W emulsions because they retain moisture and are not readily washed off with water.
   d. W/O emulsions are water washable and do not stain clothing.

10. Drugs that are administered into the eye are given by the _____ route.
    a. otic
    b. ophthalmic
    c. oral
    d. aural

Self-Assessment Answers

1. b. Isopropyl alcohol (rubbing alcohol) is not used for liquid medication.
2. a. Liquids mask tastes less effectively than other oral dosage forms, travel less conveniently, and are less precise in measurement of the dose.
3. d. The IV route is more easily contaminated and less easily reversed. Drugs given IV are immediately available to the body—not absorbed over time from muscle tissue (IM).
4. c. The ventricle of the heart (intracardiac), the eye (intravitreous), and the ventricle of the brain (intraventricular) represent other routes of administration.
5. a. Parenteral means bypassing the "enteral" or gastrointestinal system.
6. c. Intraarticular (into an artery) and intrapleural (inside the sac surrounding the lungs—the pleura) represent additional routes of administration.
7. d. Although some extemporaneously compounded liquid dosage forms, or those reconstituted immediately prior to use, may have a shorter expiration time, this is not universally true of all oral liquids.
8. a. Other extractives include fluidextracts, containing 1000 mg of crude drug per milliliter, and extracts, which are 2-6 times as potent as crude drug.
9. d. Because water is emulsed within an oil base in w/o emulsions, they resist washing with water, adhering to the skin and potentially staining clothing.
10. b. Otic and aural both refer to administration in the ear and oral administration is by mouth.

Medical Terminology and Abbreviations

LINDA Y. FRED

8

A good familiarity with, and understanding of, pharmacy terms and abbreviations is critical to the success of a pharmacy technician. A grasp of general medical terminology, although perhaps less vital, also is very beneficial and can help the technician be more helpful and productive.

Learning medical terminology may seem like learning a whole new language. Most medical terms, however, are built from a basic set of roots, prefixes, and suffixes that are easy to memorize and can be pieced together to form the words that create the body of medical text—including information found in the medication profile.

This chapter covers commonly used pharmacy terminology as well as the pharmacy abbreviations that make up the shorthand physicians use when communicating medication use directions to other health care providers. It also covers many of the word roots, prefixes, and suffixes that are combined to form some of the most useful and common medical terms.

This chapter is not a comprehensive review of the subject, but really only scratches the surface. It is, however, a good foundation on which to build and will serve the average pharmacy technician very well.

Pharmacy Terminology

Pharmacy personnel use a number of specialized terms in their work. An understanding of these terms helps make a technician efficient and capable.

Some of the terms are used to define classifications of drugs. For example, technicians must be able to differentiate between *generic* and *brand name* drugs. A generic name describes a unique chemical entity and can be applied to that entity regardless of its manufacturer. A brand name is trademarked by a manufacturer to identify its particular "brand" of that chemical entity. For example, Ancef® is a brand name product of the generic entity cefazolin.

Learning Objectives

After completing this chapter, the technician should be able to

1. Define terms unique to pharmacy practice.

2. Use abbreviations common to pharmacy practice.

3. Identify a basic set of word roots, prefixes, and suffixes with which to construct a variety of commonly used medical terms.

4. Define medical terms by breaking the words into their component parts.

5. Employ common medical terms.

Another pair of terms used to categorize drugs is *legend* and *over-the-counter*. A legend drug, also called a prescription drug, is one that may not be dispensed to the public except on the order of a physician or other licensed prescriber. The term comes from the federal legend that appears on the packaging: "Federal law prohibits dispensing this medication without a prescription." Over-the-counter medications are those that may be dispensed without a prescription.

Some terms are more typically seen in the institutional setting. For example, *D.U.E.* and *M.U.E.*, which stand for drug usage (or utilization) evaluation and medication usage (or utilization) evaluation, are organized studies of medication use that are common in hospitals but are not, in general, a part of retail practice.

The term *formulary* can be used in both institutional and retail settings. A formulary is a list of approved drugs available for use. In a hospital, it refers to the drugs that are stocked by the pharmacy and approved for use in the facility. In the retail setting, it refers to an approved drug list associated with a particular prescription benefit plan.

Pharmacy Abbreviations

Pharmacy abbreviations are commonly used as a kind of shorthand in prescriptions and medication orders to convey information about directions for use. The abbreviations are then "translated" in the prescription label. Most retail pharmacies expect their technicians to interpret prescriptions for entry into a computer system (or even a typewriter) to generate a label that the patient can read and understand. Pharmacy technicians in hospitals are often asked to interpret medication orders for entry into a patient profile. It is therefore essential that pharmacy technicians have a good grasp of this unique language pharmacists and physicians use.

The abbreviations for time and frequency of medication administration come from Latin phrases. Other commonly used abbreviations include those for routes of administration and those that designate units of measure. Lowercase Roman numerals are often used to denote a quantity, such as a number of tablets (i = one; ii = two). (See Chapter 5 for a complete discussion of Roman numerals.)

Another subset of abbreviations is called *x-substitutions* and includes the well-known and widely recognized *Rx* symbol meaning "prescription." Other

common x-substitutions are *dx* for "diagnosis" and *sx* for "symptoms."

Finally, a handful of symbols are used in prescriptions and medication orders. For example, the ° sign is used for "degree," the Greek letter delta Δ for "change," and < and > for "less than" and "greater than," respectively.

Table 8-1 lists a number of common pharmacy abbreviations, their meanings, and the Latin phrase from which the abbreviation was derived, if applicable.

Abbreviations in medical records and prescriptions are thought to be contributing factors in some medical errors. Some abbreviations should be discouraged, and, in fact, have been banned in many hospitals. One important example is the use of the letter *U* to abbreviate units. Because a *U* might be misread as a zero if sloppily written and could therefore result in a tenfold dosing error, the Institute for Safe Medication Practices recommends it never be used as an abbreviation in prescriptions or medication orders; the word *units* should always be written out in its entirety.[1] Other abbreviations that are considered unsafe by some are *q.d., q.i.d.,* and *q.o.d.,* which may be indistinguishable from each other if legibility is poor. These three abbreviations are included in this chapter, however, because they are still widely used.

The Joint Commission on Accreditation of Healthcare Organizations (JCAHO) requires hospitals to have and enforce a list of prohibited abbreviations to improve patient safety. This requirement, however, does not extend to the outpatient environment, and although some potentially "risky" abbreviations are being phased out in hospitals, they are still in common use in retail pharmacies.

Medical Terminology

Many medical terms are built from component parts called word roots, prefixes, and suffixes. The root is the base component of the word, which is modified by the addition of a prefix or suffix. Prefixes are modifying components placed in front of the word root. Examples include pre-, post-, and sub-. Suffixes appear at the end of the word root and are connected to the root by a combining vowel, for example, -ism, -itis, -ous.

Tables 8-2, 8-3, and **8-4** cover many of the most common word roots, prefixes, and suffixes that will assist the technician in understanding medical terminology. The Self-Assessment Test will help the technician practice defining words by breaking them into their component parts.

The process of defining a medical term starts with identifying and defining the components and then combining those definitions into a coherent whole. For example, consider the word *bronchoscopy*. First, divide the word into its components: "bronch/o" and "-scopy." Then, define each of the parts: *bronch/o* means bronchus, and *-scopy* means the process of viewing. Therefore, bronchoscopy means the process of viewing the bronchus.

What is the definition of *electrocardiogram*? First, break the word into its parts: "electro-," "cardi/o," and "-gram." Second, define each part: *electro-* means electricity, *cardi/o* means heart, and *-gram* means record. Finally, put the definitions together to get the complete definition of the word: recording the electrical activity of the heart.

TABLE 8-1. ABBREVIATIONS

Abbreviation	Meaning	Latin Phrase	Abbreviation	Meaning	Latin Phrase
a	before	*ante*	OS	left eye	
a.c.	before meals	*ante cibum*	OTC	over-the-counter	
ad lib	as desired	*ad libitum*	OU	both eyes	
AD	right ear		oz	ounce	
AS	left ear		p	post	*post*
AU	both ears		p.c.	after meals	*post cibum*
b.i.d.	twice a day	*bis in die*	p.o.	by mouth	*per os*
bx	biopsy		pr	per rectum	
c	with	*cum*	p.r.n.	as needed	*pro re nata*
cc	cubic centimeter		pt	pint	
dr	dram		q.	every	*quaque*
dx	diagnosis		q.a.m.	every morning	
fx	fracture		q.d.	every day	*quaque die*
g	gram		q.h.	every hour	*quaque hora*
gr	grain		q2h, q3h, etc.	every 2 hours, etc	
gtt	drop		q.i.d.	4 times a day	*quarter in die*
h	hour		q.o.d.	every other day	
hr	hour		qt	quart	
h.s.	at bedtime	*hora somni*	rx, Rx	prescription	
hx	history		s	without	*sine*
ID	intradermal(ly)		sc, S.C., s.q., subq	subcutaneous	
IM	intramuscular(ly)		ss	one half	
IU	international unit		stat	immediately	
IV	intravenous(ly)		supp	suppository	
IVPB	IV piggyback		sx	symptoms	
kg	kilogram		T, Tbsp	tablespoon	
L	liter		t, tsp	teaspoon	
lb	pound		t.i.d.	3 times a day	*ter in die*
mcg	microgram		T.O.	telephone order	
mEq	milliequivalent		tr	tincture	
mg	milligram		tx	treatment	
ml	milliliter		ung	ointment	
OD	right eye		VO	verbal order	

TABLE 8-2. PREFIXES

Prefix	Meaning	Prefix	Meaning
a-; an-; ana-	no; not; without	micro-	small
ab-	away from	multi-	many
ante-	before; forward	neo-	new
anti-	against	non-	not
auto-	self	oligo-	few; less
bi-	two; double; both	pan-	all
brady-	slow	para-	near; beside
carcin-	cancerous	per-	through
contra-	against; opposite	peri-	around; surrounding
dys-	difficult; painful	poly-	many
ect-	outside; out	post-	after
en-	within; in	pre-	before; in front of
endo-	within	primi-	first
epi-	above; upon	retro-	behind; backward; upward
ex-	out	semi-	half
gynec/o-	woman	sub-	below; under
hemi-	half	super-	above; over; excess
hyper-	above; excess	supra-	above, on top of
hypo-	below; deficient	sym-	with
infra-	below; inferior	syn-	together; with
inter-	between	tachy-	fast
intra-	within	tri-	three
iso-	same; equal	uni-	one
macro-	large	xero-	dry
mal-	bad; poor; abnormal		
meta-	change; after; beyond		

TABLE 8-3. SUFFIXES

Suffix	Meaning	Suffix	Meaning
-ac; -al; -ar; -ary	pertaining to	-globin; -globulin	protein
-algia	pain	-gram	record
-cele	hernia; herniation	-graph	instrument for recording
-centesis	surgical puncture	-graphy	process of recording
-crine	to secrete	-ia; -iac; -ic	pertaining to
-crit	to separate	-ism	condition
-cyte	cell	-itis	inflammation of
-cytosis	condition of cells	-lysis; -lytic	break down
-desis	binding together	-malacia	softening
-ectomy	surgical removal; excision	-megaly	enlargement
-emesis	vomiting	-oid	resembling; like
-emia	blood	-(o)logist	specialist
-genesis; -genic; -gen	producing; forming		

Cont'd

Table 8-3 cont'd

Suffix	Meaning	Suffix	Meaning
-(o)logy	study of	-poiesis	formation
-oma	tumor	-r/rhage; -r/rhagia	bursting forth
-osis	abnormal condition	-rrhea	flow; discharge
-ostomy	creation of an opening	-rhexis	rupture
-otomy	incision into	-sclerosis	hardening
-ous	pertaining to	-scope	instrument for viewing
-paresis	paralysis	-scopy	process of viewing
-pathy	disease	-somnia	sleep
-penia	decreased number	-spasm	twitch
-pepsia	digestion	-stasis	control; stop
-phagia	eating; swallowing	-stenosis	narrowing
-phobia	abnormal fear	-therapy	treatment
-phonia	voice; sound	-thorax	chest; pleural cavity
-phoresis	carrying; transmission	-tocia	labor; birth
-phoria	feeling; mental state	-tripsy	crushing
-plasty	surgical repair	-trophy	growth; development
-plegia	paralysis	-tropin	nourish; develop; stimulate
-pnea	breathing		

TABLE 8-4. WORD ROOTS

Root	Meaning	Root	Meaning
abdomin/o	abdomen	carcin/o	cancer
aden/o	gland	cardi/o	heart
adip/o	fat	carp/o	wrist bones
amnio	amnion	cephal/o	head
andr/o	male; man	cerebr/o	cerebrum
angi/o	vessel	chol/e	bile; gall
aque/o	watery	cholangi/o	bile duct
arteri/o	artery	cholecyst/o	gallbladder
arteriol/o	arteriole	chondr/o	cartilage
arthr/o	joint	coagul/o	clotting
ather/o	fat; fatty plaque	cochle/o	cochlea
audi/o	hearing; sound	col/o	colon
aur/o	ear	conjuctiv/o	conjunctiva
bili	bile; gall	cor/o	heart
blephar/o	eyelid	corne/o	cornea
bronch/o	bronchus	coron/o	heart
bronchiol/o	bronchiliole	cost/o	rib
bucc/o	cheek	crani/o	cranium; skull
burs/o	joint	cry/o	cold
calc/i	calcium	cut/o, cuti	skin
capnia	carbon dioxide	cutane/o	skin

Cont'd

Table 8-4 cont'd

Root	Meaning	Root	Meaning
cyan/o	blue	hydr/o	water; fluid
cyst/o	bladder, sac, urinary bladder	hyster/o	uterus
cyt/o	cell	ile/o	ileum
dacry/o	tears	ili/o	ilium
dent	tooth	immune/o	protection
derm/o	skin	is/o	equal
dermat/o	skin	jejun/o	jejunum
dipl/o	two; double	kal/i	potassium
dips/o	thirst	kinesi/o	movement
duoden/o	duodenum	lacrim/o	tears
dur/a	dura mater	lact/o	milk
electr/o	electricity	lapar/o	abdominal wall
embry/o	embryo	laryng/o	larynx
encephal/o	brain	ligament/o	ligament
enter/o	intestines	lingua	tongue
eosin/o	red	lip/o	fat
epis/i	vulva	lith/o	stone
erythr/o	red	lumb/o	lower back
esophag/o	esophagus	lymph/o	lymph
fasci/o	fascia	mamm/o	breast
femor/o	femur	mast/o	breast
fet/o; fet/i	fetus	melan/o	black
fibul/o	fibula	men/o	menses; menstruation
fund/o	fundus	metacarp/o	hand bones
gastr/o	stomach	metatars/o	foot bones
gingiv/o	gums	morph/o	form; shape
glauc/o	silver; gray	muc/o	mucus
gli/o	nerve cell	my/o	muscle
glomerul/o	glomerulus	myc/o	fungus
gloss/o	tongue	myel/o	bone marrow; spinal cord
gluc/o	glucose; sugar	miring/o	eardrum
glyc/o	glucose; sugar	narc/o	sleep
gonad/o	sex glands	nas/o	nose
gravid/a, gravid/o	pregnancy	nat/o, natal	birth, delivery
gyn/o, gyn/e	woman	nephr/o	kidney
gynec/o	woman	neur/o	nerve
hem/o	blood	noct/o	night
hemangi/o	blood vessel	nyctal/o	night
hemat/o	blood	ocul/o	eye
hepat/o	liver	onych/o	nail
hidr/o	sweat	oophor/o	ovary
humer/o	humerus	ophthalm/o	eye

Cont'd

Table 8-4 cont'd

Root	Meaning	Root	Meaning
opt/o	eye	rect/o	rectum
or/o	mouth	ren/o	kidney
orch/o	testis; testicle	retin/o	retina
orchi/o	testis; testicle	rhabdomy/o	skeletal muscle; striated muscle
orchid/o	testis; testicle	rheum	watery discharge
orth/o	straight	rhin/o	nose
oste/o	bone	salping/o	fallopian tubes
ot/o	ear	sarc/o	flesh
ovari/o	ovary	semin/o	semen
oxi	oxygen	septi	bacteria
pachy/o	thick	sial/o	saliva
pancreat/o	pancreas	sinus/o	sinus
par/o	bear; labor; childbirth	somat/o	body
part/o	bear; labor; childbirth	spermat/o	sperm
patell/o	kneecap	spher/o	round
pector/o	chest	sphygm/o	pulse
ped	children	spir/o	breathe; breath
pelv/i	pelvis	splen/o	spleen
perine/o	perineum	spondyl/o	vertebra; vertebral column
peritone/o	peritoneum	steth/o	chest
phag/o	eat	stoma, stomat/o	mouth
phalang/o	finger and toe bones	synovi/o	joint
pharyng/o	pharynx	tars/o	ankle bones
phleb/o	vein	ten/o; tend/o	tendon
phot/o	light	tendon/o; tendin/o	tendon
phren/o	diaphragm	test/o	testis; testicle
pil/o	hair	testicul/o	testis; testicle
pneum/o	lung; air	thorac/o	chest
pod/o, podi	foot	thromb/o	clot
proct/o	rectum	thyr/o	thyroid gland
psych/o, psych/i	mind or soul	trache/o	trachea
pub/o	pubis; pubic bone	tympan/o	eardrum
pulmon/o	lungs	urethr/o	urethra
py/o	pus	ur/o	urinary tract
pyel/o	renal pelvis	vas/o	vessel
quadr/i	four	ven/o	vein
radi/o	radius	xanth/o	yellow

[1]ISMP List of Error Prone Abbreviations, Symbols, and Dose Designations. November 27, 2003. ISMP Medication Safety Alert. Institute for Safe Medication Practices. As viewed 7/7/04. http://www.ismp.org/PDF/ErrorProne.pdf.

Self-Assessment Questions

1. Match the following with the correct meaning.

Abbreviations

a) bid   every
b) ac   milliliter
c) po   twice a day
d) prn   before meals
e) tid   kilogram
f) IM   by mouth
g) q   hour
h) kg   intramuscular
i) ml   three times daily
j) h   as needed

Prefixes

a) cyano   white
b) brady   fast
c) poly   difficult
d) mega   half
e) hypo   blue
f) tachy   few, less
g) semi   much; many
h) oligo   great
i) leuko   slow
j) dys   under; below

Suffixes

a) itis   lack
b) megaly   study of
c) algia   measurement
d) gram   inflammation
e) metry   blood
f) penia   process of viewing
g) rrhea   enlargement
h) emia   pain
i) logy   record
j) scopy   discharge

Word Roots

a) cephal   mind or soul
b) arthro   nose
c) mammo   nerve
d) gastro   muscle
e) nephro   gall bladder
f) hepato   cancer
g) osteo   gland
h) neuro   head
i) rhino   breast
j) thoraco   joint
k) psych   stomach
l) lacrimo   sweet; sugar
m) chole   bile
n) glyco   kidney
o) bili   electric
p) aden   chest
q) carcino   liver
r) electro   tear duct
s) vaso   bone
t) myo   vessel

2. Provide definitions for the following words by breaking them into component parts.

Skin, Skeletal, and Muscular System:

a) Dermatitis _____

b) Percutaneous _____

c) Sarcoma _____

d) Intercostal _____

e) Orthopedics _____

f) Patellectomy _____

g) Arthralgia _____

h) Bursitis _____

i) Bradykinesia _____

j) Suprapubic _____

k) Intramuscular _____

l) Epidermal _____

m) Xeroderma _____

n) Myalgia _____

Self-Assessment Questions

o) Chondromalacia _____

p) Onychomycosis _____

q) Subcutaneous _____

r) Arthritis _____

s) Tendinitis _____

t) Dermatologist _____

u) Craniotomy _____

v) Arthroscopy _____

w) Electromyogram _____

x) Osteomyelitis _____

Cardiovascular and Respiratory Systems, and Blood:

a) Cardiologist _____

b) Myeloma _____

c) Anoxia _____

d) Pulmonologist _____

e) Tachycardia _____

f) Thoracentesis _____

g) Endarterectomy _____

h) Dyspnea _____

i) Leukocytopenia _____

j) Angiography _____

k) Thrombophlebitis _____

l) Myocarditis _____

m) Cardiomyopathy _____

n) Hypoxemia _____

o) Arteriogram _____

p) Laryngoscope _____

q) Rhinoplasty _____

r) Septicemia _____

s) Pericardium _____

t) Bronchoscopy _____

u) Bradycardia _____

v) Rhinorrhea _____

w) Lymphoma _____

x) Cardiomegaly _____

Digestive and Endocrine Systems:

a) Colonoscopy _____

b) Gingivitis _____

c) Sublingual _____

d) Endocrinology _____

e) Hyperthyroidism _____

f) Endoscopic _____

g) Cholecystectomy _____

h) Hypokalemia _____

i) Dysphagia _____

j) Nasogastric _____

k) Thyroidectomy _____

l) Hepatitis _____

m) Gastroenterology _____

n) Polydipsia _____

o) Hyperglycemia _____

p) Pancreatitis _____

q) Hematemesis _____

r) Lithotripsy _____

s) Hyperemesis _____

t) Exophthalmia _____

Urinary and Reproductive Systems:

a) Nocturia _____

b) Spermatogenesis _____

c) Orchidectomy _____

d) Mammogram _____

e) Antepartum _____

f) Pyuria _____

g) Dysmenorrhea _____

h) Hysterectomy _____

i) Dysuria _____

j) Primigravida _____

k) Oliguria _____

l) Cystoscopy _____

m) Urology _____

n) Hydrocele _____

o) Nephritis _____

p) Menorrhagia _____

q) Hematuria _____

r) Gynecologist _____

s) Embryology _____

t) Amniocentesis _____

Nervous System and Sensory Organs:

a) Blepharitis _____

b) Cerebrospinal _____

c) Paraplegia _____

d) Retinitis _____

e) Hydrocephalus _____

f) Audiometry _____

g) Cerebrovascular _____

h) Myringitis _____

i) Meningitis _____

j) Conjunctivitis _____

k) Myelogram _____

l) Epidural _____

m) Intraocular _____

n) Electroencephalogram _____

o) Otalgia _____

p) Hemiparesis _____

q) Tympanoplasty _____

r) Neuralgia _____

s) Ophthalmologist _____

t) Otorhinolaryngologist _____

3. Interpret the following examples of abbreviations used prescriptions and orders.
   a) Take ii tabs tid pc
   b) Ibuprofen 200mg q4h prn temp > 101°
   c) Take i cap hs prn for sleep
   d) Cefazolin 1g IVPB q8h
   e) Mix 2 tbs in 4 oz of water and take po qid
   f) Heparin 5000 units SQ q12h
   g) Instill iii gtt OD bid
   h) Rocephin 250mg IM STAT
   i) Take i tab ac&hs
   j) Acetaminophen 10mg/kg prn pain

Self-Assessment Answers

1. Matching

Abbreviations

a) bid — twice a day
b) ac — before meals
c) po — by mouth
d) prn — as needed
e) tid — three times daily
f) IM — intramuscular
g) q — every
h) kg — kilogram
i) ml — milliliter
j) h — hour

Prefixes

a) cyano — blue
b) brady — slow
c) poly — much; many
d) mega — great
e) hypo — under; below
f) tachy — fast
g) semi — half
h) oligo — few; less
i) leuko — white
j) dys — difficult

Suffixes

a) itis — inflammation
b) megaly — enlargement
c) algia — pain
d) gram — record
e) metry — measurement
f) penia — lack
g) rrhea — discharge
h) emia — blood
i) logy — study
j) scopy — process of viewing

Word Roots

a) cephal — head
b) arthro — joint
c) mammo — breast
d) gastro — stomach
e) nephro — kidney
f) hepato — liver
g) osteo — bone
h) neuro — nerve
i) rhino — nose
j) thoraco — chest
k) psych — mind or soul
l) lacrimo — tear duct

m) chole — gall bladder
n) glyco — sweet; sugar
o) bili — bile
p) aden — gland
q) carcino — cancer
r) electro — electric
s) vaso — vessel
t) myo — muscle

2. Definitions

Skin, Skeletal, and Muscular Systems

a) Dermatitis: Inflammation of the skin; derm/a, dermat/o = skin; itis = inflammation

b) Percutaneous: Pertaining to through the skin; per = through; cutane/o = skin; ous = pertaining to

c) Sarcoma: Tumor of the flesh; sarc = flesh; oma = tumor

d) Intercostal: Pertaining to between the ribs; inter = between; cost/a = rib; al = pertaining to

e) Orthopedics: Literally means pertaining to straight foot—pertaining to the study of diseases of the skeletal and muscular system; orth/o = straight; ped = foot; ics = pertaining to

f) Patellectomy: Surgical removal of the kneecap; patell/o = kneecap; ectomy = surgical removal

g) Arthralgia: Joint pain; arthr/o = joint; algia = pain

h) Bursitis: Inflammation of the joint; burs/o = joint; itis = inflammation

i) Bradykinesia: Slow movement; brady = slow; kinesia = movement

j) Suprapubic: Pertaining to above the pubic bone; supra = above; pub/i = pubic bone; ic = pertaining to

k) Intramuscular: Pertaining to within the muscle; intra = within; muscul/o = muscle; ar = pertaining to

l) Epidermal: Pertaining to on the skin; epi = on, upon; derm = skin; al = pertaining to

m) Xeroderma: Dry skin; xero = dry; derma = skin

n) Myalgia: Muscle pain; my/o = muscle; algia = pain

o) Chondromalacia: Softening of the cartilage; chondro = cartilage; malacia = softening

p) Onychomycosis: Fungal infection of the nail; onycho = nail; myc/o = fungus; osis = abnormal condition

q) Subcutaneous: Pertaining to below the skin; sub = under; cutane/o = skin; ous = pertaining to

r) Arthritis: Inflammation of the joints; arthr/o = joint; itis = inflammation

s) Tendinitis: Inflammation of the tendon; tendin/o = tendon; itis = inflammation

t) Dermatologist: Specialist in the diseases of the skin; dermat/o = skin; ologist = specialist

u) Craniotomy: Surgical incision of the skull; crani/o = skull; otomy = surgical incision

v) Arthroscopy: Process of viewing the joint; arthr/o = joint; scopy = process of viewing

w) Electromyogram: Record of the electrical activity of a muscle; electro = electric; my/o = muscle; gram = record

x) Osteomyelitis: Inflammation of the bone and bone marrow; oste/o = bone; myel/o = bone marrow; itis = inflammation

Cardiovascular and Respiratory Systems and Blood

a) Cardiologist: Specialist in diseases of the heart; cardi/o = heart; ologist = specialist

b) Myeloma: Tumor of the bone marrow; myel/o = bone marrow; oma = tumor

c) Anoxia: Without oxygen; a = not, without; oxi/a = oxygen

d) Pulmonologist: Specialist in diseases of the lungs; pulmon/o = lungs; ologist = specialist

e) Tachycardia: Pertaining to a fast heart; tachy = fast; cardi/a = heart; ia = pertaining to

f) Thoracentesis: Surgical puncture of the chest; thora = chest; centesis = surgical puncture

g) Endarterectomy: Surgical removal of the inside of an artery; end = within; arter/o = artery; ectomy = surgical removal

h) Dyspnea: Difficulty breathing; dys = difficult, painful; pnea = breathing

i) Leukocytopenia: Too few white blood cells; leuko = white; cyt/o = cell; penia = few

j) Angiography: Process of recording a vessel (via x-ray); angio = vessel; graphy = process of recording

k) Thrombophlebitis: Inflammation of a vein due to blood clot formation; thromb/o = clot; phleb = vein; itis = inflammation

l) Myocarditis: Inflammation of the heart muscle; my/o = muscle; cardi/o = heart; itis = inflammation

m) Cardiomyopathy: Disease of the heart muscle; cardi/o = heart; my/o = muscle; pathy = disease

n) Hypoxemia: Too little oxygen in the blood; hypo = little; ox/e = oxygen; emia = blood

o) Arteriogram: Record of an artery; arteri/o = artery; gram = record

p) Laryngoscope: Instrument for viewing the larynx; laryng/o = larynx; scope = instrument for viewing

q) Rhinoplasty: Surgical repair of the nose; rhin/o = nose; plasty = surgical repair

r) Septicemia: Bacterial infection of the blood; septi = bacteria; c/emia = blood

s) Pericardium: Lining around the outside of the heart; peri = around; cardi/o = heart

t) Bronchoscopy: Process of viewing the bronchus; bronch/o = bronchus; scopy = process of viewing

u) Bradycardia: Pertaining to a slow heart; brady = slow; cardi/o = heart; ia = pertaining to

v) Rhinorrhea: Discharge from the nose; rhino = nose; rrhea = discharge

w) Lymphoma: Tumor of the lymphatic system; lymph/o = lymph; oma = tumor

x) Cardiomegaly: Enlarged heart; cardi/o = heart; megaly = enlarged

Digestive and Endocrine Systems

a) Colonoscopy: Process of viewing the colon; colon/o = colon; scopy = process of viewing

b) Gingivitis: Inflammation of the gums; gingival = gums; itis = inflammation

c) Sublingual: Pertaining to under the tongue; sub = under; lingua = tongue; al = pertaining to

d) Endocrinology: Study of the secreting glands that make up the endocrine system; end/o = within; crine = to secrete; ology = study of

e) Hyperthyroidism: Condition of too much thyroid hormone; hyper = too much; thyroid/o = thyroid; ism = condition

f) Endoscopic: Pertaining to the process of viewing within; end/o = within; scopy = process of viewing; ic = pertaining to

g) Cholecystectomy: Surgical removal of the gall bladder; chole = gall bladder; cyst/o = sac, bladder; ectomy = surgical removal

h) Hypokalemia: Low blood potassium; hypo = below or deficient; kal = potassium; emia = blood

Self-Assessment Answers

i) Dysphagia: Pertaining to difficulty in eating; dys = difficult, painful; phage = eating; ia = pertaining to

j) Nasogastric: Pertaining to the nose and the stomach (a tube that travels from the nose to the stomach); naso = nose; gastri = stomach; ic = pertaining to

k) Thyroidectomy: Surgical removal of the thyroid gland; thyroid/o = thyroid; ectomy = surgical removal of

l) Hepatitis: Inflammation of the liver; hepat/o = liver; itis = inflammation

m) Gastroenterology: Study of the stomach and intestines; gastro = stomach; enter/o = intestines; ology = study of

n) Polydipsia: Pertaining to excessive thirst; poly = much; dipso = thirst; ia = pertaining to

o) Hyperglycemia: Too much sugar in the blood; hyper = too much; glyc/o = sweet, sugar; emia = blood

p) Pancreatitis: Inflammation of the pancreas; pancreat/o = pancreas; itis = inflammation

q) Hematemesis: Bloody vomitus; heme = blood; emesis = vomit

r) Lithotripsy: Crushing of stones (such as kidney stones); lith/o = stone; tripsy = crushing

s) Hyperemesis: Excessive vomiting; hyper = too much; emesis = vomit

t) Exophthalmia: pertaining to a protuberance of the eye; ex/o = out; ophthalm/o = eye; ia = pertaining to

Urinary and Reproductive Systems

a) Nocturia: Too much urination at night; noct/o = night; uria = urine

b) Spermatogenesis: Creation of new sperm; spermat/o = sperm; genesis = new

c) Orchidectomy: Surgical removal of a testicle; orchid/o = testicle; ectomy = surgical removal

d) Mammogram: (X-ray) record of the breast; mamm/o = breast; gram = record

e) Antepartum: Before delivery; ante = before; partum = delivery

f) Pyuria: Pus in the urine; py/o = pus; uria = urine

g) Dysmenorrhea; Difficult or painful menstruation; dys = difficult, painful; men/o = menses; rrhea = discharge

h) Hysterectomy: Surgical removal of the uterus; hyster/o = uterus; ectomy = surgical removal

i) Dysuria: Difficult or painful urination; dys = difficult, painful; uria = urine

j) Primigravida: First pregnancy; primi = first; gravida = pregnancy

k) Oliguria: Too little urine; olig/o = little; uria = urine

l) Cystoscopy: Process of viewing the urinary bladder; cyst/o = sac, bladder; scopy = process of viewing

m) Urology: Study of the urinary tract; ur/o = urinary tract; ology = study of

n) Hydrocele: Accumulation of water in the scrotum; hydro = water; cele = hernia, herniation

o) Nephritis: Inflammation of the kidney; nephr/o = kidney; itis = inflammation

p) Menorrhagia: Excessive bleeding during menstruation; men/o = menses; rrhagia = bursting forth

q) Hematuria: Blood in the urine; hemat/o = blood; uria = urine

r) Gynecologist: Specialist in the diseases of the female reproductive system; gynec/o = woman; ologist = specialist

s) Embryology: Study of the growth and development of the human organism; embry/o = embryo; ology = study of

t) Amniocentesis : Surgical puncture of the amniotic sac; amnio = amnion; centesis = surgical puncture

Nervous System and Sensory Organs

a) Blepharitis: Inflammation of the eyelid; blephar/o = eyelid; itis = inflammation

b) Cerebrospinal: Pertaining to the brain and spinal cord; cerebr/o = cerebrum; spin/o = spine; al = pertaining to

c) Paraplegia: Paralysis of the lower half of the body; para = near, beside; plegia = paralysis

d) Retinitis: Inflammation of the retina; retin/o = retina; itis = inflammation

e) Hydrocephalus: Water in the brain; hydro = water; cephal/o = head

f) Audiometry: Measurement of the hearing; audi/o = hearing; metry = measurement

g) Cerebrovascular: Pertaining to the cerebrum and vessels; cerebr/o = cerebrum; vascul/o = vessels; ar = pertaining to

Self-Assessment Answers

h) Myringitis: Inflammation of the eardrum; myring/o = eardrum; itis = inflammation

i) Meningitis: Inflammation of the meninges; mening/o = meninges; itis = inflammation

j) Conjunctivitis: Inflammation of the conjunctiva; conjunctiv/a = conjunctiva; itis = inflammation

k) Myelogram: Record of a nerve; myel/o = nerve; gram = record

l) Epidural: Pertaining to above the dura mater; epi = above; dur/a = dura mater; al = pertaining to

m) Intraocular: Pertaining to the inside of the eye; intra = inside; ocul/o = eye; ar = pertaining to

n) Electroencephalogram: Record of the electrical activity of the brain; electr/o = electric; en = in; cephal/o = head; gram = record

o) Otalgia: Earache; oto = ear; algia = pain

p) Hemiparesis: Paralysis limited to one side; hemi = half; paresis = paralysis

q) Tympanoplasty: Surgical repair of the eardrum; tympan/o = eardrum; plasty = surgical repair

r) Neuralgia: Nerve pain; neur/o = nerve; algia = pain

s) Ophthalmologist: Specialist in diseases of the eye; ophthalm/o = eye; ologist = specialist

t) Otorhinolaryngologist: Specialist in the diseases of the ear, nose, and throat; oto = ear; rhino = nose; laryng/o = larynx (throat); ologist = specialist

3. Abbreviations used in prescriptions and orders

a) Take two tablets 3 times daily after meals

b) Ibuprofen 200 milligrams every 4 hours as needed for temperature greater than 101 degrees

c) Take one capsule at bedtime as needed for sleep

d) Cefazolin 1 gram intravenous piggyback every 8 hours

e) Mix 2 tablespoons in 4 ounces of water and take by mouth 4 times daily

f) Heparin 5000 units subcutaneously every 12 hours

g) Instill three drops in right eye 2 times daily

h) Rocephin 250 milligrams intramuscularly immediately

i) Take one tablet before meals and at bedtime

j) Acetaminophen 10 milligrams per killigram as needed for pain

Interpreting Medication Orders and Prescriptions

LINDA Y. FRED

This chapter will describe the technician's role in evaluating and processing medication orders and prescriptions from the time they are received until the medications leave the pharmacy. The differences between the process in the inpatient and outpatient settings will be discussed as well. The differences will be covered in separate sections on inpatient and outpatient settings, but for a complete understanding of the topic, it is recommended that both sections be reviewed. Additional information specific to one setting or the other is offered in the Institutional Pharmacy Practice and Ambulatory Pharmacy Practice chapters.

Typically, the term *medication order* refers to a written request on a physician's order form or a transcribed verbal or telephone order in an inpatient setting. This order becomes part of the patient's medical record. The term *prescription* refers to a medication order on a prescription blank to be filled in an outpatient or ambulatory care setting. Medication orders and prescriptions both represent a means for the prescriber to give instruction to the dispenser of the medication and those who will be administering it.

The specific roles fulfilled by technicians will vary from practice site to practice site. This text assumes that technicians will perform all processes they may legally be allowed to perform.

INPATIENT PHARMACY

Receiving Medication Orders

Medication orders come to the pharmacy in various ways. (See **Figure 9-1** for an example of a medication order.) They are hand-delivered to the pharmacy or one of its satellites or sent via some mechanical method, such as fax transmission or a pneumatic tube system. Orders may also be telephoned to the pharmacy by either the prescriber or an intermediary,

After completing this chapter, the technician should be able to

1. Identify the components of a complete prescription or medication order.

2. Prioritize prescriptions and medication orders on the basis of pertinent criteria.

3. Identify the necessary steps in processing a prescription or medication order.

4. List the information normally contained in a patient profile.

5. List the information needed to make a medication label complete.

6. Identify communication requirements related to processing an order or prescription.

Achieving these objectives will give the reader a basic understanding of medication order processing activities. However, actually performing these functions requires specialized training in the procedures of the specific practice site, such as the use of the organization's computer system or manual record-keeping system.

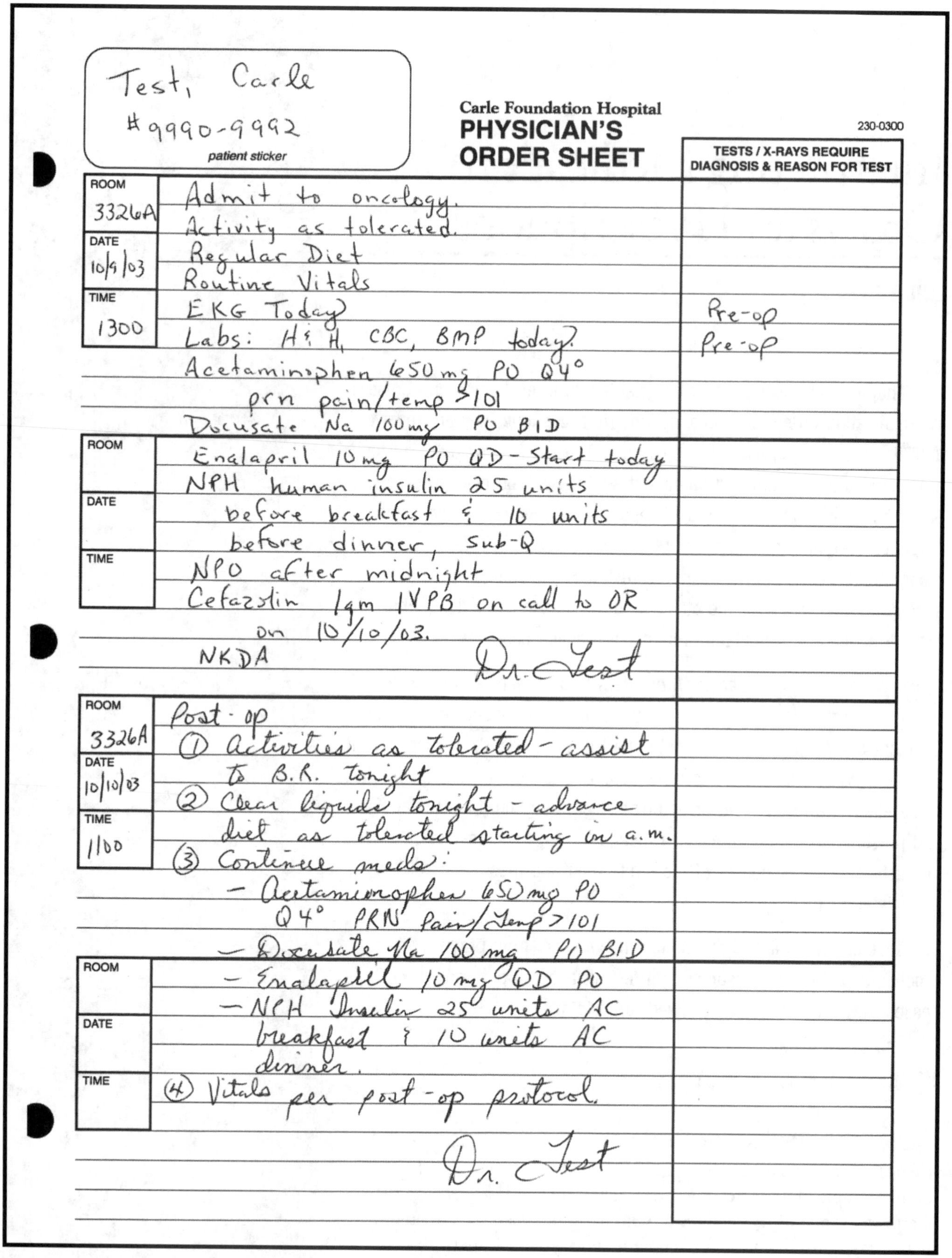

Test, Carle
#9990-9992

patient sticker

Carle Foundation Hospital
PHYSICIAN'S
ORDER SHEET

230-0300

	TESTS / X-RAYS REQUIRE DIAGNOSIS & REASON FOR TEST

ROOM 3326A
DATE 10/9/03
TIME 1300

Admit to oncology.
Activity as tolerated.
Regular Diet
Routine Vitals
EKG Today   Pre-op
Labs: H&H, CBC, BMP today.   Pre-op
Acetaminophen 650 mg PO Q4°
　　　prn pain/temp >101
Docusate Na 100 mg PO BID

ROOM
DATE
TIME

Enalapril 10 mg PO QD - Start today
NPH human insulin 25 units
　　before breakfast & 10 units
　　before dinner, sub-Q
NPO after midnight
Cefazolin 1 gm IVPB on call to OR
　　on 10/10/03.
NKDA   Dr. Test

ROOM 3326A
DATE 10/10/03
TIME 1100

Post-op
① Activities as tolerated - assist
　　to B.R. tonight
② Clear liquids tonight - advance
　　diet as tolerated starting in a.m.
③ Continue meds:
　　- Acetaminophen 650 mg PO
　　　Q4° PRN Pain/Temp >101

ROOM
DATE
TIME

　　- Docusate Na 100 mg PO BID
　　- Enalapril 10 mg QD PO
　　- NPH Insulin 25 units AC
　　breakfast & 10 units AC
　　dinner.
④ Vitals per post-op protocol.

　　　　　　　Dr. Test

Figure 9-1. Sample inpatient medication order from the medication chart.

such as a nurse. There are some legal restrictions on who may telephone in an order or a prescription and who may receive that information in the pharmacy, particularly when controlled substances are involved. Technicians should consult their employer's policies and procedures or their job descriptions to see what restrictions apply in their practice setting. Many states require that prescriptions be phoned in by the prescriber or licensed professional operating under the prescriber's authority. It is also commonly required that telephone prescriptions be received by a pharmacist or another licensed professional.

Upon receipt of a medication order, two steps should be taken. The first is to review the order for clarity and completeness. The second is to prioritize the order on the basis of a number of factors, including the time the medication is needed, the seriousness of the condition that is being treated, and the urgency of the other medication orders waiting to be processed.

Clarity and Completeness

When a new order is received, the first step is to ensure the order is clear and complete. Ideally, every medication order should contain the following elements:

- Patient name, hospital identification number, and room/bed location

- Generic drug name (it is recommended that generic drug names be used, and many institutions have policies to this effect)

- Brand drug name (if a specific product is required)

- Route of administration (with some orders, the site of administration should also be included)

- Dosage form

- Dose/strength

- Frequency and duration of administration (if duration is pertinent—may be open-ended)

- Rate and time of administration, if applicable

- Indication for use of the medication

- Other instructions for the person administering the medication, such as whether it should be given with food or on an empty stomach

- Prescriber's name/signature and credentials (some hospitals require a printed name, physician number, or pager number in addition to the signature to assist with identification)

- Signature and credentials of person writing the order, if other than prescriber

- Date and time of the order

Some of this information is required by state law or by policy. As shown in Figure 9-1, however, not all of the elements are included in every order.

If information is missing—for example, the room number—the technician may be able to clarify the order without pharmacist intervention. However, some clarifications should involve the pharmacist. The pharmacist may wish to discuss with the prescriber the choice of medication or a potential interaction, for example. When an order is deferred for clarification, it is important to make sure the other caregivers (e.g., the nurse waiting to administer the medication) are aware of any anticipated delays.

Prioritization

Once orders are deemed clear and complete, they must be prioritized so that the most urgent orders are filled first. Prioritizing orders means comparing the urgency of new orders against the urgency of all the orders requiring attention. Prioritizing ensures that the most-needed orders will be processed first. Technicians can prioritize orders by evaluating the route, time of administration, type of drug, intended use of the drug, and patient-specific circumstances.

Additional clues about urgency can be gleaned from orders. For example, when surgery or some diagnostic procedure is indicated, such as in this order: "Give 1 g cefazolin IVPB 30 minutes prior to incision," the technician might consult the operating room schedule to determine the priority of the order. Some orders are designated as "stat" (abbreviation of *statim*, Latin for *immediately*), which indicates an urgent need. A prescriber may also designate that a medication is to be started "now" or "ASAP" (as soon as possible), or simply state "start today" or "start this morning." It is also necessary to consider whether a medication might already have been started prior to the pharmacy's receipt of the order—a first dose of an antibiotic administered in the emergency room prior to the patient's admission, for example. If no apparent urgency or specific time is denoted in the order, it may receive a lower priority. Most pharmacies, however, designate a standard amount of time it should take to process and deliver an order. A typical turnaround time for filling an order in an institutional setting might be 10 to 15 minutes for a stat order and 1 hour for a routine order.

If no specific designation about the urgency of a medication is given in the body of the order, technicians can use some assumptions to prioritize orders. Medications ordered for the initial treatment of pain, fever, or nausea and vomiting are generally high priority because of the desire to relieve the patient's discomfort. A regularly scheduled vitamin, on the other hand, would be a lower priority. Most of the decisions involved in prioritizing orders require some basic knowledge of the drugs and common sense. It is also helpful for technicians to be familiar with their hospital's specific policies regarding prioritization of orders. Some hospitals, for example, treat all orders from a particular unit—such as an intensive care unit—as urgent. Many hospitals have designated administration times for certain drugs, such as warfarin, that may alter prioritization of the order depending on the time the order is received. Policies vary from pharmacy to pharmacy, and technicians need to become familiar with the system of prioritization used at their institution.

Processing Medication Orders

After the order has been received, determined to be clear and complete, and prioritized, it is ready to be processed. Processing usually involves a computer, but some pharmacies still use a manual system (typewriters, pen and paper, profile cards, or notebooks). The discussion in this chapter will focus on computerized operations.

A number of steps are involved in processing an order. First, the patient must be positively identified to avoid dispensing medication for the wrong patient. Second, the order typically is compared against the patient's existing medication profile, or a new profile is created for the patient. Then, a number of order entry steps occur to update the patient's medication profile. These steps include such tasks as choosing the correct medication from the database, identifying the administration schedule, and entering any special instructions. (Later in this section, a step-by-step procedure walks the technician through the order entry process.) Finally, the medication must be selected, prepared, or compounded, checked, and dispensed for use.

Identifying the Patient

Identifying the patient entails comparing the patient identification on the medication order against the one in the patient profile system (i.e., the patient's computer record) to make sure they match. Although it

sounds like a very elementary task, its importance cannot be overstated, and the technician must pay an appropriate level of attention to this detail—particularly when dealing with very common names.

In an institutional setting, patient identification numbers are generally used. Most commonly, patients are identified by two numbers: a unique medical record number that distinguishes patients from one another and an account number that is specific to a transaction or set of transactions, such as an individual hospitalization. A patient's medical record number never changes, but account numbers change every time a patient is admitted to an institution. The account number may also be known by other names, such as a billing number, a financial number, or an admission number.

Some institutions are now using bar codes or magnetic strips to facilitate accuracy in verifying patient identification. As more hospitals employ electronic charting, the use of bar-coded or magnetic strip patient identifiers will play a larger role. In the meantime, many hospitals rely on a computer-generated adhesive label that is affixed to the documents or a printed name that is generated by an addressograph (a raised-letter registration card similar to a credit card).

When entering the order into the computer or other patient record, it is important to make sure the patient name matches the number and vice versa. It is easy to make errors when keying numbers, and some patients may have the same or very similar names. Occasionally, orders get marked with the wrong patient name, and checking the profile may prevent this error from causing any harm to the patient. Because of the possibility of an order being marked with a wrong patient name, it is also vital to ensure that each order makes sense for the patient by checking the order against the patient profile.

Creating, Maintaining, and Reviewing Patient Profiles

The pharmacy's patient profile is a fundamental tool that pharmacists use in reviewing orders. It is vital that pharmacists and technicians build and review patient profiles while they are processing medication orders. The following information is generally found in the hospital pharmacy's patient profile, although system capabilities may limit access to some components:

- Patient name and identification numbers
- Date of birth or age

- Sex
- Height and weight
- Certain lab values, such as creatinine clearance
- Admitting and secondary diagnoses (including pregnancy and lactation status)
- Name of parent or guardian, if applicable
- Room and bed number
- Names of admitting and consulting physicians
- Medication allergies; latex allergy; pertinent food allergies
- Medication history (current and discontinued medications; medications from a previous admission in some instances)
- Special considerations (e.g., foreign language, disability)
- Clinical comments (e.g., therapeutic monitoring, counseling notes)

Before orders are entered into a patient's profile, the profile should be reviewed in relation to the changes indicated on the new orders. In some cases, information in the profile may raise questions about whether the patient should receive the medication as it is prescribed. For example, the patient may be allergic to the medication or may already be on a similar medication. In addition, the profile may contain information that changes how the order will be processed or prioritized. For example, a new order may simply represent a change in administration time that does not require any additional dispensing. A technician who suspects that the prescribed medication is inappropriate for the patient should consult the pharmacist or follow the pharmacy's standard procedure for order clarification.

Processing medication orders involves adding a medication to a patient's regimen or modifying or discontinuing a previously ordered medication. Computerized systems make processing orders faster and more accurate because patient profiles can be created or modified easily and medication labels can be printed quickly, all within a single step. In manual systems, two separate steps are needed: the patient's profile is modified, and the medication labels are typed or handwritten separately. Generally, for safety reasons, labels and medication administration records (MARs; discussed later in the chapter) are not produced until the medication order entry/transcription process has been completed and verified.

Order Entry Steps

Selecting the Drug Product

Once the order has been compared against the profile, the technician can proceed with selecting the drug product indicated on the medication order. It is recommended that prescribers order drug products by generic name instead of brand name. However, drug products are often prescribed by either or both names, which can result in confusion. Abbreviations, although best avoided, are also sometimes used in ordering medications. Selecting drug products requires a working knowledge of both brand names and generic names—although most computer systems can search for either name—and a sensible approach to interpreting orders when abbreviations are used. When in doubt about a drug name or an abbreviation, however, it is always better to clarify the order with the prescriber, or the person who wrote the order if it was someone other than the prescriber. Patient safety must be protected, and making assumptions when interpreting orders is dangerous. Most pharmacies take special precautions to ensure accurate interpretation of prescriptions and medication orders involving look-alike and sound-alike drugs. For example, drugs that look alike are often stored in separate locations in the pharmacy.

With most pharmacy computer systems, drug products can be reviewed by scrolling through an alphabetical listing of the brand or generic names or by entering a code or mnemonic that is associated with the product name in the computer. For example, to enter an order for ampicillin 250 mg, the technician might enter the mnemonic, or drug code, "amp250," at the drug name prompt, and the following choices would appear:

1. amp250c ampicillin 250 mg capsule
2. amp250s ampicillin 250 mg/5 ml oral suspension
3. amp250i ampicillin 250 mg injection

Note that once the correct drug and strength are located, the correct dosage form for the route of administration must be selected. If the order were for a 250 mg/5 ml suspension, the proper choice would be number two. Not only is it important that the correct dosage form be chosen for the purposes of dispensing, but the dosage form often determines the type of label that prints from the pharmacy computer system— an IV label format is generally very different from a unit dose label format and includes different information (such as an expiration date for IVs).

Multiple dosage forms of the drug may make sense for an order. For example, the order "ampicillin 250mg po q6h" could be entered using either the "amp250c" mnemonic or the "amp250s" mnemonic. Patient and caregiver considerations must be taken into account when choosing the form of the drug to dispense. For example, when providing an oral medication, checking with the nurse or parent to determine if a young adolescent would prefer to swallow tablets or take a liquid medication is a common practice in the institutional setting. Providing liquid forms of oral medications when patients are receiving drugs through tubes (nasogastric tubes, gastric tubes, etc.) is another opportunity to tailor dispensing to the needs of patients and caregivers.

In some institutions, the technician may enter only those drugs approved for use in the institution (i.e., formulary drugs). Input from the pharmacist is often required to process an order for a medication not approved for use in the institution (nonformulary drugs).

Many computer systems alert the operator if he or she attempts to enter medications that interact with pre-existing orders, conflict with the patient's drug allergies, represent therapeutic duplications, or are nonformulary drugs. Many systems also check the dosage range and alert the operator if he or she enters a dose that exceeds the recommended dose for that patient. Although these alert systems help prevent errors, they are not always relevant to the patient's situation. Therefore, the technician should consult the pharmacist when the alert is posted. The pharmacist may bypass the alert on the basis of his or her professional judgment, or may call the prescriber and ask to change the order. Technicians should know and follow the procedure at their practice site regarding computer alerts.

Besides just choosing the "correct drug" as has been outlined in this section, some other related choices are included in this step. For example, if an IV medication is being entered, it might be necessary to choose the correct diluent into which the drug is to be mixed. Most hospitals have standard diluents that are used for IV compounding, and in a computerized system, the diluent will often automatically load with the drug.

Another decision is the choice of the correct package type and size, such as bulk or unit dose, 15 gram tube or 30 gram tube, 100 ml bottle or 150 ml bottle.

Scheduling Medication Administration Times

Scheduling medication administration times can have an impact on drug efficacy or other treatment factors, such as diagnostic laboratory testing, and this impact can be important for some medications. The timing of gentamicin in relation to a laboratory test to measure the amount of drug circulating in the blood, for example, might effect a dose adjustment by the pharmacist or physician. Many drugs should be given at specific times in relation to meals for the best effect. In institutions, standard medication administration times are generally set. These times are often defined by institutional policy or by a drug therapy protocol. Such policies and protocols may define times for common dosing frequencies, such as "every day" (e.g., qd = 0800, bid = 0900 and 1700), or a specific administration time for certain drugs (e.g., warfarin may be administered at a set time to coincide with laboratory blood draws). These schedules are usually based on therapeutic issues, nursing efficiency, or coordination of services. Pharmacy, nursing, and the hospital's medical staff usually agree on standard administration schedules and protocols. Many pharmacies have a written document that staff can refer to when the appropriate administration time is unclear. These times are usually conveyed on the pharmacy's patient profile, on medication labels, and on the MAR. Pharmacy technicians should be sure to choose the correct medication administration schedule.

Standardized administration times usually appear as default entries associated with a particular drug or administration schedule that was selected in the computer during the order entry process. This means that if a "bid" administration schedule were entered for a particular drug, the computer would automatically assign its standard administration times, which could be 0900 and 1700.

Default time schedules may differ on some specialized nursing units. For example, scheduling for "q12h" may default to 0900 and 2100; however, a pediatrics unit might require administration to start when the order is received and then every 12 hours thereafter. During order entry, the technician must be aware of such exceptions and change the default entries when necessary.

When scheduling medication administration times for a new medication, pharmacists also consider other medications the patient is taking. This consideration is critical. For example, if a patient is taking both digoxin and milk of magnesia, there must be an adequate amount of time between the doses of each agent. If these medications are taken too close together, the milk of magnesia can reduce the amount of digoxin the patient absorbs. The resulting reduced absorption of digoxin could render therapy ineffective.

Another consideration is day or days of the week that a medication is due. Medications are sometimes ordered to be given every other day, every 3 days, or 3 days a week. In these instances, it is important to coordinate with the patient's home schedule if this is a continuation of home therapy. One must also be careful with every other day orders and advising the caregiver to give the medication on odd days or even days. Depending on the number of days in a month, every other day will change with respect to odd/even. Another example is estrogen and progesterone hormone replacement therapy in postmenopausal women. The start and stop dates for both medications must be clear. An example of a good approach is, "Take conjugated estrogens 0.625 mg by mouth on days 1–25 of each calendar month. Take medroxyprogesterone 5 mg by mouth on days 16–25 of each calendar month." Note how this set of instructions differs from "Take conjugated estrogens 0.625 mg for 25 days each month and medroxyprogesterone 5 mg for 10 days each month."

Special Instructions

The prescriber's directions for proper use of the medications must be conveyed clearly and accurately. In the hospital setting, the style used to convey the prescriber's directions is geared toward another health care professional at the bedside. More medical abbreviations are used, and information may be in a kind of shorthand that might be difficult for a patient to interpret. As shown later in this chapter in the discussion of ambulatory care, the style is vastly different when the end user is a patient or family member.

In institutions, physicians' orders are input into the patient profile in the pharmacy information system. Then pharmacy technicians generate MARs for nursing documentation (see **Figure 9-2**), medication profiles and fill lists (for pharmacy use), and labels for medications to be issued to patient care areas (see **Figure 9-3**). Because only health care personnel will use this information, the directions for use may contain only the name of the medication, strength, dose and schedule, and administration times, much of which may be written using medical terminology and Latin abbreviations. It is important to note that MARs may be either paper or electronic. Electronic systems are becoming more common and allow more efficient transfer and

sharing of information between the physician, the pharmacist, and the bedside nurse. For example, in an electronic system, it may be possible for the prescriber and pharmacist to tell from the record exactly when a medication has been administered simply by pulling it up on the computer. A traditional paper system would require going to the bedside to review the record.

Additional instructions for the caregiver are often entered into the pharmacy information system for presentation on one of the many documents printed from the profile (or for the nurses' use in an electronic system) or simply as additional information for the pharmacists' use at a later time. These special instructions might include storage information, such as the need to refrigerate, or special instructions, such as for chemotherapy drugs. Another example would be physician-specified parameters for use, such as "hold if systolic BP less than 100 mm Hg" or "repeat in 1 hour if ineffective." These types of instructions would typically be displayed on the MAR and also on the medication label.

Many pharmacy systems also allow for notes between the pharmacist and the technician to be displayed only on a fill list or work list. These instructions might include something like "reconstitute with normal saline only."

Most systems have a field or location in the pharmacy patient profile system where pharmacists can note clinical comments. Such comments may include indications for use, incidents of adverse drug reactions, laboratory values, or any other information that may

Figure 9-3. Sample inpatient labels to be used on a medication container sent to the patient care area or to update the MAR. (Note that these labels are for use by health care personnel and contain abbreviations, such as "ac," that a patient would not be likely to understand.)

MEDICATION ADMINISTRATION RECORD

SCHEDULED

DIAGNOSIS:
ALLERGIES: fta:DEMEROL INTOLERENCE,
fta:ERYHTROMYCIN CAUSES NAUSEA, SULFA,
PENICILLIN AND DERIVATIVES, SULFITES

ISOLATION: _____

Patient: **TEST, CARLE/OMNICELL**
Patient ID: 9990-9992
Admitted: 09/05/02
Physician: TEST, CERNER
Med Rec #: (00000)999-9999
Room: **3326-A**
Ht: 72.0 in Wt: 212.0 lb
Age: 44 yrs Sex: M

Start/Stop	Medication	Dose Route Freq	Time	NIGHT	DATE: 10/08/03 DAY	EVENING
10/08/03 1800	DOCUSATE SODIUM CAPSULE (COLACE 100MG CAPSULE) CATHARTICS AND LAXATIVES	100 MG / 1 CAP ORAL 2 TIMES A DAY	1800		OMNICELL	
10/08/03 1300	ENALAPRIL MALEATE 10MG TABLET (VASOTEC 10MG TAB) CARDIAC DRUGS	10 MG / 1 TAB ORAL EVERY DAY	1300			
10/08/03 1600	INSULIN HUMAN NPH INJECTION (NOVOLIN-N INSULIN) INSULINS 25 UNITS AC BREAKFAST; 10 AC DINNER ** USE FROM FLOOR STOCK **	25-0-10-0 S.C. 2 TIMES A DAY BEFORE MEALS	1600			

OMISSION CODES
1-NPO
2-N/V
3-GONE FROM UNIT
4-REFUSED

5-IV INCOMPAT
6-CHEMO/BLOOD
7-ON HOLD
8-CONDITION

9-MED NOT AVAILABLE
10-NO SITE
11-ABNORMAL VS/LAB VALUES
12-OTHER_____

SIGN RN

RN

SITE CODES

GLUTEAL	UPPER ARM	VENTRAL GLUTEAL	RECTUS FEMORIS	NOSTRIL
RIGHT-RG	RIGHT-RUA	RIGHT-RVG	RIGHT-RFR	RIGHT-RNOS
LEFT-LG	LEFT-LUA	LEFT-LVG	LEFT-RFL	LEFT-LNOS

US

DELTOID	VAS LATERALIS	UPPER THIGH	ABDOMINAL
RIGHT-RD	RIGHT-RVL	RIGHT-RUT	RIGHT-RUQ, RLQ
LEFT-LD	LEFT-LVL	LEFT-LUT	LEFT-LUQ, LLQ

Figure 9-2. Sample medication administration record (MAR).

Cont'd

MEDICATION ADMINISTRATION RECORD

PRN

Patient: **TEST, CARLE/OMNICELL**
Patient ID: 9990-9992
Admitted: 09/05/02
Physician: TEST, CERNER
Med Rec #: (00000)999-9999
Room: **3326-A**
Ht: 72.0 in   Wt: 212.0 lb
Age: 44 yrs   Sex: M

DIAGNOSIS:
ALLERGIES: fta:DEMEROL INTOLERENCE,
fta:ERYHTROMYCIN CAUSES NAUSEA, SULFA,
PENICILLIN AND DERIVATIVES, SULFITES

ISOLATION: _____

DATE: 10/08/03

Start/ Stop	Medication	Dose Route Freq	Time	NIGHT	DAY	EVENING
10/08/03 1253	ACETAMINOPHEN TABLET (TYLENOL 325MG TABLET) MISC ANALGESICS & ANTIPYRETICS DO NOT EXCEED 4GM ACETAMINOPHEN/24H PRN PAIN/TEMP>101	650 MG / 2 TAB ORAL EVERY 4 HOURS AS NEEDED	prn		OMNICELL	

OMISSION CODES
1-NPO   5-IV INCOMPAT   9-MED NOT AVAILABLE
2-N/V   6-CHEMO/BLOOD   10-NO SITE
3-GONE FROM UNIT 7-ON HOLD   11-ABNORMAL VS/LAB VALUES
4-REFUSED   8-CONDITION   12-OTHER_____

SIGN RN

RN

US

SITE CODES

GLUTEAL	UPPER ARM	VENTRAL GLUTEAL	RECTUS FEMORIS	NOSTRIL
RIGHT-RG	RIGHT-RUA	RIGHT-RVG	RIGHT-RFR	RIGHT-RNOS
LEFT-LG	LEFT-LUA	LEFT-LVG	LEFT-RFL	LEFT-LNOS
DELTOID	VAS LATERALIS	UPPER THIGH	ABDOMINAL	
RIGHT-RD	RIGHT-RVL	RIGHT-RUT	RIGHT-RUQ, RLQ	
LEFT-LD	LEFT-LVL	LEFT-LUT	LEFT-LUQ, LLQ	

Figure 9-2. Sample medication administration record (MAR).

Cont'd

MEDICATION ADMINISTRATION RECORD

LVP

DIAGNOSIS:
ALLERGIES: fta:DEMEROL INTOLERENCE,
fta:ERYHTROMYCIN CAUSES NAUSEA, SULFA,
PENICILLIN AND DERIVATIVES, SULFITES

ISOLATION: _____

Patient: **TEST, CARLE/OMNICELL**
Patient ID: 9990-9992
Admitted: 09/05/02
Physician: TEST, CERNER
Med Rec #: (00000)999-9999
Room: **3326-A**
Ht: 72.0 in   Wt: 212.0 lb
Age: 44 yrs   Sex: M

DATE: 10/08/03

Start/Stop	Medication	Dose Route Freq	Time	NIGHT	DAY	EVENING

OMISSION CODES
1-NPO
2-N/V
3-GONE FROM UNIT
4-REFUSED
5-IV INCOMPAT
6-CHEMO/BLOOD
7-ON HOLD
8-CONDITION
9-MED NOT AVAILABLE
10-NO SITE
11-ABNORMAL VS/LAB VALUES
12-OTHER_____

SIGN RN

RN

US

SITE CODES

GLUTEAL	UPPER ARM	VENTRAL GLUTEAL	RECTUS FEMORIS	NOSTRIL
RIGHT-RG	RIGHT-RUA	RIGHT-RVG	RIGHT-RFR	RIGHT-RNOS
LEFT-LG	LEFT-LUA	LEFT-LVG	LEFT-RFL	LEFT-LNOS

DELTOID	VAS LATERALIS	UPPER THIGH	ABDOMINAL
RIGHT-RD	RIGHT-RVL	RIGHT-RUT	RIGHT-RUQ, RLQ
LEFT-LD	LEFT-LVL	LEFT-LUT	LEFT-LUQ, LLQ

Figure 9-2. Sample medication administration record (MAR).

help the pharmacist provide pharmaceutical care. During the initial screening and evaluation of the drug order, for example, the pharmacy technician might notice in the clinical comments field that therapeutic monitoring may be needed or that recent monitoring parameters are outside normal limits. To ensure optimal safety and efficacy of drug therapy, the technician should alert the pharmacist to such situations as early as possible.

The last step in the order entry process is generally an acceptance (also called verification or validation) function when the pharmacist verifies that the order is correctly entered for the right patient. This occurs as a last checking step for the pharmacist when he or she has completed the order entry process personally, or if a pharmacy technician entered the order, as a formal, legal check of the technician's work by the pharmacist. This is generally the point at which labels and other documents are generated, although some systems allow printing prior to pharmacist validation.

Sample Inpatient Order Entry

Inpatient order entry usually goes as follows (using the enalapril example from Figure 9-1):

1. *Enter the patient's name or medical record number and verify them.* To begin, key in the medical record number or the name. Compare the patient profile with the written medication order to verify that the patient represented on the screen is the one for whom the order was written.

2. *Compare the order with the patient profile in detail.* The order to be entered is "Enalapril 10 mg QD PO." Check for general appropriateness of the order; it should make sense in regard to patient profile information, such as the patient's age, allergy profile, and drugs currently being taken. Note that the patient's allergies are sometimes listed on the physician's order form. It is useful to check this information against the patient's profile to make sure they agree.

3. *Enter the drug.* Go into the order entry mode and type in the drug mnemonic or find the drug in an alphabetical listing. For example, typing "enal" might result in a short list of enalapril products to select from, whereas typing "enal10" (the mnemonic for enalapril 10 mg tablets, as in the example) might result in a match for the specific product. After the product has been selected (enalapril 10 mg tablet), most systems check for drug interactions, therapeutic duplication, and

drug allergies. At this point, department policy determines what action the technician should take if an alert occurs. Once interaction checks are cleared, the computer will show the drug on the screen, and order entry may proceed.

4. *Verify the dose.* Check the dose on the order against the drug product entered. Most computer systems have a field that allows for some modifications here. In the enalapril example, the drug product chosen was a 10 mg tablet, and the dose is 10 mg, so no adjustments are necessary. However, if entering the Tylenol (acetaminophen) order (Figure 9-1), the technician would find only a 325 mg tablet in the computer. Therefore, the dose field would have to be modified to 650 mg, or two tablets. It is important to review all the available products and become familiar with available drug product dosages. For example, if a patient needs 100 mg of a drug and it comes in 10, 25, and 50 mg tablet strengths, it would be preferable to give the patient two 50 mg tablets rather than ten 10 mg tablets. Also, the technician should be aware that odd dosages may indicate a prescribing error. In the previous example, if the only available tablet strength were 10 mg, a 100 mg dose would be odd and should be verified by the pharmacist.

5. *Enter the administration schedule.* Type in the scheduling mnemonic (qd). Verify that the default administration time is appropriate for the patient and medication.

6. *Enter any comments in the clinical comments field.* There may be nothing to add for enalapril. In the Tylenol example, an entry of "for temp > 101" would be appropriate.

7. *Verify the prescriber name.* Depending on the computer system, the accuracy of the prescriber name may need to be verified. Most systems default to the admitting or attending physician, but some allow or require changing to the actual prescriber.

8. *Fill and label the medication.* The correct product (e.g., enalapril 10 mg tablets) must be obtained and supplied in the correct quantity with proper labeling. In this case, one or two tablets might be sent in a traditional inpatient setting, depending on the time of day, the time the next dose was due, and the next scheduled filling time. This would vary dramatically, however, depending on

the degree and type of automation. Whether dispensing happens on a patient-specific basis or as part of a batch automated system fill, however, this is the final opportunity for the technician to check the medication against the label, the fill list, or the order to ensure accuracy.

Filling, Labeling, and Checking Medications

Once the computer entry has been completed and labeling materials generated, the medication order must be filled with the correct quantity of the correct drug. During this step, it is important to review the label carefully against the order and the product to be used to make sure the correct product has been chosen. This is the final opportunity for the pharmacy to catch an error prior to dispensing to a patient care area.

The accuracy of the label should be checked before the medication order is filled. If a label doesn't look right, it may not be right. If an order is filled from an inaccurate label and the pharmacy system of checking fails, the wrong product could be dispensed and given to the patient.

When a label seems to indicate an error, the first step is to review the label against the order and profile. From the example in Figure 9-1, if the label indicated a 100 mg enalapril dose, and it was reviewed against the original order, it would be clear that an error was made when the order was entered. The label would be discarded and the entry in the computer would have to be corrected. If, however, the original order did specify a 100 mg dose, the order should be brought to the attention of the pharmacist. The pharmacist can then evaluate the order and take action to get it corrected if necessary.

Finally, the medication order is filled and left for the pharmacist to check. This pharmacist check is legally required in most cases, and must occur before any drug is dispensed to a patient care area.

Medication orders may need to be filed after they are filled. Policies and legal requirements differ as to how orders are filed and how long the files have to be maintained. Consult state and federal law and your organization's policies with regard to these rules.

Special Considerations in Hospital Order Processing

"Charge-Only" and "No-Charge" Entries

In some situations, order entry into the pharmacy computer system is done for record-keeping or billing purposes only. Technicians are often involved in these practices when charging patients for medications used

from floor stock, for example. Most hospitals keep some inventory in floor stock (inventory kept in a controlled space in the patient care areas) for use as first doses, emergency doses, or convenience medications. When these drugs are used, the pharmacy is generally notified for the purposes of patient charging and floor stock replenishment.

Another situation is the dispensing of medication for which there is no charge but still a record-keeping requirement or need. An example would be investigational medications, which are often provided free of charge but still need to be accounted for.

A similar situation would be the case of medications brought in from home to be used while a patient is in the hospital. Because they are the patient's property, there is typically no charge for the drugs, but it is important for the medications to show up on the MAR and in the patient profile so that all caregivers are aware that the patient is receiving the medication.

Diagnostic Preparation Orders

Many hospitals (as well as some retail pharmacies affiliated with a physician's office practice) dispense "preparations" (or preps) for diagnostic tests. Sometimes these orders are very vague (e.g., "routine prep for colonoscopy"), and the pharmacists and technicians are expected to follow a specific protocol for dispensing medications. These protocols are generally agreed upon by the individual hospital's medical staff and are recorded in policies for everyone's reference.

Physician Order Entry

In some hospitals, physicians enter orders directly into the hospital's computer system instead of writing orders and sending them to nursing or pharmacy to be entered into the computer system. In this situation, a pharmacist still reviews the order before dispensing the medications. Generally, physician order entry is advantageous, because it promotes the submission of more complete orders and prevents errors caused by illegible handwriting, among other reasons. When physician order entry is used, technicians may not be involved in the order entry process at all, but still fulfill many of the same dispensing roles.

Automated Dispensing Technology

Automated dispensing technology may have a profound effect on the filling, labeling, and checking functions performed in the pharmacy. There are two basic approaches to automation: centralized dispensing automation in the pharmacy and decentralized automation at the point of care. The two approaches may be employed independently of each other or may be combined in some institutions.

Centralized dispensing automation generally takes the form of robotics. Robotic systems use bar codes to identify medications accurately during filling. In a fully automated example, a technician might take the following steps:

1. Scan a bulk container's bar code to fill a bulk bin in an automated packaging device. Because an error at this point in the process might result in many patients getting an incorrect medication, this is often a checkpoint for a pharmacist.

2. Package the drug into robot-friendly containers via the packaging device (which may include a hole at the top to fit on spindles on the robot and a bar code imprint on the package for product identification).

3. Restock the robot. This process is automated as well. The technician puts all individual containers to be stocked into the machine on a single spindle, and the machine reads the bar code on each package and places the drug in the correct location on the robot.

4. Enter the order into the pharmacy's computer. When an order is entered into the pharmacy's computer, the information passes to the robot and the correct drug is pulled for a first dose—again, by matching the drug order to the correct bar code.

5. Remove each patient's drugs from the machine and distribute them to the patient care area by whatever distribution method is used. Some type of random check is often applied here, but because of the inherent accuracy of these systems, a routine check of all dispensed drugs is not typical. State law may determine the amount of checking that is required.

6. A batch fill of patient medications is scheduled at some point during the day. When this happens, the robot does a complete (24-hour) fill of medications by patient and unit. Again, a random checking procedure may occur at this point.

In decentralized automation systems, distribution devices are placed in the patient care areas. These devices may be used for floor stock distribution and narcotic control only or for the majority of drug distribution in a facility. When used for the majority of the drug distribution, point-of-care automation makes

distribution more of a batch system. In a traditional (nonautomated) system—as has been described—most of the dispensing is "on demand," which means an order comes to the pharmacy by some means and is entered and filled at the time. When decentralized automation is used, orders are entered upon receipt, but the drugs are already "distributed" to the automation devices. A fully implemented decentralized system would work something like this:

1. An order is received in the pharmacy and is entered into the pharmacy computer.

2. Once order entry is completed, a computer interface sends the information to the automation device, effectively "releasing" the medication for use for a specific patient.

3. The nurse can then go to the machine and key in the patient's name and the drug name, and the appropriate location in the device "unlocks" so the medication can be removed.

4. For continuing medications (e.g., a TID medication), the nurse can go back to the device at designated times (standard administration times) throughout the day and remove the medication for administration to the patient.

5. When it is time to restock the machine, the technician prints a batch restock report that is filled by a technician and then checked by a pharmacist. The technician then makes a delivery to each unit and restocks the medications into the machines. Some devices allow for bar code verification of the medication to ensure that the correct medication goes to the correct bin, but that is not a feature of all systems at this time.

Both types of automation allow for some efficiencies. For example, with point-of-care automation, medication orders must still be filled, but by moving that function to a batch report, all the orders for all the patients on a particular floor can be filled at the same time, and the filling can be scheduled at a time that is convenient for the pharmacy instead of on demand at the convenience of the prescriber. Centralized automation makes the filling process more efficient by automating the filling act itself. The machine does the filling—no more walking around the pharmacy to pull inventory from different locations.

AMBULATORY PHARMACY

Receiving Prescriptions

Traditionally, prescriptions are presented to the pharmacy in person after having been written by the prescribing physician on a prescription blank. It is now possible, however, for prescriptions to come in to the pharmacy by a number of other means. Many prescriptions are telephoned in from the prescriber's office to the pharmacy. As in the inpatient setting, there are regulatory restrictions on who can receive a telephone order, and the technician should refer to state laws for specific information. Other means of communication include facsimile and electronic transmission. These methods are also regulated, with state-by-state variations, especially as related to electronic signatures and controlled substance prescribing. Many pharmacies also accept refill requests over the Internet through a pharmacy Web page. Patients eventually may use these Web pages routinely to log in to their own accounts to view a refill history, print an insurance receipt, or access drug information online.

Obtaining payer information is an important step in receiving a prescription in the outpatient setting. This information is used for a number of purposes, including establishing the primary payer for the prescription, the patient's portion of the reimbursement (copay), and, in some instances, the drug formulary. Most prescriptions are now electronically filed with a third party payer at the time they are entered into the pharmacy information system. This process is called electronic adjudication. If the information is not available when the prescription is received, it may be held until the patient is present. This is generally an issue only the first time a pharmacy fills a prescription for a patient because the information typically is then held as part of the patient's profile.

However a prescription comes in to the pharmacy, a technician is often the first person to handle it. The initial treatment, as in an inpatient pharmacy, must include screening for completeness and clarity. Then the order is prioritized for processing.

Clarity and Completeness

Reviewing a prescription for clarity and completeness is similar in the outpatient and inpatient settings. The following prescription elements are typically present:

- Patient name
- Patient home address
- Date the prescription was written
- Drug name—either generic or brand
- Drug strength and dose to be administered
- Directions for use, including route of administration, frequency, and duration of use as applicable (some durations are open-ended)
- Quantity to be dispensed
- Number of refills to be allowed
- Substitution authority or refusal
- Signature and credentials of the prescriber and DEA number if required
- Reason for use, or indication (not generally required)

An example of an outpatient prescription is presented in **Figure 9-4**.

In an ambulatory practice, some special clarity and completeness issues must be considered. When the prescriber uses "Dispense As Written," or DAW, on the prescription blank, the brand name drug written on the prescription must be dispensed. Substituting the generic equivalent is not allowed. Depending on state law, pharmacy policy, or both, some prescription

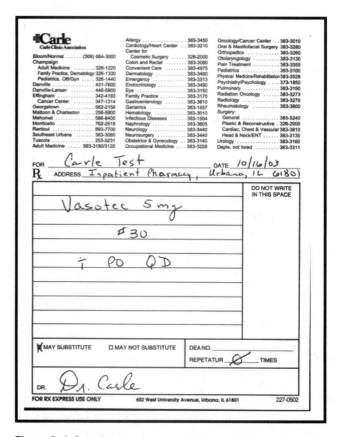

Figure 9-4. Sample outpatient prescription.

blanks come preprinted with areas the prescriber can use to designate DAW or, alternatively, "generic substitution acceptable." In some practice settings, the prescriber must write DAW, and preprinted prescription blanks are not recognized as official.

Another outpatient issue is prescription forgeries. Screening prescriptions, particularly those for controlled substances, for potential forgeries should be part of the technician's routine. Some prescription forgeries may be fairly easy to identify, such as erasure or overwriting of the strength or dispensing quantity of the drug (e.g., changing a 3 to an 8). Some forgeries are much more subtle and may involve, for example, theft of preprinted prescription pads and legitimate-looking prescriptions. Forged prescriptions may also be telephoned in to the pharmacy. The technician should screen prescriptions for anything that looks unusual, such as a dispense quantity in excess of normal quantities or an unrecognizable signature. Any suspicious prescription should be *discreetly* presented to the pharmacist for further evaluation. A telephoned prescription that is suspected of "forgery" should be validated with the prescriber. Forgeries are not typically a concern for inpatient pharmacies because of their much more controlled environment.

Checking for clarity and completeness includes considering legibility problems and interpreting abbreviations. If there is any doubt, the prescribing physician must be contacted for clarification. Making assumptions in either of these instances might compromise patient safety.

As is true for inpatient orders, it is important to communicate fully when clarification is expected to result in delays in order processing. The prescribing physician may wish to make a short-term change in therapy while waiting for a product to be ordered or may change the prescription altogether. The patient should be made aware if the problem cannot be readily resolved with the prescriber, resulting in a delay in filling the prescription.

Prioritization
Prioritization of prescription processing in the outpatient pharmacy is generally an issue of customer service as opposed to patient care. Although some outpatient pharmacies may experience the equivalent of the inpatient stat order—if they provide preps for procedures for a physicians' office practice, for example—most outpatient pharmacy prioritization is based on the customer's needs. In general, prescriptions are filled in

the order in which they are presented to the pharmacy, and many pharmacies use some sort of "take-a-number" system. Some common sense judgment does apply, however. Prescriptions are generally filled first for customers who are waiting—as opposed to prescriptions to be mailed the next day, for example—regardless of the order in which they were presented.

Processing Prescriptions
Prescription processing involves many of the same steps as medication orders in the inpatient setting. There are some differences, however, that will be covered in this section.

Identifying the Patient
Patient identification in the outpatient pharmacy, although not generally as complex as it is for inpatient pharmacies, is still an important step. Making sure prescriptions are filled for and dispensed to the correct patient is important. Proper attention needs to be paid to similar or same names to make sure the medication is profiled on the right patient profile. Another important concern at this stage is to ensure that there is no forgery and that the individuals obtaining controlled substances are lawfully entitled to do so.

Most outpatient pharmacies use some type of patient identification system—often a numeric identifier that is unique to the patient, such as an account number. These systems are used to ensure accurate identification of patients for profiling and billing purposes.

Creating, Maintaining, and Reviewing Patient Profiles
Patient profiles are just as important in outpatient sites as they are in inpatient pharmacies. There are legal requirements for profiling just as there are for hospital pharmacies. More important, however, patient profiles serve as a basis for providing patient care. The pharmacist is an integral participant in outpatient health care. The pharmacist is often the first provider to interact with a patient who is ill and intends to self-medicate and also the last professional to interact with a patient who has been prescribed medication prior to implementation of the treatment plan. The pharmacist has a tremendous opportunity and responsibility to help patients use their medications safely and effectively. Patient profiles are an important tool in supporting that care.

A number of pieces of information are typically collected in the patient profile—some according to law (which varies from state to state) and some for efficiency and convenience purposes for both the pharmacy and the patient. They include the following:

- Patient's name and identification number
- Age or date of birth
- Home address and telephone number
- Allergies
- Principal diagnoses
- Primary health care providers
- Third-party payer(s) and other billing information
- Over-the-counter medications and herbal supplements used by the patient
- Prescription and refill history
- Patient preferences (e.g., child-resistant packaging waiver, prefers prescriptions be mailed)

Maintaining patient profiles is a function technicians commonly perform in the ambulatory setting. For this reason, technicians must be aware of the types of information that should be obtained from the patient to create and update the profile and should bring any profile issues to the attention of the pharmacist. For example, the technician should notify the pharmacist if a medication is a duplication of something the patient has already been taking. As is true of the inpatient setting, outpatient pharmacy computers generally screen for many potential medication problems at the time of order entry. These alerts should be given to the pharmacist for follow-up according to the pharmacy's policies.

Prescription Entry into the Computer

Selecting the appropriate drug product is the first step in the order entry process, once the patient's profile is located or created. Most outpatient computer systems, like inpatient systems, allow drug product choice by typing in a mnemonic or by accessing an alphabetical listing of some sort. It may also be possible to access the drug by National Drug Code (NDC) number.

Selecting the correct drug is not just a matter of choosing the correct product by name. It is also important to choose the correct strength and

package size to match the NDC number with the product dispensed, especially when generic products are used. Accuracy ensures correct billing as well as correct dispensing and is important in regulatory compliance and in protecting the pharmacy against accusations of fraud.

Keying in a mnemonic will generally result in a short list of options from which the correct drug is then chosen. It is important to pick the correct dose, dosage form, and—in the case of a bulk item—the correct package size at this step.

A variety of information must be entered into the computer at this point, and systems differ as to the order in which it is entered. Required elements include the following:

- Physician's name
- Directions for use
- Fill quantity
- Initials of the pharmacist checking the prescription
- Number of refills authorized

Once this information is entered into the computer, the technician accepts the prescription and, if applicable, the prescription entry is electronically submitted to the patient's insurance carrier for adjudication. Drug formularies were mentioned earlier in relation to choosing drug products in an institutional setting. Outpatient dispensing may be governed by numerous formularies because each third-party payer has the option of identifying a formulary for its patients.

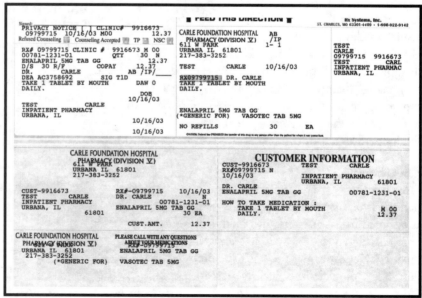

Figure 9-5. Sample outpatient prescription label.

Unfortunately, identification of a nonformulary medication does not generally happen until this step in the process. If a product is not covered by a patient's insurance, it is important to bring this fact to the pharmacist's attention so that the pharmacist can discuss the issue with the patient. Because nonformulary costs may be prohibitive for some patients, many will want the pharmacist to contact the prescriber to see if a formulary product might be an option.

Filling, Labeling, and Checking Prescriptions

The prescription entry process typically generates a label (see **Figure 9-5**) and may also produce additional documents, such as the patient's insurance receipt, a mailing label, and a drug information sheet for the patient. At this point, the technician fills the prescription and labels the container.

The following components must generally appear on a prescription label, whether typed or computer-generated (information may vary by state):

- Patient's name
- Date the prescription is being filled (or refilled)
- Prescriber's name
- Sequential prescription number
- Name of the drug (including manufacturer, if filled generically)
- Quantity to be dispensed
- Directions for use
- Number of refills remaining (or associated refill period)

Labeling includes more than just the actual prescription label. The inpatient section of the chapter noted that labeling for inpatient use is often abbreviated or in a form of shorthand. For home use, however, this is not acceptable. Beyond the prescription label itself, auxiliary information is often included in the form of special labels affixed to the container or written drug information leaflets for patients to read at home (see **Figure 9-6**).

Of primary importance is that the instructions for use be presented very clearly on the label or within the auxiliary labeling. This information also is commonly shared verbally with the patient at the time of dispensing. Instructions for use must include at least the following:

- Administration directions (e.g., "Take," "Insert," "Apply")

- Number of units constituting one dose and the dosage form (e.g., two tablets)
- Route of administration (e.g., "by mouth," "vaginally")
- How frequently or at what time (e.g., "twice daily," "daily at 9 a.m.")
- Length of time to continue, if applicable (e.g., "for 10 days," "until finished")
- Indication, or purpose, if applicable (e.g., "for pain," "for blood pressure")

At the time of dispensing, it is important to be sure the patient fully understands how to use the medication. This is an appropriate time to consider language barriers, such as illiteracy or English not being the patient's primary language. Many pharmacies now have interpreters available if they serve a large non-English-speaking population, and some pharmacies translate prescription labels and offer educational materials in languages other than English.

This is also the point at which the pharmacist generally offers to counsel the patient if he or she has any questions.

Sample Outpatient Prescription Process

This section highlights how the outpatient order entry process differs from the inpatient order entry process.

Refer to the prescription in Figure 9-2.

1. *Enter the patient's medical record number or name and verify them* (same as for inpatients). On the basis of the prescription or by questioning the patient directly, verify that the rest of the patient information (address, date of birth, allergies, insurance information, etc.) is correct.

2. *Enter or verify existing third-party billing information.* Accurate third-party billing information is essential. Often, drug product choices must coincide with the payer's formulary for the patient's medication to be covered. If third-party payer information is incorrect, the patient may have significant out-of-pocket expense or may choose not to use the medication because of the expense.

3. *Compare the order with the patient profile in detail* (same as for inpatients).

4. *Enter the drug* (same as for inpatients).

5. *Enter the label direction mnemonic.* This step will encompass steps four and five of the inpatient procedures. Remember, outpatient directions

CARLE RX-EXPRESS
611 W PARK
URBANA IL 61801
217-383-3252

== CUSTOMER ===
== INFORMATION ==
10/16/03
ENALAPRIL 5MG TAB GG

*** IF YOUR PHYSICIAN HAS PRESCRIBED THIS MEDICATION FOR A USE BEYOND ITS LISTED ***
INDICATION, THE FOLLOWING INFORMATION MAY NOT BE COMPLETELY RELEVANT FOR YOU
*** PLEASE CONSULT YOUR PHYSICIAN OR PHARMACIST WITH ANY QUESTION. ***

ENALAPRIL MALEATE - ORAL
(e-NAL-a-pril)

COMMON BRAND NAME(S): Vasotec

WARNING: This drug can cause serious fetal harm (possibly death)
if used during the last six months of pregnancy. If you become
pregnant or think you may be pregnant, contact your doctor
immediately.

USES: This drug belongs to a group of medications called ACE
inhibitors. It is used to treat high blood pressure
(hypertension) in adults and children. It works by relaxing blood
vessels, causing them to widen. High blood pressure reduction
helps prevent strokes, heart attacks and kidney problems.
    This medication is also used with other drugs (e.g., "water
pills"/diuretics, digoxin) to treat congestive heart failure.

OTHER USES: This medication may also be used to help protect the
kidneys from damage due to diabetes.

HOW TO USE: Take this medication by mouth, usually once or twice
a day; or as directed by your doctor. You may take this drug with
or without food. Use this medication regularly in order to get
the most benefit from it. To help you remember, use it at the
same time(s) each day.
    If you are taking this drug in the liquid suspension form,
shake the bottle well before each use. Measure the dose out
carefully.
    Do not take potassium supplements or salt substitutes
containing potassium without talking to your doctor or pharmacist
first. This medicine can raise your potassium levels, which
rarely can cause serious side effects such as muscle weakness or
very slow heartbeats. Tell your doctor immediately if these
effects occur.
    The dosage is based on your medical condition and response to
therapy. For the treatment of high blood pressure, it may take
several weeks before the full benefit of this drug occurs. It may
take several weeks or months to see the full benefit when this
drug is used for congestive heart failure.
    It is important to continue taking this medication even if you
feel well. Most people with high blood pressure do not feel sick.

SIDE EFFECTS: You may experience headache, dizziness,
lightheadedness, weakness, nausea, dry cough or blurred vision as
your body adjusts to the medication. If any of these effects
persist or worsen, notify your doctor or pharmacist promptly.
    Tell your doctor immediately if any of these unlikely but
serious side effects occur: fainting, decreased sexual ability.
    Tell your doctor immediately if any of these highly unlikely
but very serious side effects occur: change in the amount of
urine, signs of infection (e.g., fever, chills, persistent sore
throat).
    This drug may rarely cause serious (possibly fatal) liver
problems. If you notice any of the following highly unlikely but
very serious side effects, seek immediate medical attention:

Figure 9-6. Sample drug information sheets to be given to the patient at the time of dispensing.

Cont'd

yellowing of the eyes or skin, dark urine, stomach/abdominal pain, persistent fatigue, persistent nausea.

An allergic reaction to this drug is unlikely, but seek immediate medical attention if it occurs. Symptoms of an allergic reaction include: rash, itching, swelling (especially of the face, lips, tongue, or throat), severe dizziness, trouble breathing.

If you notice other effects not listed above, contact your doctor or pharmacist.

PRECAUTIONS: This medication should not be used if you have certain medical conditions. Before using this medicine, consult your doctor or pharmacist if you have: allergies to other ACE inhibitors (e.g., benazepril, captopril), history of an allergic reaction which included swelling of the face/lips/tongue/throat (angioedema).

Before using this medication, tell your doctor or pharmacist your medical history, especially of: kidney disease, liver disease, high blood levels of potassium, heart problems, severe dehydration (and loss of electrolytes such as sodium), diabetes (poorly controlled), strokes, blood vessel disease (e.g., collagen vascular diseases such as lupus, scleroderma), any allergies in addition to those listed above (including allergies to bee or wasp stings, or exposure to certain membranes used for blood filtering).

This drug may make you dizzy; use caution engaging in activities requiring alertness such as driving or using machinery. Limit alcoholic beverages.

To minimize dizziness and lightheadedness due to lowering of your blood pressure, get up slowly when rising from a seated or lying position. Serious loss of body fluids can also lower your blood pressure and worsen dizziness. Drink adequate fluids to prevent from becoming dehydrated. If you are on restricted fluid intake, consult your doctor for further instructions. Be careful not to become too overheated during exercise which can lead to excessive sweating. Consult your doctor if you experience severe vomiting or diarrhea.

Before having surgery, tell your doctor or dentist that you are taking this medication.

Caution is advised when using this drug in the elderly because they may be more sensitive to the effects of the drug, especially the dizziness effect.

Caution is advised when using this drug in children because they may be more sensitive to the effects of the drug.

This medication should be used only when clearly needed during the first three months of pregnancy. It is not recommended for use during the last six months of the pregnancy due to the risk for fetal harm. Discuss the risks and benefits with your doctor. See also the Warning section.

This drug passes into breast milk. While there have been no reports of harm to nursing infants, consult your doctor before breast-feeding.

DRUG INTERACTIONS: Before using this medication, tell your doctor or pharmacist of all prescription and nonprescription products you may use, especially of: potassium-sparing "water pills" (diuretics such as amiloride, spironolactone, triamterene), "water pills" (diuretics such as furosemide), potassium supplements (e.g., potassium chloride) or salt substitutes, non-steroidal anti-inflammatory drugs (e.g., celecoxib, ibuprofen, indomethacin), lithium, drugs that suppress the immune system (e.g., azathioprine), other high blood pressure medications, other heart drugs (e.g., digoxin).

Check the labels on all your medicines (e.g., cough-and-cold products, diet aids) because they may contain ingredients that could increase your heart rate or blood pressure. Ask your

Figure 9-6. Sample drug information sheets to be given to the patient at the time of dispensing.

Cont'd

pharmacist about the safe use of those products.

Do not start or stop any medicine without doctor or pharmacist approval.

OVERDOSE: If overdose is suspected, contact your local poison control center or emergency room immediately. Symptoms of overdose may include: unusually fast or slow heartbeat, severe dizziness, or fainting.

NOTES: Do not share this medication with others. Lifestyle changes such as stress reduction programs, exercise and dietary changes may increase the effectiveness of this medicine. Talk to your doctor or pharmacist about lifestyle changes that might benefit you.

Laboratory and/or medical tests (e.g., kidney function, potassium blood level) should be performed periodically to monitor your progress or check for side effects. Consult your doctor for more details.

Have your blood pressure checked regularly while taking this medication. Learn how to monitor your own blood pressure at home. Discuss this with your doctor.

MISSED DOSE: If you miss a dose, use it as soon as you remember. If it is near the time of the next dose, skip the missed dose and resume your usual dosing schedule. Do not double the dose to catch up.

STORAGE: Store tablets at room temperature below 86 degrees F (30 degrees C) away from light and moisture. Do not store in the bathroom. Refrigerate the liquid suspension between 36 to 46 degrees F (2 to 8 degrees C). Discard any unused suspension after 30 days. Keep all medicines away from children and pets.

MEDICAL ALERT: Your condition can cause complications in a medical emergency. For enrollment information call MedicAlert at 1-800-854- 1166 (USA) or 1-800-668-1507 (Canada).

Figure 9-6. Sample drug information sheets to be given to the patient at the time of dispensing.

must be in a language the patient can understand, so they must go beyond giving a milligram dose and a scheduled time to take the medication. The dosing mnemonic for the enalapril prescription might be t1tpoqd, which consists of encoded characters for all of the major elements of the directions ("sig" text): *t* = take, *1* = one, *t* = tablet, *po* = by mouth, *qd* = daily. The translation onto the patient label is "Take one tablet by mouth each day."

6. *Enter comments.* Comments, such as "to control blood pressure," are added to the label and the medication profile at this point.

7. *Enter the prescriber's name.* Depending on the computer system, the technician might enter the full name, a mnemonic, or a numeric code.

8. *Enter the amount to dispense and the refill information.* In the example, the amount dispensed is 30 and no refills are authorized.

9. *Fill and label the prescription.* The correct medication must be chosen, the fill quantity counted and packaged, and the appropriate labeling applied. As in the inpatient setting, this is the final opportunity for the technician to ensure the accuracy of the process by checking the chosen product against the original order—not just against the label.

Conclusion

As a member of the health care team, the technician provides considerable assistance in operations of the pharmacy. The technician's ability to evaluate and assist in processing orders and prescriptions adds another measure of safety and efficiency to the system and is an opportunity for the technician to contribute significantly to the welfare of patients.

Recommended Reading

1. Employer's policy and procedure manual and orientation materials regarding receiving and processing orders, filling and labeling medication orders, using the computer system, preventing errors, standard administration times, delivery expectations and turnaround time, and duties of the technician involved in dispensing functions.

2. Rules and Regulations for the Administration of the Pharmacy Practice Act for the state in which the technician is employed. (These may generally be obtained from the regulating body in the state.)

Footnote

The contributions of Robert S. Guynn and Kevin W. Zajac to this chapter are gratefully acknowledged.

Self-Assessment Questions

1. Anyone who has worked in a pharmacy for a minimum of 1 year may receive a telephone prescription from a physician.
   a. True
   b. False

2. Generally, the first step when a prescription is received is a review of the prescription for completeness and accuracy, and the second is to prioritize the prescription in relation to the other work to be done.
   a. True
   b. False

3. An outpatient pharmacy generally has a single formulary that is used for all patients, regardless of the third-party payer.
   a. True
   b. False

4. Which of the following pieces of information should be on a prescription in an outpatient pharmacy but would *not* be required on a medication order for a hospitalized patient?
   a. patient's address
   b. physician's address and telephone number
   c. refill information
   d. all of the above

5. What does "dispense as written" on a prescription mean?
   a. The brand name product ordered by the physician must be used to fill the prescription.
   b. Generic substitution is prohibited, but an alternative brand name product may be used if the one ordered is not available.
   c. Generic substitution may occur only if the patient insists on it.
   d. none of the above

6. Any suspicious prescription should be brought to the attention of the pharmacist because it may be a forgery.
   a. True
   b. False

7. Considerations in determining an order's priority include all of the following *except:*
   a. the type of medication prescribed and what it is used to treat
   b. the type of patient identification used
   c. the patient's or caregiver's expectation for the time of delivery

   d. specific instructions from the prescriber as to the delivery time

8. A typical "turnaround time" for a stat order in a hospital is 10 to 15 minutes.
   a. True
   b. False

9. Common methods of identifying patients on medication orders in institutional settings include:
   a. addressograph cards
   b. bar-coded name labels
   c. patient account number
   d. all of the above

10. Patient identification is not a concern in an outpatient pharmacy because the technician has no control over who actually takes the medication.
    a. True
    b. False

11. Once a bar-coded account number system is instituted in an organization, less attention needs to be paid to patient identification because these systems are basically foolproof.
    a. True
    b. False

12. A thorough review of a well-kept patient profile in an ambulatory pharmacy will generally allow the technician to identify all the following problems *except:*
    a. existing orders for the same medication
    b. allergies that may indicate that the medication should not be used
    c. a disability, such as blindness, that requires special attention
    d. how the patient will pay for the amount the insurance company does not pay (i.e., the copay)
    e. the patient's date of birth or age

13. Which of the following drug file options would be the best choice for an outpatient prescription for 250 mg of cephalexin suspension four times daily for 10 days?
    a. cep125s100—cephalexin suspension 125 mg/5 ml, 100 ml
    b. cep125s150—cephalexin suspension 125 mg/5 ml, 150 ml
    c. cep250c—cephalexin capsules 250 mg
    d. cep250s100—cephalexin suspension 250 mg/5 ml, 100 ml

e. cep250s150—cephalexin suspension 250 mg/5 ml, 150 ml

14. Besides choosing the correct drug entity, which of the following decisions must be made at the time an IV drug is being chosen during a computerized order entry process in a hospital?
    a. the correct diluent solution
    b. the correct package size for the amount being prepared
    c. the correct dosage form for the route of administration
    d. all of the above

15. Common screening options during a pharmacy- or nursing-operated computerized order entry process in a hospital include all of the following *except*:
    a. therapeutic duplication
    b. price range checking
    c. allergy screening
    d. dose range checking
    e. drug interactions with existing orders

16. Medication administration times are generally standardized without exception within hospitals.
    a. True
    b. False

17. In the outpatient setting, appropriate medication administration times must be discussed with the patient or family member to ensure optimal benefit.
    a. True
    b. False

18. In the case of a prescription with complex directions, such as "tid for 3 days, bid for 3 days, qd for 3 days and dc," it is acceptable to use the Latin abbreviations on the label as long as they are carefully explained to the patient.
    a. True
    b. False

19. Which of the following statements about prescription labeling is *false*?
    a. Some prescriptions require labeling beyond what will fit on the label itself.
    b. Auxiliary labels are often used to clarify or elaborate on directions for use.
    c. If the patient is in a hurry, it is acceptable to dispense the prescription without an affixed label as long as you talk to the patient about how to use the medication

and he or she understands.
    d. Most states have specific requirements about what information must be included in prescription labeling.

20. Which of the following best incorporates all recommended components of label directions for outpatient use?
    a. Take one tablet three times daily.
    b. Take one tablet by mouth three times daily.
    c. Take one tablet three times daily for pain.
    d. Take one tablet by mouth three times daily for 10 days.
    e. Take one tablet by mouth three times daily for 10 days for infection.

21. In some hospitals, physicians enter medication orders into the hospital's computer system instead of writing orders on paper.
    a. True
    b. False

22. Inpatient pharmacies may become more efficient by implementing decentralized dispensing automation, thereby moving more of the filling functions to batch runs.
    a. True
    b. False

23. Which of the following is *not* true of hospital pharmacy dispensing automation?
    a. Dispensing automation may be centralized in the pharmacy or decentralized at the point of care.
    b. Decentralized automation is superior to centralized automation.
    c. Both centralized and decentralized automation make dispensing more efficient.
    d. Some institutions combine both centralized and decentralized automation to incorporate advantages of both systems.

24. When a filling label seems to indicate an error, which of the following would be an appropriate initial action for the technician?
    a. Alert the pharmacist that an error has been made.
    b. Check the label against the original order to determine if an error was made.
    c. Call the physician to clarify the order.
    d. Call the nursing unit (institutional setting) or notify the patient (outpatient setting) that an

error was made on the prescription order and that delays will result.
e. Any of the above

25. The final step in processing a prescription or medication order is filing the order in compliance with the requirements of the state in which the pharmacy is located and the policies of the organization.
a. True
b. False

Self-Assessment Answers

1. b. State laws vary in their requirements for telephone prescriptions—particularly when controlled substances are involved. In many states, only a pharmacist is allowed to receive telephone prescriptions.

2. a. An initial review of the prescription for completeness and accuracy will identify problems and facilitate their efficient resolution. Prioritization will help ensure that the most urgent work is done first.

3. b. An outpatient pharmacy generally does not have a single formulary as a hospital pharmacy might, but must conform to the various formularies of all the different third-party payers its customers use.

4. d. All the listed information would appear on an outpatient prescription but not on an inpatient order. Several other pieces of information would appear on inpatient orders but not outpatient prescriptions—most commonly a room and bed location for the patient and an admission number or account number of some type.

5. a. A "dispense as written" order must be filled with the brand listed by the prescriber.

6. a. Prescription pads may be lost or stolen and can then be used in attempts to obtain controlled drugs. It is also possible for forged prescriptions to be called in to the pharmacy. Although telephone forgeries may be more difficult to spot than written forgeries, the technician should consider anything unusual in a phone order as potentially indicating an attempt to obtain medications illegally. These calls should be directed to the pharmacist.

7. b. The type of identification offered or placed on the order does not influence priority.

8. a. Stat is derived from the Latin word *statim*, meaning immediately. Most hospitals have a designated time limit on these orders—typically 10 to 15 minutes.

9. d. Institutions rely heavily on a patient account number that is reproduced by an addressograph system or on a self-adhesive label that may be bar coded.

10. b. Although the person picking up the prescription may not be the one who will ultimately be using it, patient identification is still an important function. The technician must always make sure prescriptions are filled for the correct patient and that the pharmacy's dispensing records are correct.

11. b. No identification system is completely free from potential error. Patient identification is one of the most important steps in the order processing sequence.

12. d. The patient profile should contain a full range of patient information, including patient demographics, such as date of birth, allergies, medical conditions, and disabilities, as well as a complete list of currently prescribed medications. Although it would typically contain information regarding the type of insurance coverage the patient has and the amount of any required deductible or copay, how the patient chooses to meet that requirement would not usually be indicated.

13. d. The best choice in this example would be the 100 ml bottle of 250 mg/5 ml suspension. Two full bottles would be required and would have to be transferred to another properly labeled container.

14. d. All three of the answers are integral to entering an IV order correctly.

15. b. There is no screening for prices of drugs, although price information may be available. Some outpatient systems may offer price information for generic equivalents.

16. b. Although the majority of administration times are standardized, there may be numerous exceptions to such a policy. For example, pediatric or neonatal units may have specialized administration schedules that differ from other units. This is also true of many intensive care areas. Exceptions may be based on individual drug characteristics as well. One example is a "tid" order for a medication that should be given before meals. Standard "tid" administration times may be 0900, 1300, and 1800. The schedule might automatically be altered to 0730, 1130, and 1700 to be timed for 30 minutes before each meal.

17. a. Because there are fewer controls on medication administration in the outpatient setting,

scheduling should be discussed with the patient or a family member to make sure the instructions are clear and the patient will not have difficulty using the medication as intended.

18. b. Latin abbreviations should never be used on labeling for home use. Although patients may fully understand the directions when they leave the pharmacy, they may forget by the time they get home. If detailed instructions do not fit on the prescription label itself, it would be more appropriate to give the patient a separate piece of paper with instructions written in plain English.

19. c. There are legal requirements for labeling that must be met, including a label affixed to the prescription itself.

20. e. Six pieces of information are recommended for inclusion in outpatient labeling: (1) the administration direction, (2) the number and type (dosage form) of units constituting one dose, (3) the route of administration, (4) frequency of administration, (5) duration of therapy, and (6) indication or purpose.

21. a. Physician order entry is not yet widespread but is becoming more common. It offers some advantages because it allows that physician to make timely responses to potential problems with the order without having to wait for the technician to discover the issue and refer it to the pharmacist, who must then contact the prescriber for clarification.

22. a. One way of improving efficiency through automation is to decentralize the inventory into automated dispensing machines. This allows more of the work to be completed on a batch basis as opposed to "on demand" filling in response to a physician's order.

23. b. Both centralized and decentralized automation offer efficiencies, although at different points in the dispensing system. They represent different choices, but one is not inherently superior to the other. The choice of which system to use is a matter of organizational fit and determining which system best achieves the organization's objectives.

24. b. Checking the label against the original order is a good initial step because the error may have been a simple keystroke error in the computer, which could be easily corrected, eliminating the need for many of the other options listed.

25. a. Once the dispensing activities have been completed, the order should be filed. State laws differ in their requirements for filing. Individual organizations will develop their own policies dictating how orders are to be filed and for how long. The technician should be familiarized with those requirements during training and orientation.

Understanding Physiology

10

ALICE J. A. GARDNER, DIANE F. PACITTI

Human physiology is the study of how the major organ systems of the body work. To understand how these systems function, it is essential to first study the components of each of the organ systems, that is, their anatomy. Anatomy provides a framework for understanding their physiological functions and how the organ systems are dependent on each other. Normal functioning of the organ systems is required to bring about a balanced internal environment. When damage to, or an imbalance in, any of these systems occurs, the normal physiological functions are disrupted, which leads to the development of disease states, or pathophysiological conditions.

In this chapter, we will present and discuss 10 body systems. We will discuss the anatomy, physiology, and pathophysiology for each system. None of these body systems works alone; to maintain a stable internal environment, each system requires and depends on the proper functioning of one or more of the other body systems.

Nervous System

What Is It? (Anatomy)

The nervous system is comprised of the brain, the spinal cord, and a system of nerve cells (neurons) that connect to organs and tissues throughout the body (see **Figure 10-1**). The nervous system has two major parts: the central nervous system and the peripheral nervous system. The central nervous system consists of the brain and the spinal cord, and the peripheral nervous system consists of a network of nerve cells that exit from the spinal cord and extend throughout the body.

Further divisions occur within the peripheral nervous system: the afferent division and the efferent division. Functionally, the afferent division of the peripheral nervous system brings information about the external environment, such as temperature, as well as information on the status of internal organs, such as heart rate, to the brain. The efferent division delivers signals from the brain to the organs and tissues of the

After completing this chapter, the technician should be able to

1. Identify the major **structures** of each of the body systems presented.

2. Understand the major **functions** of each of the body systems presented.

3. Identify the key **pathophysiological conditions** and understand how they develop when something goes wrong within the body systems.

body. The efferent division is divided into the somatic and autonomic nervous systems.

The somatic nervous system transmits signals, via nerve cells, only to the skeletal muscles of the body, which are under voluntary control (see **Figure 10-2**). In contrast, the autonomic nervous system communicates with many different organs, such as the heart, muscles, and glands; this system is not under voluntary control, but is under the control of the brain. The autonomic nervous system is divided into the sympathetic and parasympathetic divisions, and each division, in general, has opposite effects on organs.

What Does It Do? (Physiology)

The nervous system is the major communication system in the body. It receives signals from, and transmits signals to, different organs to regulate their activities. Communication by the nervous system is rapid, and the resulting changes in the body can take place quickly. The function of the central nervous system is to receive, interpret, and process information from the organs and, in turn, send information back to the organs to perform a function. For example, the brain may receive informa-

tion from sensors in the skin indicating that the temperature of the skin is too hot; consequently, the brain transmits a signal via the afferent division to blood vessels near the surface of the skin telling them to open. As a result, heat is lost and the skin is cooled. In addition to regulating everyday functions, the central nervous system controls complex functions, such as formation and storage of memories, learning, emotions, motivation, and sleep.

In the autonomic nervous system, the sympathetic and parasympathetic divisions are responsible for regulating the internal organs of the body, such as the sweat glands, smooth muscle, heart, lung, eye, kidney, and sexual organs. For example, the brain may receive information that the heart is beating too rapidly, and consequently nerve cells of the parasympathetic nervous system will transmit signals to the heart to slow its rate. In contrast, the somatic nervous system is solely responsible for regulating the contractions of the skeletal muscle.

The central and peripheral nervous systems communicate with and regulate the function of organs in the body through the release of chemical messengers called neurotransmitters. These messengers are produced and stored in the nerve cells and are released only when an appropriate signal is transmitted (see **Figure 10-3**).

Nervous System

Brain

Spinal cord

Nerves

Figure 10-1. The nervous system. The nervous system is comprised of the brain, the spinal cord, and an extensive network of nerves. The system controls many activities of the body by transmitting electrical signals via neurons and the release of chemical signals known as neurotransmitters.

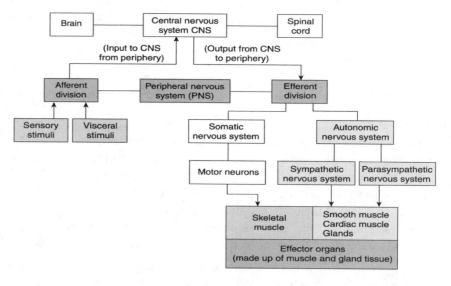

Figure 10-2. The nervous system is a highly organized network. The two major divisions are the central nervous system, which is comprised of the brain and spinal cord, and the peripheral nervous system, which is comprised of a network of nerves outside the spinal cord. The peripheral nervous system is divided into the afferent division, which carries sensory information to the brain, and the efferent division, which carries information from the brain to organs. The efferent division is divided into the autonomic and somatic nervous systems.

What Happens When It Goes Wrong? (Pathophysiology)

Many clinical problems, such as the following, can occur when the communication processes within the nervous system break down or are disrupted.

Depression: Depression is characterized by lack of energy, problems with sleeping, feelings of poor self-worth, poor eating habits, anger, withdrawn behavior, and suicidal thoughts. Research suggests that depression is the result of a deficiency of neurotransmitters—serotonin and norepinephrine—in the brain.

Parkinson's disease: In Parkinson's disease, the nerve cells in the brain, which control motor function, begin to degenerate and gradually lose their ability to release the neurotransmitter dopamine. The symptoms include problems with movement, that is, initiating and controlling the process. A person with Parkinson's disease, for example, has a stooped, slow, stiff, shuffling-style walk. Tremors while at rest are also common.

Alzheimer's disease: This is a progressive, degenerative neurological disorder in which brain tissue in specific areas of the brain begins to shrink and nerve cells are lost. Plaques and tangles are present in the brains of people with the disease. The primary nerve cells that are lost are those that produce the neurotransmitter acetylcholine. Eventually, the condition leads to impairments in memory, thinking, reasoning, and the ability to communicate. These symptoms slowly become more pronounced over time. Accompanying problems include depression and paranoia.

Schizophrenia: A type of psychosis, schizophrenia is a chronic, disabling brain disorder that alters the way an individual thinks, behaves, expresses emotions, perceives reality, and interacts with people. The symptoms of the disease are delusions, hallucinations, disturbed thought disorders, withdrawal, and lack of emotional responses. The cause of schizophrenia is unclear, but several factors are believed to be involved: heredity (genetics), imbalance of the neurotransmitter dopamine in the brain, abnormal brain structure and function, and environmental factors.

Myasthenia gravis: In this disease, communication between the somatic nervous system and the muscles is disrupted. Special proteins, called receptors, that are found in the skeletal muscle are destroyed by the body's own defense systems, and the neurotransmitter acetylcholine can no longer function to contract the muscle. The symptoms are difficulty in speaking, swallowing, and breathing; extreme fatigue; and drooping eyelids, because muscle contractions that maintain these functions are reduced.

Cardiovascular System

What Is It? (Anatomy)

The cardiovascular system is comprised of the heart; blood vessels called arteries, capillaries, and veins; and the blood (see **Figure 10-4**). Blood contains red blood cells (erythrocytes) and white blood cells. Red blood cells are responsible for transporting oxygen to, and carbon dioxide away from, cells. White blood cells help the body fight against invading microorganisms. Blood is also responsible for carrying nutrients to cells and break down products

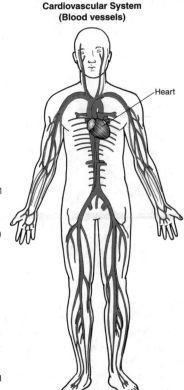

Cardiovascular System (Blood vessels)

Heart

Figure 10-4. The cardiovascular system. The cardiovascular system is comprised of the heart and an extensive system of arteries and veins that transports blood, nutrients, and gases to and from organs. In general, arteries carry blood rich in oxygen away from the heart, except the pulmonary artery, which carries blood low in oxygen to the lungs. In general, veins carry blood low in oxygen to the heart, except the pulmonary vein, which carries oxygenated blood from the lungs.

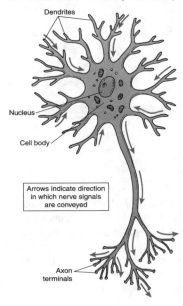

Dendrites

Nucleus

Cell body

Arrows indicate direction in which nerve signals are conveyed

Axon terminals

Figure 10-3. The neuron. The neuron is the major cell of the nervous system and is important in communication. It communicates by transmitting electrical signals by way of its axon and releasing chemical messengers from the axon terminal to organs.

away from them. Blood vessels function to transport blood throughout the body. The heart is a muscular pump that sends blood through the blood vessels and around the body.

The heart is a fist-sized, hollow muscular organ, located in the center of the chest (thoracic) cavity between the lungs and behind the breastbone (sternum). In the chest cavity, the bottom (apex) of the heart is tilted toward the left side of the body (see **Figure 10-4, 10-5A**). Surrounding the heart is a protective covering that is attached to the chest wall. Beneath the covering is the outside layer of the heart, which contains the blood vessels of the heart (coronary arteries), nerve fibers, and fat. Underneath this is the middle layer of the heart, which is made up of specialized muscle, comprised primarily of heart tissue. This muscular tissue is responsible for contracting the heart. The inside of the heart and its structures is lined with a special membrane, which allows for the smooth flow of blood. Throughout the heart muscle tissue is a fibrous network of connective tissue, which adds structure to the heart.

The heart is separated into four chambers. The two upper chambers, called the atria, are found on the left and right sides of the heart. Below the atria are two chambers called the ventricles, which are also on the left and right sides of the heart. The right and left sides of the heart comprise two functional pumps—the right atria and the right ventricle work together as a low-pressure pump, and the left atria and left ventricle work together as a high-pressure pump.

Blood vessels bring blood to the heart and take it away. Veins bring blood to the organ. Veins enter both atria. The superior and inferior vena cava enter the right atria, and the pulmonary veins enter the left atria. Arteries take blood away from the heart. Arteries exit both ventricles. The pulmonary artery exits the right ventricle, and the aorta exits the left ventricle.

Located in the heart are four valves, which ensure that blood travels in one direction as it flows through the organ. Two valves are found between the atria and the ventricles on each side of the heart, and the remaining two between the ventricles and the arteries—one between the left ventricle and the aorta and the other between the right ventricle and the pulmonary artery.

What Does It Do? (Physiology)

The cardiovascular system pumps oxygenated (high in oxygen, low in carbon dioxide) blood to every part of the body and transports deoxygenated (low in oxygen, high in carbon dioxide) blood from the cells (see **Figure 10-5B**). Blood that is low in oxygen enters the right atrium from the superior and inferior vena cava and flows through the valves separating the two chambers into the right ventricle. From there it is pumped through the pulmonary veins into the lungs. In the lungs, carbon dioxide is exchanged for oxygen (see **Figure 10-6**).

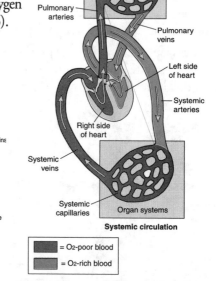

Figure 10-6. **How blood flows through the circulatory system.** There are two major divisions that transport blood throughout the body. In the pulmonary circulation, blood is pumped between the heart and the lungs to carry out gas exchanges. In the systemic circulation, blood is pumped between the heart and the organs and tissues of the upper and lower body.

Figure 10-5 A & B. **The anatomy of the heart. (A)** The heart has its own blood vessels, the coronary artery and veins, which supply blood to and from the heart. **(B)** The structure is divided into four chambers. The upper chambers are called atria and the lower chambers are called ventricles. On the right side of the heart, the superior and inferior vena cava enter the right atrium, and the pulmonary artery leaves the right ventricle. On the left side of the heart, the left and right pulmonary veins enter the left atrium, and the aorta leaves the left ventricle.

The oxygen-rich blood then returns to the left atrium and flows through the valve into the left ventricle, from which it is pumped throughout the body. The blood also delivers nutrients to cells and carries away waste products.

The cardiovascular system is also involved in maintaining blood pressure. Blood is pumped through the chambers of the heart in a continuous and repetitive cycle. During this cardiac cycle, the pressure in the heart rises and falls. When the atria and ventricles of the heart contract and consequently eject blood from the heart, the pressure rises. This phase in the cycle is called systole. When the atria and ventricles are relaxed and filling with blood, the pressure falls. This phase in the cycle is called diastole. The pressure changes during systole (systolic pressure) and diastole (diastolic pressure) can be measured by a sphygmomanometer, and these two measurements are called blood pressure. **Figure 10-7** illustrates the technique for measuring arterial blood pressure. The heart contains specialized cells, called pacemaker cells, that can generate electrical signals that trigger contraction of the heart and set the heart rhythm. In addition, the rate and force with which the heart pumps blood is regulated by the sympathetic and parasympathetic divisions of the autonomic nervous system. The sympathetic nervous system increases the heart rate and the force with which it contracts. The parasympathetic division slows the heart rate. Alteration of the rate and force of contraction of the heart can affect blood pressure.

What Happens When It Goes Wrong? (Pathophysiology)

When the regulation of the cardiovascular system is disrupted, a number of clinical problems can occur.

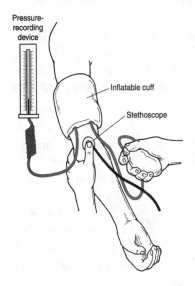

Pressure-recording device

Inflatable cuff

Stethoscope

Figure 10-7. The sphygmomanometer. This instrument accurately measures arterial blood pressure. The inflatable cuff is placed over the brachial artery and the pressure in the cuff is varied to determine systolic and diastolic readings of blood pressure.

Stroke: Stroke is an acute decrease or stoppage of blood flow to a part of the brain. The cause of a stroke can be a blood clot, which blocks the flow of blood in the vessels. Conditions that can lead to the development of a stroke are arteriosclerosis, which is caused by fatty deposits in the inside of blood vessels; aneurysm and high blood pressure.

Heart failure: In heart failure, the heart cannot eject enough blood from its ventricles. One or both sides of the heart can be affected. If it occurs in the left side of the heart, sufficient oxygenated blood cannot be pumped around the body, and the individual shows symptoms of tiredness, a blue tint to the skin, and a weak pulse. In addition, fluid builds up in the lungs, which decreases the exchange of gases in the lungs, and consequently, shortness of breath occurs. Heart failure can be caused by a heart attack, heart block, and bacterial or viral infections.

Hypertension: Hypertension develops when the normal regulation of blood pressure is disrupted and the diastolic pressure remains chronically elevated, higher than 90 mm Hg, and is accompanied by an increased systolic pressure of higher than 140 mm Hg. Uncontrolled blood pressure can increase the risk for stroke, heart attack, heart failure, and kidney and retinal damage.

Arrhythmias: Arrhythmias are abnormal rhythms of the heart. Some arrhythmias can cause the heart to beat too slowly or too rapidly, whereas others produce abnormal electrical activity in the organ. In some cases, arrhythmias can be life threatening, and in others, they are risk factors for stroke.

Respiratory System

What Is It? (Anatomy)

The respiratory system is comprised of the upper airways, the respiratory tract, and the lungs. The nasal and oral cavity and a muscular tube called the pharynx form the upper airways (see **Figure 10-8**). When air is breathed in, it enters the body through the nasal and oral cavity into the pharynx. From there it travels to the structures of the respiratory tract, namely the larynx, which also contains the vocal cords. Attached to the larynx is the epiglottis, a flap-like structure that prevents food and water from entering the respiratory tract. After traveling to the larynx, air enters the trachea, which is a rigid tube held open by C-shaped rings of cartilage. The trachea divides into smaller

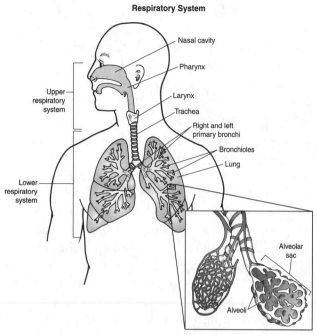

Figure 10-8. Anatomy of the respiratory system. The upper respiratory system is comprised of structures that bring air into the lungs. The lower respiratory system contains the bronchi, bronchioles, and the lungs. At the terminal end of the bronchioles are the alveolar sacs where the exchange of gases takes place.

airway passages called bronchi. Two major bronchi conduct air to the left and right lung. Inside each of the lungs, the bronchi divide into primary, secondary, and tertiary bronchi, becoming progressively smaller as they divide. The bronchi divide into even smaller tubes that have no cartilage, called bronchioles, and they terminate in single-layered cell structures called alveoli. Alveoli group in clusters known as alveolar sacs (Figure 10-8), and it is at this level that exchange of gases takes place between the lungs and the blood. Breathing, and therefore exchange of gases, can occur because movement of the muscles of the chest wall creates pressure changes that cause air to move into the lungs (inspiration) and out of the lungs (expiration).

Lining the larynx and trachea are specialized cells that secrete mucous, which traps particles and dust from the air breathed into the lungs. The mucous and trapped particles are then propelled by the beating action of cilia (hair-like projections) toward the pharynx, where they are swallowed.

What Does It Do? (Physiology)

The respiratory system is responsible for gas exchange, which ultimately allows oxygen to be taken to cells in the body and carbon dioxide to be removed from the cells. Gas exchange occurs at two levels: in the lungs between the alveoli and the blood and at the cellular

level between the blood and the tissues. In the blood, a molecule called hemoglobin carries oxygen. Carbon dioxide is also carried in the blood, some attached to hemoglobin, and the rest dissolved in the blood.

Deoxygenated blood (low in oxygen and high in carbon dioxide) travels from the right side of the heart to the lungs. At the level of the alveoli, carbon dioxide is released from the red blood cells into the lungs and exchanged for oxygen that has been brought into the lungs by the process of inspiration. The lungs release carbon dioxide through the nose or mouth by the process of expiration. The blood, rich in oxygen, then travels to the left side of the heart, where it is pumped to cells of the various tissues and organs where gas exchange continues.

Another function of the respiratory system is maintaining the acid–base balance of the blood. The blood is kept at a pH of 7.4. The pH must be maintained at this level, otherwise critical proteins, such as receptors and enzymes, can lose their ability to function. If the blood becomes too acidic, a condition called acidosis develops, which can affect the functioning of the nervous system and, in severe cases, can cause respiratory failure. If the blood becomes too basic, a condition called alkalosis develops, which can also affect the nervous system. In this case, the nervous system becomes overactive, resulting in seizures and convulsions.

Other functions of the respiratory system involve filtering out irritants in the air breathed and protecting the body from invading pathogens.

What Happens When It Goes Wrong? (Pathophysiology)

Asthma: Asthma is a disease of the lungs characterized by inflammation of the bronchioles, increased mucous secretion, and abnormal contractions of the smooth muscles in the bronchioles that lead to narrowing of the airway passages. The symptoms of the condition are difficulty breathing, wheezing, and coughing. The cause is often an allergic response to fungi, dust mites, or pet dander. Other factors, such as exercise, stress, and cold air, can also induce asthma.

Emphysema: Emphysema is the destruction of the airway walls. In the process of this destruction, airway spaces in the lungs enlarge, which makes it difficult to exchange gases between the blood and the air entering the lungs. The symptoms of the disease are difficulty breathing, coughing, and lung infections. The disease is believed to be caused by such factors as smoking, other environmental hazards, such as air pollutants, and occupational hazards, such as coal or stone dust.

Bronchitis: In bronchitis, the bronchi of the lungs become inflamed. A persistent cough is the major symptom. Bronchitis can last for a short time, in which case it is called acute bronchitis, or it can last for a longer time, in which case it is called chronic bronchitis.

Pulmonary edema: Pulmonary edema is characterized by excess fluid accumulating in the lungs. Eventually, fluid accumulates in the alveoli, where it interferes with gas exchange in the lungs and makes breathing difficult. The condition is characterized by rapid, shallow breathing, respiratory distress, and a blue tinge to the skin and mucous membranes. If left untreated, the condition can be life threatening.

Anemia: Anemia is characterized by a decreased oxygen-carrying capacity of the red blood cells. The condition can result from dietary deficiencies in iron, folic acid, or vitamin B12. When vitamin B12 is deficient, the condition is called pernicious anemia. Other types of anemia can be caused by a defective bone marrow, kidney failure, rupture of red blood cells, or loss of blood.

Musculoskeletal System

What Is It? (Anatomy)

This system is comprised of first a framework of individual bones called the skeleton. The skeleton is made up of 206 bones of different sizes and shapes. The bones are connected by joints (see **Figure 10-9**). Joints can be *fixed* to hold bones together, such as those holding the skull bones together, *partially moveable* to allow some flexibility, such as those in the spine, or *freely moveable*, such as those in the hipbones, arms, and legs. The skeletons of a man and woman are almost identical, with only small differences between the sexes. For example, the bones in the arms and legs are denser in the male, whereas the hipbones are wider in the female.

Covering the skeleton are the skeletal muscles, most of which are joined to the bones by tendons, although some, such as the facial muscles, are attached to the skin. The skeletal muscle is the largest tissue in the body, and the body has more than 600 muscles, which vary in length (see **Figure 10-10**). Each muscle is comprised of numerous individual muscle cells, called muscle fibers, that are highly elongated in shape and, in many cases, can run the length of the bone they are covering (see **Figure 10-11**). The muscle fibers are made up of thick and thin filaments that contain specialized proteins, called actin and myosin. Actin and myosin are responsible for making a muscle contract and relax. The orderly arrangement of actin and myosin in the muscle fibers gives skeletal muscle its character-

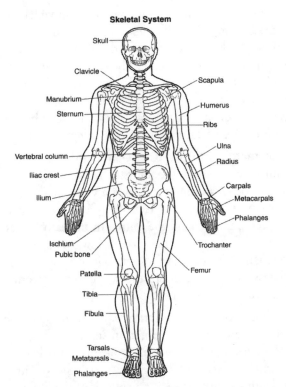

Figure 10-9. The skeletal system anterior view. The skeletal system is an extensive system of large and small bones that supports the muscle and protects the internal organs.

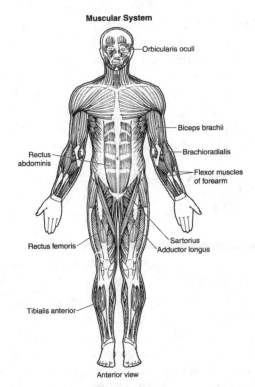

Figure 10-10. The skeletal muscles of the body. The skeletal muscles of the body attach to the skeleton via ligaments and tendons. When they contract, they can move or restrain parts of the body.

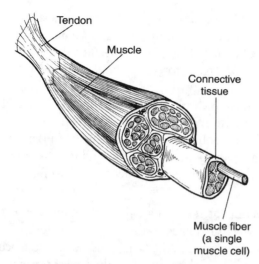

Figure 10-11. The structure of skeletal muscle. Each muscle is comprised of single muscle cells known as muscle fibers. The muscle fiber is formed from bundles of myofibrils that are surrounded by a specialized membrane known as the sarcolemma, which contains the sarcoplasmic reticulum and T-tubules. Each myofibril is composed of thick and thin filament, and their arrangement gives skeletal muscle its striated appearance.

istic striped appearance when viewed under the microscope. Skeletal muscle is under voluntary control.

In addition to skeletal muscle, two other types of muscle are found in the body: smooth muscle and cardiac muscle. These types of muscle are not under voluntary control. Smooth muscle is the primary muscle found in the internal organs of the body, such as the stomach, gut, glands, and blood vessels. Smooth muscle also contains actin and myosin. However, the actin and myosin are arranged in layers, which allow this muscle to stretch and expand, as, for example, the muscle of the bladder does. Cardiac muscle is found only in the heart. Like skeletal muscle, it has a characteristic striped appearance.

What Does It Do? (Physiology)

The skeleton functions as a dense, protective framework to shield internal organs, in addition to forming a structure to which other tissues, such as muscle, can attach. The skeleton also supports the weight of the body. Moreover, most bones contain red bone marrow, which produces red and white blood cells.

The skeletal muscles move the body by contracting and relaxing in a synchronized fashion. When the somatic nervous system sends a signal to a muscle, it contracts. Some muscles contract and relax quickly, such as the eyelid muscles, whereas others contract and relax for longer periods, such as the muscles in the back that control posture. The proper functioning of muscles allows an individual to carry out a wide range

of complex movements, from the gross motor control movements required for running to the fine motor control movements required for playing the piano.

Skeletal, smooth, and cardiac muscles are regulated by the nervous system. However, smooth and cardiac muscles have their own ability to initiate electrical signals, and therefore muscle activity, without input from the nervous system. This type of function is called *pacemaker activity*.

What Happens When It Goes Wrong? (Pathophysiology)

Osteoporosis is a condition that affects the bones. The bone structure changes from dense and heavy to thinner and lighter because of loss of proteins and minerals such as calcium and phosphate. In this condition, bone loss occurs faster than bone replacement, and the bones become fragile and prone to fractures.

The symptoms of osteoporosis are "silent," and often it is not diagnosed until a fracture occurs, a characteristic rounding of the back is evident, or a person becomes shorter. Certain diseases, such as Cushing's syndrome, can cause this condition. Women who have undergone menopause, artificial or natural, are prone to developing osteoporosis.

Osteomalacia: This is a rare condition in which the bones become soft and structurally weakened because the body is unable to absorb calcium or deposit minerals into the bone. The cause of the disease is vitamin D deficiency. Vitamin D deficiency can result from inadequate dietary intake, renal disease, celiac disease, malabsorption conditions in the gut, or prolonged treatment with certain epilepsy drugs.

Rheumatoid arthritis: Rheumatoid arthritis is an inflammatory disease of the joints. The cause is believed to be an autoimmune disease whereby the body produces antibodies that cause inflammation of a special membrane around the joints. In the early stages of the disease, the person may have a low-grade fever, lack of energy, loss of appetite, and a general feeling of unwellness. As the disease advances, the joints become swollen, red, painful, and stiff.

Osteoarthritis: In osteoarthritis, the cartilage of the joint deteriorates. This deterioration starts to affect the bone underneath, which eventually begins to thicken and distort. Osteoarthritis generally affects the weight-bearing joints—hips, knees, and spine—of the body. Pain, swelling, and stiffness of the joints are characteristic symptoms of this condition.

Endocrine System

What Is It? (Anatomy)

The endocrine system is made up of a group of glands that release chemical substances into the blood. The glands that make up the endocrine system are widely dispersed throughout the body and are not structurally related to each other. Even though the endocrine glands are not connected to each other, they make up a system in a functional sense; that is, they all perform the same role: They secrete chemical messengers into the bloodstream. These chemical messengers, called hormones, circulate in the bloodstream and affect many types of body cells.

These are the major endocrine glands (see **Figure 10-12**):

Hypothalamus
Pancreas
Posterior pituitary
Adrenal glands (medulla and cortex)
Anterior pituitary
Thymus
Pineal gland
Testis

Endocrine System

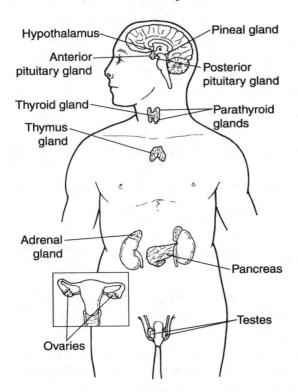

Figure 10-12. The major glands of the endocrine system. The endocrine system is made up of a group of glands that secrete chemical substances, known as hormones, into the bloodstream. The endocrine glands are widely dispersed throughout the body and are not structurally related to each other.

Thyroid
Ovary
Parathyroid

How Does It Work? (Physiology)

The endocrine system is made up of three parts: (1) the endocrine glands, (2) the hormone(s) they secrete into the bloodstream, and (3) the hormone's target tissue or cells (Figure 10-12). These three parts work together to relay information and instructions throughout the body.

The purpose of the secreted hormones is to bring on a specific response in *other* cells of the body. Some hormones function only to regulate the production of other hormones. Other hormones exert their effects on the target tissues themselves. Because the hormones are secreted into the bloodstream, they can reach all the cells of the body.

The endocrine system works to do the following:

- Maintain the body's internal state.
- Help the body deal with stressful situations.
- Regulate growth and development.
- Control reproduction.
- Produce, use, and store energy.

It happens like this:

1. Glands and nerve cells signal endocrine glands about temperature changes, hunger, fear, growth needs, or other stimuli.

2. In response, endocrine glands release hormones to carry instructions to specific cells. These chemical messengers travel throughout the bloodstream until they reach and lock onto special binding proteins, known as receptors, located in and on the target cells.

3. Once bound, the receptor reads the hormone's message and carries out its instructions by starting one of two distinct cellular processes. The receptor can (1) turn on genes to make new proteins, which causes *long-term* effects, such as growth and sexual and reproductive maturity or (2) alter the activity of existing proteins inside the cell, which produces *rapid* responses, such as a faster heartbeat or varied blood sugar levels.

The endocrine glands are characterized by the hormone(s) that they secrete and the target tissue(s) that the hormone affects. Because of the large number of endocrine glands (listed above), the best way to understand the endocrine system is to view the effects that each hormone has on the body. **Table 10-1** lists

TABLE 10-1. ENDOCRINE GLANDS AND HORMONAL PHYSIOLOGIC EFFECTS ON THE BODY

Endocrine Gland	Principal Hormone(s) Secreted	Target Tissue(s)	Physiologic Effect of Hormone
Hypothalamus	Releasing and inhibiting hormones	Anterior pituitary	Controls release of anterior pituitary hormones
Anterior Pituitary	Thyroid-stimulating hormone (TSH)	Thyroid	Production of thyroid hormone
	Adrenocorticotropic hormone (ACTH)	Adrenal cortex	Secretion of cortisol
	Growth hormone	Bones; soft tissues	Stimulates growth of bones and soft tissues
	Follicle-stimulating hormone (FSH)	Females: ovary	Promotes growth of ovarian follicle; stimulates estrogen secretion
	Luteinizing hormone (LH)	Males: testes	Stimulates sperm production
		Females: ovary	Stimulates ovulation; stimulates estrogen and progesterone secretion
	Prolactin	Males: testes	Stimulates testosterone secretion
		Females: breast	Promotes breast development; stimulates milk secretion
Posterior Pituitary	Vasopressin (antidiuretic hormone)	Kidney	Causes water retention
	Oxytocin	Uterus	Causes contractions
		Breasts	Causes ejection of milk
Pineal	Melatonin	Brain; anterior pituitary; reproductive organs; possibly other sites	Sets the body's "time clock"; causes sleep in response to darkness
Thyroid	Thyroid hormone (T_3 and T_4)	Most cells	Increases the metabolic rate; necessary for normal growth and development
Parathyroid	Parathyroid hormone	Bone; kidney; intestine	Increases amount of calcium in the bloodstream; decreases amount of phosphate in the bloodstream
Thymus	Thymosin	T lymphocytes	Enhances the production of T lymphocytes
Pancreas	Insulin	Most cells	Promotes use and storage of nutrients, particularly glucose, after eating
	Glucagon	Most cells	Maintains glucose levels in the bloodstream during periods of no food
	Somatostatin	Digestive system	Inhibits digestion and absorption of nutrients
Adrenal Medulla	Epinephrine and norepinephrine	Nervous system sites throughout the entire body	Reinforces the nervous system; "fight or flight" system
Adrenal Cortex	Aldosterone	Kidney	Increases sodium retention and potassium secretion
	Cortisol	Most cells	Increases glucose in the bloodstream
	Androgens	Females: bone and brain	Puberty growth spurt and sex drive in females
Testes (male)	Testosterone	Male sex organs; body as a whole	Stimulates production of sperm; responsible for development of sex characteristics; promotes sex drive
Ovaries (female)	Estrogen	Female sex organs; body as a whole	Stimulates uterine and breast growth; responsible for development of sex characteristics
	Progesterone	Uterus	Prepares for pregnancy

each endocrine gland, the hormone(s) it produces, and the hormone's *main* physiologic effect.

What Happens When It Goes Wrong? (Pathophysiology)

Because the number of endocrine glands, hormones, and target cells throughout the body is so large, when something in one of the endocrine glands goes wrong, it has a profound impact on a number of other bodily functions. Generally, problems within the endocrine system are due to either too little or too much hormone being produced. Disorders resulting from a decreased production of hormone are treated by giving the patient a prescription of replacement hormone. Disturbances within the endocrine system may also occur from damage done directly to the endocrine gland or, less commonly, from a decreased sensitivity of the target tissue to the hormone. Because the actions of hormones are so extensive, the following review focuses only on the most common endocrine disorders.

Diabetes: Diabetes is characterized by high levels of glucose (sugar) in the bloodstream and urine. Diabetes results from either a decreased production of insulin by the pancreas (Type I diabetes) or a decreased sensitivity of target tissues to insulin (Type II diabetes). Treatment depends on the type of diabetes diagnosed. Type I diabetics are typically treated with replacement insulin therapy, whereas Type II diabetics usually benefit from oral medication that decreases blood sugar levels.

Acromegaly: In acromegaly, the production of too much growth hormone in childhood results in a rapid growth in height. Although this happens without disfiguring the rest of the body, an individual may reach a height of 8 feet or more if not treated with a growth hormone blocker. If the overproduction of growth hormone occurs after the growth plates have closed (typically after adolescence), the resulting condition is not an increase in height, but rather a thickening of the bones and soft tissues. This results in a disfiguring condition known as gigantism.

Dwarfism: Underproduction of growth hormone in childhood can result in dwarfism, which is characterized by short stature and retarded growth of the skeleton.

Thyroid disease: Thyroid disease can result from the production of too little thyroid hormone (hypothyroidism) or too much thyroid hormone (hyperthyroidism). An individual suffering from hypothyroidism can be treated with a prescription of replacement thyroid hormone. Hyperthyroidism is not as easily treated. Depending on the cause of increased thyroid levels, treatment may range from a thyroid hormone blocker

to treatment of the thyroid gland with radioactivity to destroy part of the gland itself.

Gastrointestinal System

What Is It? (Anatomy)

At its simplest, the gastrointestinal (GI) tract is a hollow tube running through the body from the mouth to the anus. The adult GI tract (also known as the digestive tract) is about 30 feet long. The basic components of the GI system are described below (see **Figure 10-13**):

- **Mouth:** The mouth, or oral cavity, is the entrance to the digestive tract. Food is broken down mechanically by chewing, and saliva is added as a lubricant.

- **Pharynx:** The pharynx, which is about 5 inches long, is a cavity located at the rear of the throat. It serves as a shared passageway for food and air. A flap called the epiglottis reflexively closes the windpipe while food is being swallowed.

- **Esophagus:** The esophagus is a fairly straight muscular tube that extends between the pharynx and the stomach; it serves simply to connect the mouth with the stomach. It is the least complex section of the GI tract. The esophagus is guarded at both ends by sphincters (rings of muscle that control passage of contents through an opening

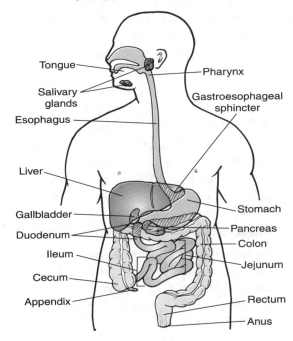

Figure 10-13. Anatomy of the major components of the gastrointestinal tract. The gastrointestinal tract can be thought of as a long, hollow tube running through the body from the mouth to the anus. Shown are the basic components of the gastrointestinal tract, which function to transfer energy from ingested food to the internal cells of the body and rid the body of undigested waste.

into, or out of, a hollow organ; when closed, a sphincter prevents passage through the tube). The upper sphincter is the *pharyngoesophageal* sphincter, and the lower sphincter is the *gastroesophageal* sphincter.

- **Stomach:** The stomach is a pouch-like chamber located in the upper middle of the abdomen, between the esophagus and the small intestine. The stomach stores food while thoroughly mixing it with acids and enzymes, breaking it into much smaller, digestible pieces. When empty, an adult's stomach has a volume of one-fifth of a cup, but it can expand to hold more than 8 cups of food. Chemical digestion of food begins in the stomach, where food particles are reduced to a liquid form.

- **Small intestine:** The small intestine is a coiled tube nearly 10 feet long. The final stages of chemical digestion occur in the small intestine, where almost all nutrients from the ingested food are absorbed. The inner wall of the small intestine is covered with microscopic fingerlike projections called *villi*. The villi are where nutrients are absorbed into the body.

- **Large intestine:** The large intestine is mainly a drying and storage organ. It is made up of three parts: (1) the *cecum*, a small sac-like section of bowel, at the end of which the appendix hangs; (2) the *colon*, which extends from the cecum, up the right side of the abdomen, across the upper abdomen, and then down the left side of the abdomen, finally connecting to the rectum; and (3) the *rectum*, which terminates at the anus. The cecum and colon are about 5 feet long, while the rectum is only 5 inches long.

- **Liver:** The liver is located beneath the ribcage of the right upper part of the abdomen. It is the center of metabolic activity in the body and also plays a large role in the digestion and absorption of nutrients.

- **Pancreas:** The pancreas is located beneath the stomach. It serves an important role, providing to the small intestine a potent mixture of digestive enzymes that are critical for digestion of food, in addition to its role in insulin production and glucose regulation.

What Does It Do? (Physiology)

The GI tract functions to transfer energy from food to the cells of the body. This system also eliminates undigested food residues to the external environment.

Plants can transfer the energy from the sun into usable forms of energy; humans cannot. Humans must rely on ingested food as an energy source for the cells of the body to use to carry out energy-dependent activities. The breakdown of food is accomplished through a combination of mechanical and chemical (enzymatic) processes. To accomplish this breakdown, the digestive tube requires considerable assistance from accessory digestive organs, such as the salivary glands, liver, and pancreas, which dump their secretions into the tube. The main function of the tube is to break down food (proteins, fats, and carbohydrates), which cannot be absorbed whole, into smaller molecules (amino acids, fatty acids, and glucose) that can be absorbed across the wall of the tube and into the circulatory system for distribution around the entire body. Some of the molecules are used for energy, some as building blocks for tissues and cells, and some are stored for future use.

The first step in the digestive process is the chewing and mixing of ingested food by the teeth. The purposes of chewing are (1) to tear, grind, and break down food particles into smaller pieces to facilitate swallowing and (2) to mix food with saliva. Saliva is produced by salivary glands located outside the mouth and is secreted into the mouth by small ducts. The mass of chewed, moistened food (known as a *bolus*) is moved to the back of the mouth by the tongue. In the pharynx, the bolus triggers an involuntary swallowing reflex that prevents food from entering the lungs and directs the bolus into the esophagus. Muscles in the esophagus propel the bolus by waves of involuntary muscular contractions (peristalsis) of the muscle lining the esophagus (see **Figure 10-14**). The bolus then passes

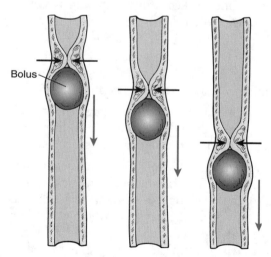

Bolus

Figure 10-14. Peristalsis. Waves of involuntary muscular contractions propel boluses of food along the esophagus down toward the stomach.

through the gastroesophogeal sphincter into the stomach.

The stomach provides four basic functions: (1) it serves as a short-term storage site, allowing a rather large meal to be consumed quickly and dealt with over an extended period; (2) it starts substantial chemical and enzymatic digestion; (3) it mixes food with acidic stomach secretions by vigorous contractions of the stomach muscles, resulting in liquefaction of food, which must occur before food can be delivered to the small intestine; and (4) it slowly releases food, as it is liquefied, into the small intestine for further processing. By the time food is ready to leave the stomach, it has been processed into a thick liquid called *chyme* (see **Figure 10-15**). The outlet of the stomach—a small muscle called the *pylorus*—keeps the chyme in the stomach until it reaches the right consistency to pass into the small intestine. Chyme is then squirted down into the duodenum of the small intestine by the action of peristalsis.

In the small intestine, where most nutritional absorption occurs, digestive chemicals work on the partially digested food. The pancreas and liver connect with the small intestine and send secretions into it to aid digestion. These secretions include *pancreatic juice*, which contains enzymes that help digest carbohydrates, proteins, and fats; and *bile*, which breaks down and aids in the absorption of fat. Though bile is produced in the liver, it is stored in the gallbladder and sent into the small intestine through the bile duct. Once broken down, these now-soluble food products, along with vitamins and minerals, are dissolved and absorbed

directly into the bloodstream through the walls of the small intestine. This process is called *absorption*. By the time the food reaches the large intestine, the work of digestion is almost finished.

The main function of the large intestine is to remove water from the undigested matter and form the matter into feces that will be eliminated from the body by excretion. Bacteria in the colon aid digestion of the remaining food products. The final waste product, the feces, is stored in the rectum until it exits the body through another sphincter at the anus.

What Happens When It Goes Wrong? (Pathophysiology)

If the normal function of the GI tract is disrupted, a number of different clinical situations may occur, such as the following. They differ depending on the site of the malfunction or disease.

Ulcers: The stomach contains strong acids to aid in the breakdown of foods. Under normal conditions, the stomach and small intestine are extremely resistant to irritation by the strong acids they contain. A bacterium (most commonly *helicobacter pylori*) or the chronic use of certain medications may weaken the protective coating of the stomach and duodenum and allow acid to get through to the sensitive lining beneath. Both the acid and the bacteria can irritate and inflame the lining (a condition known as *gastritis*) or cause peptic ulcers, which are sores or holes that form in the lining of the stomach or the duodenum and cause pain or bleeding. Medications are used to treat these conditions, including a course of antibiotics if *helicobacter pylori* is involved.

Esophageal disorders: Inflammation of the esophagus (*esophagitis*) can be caused by complications of certain medications or infection. Esophagitis is also commonly caused by a condition in which the lower esophageal sphincter is weakened and thus allows the acidic contents of the stomach to move backwards, or reflux, up into the esophagus. The result is inflammation and tissue damage of the esophagus. This condition is known as gastroesophageal reflux disease (GERD). Medications that reduce the production of stomach acid are used to protect the tissue lining the esophagus.

Gastrointestinal infections: Infections of the gastrointestinal tract are quite common and are caused most commonly by viruses (such as enterovirus or rotavirus), bacteria (such as salmonella, shigella, or *E. coli*), or parasites or protozoan organisms. The microor-

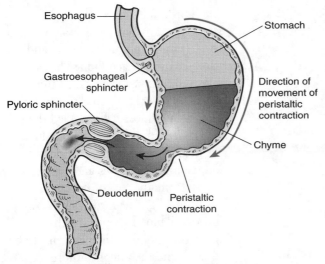

Figure 10-15. Gastric emptying. Peristaltic contractions originate in the upper portions of the stomach and gain strength as they near the pyloric sphincter. These contractions function to mix and propel chyme (liquid stomach contents) toward the pyloric sphincter and are responsible for pushing small quantities of chyme through the sphincter into the duodenum.

ganisms that cause GI infections often increase the muscle contraction (peristaltic) activity of the gastrointestinal tract; this results in vomiting and diarrhea.

Diarrhea: Diarrhea is a condition in which bowel movements are abnormally frequent and feces are loose and watery. It occurs when the muscle contractions (peristalsis) of the intestines move the fecal material along too quickly, not allowing enough time for the water content to be absorbed into the body. In addition to bacterial and viral infections, diarrhea can be caused by food poisoning (when food is infested with harmful bacteria), drinking contaminated water, lactose intolerance, and stress. If diarrhea lasts for more than a couple of days, the body may lose too much water and become dehydrated.

Appendicitis: Appendicitis is inflammation of the appendix, the finger-like appendage of the colon that sits on the lower right side of the abdomen. The common symptoms of appendicitis are abdominal pain, fever, and vomiting.

Inflammatory bowel disease: Inflammatory bowel disease is a chronic inflammation of the intestines. There are two types: *ulcerative colitis*, which affects just the rectum and the large intestine, and *Crohn's disease*, which can affect the whole GI tract, from the mouth to the anus. The most common symptoms of inflammatory bowel disease are chronic abdominal pain; intermittent, severe diarrhea, which may be bloody; and weight loss. Flare-ups of inflammatory bowel disease can occur at any time but are especially common during times of stress.

Constipation: In this condition, the contents of the intestines do not move along fast enough, resulting in an infrequent and painful emptying of the intestines. Waste materials stay in the large intestine so long that too much water is removed and the feces become hard.

Urinary Tract System

What Is It? (Anatomy)

The structures of the urinary tract system are the kidneys, ureters, bladder, and urethra. The two kidneys, bean-shaped organs that produce urine, are toward the back of the mid-abdominal cavity (see **Figure 10-16**). Each of the kidneys receives a large supply of blood that enters the organs by the right and left renal artery. The kidneys filter this blood to remove waste products and supply the kidneys with oxygen. Once the blood has been filtered, it leaves the kidneys via the renal veins and returns to the right side of the heart. The two ureters—one running from each kidney—are responsible for transporting urine to the bladder. The bladder is a small, muscular ball that can expand to a large volume to store urine until it is ready to be excreted from the body via the urethra.

The kidneys have a highly specialized anatomy, which allow them to filter huge volumes of blood and produce urine. Each kidney has a special outermost layer called the *cortex*, an inner layer called the *medulla*, and an innermost region called the *renal pelvis*. In the cortex and medulla are the functioning units of the kidney, called *nephrons*, and each kidney contains tens of thousands of nephrons. Each nephron has its own individual blood supply, which transports blood to the nephrons to be filtered, and each nephron forms urine (see **Figure 10-17**). All the urine that has been formed by the nephrons is collected in the renal pelvis and then transported to the ureter.

Figure 10-16. The anatomy of the urinary tract system. The urinary tract system is comprised of the right and left kidney and ureters, the bladder, and the urethra. The kidney has two major layers of tissue—renal cortex and renal medulla—and an inner structure—renal pelvis. Urine collects in the renal pelvis and flows from the kidneys, via the ureters, to the bladder, where it is stored until emptied outside the body by way of the urethra.

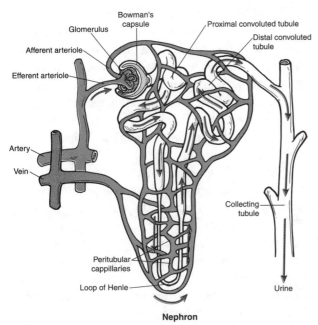

Figure 10-17. The nephron. The nephron is the basic functioning unit of the kidney. It processes blood plasma and produces urine. Fluid flows through the nephron in the following order: Bowman's capsule, proximal convoluted tubule, loop of Henle, distal convoluted tubule, collecting duct.

What Does It Do? (Physiology)

The kidneys perform many important functions. One is to filter the blood as it passes through the nephrons removing waste products, such as products from protein breakdown, while reabsorbing important substances, such as glucose and protein, and returning them into circulation for use by the cells of the body. In the process of filtering the blood, urine is formed. The kidneys also play a critical role in regulating the volume of the plasma, and therefore blood volume, which affects blood pressure. Another function of the kidneys is regulating the concentration of ions in the plasma, which are important for maintaining the healthy functions and processes of cells. This is possible because the kidneys are able to excrete or reabsorb ions, such as sodium, potassium, calcium, magnesium, phosphate, bicarbonate, and chloride, and thus maintain the balance of these ions in the blood. Additional functions of the kidneys include maintaining the pH of the blood and excreting drugs and pesticides. The kidneys are involved in the production of an important hormone that stimulates production of red blood cells, and they also activate vitamin D3.

What Happens When It Goes Wrong? (Pathophysiology)

Kidney stones: Kidney stones are formed when the substances that are normally excreted in the urine crystallize in the pelvis of the kidney and form into small masses called stones. They can be formed from such substances as calcium, phosphate, or uric acid. Small stones are excreted in the urine unnoticed. Larger stones can lodge in the kidney or the bladder, and if they move, they cause excruciating pain. In most cases, the reason for the formation of kidney stones is unknown. Certain diseases, however, such as gout and urinary tract infections, can precipitate the condition. Also, certain environments, such as hot climates where dehydration can easily occur, can promote kidney stones. Men are affected more than women, and young people are affected more than the elderly.

Kidney disease: Many conditions can seriously damage the kidney. Most kidney diseases attack the nephrons, causing them to lose their filtering function. Damage to the nephrons can happen quickly, with the kidney function recovering after a few weeks. For example, in acute nephrotic syndrome, which can occur after tonsillitis or certain types of streptococcal bacterial infection, damage to the filtering component of the nephron occurs. Most kidney diseases destroy the nephrons slowly, and the kidneys ultimately fail. For example, diabetic nephropathy, uncontrolled high blood pressure, and polycystic kidney disease lead to kidney failure.

Diabetes insipidus: In this condition, the kidneys do not respond to the hormone vasopressin or an antidiuretic hormone. As a result, the kidneys are unable to reabsorb water, which leads to high volumes of urine being excreted.

Reproductive System

What Is It? (Anatomy)

Unlike the body systems discussed so far, which are essentially identical in males and females, the reproductive system is vastly different in the two sexes. The primary reproductive organs, or gonads, consist of a pair of testes in the male and a pair of ovaries in the female (see **Figure 10-18**). In both sexes, mature gonads perform two functions: (1) the production of reproductive cells, called gametes (sperm in males and eggs in the female) and (2) the production of sex hormones (testosterone in males and estrogen and progesterone in females).

Although an individual can survive without reproducing, the human species needs the reproductive system to continue to exist.

Male System

The male reproductive system enables a man to have

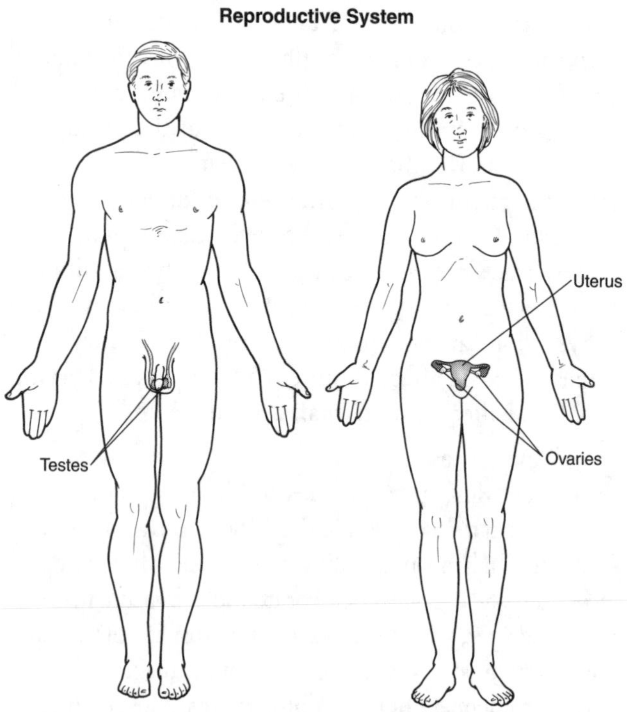

Reproductive System

Figure 10-18. Reproductive organs in the male and female. The anatomy and physiology of the reproductive systems are vastly different in the male and the female.

sexual intercourse and to fertilize eggs (ova) with sperm (male sex cells). Sperm, along with male sex hormones, are produced in the testes, a pair of oval-shaped glands that are suspended in a pouch called the scrotum. The sexual organs of the male are in part external and in part internal. The visible parts are the penis and the scrotum. Inside the body are the prostate gland and tubes that link the system together. The male organs produce and transfer sperm to the female.

Female System

The female reproductive system consists of organs that enable a woman to produce eggs (ova), to have sexual intercourse, to nourish and house the fertilized egg until it is fully developed, to give birth, and to be the sole source of nutrition for a newborn baby. The female sexual organs are almost entirely internal. The female organs are the vulva, the vagina, the uterus (or womb), the fallopian tubes, and the ovaries. The breasts are also included in the reproductive system of the female because they develop to become the feeding source of a newborn baby.

What Does It Do? (Physiology)

The reproductive capability of an individual depends on a complex relationship between the hypothalamus, anterior pituitary, reproductive organs, and target cells of sex hormones.

The reproductive organs, or gonads, produce sex hormones (estrogen and progesterone in the female, testosterone in the male). These hormones are responsible for the development of secondary sex characteristics when an individual reaches puberty. The ultimate consequence of sexual development is the production of reproductive cells that will pass genes on to the next generation. In addition to producing sex hormones, the gonads produce reproductive cells. Both sexes produce reproductive cells: sperm in males and ova (eggs) in females. Each individual produces an enormous amount of reproductive cells; the sexes differ, however, as to when the reproductive cells are produced. The female possesses all her several million reproductive cells at birth; only several hundred, however, will develop to the point where they will have the chance to be fertilized—the rest will degenerate over time. She will not produce any more during her lifetime. The male produces his reproductive cells continuously after reaching sexual maturity, and each ejaculation releases perhaps a hundred million sperm.

What Happens When Something Goes Wrong? (Pathophysiology)

The gonads are responsible for producing the sex hormones; if there is a problem with this production, a number of conditions may occur. If the individual (male or female) is deficient in the amount of sex hormone during growth and development, secondary sex characteristics may not develop, and the individual may not develop a mature reproductive system. This would mean that the gonads would not fully develop, and the individual would not produce either sex hormone or reproductive sex cells.

Immune System

What Is It? (Anatomy)

The body is equipped with a complex defense system—the immune system—which provides constant protection against foreign invaders. The immune system is a collection of molecules, cells, and organs whose complex interactions form an efficient system to usually protect the body from both outside invaders and its own altered cells and also rid the body of unwanted cellular debris.

The immune system is composed of the cells in the bone marrow; the thymus; and the lymphatic system of ducts and nodes, spleen, and blood that function to protect the body (see **Figure 10-19**).

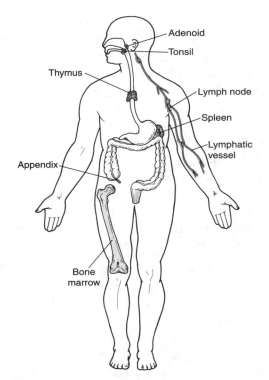

Figure 10-19. Tissues of the immune system. The immune system is composed of the cells of the bone marrow, the thymus, and the lymphatic system of ducts and nodes, spleen, and lymphoid tissue (tonsils, adenoids, appendix), which protect the body against foreign materials. Note that the components of the immune system are widely dispersed throughout the body.

The "worker" cells of the immune system, which are responsible for the various immune defenses, are found in the bloodstream and known as white blood cells (leukocytes) and the cells that are made from them (see **Figure 10-20**). All blood cells, including those destined to become immune cells, arise in the bone marrow from stem cells.

Numerous cell types function in the immune system. Phagocytes are large white blood cells (including monocytes, macrophages, and neutrophils) that devour cells and particles. Eosinophils and basophils are granule-containing inflammatory cells. The only immune cells that are not derived from stem cells are the lymphocytes, which are white blood cells that provide immune defense against specific targets. The two types of lymphocytes are called B cells and T cells.

The organs of the immune system are found throughout the body. They are known as *lymphoid* organs because they are concerned with the growth, development, and deployment of lymphocytes, the white blood cells discussed above. The organs of the immune system are connected with one another and with other organs of the body by a network of lymphatic vessels similar to blood vessels. Immune cells

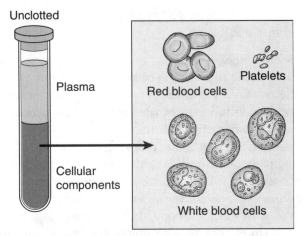

Figure 10-20. Components of blood. Cellular components found in the blood.

and foreign particles are transported through the lymphatic vessels in lymph, a clear fluid that bathes the body's tissues. The major lymphoid organs are lymph nodes, tonsils, adenoids, the appendix, the spleen, and the thymus. Lymph nodes are small, bean-shaped structures that are located throughout the body along the lymphatic routes. Lymph nodes contain specialized compartments where immune cells congregate.

What Does It Do? (Physiology)

When the body is threatened by microorganisms, viruses, or cancer cells, the action of the immune system, known as an immune response, provides protection by destroying the threatening organism. Normally, the immune system does not mount a response against itself. This lack of an immune response is called *tolerance*. It is vital that the immune response is able to distinguish between "self" and "nonself." Every body cell carries distinctive molecules that distinguish it as self; immune cells do not attack tissues that carry a self marker.

Foreign molecules carry distinctive markers as well—characteristic shapes that allow the immune system to recognize them as foreign and initiate an immune response. Any substance capable of triggering an immune response (and carrying a nonself marker) is known as an *antigen*. An antigen can be a bacterium, a virus, or even a portion or product of one of these organisms. Tissues or cells from another individual also act as antigens, which is why transplanted tissues are rejected as foreign without preventative drug therapy.

Invading microorganisms attempting to get into the body must first get past the the skin and mucous membranes. If the invader gets past these physical barriers, the activities of the immune system come into play. The primary defensive cells are neutrophils, eosinophils, basophils, B lymphocytes, T lymphocytes, and macrophages.

The Immune Response

The immune response can occur in a number of different ways. These mechanisms, known together as *immunity*, include both innate and adaptive, or acquired, immune responses. Innate immune responses are nonspecific responses that defend against foreign material nonselectively, even the first time the body is exposed to it. Adaptive, or acquired, immune responses are specific responses that target specific invaders to which the body has been exposed at least once before. In an adaptive immune response, the body is ready because it has been specially prepared for the invader to return.

The immune response is initiated once the immune system recognizes a foreign molecule. The first immune system cells called the invader encounters are cells circulating in the bloodstream: a series of nonspecific (innate) defenses—cells and substances that attack all invaders regardless of the antigens they carry. One example of an innate immune response is the inflammation response. Inflammation is a nonspecific response to foreign invasion or tissue damage that occurs when neutrophils and macrophages destroy foreign or damaged cells. Neutrophils and macrophages attack invaders by phagocytosis (a cell "eats up" the foreign cell) and by releasing chemicals that attract more cells of the immune system to the area of inflammation. The ultimate goal of inflammation is to bring more help from the immune system to destroy the invaders, remove the dead cells, and begin the process of tissue healing and repair. These actions are responsible for the visible effects of inflammation: swelling, redness, heat, and pain.

Following the first exposure to a microorganism, specific players of the adaptive (or acquired) immune system become specially prepared to attack the invading microorganism should it invade again. The cells of the adaptive immune system are the lymphocytes, and they are prepared to attack the invader by carrying special markers on their surface that seek out the antigen of that specific microorganism. B lymphocytes generally attack bacteria, and T lymphocytes attack viruses. Once the lymphocyte encounters its specific antigen, the microorganism is either directly or indirectly destroyed. B lymphocytes secrete antibodies that indirectly lead to the destruction of foreign material. Antibodies are proteins known as *immunoglobulins* that are produced by a specific B cell against a particular antigen. Antibodies do not directly destroy the invader. Instead, they bind to the antigen against which they are produced and intensify the nonselective immune responses that are already initiated against the antigen. The T lymphocytes are responsible for the direct destruction of virus-invaded cells.

What Happens When It Goes Wrong? (Pathophysiology)

A number of clinical problems can occur when something within the immune system goes wrong. If the immune system produces too few T cells, viral defenses fail. If the immune system produces too few B cells, bacterial defenses fail.

Allergy: One of the most well-known disorders of the immune system is allergy. Allergies occur when the body mounts an immune response against a normally harmless substance, such as grass pollen. In this case, the offending agent is called an allergen. Allergies such as hay fever and hives are related to an antibody known as IgE. The first time an allergy-prone individual is exposed to an allergen (for example, grass pollen), the individual's B cells make large amounts of grass pollen IgE antibody. These IgE molecules attach to granule-containing cells known as mast cells, which are plentiful in the lungs, skin, tongue, and linings of the nose and GI tract. The next time the individual is exposed to grass pollen, the IgE-primed mast cell releases powerful chemicals that cause the wheezing, sneezing, and other symptoms of allergy.

Autoimmune disease: In an autoimmune disease, the immune system destroys the body's own normal cells. When the body loses its ability to correctly identify body cells belonging to self, it can mount immune responses against its own cells and organs. In this case, antibodies produced by B or T cells are called autoantibodies. Autoimmunity can cause a broad range of human illnesses. For instance, T cells that attack pancreas cells contribute to diabetes, and an autoantibody known as *rheumatoid factor* is common in persons with rheumatoid arthritis.

AIDS: AIDS stands for acquired immunodeficiency syndrome. AIDS is caused by infection with a virus called human immunodeficiency virus (HIV). This virus is passed from one person to another through blood-to-blood and sexual contact. HIV destroys T-helper cells, which are essential to the normal function of the immune system. Infection with HIV can weaken the immune system to the point that it has difficulty fighting off certain other infections. These types of infections are known as "opportunistic" infections because they take the opportunity a weakened immune system gives to cause illness. Many of the infections that cause illness or may be life threatening for people with AIDS are usually controlled by a healthy immune system.

Most people infected with HIV carry the virus for years before enough damage is done to the T-helper cells and the immune system for AIDS to develop. A strong connection exists between the amount of HIV in the blood and the decline in T-helper cells, leading to the development of AIDS. Therefore, drug therapy has been targeted to reducing the amount of virus in the body with anti-HIV medications to slow the immune system destruction and progression of the disease.

Special Senses

What Is It? (Anatomy)

To maintain a stable internal environment, an individual must be equipped to deal with fluctuations in the external environment and continually adapt to ever-changing circumstances. Somehow, information from the external environment, or outside world, must be communicated to the internal environment, or brain, of a human being for the individual to perceive the world and its surroundings. The skin and special senses make up a functional system of perception that allows an individual to perceive his or her surroundings for the purpose of adaptation to the environment. Organs known as sensory organs sense information on the exterior of the body and transmit it to the brain, where the information can be processed. Specialized sites, called receptors, on the sensory organs pick up information about the external surroundings (see **Figure 10-21**). Each of the sensory organs has receptors that can detect changes in the exterior environment and transmit this information to the brain.

Transmitting signals from the outside to the inside involves a number of players: receptors, nerve cells, and the brain. Receptors are protein molecules located on the outside of a cell capable of sensing change. The different types of receptors are characterized by what they are capable of detecting. For example, receptors on the skin that are sensitive to temperature changes are called thermoreceptors. Receptors have been identified that are responsive to changes in light (photoreceptors), mechanical energy (mechanoreceptors), chemicals (chemoreceptors), and pain and damage to tissue (nociceptors).

The primary sensory organs are the skin (nociceptors), the eyes (photoreceptors), the ears

(mechanoreceptors), and the nose and tongue (chemoreceptors). See Figure 10-21. The actions of these sensory organs create the abilities known as the senses: touch, vision, hearing, taste, and smell.

What Does It Do? (Physiology)

This information about the outside world is transmitted to the inside through a complex process that involves the nervous system. Through the receptors, information is "picked up" and relayed to the brain, where the information is processed. The human reacts, either consciously or unconsciously, to the situation. These signals are transmitted almost continually, in fractions of a second. When an individual's hand gets too close to a flame, for example, it only takes a fraction of a second to move it. The signal to move the hand is carried on long nerve fibers to the brain, where the information is processed. Depending on the type of receptor that is activated, the brain may send a signal back to the body with a message. For example, the hand placed too close to the flame activates both nociceptors and thermoreceptors located on the skin of the hand. Signals are transmitted to the brain; the brain then tells the muscles of the arm to remove the hand from the flame as quickly as possible. This type of action is known as a reflex.

Researchers are just beginning to understand the complex communication signals that take place to transmit this information accurately to the brain. Scientists have found that perception depends on the simultaneous, cooperative activity of millions of nerve cells spread throughout expanses of the cortex region of the brain. Which area of the brain processes the

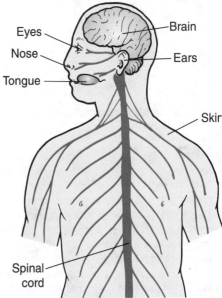

Sensory Nervous System

Figure 10-21. **The sensory nervous system.** The sensory organs of primary importance are the skin, eyes, ears, nose, and tongue. From the actions of these sensory organs, individuals have the abilities known as the *senses*: vision, hearing, taste, smell, and touch.

sensory input depends on which sensory organ sends the information, as described in the following examples (see **Figure 10-22**).

Pain: Pain is primarily a protective mechanism that is meant to bring awareness of the fact that tissue damage or injury is occurring. Stimulation of the pain receptors (nociceptors) elicits the perception of pain and causes a reaction to stop or prevent the pain. The pain receptors not only detect such damage as pinching, cutting, and crushing of tissue but also detect changes in temperature or damage from irritating chemicals. Once the pain receptors sense damage of any type, they send their message via long nerve fibers to the brain, where the information is processed.

Vision: The ability to see requires at least one functional eye. The anatomy of the eye allows light to pass through to the back of the eye, where it reaches a structure called the retina. Light must then pass through several layers of the retina before it reaches the rods and cones, the parts of the eye that contain the light receptors (photoreceptors). The main function of the eye is to focus light rays from the environment onto the photoreceptors. The photoreceptors then change the light energy into energy that can be carried on a nerve cell. Once this energy change occurs, the nerve cell carries information collected from the eye to the brain, where the information is processed.

Hearing: The ability to hear is a complex process that requires an intact anatomy of the ear. The ear detects sound waves, which are traveling vibrations of air. The external and middle parts of the ear convert sound waves into vibrations of fluid located in the inner part of the ear. Receptors located on little hairs inside the inner ear (mechanoreceptors) communicate the vibration energy to the nervous system. Similar to the eye, which converts light energy into a form of energy that can be carried on a nerve cell, the ear converts sound wave energy into a form that the nervous system can transmit to the brain, where the information is processed.

Taste: The taste receptors (chemoreceptors) are located on taste buds on the tongue. There are four primary tastes—salty, sour, sweet, and bitter—and all other tastes are various combinations of the four. Chemical molecules bind with the taste receptors and cause a physical change within the receptor. This receptor change "excites" the nerve cells around it, and this excited energy is carried by the nervous system to the brain, where the information is processed. The perception of taste can be affected by other senses, particularly the sense of smell.

Smell: The smell receptors (chemoreceptors) are located in the nose. For a substance to be smelled, it must be volatile enough so that some of its molecules can enter the nose, and it also must be able to dissolve in the tissue lining of the nose to be able to reach the receptors. If a chemical is unable to do this, it is said to have "no smell." If a substance binds with the smell receptor in the nasal passage, then a physical change within the receptor takes place, as in the case of taste. The transmission of the signal occurs similarly to taste, and the information from the smell receptor is processed by the brain.

What Happens When It Goes Wrong? (Pathophysiology)

When any portion along the pathway of information transmission from a sensory organ is disrupted, then the ability to process information will be faulty. If damage occurs to the sensory organ itself or to the nerve that carries information to the brain, then the individual will lose the sensory capacity of that organ. A number of clinical conditions can occur from such disruption, the most serious of which are blindness and deafness—a complete loss of the ability to see and hear.

Summary

Controlling and coordinating the function of the major body organs are the nervous and endocrine systems.

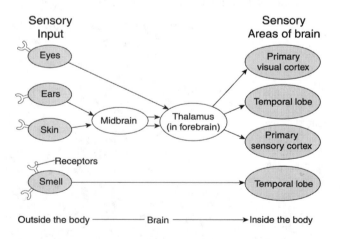

Figure 10-22. Sensory perception and the brain. Sensory input is processed through various structures in the brain. Transmitting the signals from the outside to the inside involves a number of players: receptors, nerve cells, and the brain. Each of the sensory organs has receptors that are able to detect changes in the exterior environment and transmit this information to the appropriate brain region.

The nervous system communicates with organs through chemical messengers called neurotransmitters. Changes in the nervous system can take place within seconds. In contrast, the endocrine system communicates with organs through chemical substances called hormones, which produce changes over hours or days.

Although each of the body systems has different functions—for example, the cardiovascular system pumps deoxygenated blood to the lungs, whereas the lungs are responsible for exchanged gases in the deoxygenated blood—each is dependent on the others to maintain normal physiological balance in the body. For example, the cardiovascular system and the kidney control blood pressure, and the gastrointestinal system and the endocrine system control blood sugar.

When one of the systems is damaged and normal function is disrupted, disease states can occur. Some disease states, such as Type I diabetes, develop rather quickly, whereas others, such as high blood pressure (hypertension), can take years to develop,. When pathophysiological conditions occur in one system, this imbalance can affect other body systems as well. For example, hypertension can damage the kidneys, blood vessels, and heart; diabetes can damage the kidneys, eyes, circulation, and nerves.

Normal functioning of the organ systems is therefore required to bring about a balanced internal environment.

Recommended Reading

Austgen L, Bowen RA, Rouge M. Pathophysiology of the digestive system. http://arbl.cvmbs.colostate.edu/hbooks/pathphys/digestion/index.html (last updated 2001 May 22).

Crimando J. "Anatomy and Physiology Tutorials" WebSite images and text created and © GateWay Community College; Phoenix, AZ; Orig. created Fall 1997. http://www.medterms.com/script/main/hp.asp (accessed 2003 Oct 29).

Germann WJ, Stanfield CL. Principles of human physiology. 1st ed. San Francisco: Benjamin Cummings Publications; 2002

Grayson CE. Alzheimer's disease research. *WebMD Health.* http://my.webmd.com/content/article/46/1626_50823.htm (accessed 2003 Jan 10).

Grayson CE. Schizophrenia. *WebMD Health.* http://my.webmd.com/content/article/60/67143.htm (accessed 2003 Jan 7).

Harley JP. Study guide for Sherwood's human physiology: from cells to systems. 4th ed. Pacific Grove, CA: Brooks Cole Publications; 2001.

MedTerms.com medical dictionary. http://www.medterms.com/script/main/hp.asp (accessed 2003 Oct 29).

Moffett DE, Moffet SB, Schauf CL. Human physiology: foundations and frontiers. 2nd ed. St. Louis: Mosby-Year Book, Inc.; 1993.

Sherwood L. Human physiology: from cells to systems. 4th ed. Pacific Grove, CA: Brooks Cole Publications; 2001.

Stedman TL. Stedman's medical dictionary. 27th ed. Philadelphia: Lippincott, Williams & Wilkins; 2000.

Vogin, G. All about kidney stones. *WebMD Health.* http://my.webmd.com/content/article/7/1680_54072.htm (accessed 2003 Jan 15).

Self-Assessment Questions

Answer True or False to the following questions.

Nervous System

1. The autonomic nervous system is under voluntary control.
2. The somatic nervous system is solely responsible for contracting skeletal muscle.
3. The central nervous system consists of the brain, spinal cord, and nerves that leave the spinal cord.
4. Parkinson's disease is characterized by delusional thought.

Cardiovascular System

5. Blood transports oxygen and nutrients to cells in the body.
6. The right side of the heart transports oxygenated blood to the lungs.
7. A chronically elevated systolic pressure of greater than 140 mm Hg and diastolic pressure of greater than 90 mm Hg is classified as hypertension.
8. The left atrium of the heart is responsible for pumping blood to the lungs.

Musculoskeletal System

9. Muscles are made up of muscle fibers.
10. Actin and myosin are not involved in muscle contraction.
11. Skeletal muscles are under voluntary control.
12. Cardiac muscle and smooth muscle have a striped appearance.

Endocrine System

13. One endocrine gland may influence more than one target tissue.
14. One endocrine gland may secrete more than one hormone.
15. The purpose of hormones is to affect cells that are located next to each other.
16. Treatment of endocrine disorders may be as simple as replacement of the hormone.

Gastrointestinal Tract

17. Food is converted into chyme in the large intestine.
18. GERD can result from a faulty pyloric sphincter.
19. Peptic ulcers may result from a bacterium.
20. The esophagus is the most complex portion of the gastrointestinal tract.

Respiratory System

21. Gas exchange occurs at the alveoli.
22. Oxygenated blood travels from the lungs to the left side of the heart.
23. Blood that is too acidic results in a condition called alkalosis.
24. Asthma is an inflammatory disease of the bronchioles.

Urinary Tract System

25. The nephron is the functional unit of the kidney.
26. The kidney can produce hormones.
27. Diabetes insipidus is a condition in which the kidneys respond to vasopressin.
28. The kidneys are responsible for regulating blood volume.

Reproductive System

29. The reproductive system is the same in both males and females.
30. The term for the primary reproductive organs is *gonads*.
31. Sex hormones are responsible for the development of secondary sexual characteristics.
32. A female possesses all her reproductive cells at birth and will not produce any more.

Immune System

33. An antigen is anything that elicits an immune response.
34. The lack of an immune response to self is called autoimmunity.
35. A lymphocyte is a type of white blood cell.
36. T lymphocytes attack cells infected with virus.

Special Senses

37. The body has a system that can sense changes in the external environment.
38. An individual does not require two functional eyes to have vision.
39. Pain is a response to damage or tissue injury and does not require the brain for perception.
40. Mechanoreceptors can sense changes in light energy.

Self-Assessment Answers

1. **False.** The autonomic nervous system is not under voluntary control. The actions are carried out without the individual being consciously aware of the changes.
2. **True.** The somatic nervous system has the sole responsibility of contracting skeletal muscle. The organization does not allow it to impinge on any other nervous system.
3. **False.** The central nervous system consists of the brain and spinal cord. Nerves that leave the spinal cord are the peripheral nervous system.
4. **False.** Parkinson's disease is a disease that affects movement and does not affect the way a person thinks. Delusional thoughts are among the symptoms of schizophrenia.
5. **True.** The function of blood is to take oxygen and vital nutrients to the cells.
6. **False.** The right side of the heart pumps deoxygenated blood, low in oxygen, to the lungs to allow gas exchange and oxygenation of the blood.
7. **True.** These are the measurements recommended by the American College of Cardiology to denote hypertension.
8. **False.** The right ventricle of the heart is responsible for pumping blood to the lungs. The atrium is the chamber above the ventricle, and blood flows from the atrium to the ventricle. The right side of the heart always takes blood to the lungs.
9. **True.** Muscle fibers are the components of muscle.
10. **False.** Actin and myosin are the contractile elements that bring about muscle contraction.
11. **True.** A person can voluntarily move skeletal muscles.
12. **False.** Cardiac muscle has a striped appearance under the microscope as does skeletal muscle, but smooth muscle does not.
13. **True.** The table shows that an endocrine gland, by the one or more hormones that it can secrete, can influence one or more target tissues.
14. **True.** An endocrine gland is often responsible for the synthesis and secretion of more than one hormone.
15. **False.** The purpose of hormones is to affect organs at a distance. This is why they are secreted into the bloodstream to travel to distant tissues and organs.
16. **True.** Often endocrine disorders result from a hormone deficiency, and hormone replacement therapy is available by prescription.
17. **False.** Food particles are converted to chyme, the liquefied form of food, in the stomach.
18. **False.** GERD is caused by a faulty esophageal sphincter, resulting in the reflux of acid into the esophagus.
19. **True.** Bacterial infection of *heliobacter pylori* can result in the formation of peptic ulcers.
20. **False.** The esophagus is the simplest anatomical and functional portion of the GI tract. The small intestine is the most complex portion of the GI tract.
21. **True.** Gas exchange occurs between the blood and the alveoli, which are located at the ends of the smallest bronchioles in the lungs.
22. **True.** Once oxygen is exchanged for carbon dioxide in the lungs, the oxygenated blood travels back to the left side of the heart to be pumped around the body.
23. **False.** Blood that is too acidic results in a condition known as acidosis.
24. **True.** Symptoms of asthma are initiated when the bronchioles become inflamed.
25. **True.** Tens of thousands of nephrons are the functioning units of the kidney.
26. **True.** The kidney produces an important hormone called erthryopoetin.
27. **False.** In diabetes insipidus the kidneys do not respond to vasopressin, and the person loses large volumes of urine.
28. **True.** Regulating blood volume is one of the functions of the kidney.
29. **False.** The reproductive system is one of the few anatomically and functionally different systems in males and females.
30. **True.** The gonads are known as the *testes* in males and the *ovaries* in females.
31. **True.** Without sex hormones, an individual would be unable to reach sexual maturity.
32. **True.** Unlike males, who produce sperm throughout their adult life, females are born with all the eggs they will ever produce.

33. **True**. An antigen may be a bacterium, a virus, or a cancer cell.

34. **False**. The lack of an immune response to self is called tolerance. Autoimmunity is an immune response against self.

35. **True**. A lymphocyte is a type of white blood cell that is produced outside of the bone marrow.

36. **True**. Attacking cells infected with a virus is the function of a T lymphocyte.

37. **True**. This is the system commonly referred to as *perception*.

38. **True**. An individual requires only one functional eye to have the sense of vision.

39. **False**. The transmission of pain requires the brain to process the information that the nerve cells carry to it.

40. **False**. Mechanoreceptors sense changes in mechanical energy and result in hearing; the receptors that sense changes in light energy are called photoreceptors.

Basic Biopharmaceutics, Pharmacokinetics, and Pharmacodynamics

TANYA C. KNIGHT-KLIMAS

The purpose of this chapter is to aid the pharmacy technician in understanding the basic elements of biopharmaceutics, pharmacokinetics, and pharmacodynamics. These subjects are useful in correlating the physical and chemical properties of medications with their clinical effects. Biopharmaceutics is the understanding of how specific medications are produced and formulated in the laboratory such that delivery of the medications yields a predictable response. Pharmacokinetics is the understanding of absorption of medication into the systemic bodily circulation, distribution of medication to various body tissues, breakdown of medication by the body, and finally, elimination of medication from the body. Pharmacodynamics is the study of therapeutic and adverse effects medications may exert on the body.

The pharmacy technician is often the first person in the pharmacy to handle a patient's medication, and the technician often fills multiple prescriptions for a single patient. Thus, the pharmacy technician who prepares prescriptions for dispensing should have a basic understanding of biopharmaceutics, pharmacokinetics, and pharmacodynamics, which collectively describe how a particular medication is prepared, is handled by the body, and affects the body. Having this understanding can help avoid adverse drug events, because polypharmacy and pharmacokinetic and pharmacodynamic alterations have been shown to be risk factors for adverse drug events in the elderly population.[1-5] For example, a prescriber may write for a particular prescription medication to be crushed before taken; however, a knowledgeable pharmacy technician may identify that particular medication as one that is formulated such that crushing adversely alters its effects on the body. Likewise, a pharmacy technician knowledgeable about the absorption of a particular medication may know that it should not be taken with dietary agents or other medications that could affect its absorption. An understanding of basic biopharmaceutical, pharmacokinetic, and pharmacodynamic principles

Learning Objectives

After completing this chapter, the technician should be able to

1. Define the study of biopharmaceutics, and list some of the properties, advantages, and disadvantages of different formulations and their routes of administration.

2. List and describe the four major processes that make up the study of pharmacokinetics.

3. Describe factors that may alter the absorption of a medication.

4. Describe how medications are distributed within the body, and list factors that affect medication distribution in the body.

5. Describe how medications are eliminated from the body, and list factors that may increase or decrease elimination of a medication.

6. Define pharmacodynamics and describe the steps that must occur before a medication can exert its effect on the body.

7. Integrate the above objectives by describing potential problems that can occur when a product formulation is disrupted or when absorption, distribution, metabolism, or elimination is altered, and how these alterations may affect the pharmacodynamics of a medication.

can aid the clinician in appropriately monitoring medication therapy, and the pharmacy technician can aid the pharmacist in such surveillance.

Biopharmaceutics

Biopharmaceutics is defined as the study of the "interrelationship of the physicochemical (physical and chemical) properties of a drug, dosage form in which the drug is given, and the route of administration on the rate and extent of drug absorption."[6] It has long been recognized that the method by which a medication is prepared and formulated can affect its action.[6] The study of biopharmaceutics led to the rational design of drug products to enhance the delivery of medication and ultimately to optimize the clinical effect of medication.[6]

Medications can be formulated and administered in many different ways. Common formulations include tablets, capsules, solutions, suspensions, suppositories, transdermal patches, creams, nasal sprays, and aerosolized medications. Routes of administration include oral, intra-ocular, rectal, sublingual (under the tongue), buccal (cheek), topical, transdermal, injectable, intravaginal, and inhaled. Different medications are formulated and administered differently for several reasons. In some instances, a particular medication is available via multiple routes, and choosing one over the other may simply be a matter of preference or convenience. For instance, acetaminophen is available in many different dosage forms, including tablets, capsules, caplets, elixirs, and suppositories. For small children, administration via elixir or suppository will likely be easier than by a tablet. In other instances, however, different formulations and routes of administration are used because they can influence the rate, duration, or even extent of drug effect. Therefore, using the correct or optimal formulation is important and often has a bearing on the clinical effect of the medication.

Before most medications can exert a pharmacological response, they need to be absorbed (taken up by the bloodstream), and before they can be absorbed, they need to be manipulated and released from their formulations. A medication in a tablet formulation, for instance, is more than just the active drug. Any given tablet will contain not only active drug but also binders that keep the tablet from falling apart, fillers that add bulk to the tablet, and preservatives. Two processes—disintegration and dissolution, in that order—usually

need to occur to prepare the medication for absorption. Disintegration is the breakdown of the medication from the original solid formulation, and dissolution is the dissolving of medication into solution, usually in the gastrointestinal tract. Disintegrating aids dissolution, as smaller particles dissolve more easily than larger particles. Once a medication is disintegrated and dissolved, it can be absorbed into the bloodstream (see **Figure 11-1**). Some product formulations are disintegrated and dissolved more slowly or more rapidly than others, which may ultimately affect the rate of onset of therapeutic effect.

Oral Agents

Oral agents can be manufactured in many different ways. Immediate-release products release medication into the system all at once, so the effects are faster and the duration of action is shorter. Sustained-release products release a smaller amount of medication consistently over time so the effects are sustained over a longer period. Such formulations can usually be given less frequently and side effects may be lessened because the body is exposed to a smaller amount of medication at any given time. It is important to note that enough medication must be released per unit time to make it effective. An example of a medication formulated as an immediate-release product and a sustained-release product is verapamil, an antihypertensive. The original, immediate-release verapamil needs to be given three times daily, whereas the sustained-release product can be given once daily and maintain blood pressure control throughout the day.

Because sustained-release, timed-release, and controlled-release products are formulated so medication is delivered over time, altering the formulation will disrupt the intended release of medication from the product. Therefore, it is important to label these medications with a "do not crush or chew" sticker. If crushed or chewed, all the medication will be released

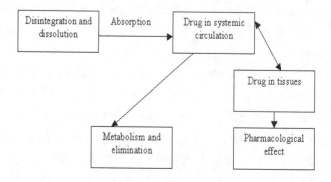

Figure 11-1. Relationship between drug and effect.

at once, which may lead to serious side effects. Some timed-release medications in capsule form can be opened and either sprinkled onto food or mixed with certain liquids without disrupting the timed-release structure, as long as the pellets inside the capsule are not chewed or altered. Examples are omeprazole and lansoprazole, agents used for peptic ulcer disease and gastroesophageal reflux disease, respectively. These medications are acid-labile, which means they are subject to destruction by stomach acid. They are thus formulated such that the pellets inside the capsule are coated with a "seal" that withstands stomach acid, and the coated pellet remains intact until it enters the intestine, where the coating dissolves and the medication is absorbed into the bloodstream[7] (see **Figure 11-2**). The technician should check with the manufacturer of a particular medication if unsure whether the medication dosage form may be altered.

Injectable Agents

Injectable medications may be administered intramuscularly, intradermally (in the dermis layer of the skin), subcutaneously (in the fatty tissue), or intravenously. Medications that are administered intramuscularly must be released from the muscle, migrate to surrounding tissue, and then enter the bloodstream; this process often occurs slowly and erratically. Medications that are given intravenously have a very rapid onset of action because the medications are already in solution (therefore disintegration and dissolution do not need to occur) and are placed directly in the vein and therefore in the bloodstream.

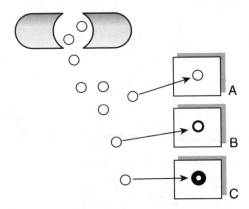

Figure 11-2. Timed-release capsule. This figure generically represents how a particular timed-release capsule may be formulated. This type of timed-released capsule can be opened as long as the pellets inside are unaltered. The thinly coated pellet in A is designed to disintegrate and dissolve faster than the thicker coated pellets. The thickest coated pellet in C is designed to disintegrate and dissolve slower than the pellets depicted in A and B. This staggered release rate is what makes this type of formulation *timed-release*.

Rectal Agents

Rectal agents are convenient to give to patients who are experiencing nausea and vomiting. Some rectal agents are better absorbed than the same agent given orally because some oral agents are broken down in the liver before they can be absorbed into the bloodstream. Breakdown of medication by the liver, called *first-pass metabolism*, does not occur with rectally administered agents.

Sublingual and Buccal Agents

Sublingual agents are placed under the tongue, where they dissolve rapidly. A common example of a sublingual medication is nitroglycerin SL, which is used for angina. A patient who experiences anginal chest pain can place a tablet under the tongue and let it dissolve. Chest pain should subside within approximately 5 minutes.[8] Buccal agents are placed between the molars and cheek and are also absorbed rapidly. Buccal agents, like rectal and sublingual agents, avoid first-pass metabolism.

Transdermal Agents

Transdermal medications such as the nicotine patch, are often formulated in a patch that releases medication that is absorbed through the skin. Medication is released slowly over a period of time and may be associated with less gastrointestinal side effects than oral agents. One minor side effect of patches is local irritation that is often due to the adhesive used. Counseling patients about proper patch application is important. A patch should usually be applied to dry, hairless, intact skin. When applied to skin broken from minor cuts or rashes, too much medication may be absorbed. Most patches should not be cut, because doing so may cause the medication to be released too quickly.

Local Agents

Some agents are formulated to provide a local effect only. Most topical creams and ointments are intended to act locally on the skin to relieve itching, burning, acne, and minor rashes. In this instance, only medication that comes in direct contact with the skin will be effective. Therefore applying a thick coating of the product is usually not necessary, because the top layers will not contribute to the therapeutic effect. Intraocular medications are intended to provide a local effect to the eye only. Some medication may be absorbed systemically (throughout the body), but most of the medication remains in the eye, where it exerts its effect. Aerosolized medications also provide a largely local effect. Medication for asthma and chronic obstructive pulmonary disease is often aerosolized. The advantage of aerosolization is that medication is dispersed into the lungs more quickly than when given orally. Medications that act locally tend to have fewer systemic (bodywide) side effects than orally administered medications.

Suspensions and Solutions

Suspensions and solutions can be administered orally, subcutaneously in the case of insulin, or topically in the case of eyedrops and eardrops. One very important difference between suspensions and solutions must be recognized: Oral and ocular suspensions need to be shaken before dispensing and with each dosing administration because heavy drug particles in suspensions settle to the bottom, which may lead to an underdose if dispensing or administering from a full bottle or an overdose if dispensing or administering from an almost empty bottle. Products in solution do not need to be shaken (see **Figure 11-3**). Short-acting insulin (R insulin) and rapid-acting insulins (insulin lispro and aspart) are available as clear solutions, while intermediate and most long-acting insulins, such as insulin NPH and ultralente, are cloudy suspensions. One exception is insulin glargine, which is a long-acting, once-daily insulin available as a clear solution.[9,10] Insulins in suspension must be gently rolled in the palms of the hands to ensure dispersion of suspended particles, while insulins in solution need not be. Insulin suspensions should not be shaken vigorously because proteins may be denatured (permanently altered) and air bubbles may develop, leading to inaccurate dosing.

Pharmacokinetics

Pharmacokinetics often is described simply as "what the body does to the drug." The body (1) *absorbs* the medication, (2) *distributes* it to different tissues, (3) *metabolizes* it (breaks it down), and (4) *eliminates* it.

Absorption

Medication that is absorbed is not merely the amount administered by pill or capsule that enters the gastrointestinal tract or the amount injected into the muscle. Absorption specifically refers to the amount of medication that enters the bloodstream, or systemic circulation. Not all the medication in a tablet, capsule, suppository, inhaler, or intramuscular or subcutaneous syringe enters the bloodstream, and therefore not all of it is absorbed. Only absorbed medication has the potential to exert a pharmacologic effect. The term *bioavailability* refers to the percentage of an administered dose of a medication that reaches the systemic circulation.[11] The bioavailability of an agent depends on many factors, including its (1) dissolution ability (ability of the drug to dissolve) (2) dosage form (tablet, solution), and (3) route of administration (oral, intravenous).[11]

Some medications are metabolized before they can be absorbed; this is called *first-pass metabolism* because a percentage of those medications is metabolized on their first pass through the body (see **Figure 11-4**). Medications that undergo a high first-pass metabolism have a high metabolized percentage, and therefore a lower percentage is absorbed. Medications can also be metabolized by bacteria in the gastrointestinal tract or by the gastrointestinal tract itself.

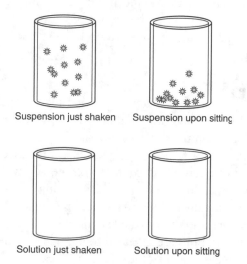

Suspension just shaken   Suspension upon sitting

Solution just shaken   Solution upon sitting

Figure 11-3. Drug particles in suspension sink down to the bottom when the suspension is at rest, whereas particles in solution are dissolved and are homogenous with the solution.

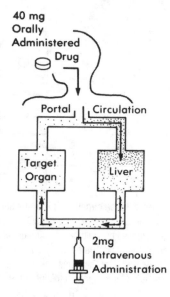

Figure 11-4. First-pass metabolism.

Medications given intravenously are administered directly into the vein and therefore enter the bloodstream directly. Thus, they are 100 percent bioavailable, which means 100 percent of the administered dose has the *potential* to exert a pharmacologic effect. This is why medications that are available orally and parenterally have different doses. Usually, the dose needed orally is more than the dose needed intravenously because the bioavailability of the intravenous formulation is 100 percent, whereas the bioavailability of the oral form is often less than that. For example, levothyroxine, used for hypothyroidism, has an intravenous dose that is half that of the oral dose but will produce the same pharmacological response.[8] In other instances, the oral bioavailability of an agent is so poor that it is not normally given orally; rather, it is usually given intravenously. Vancomycin is an example of an antibiotic that is normally used intravenously for systemic infections because it is so poorly absorbed orally. As will be covered in this chapter, however, absorption is not the only factor that can affect the amount of medication able to elicit a response.

Once absorbed into the systemic circulation (bloodstream), medication can either leave the bloodstream and travel to tissues—including, but not limited to, the site of action (the tissue organ site where the medication is to exert its intended pharmacologic response)—or it can remain in the plasma and can bind to plasma proteins. Therefore, for any given dose of medication, some of it will travel to tissues and some of it will remain in the bloodstream. Some medications are highly protein bound, so that more than 80 or 90 percent of the administered dose is bound to plasma proteins. The medication bound to proteins is inactive and does not exert any effect because it is *tied up*, or physically bound, to plasma protein. Only medication that is *free*, or not bound to proteins, can exert a pharmacological effect. Of the percentage that is free, or circulating to tissues, only the amount that reaches the target site will exert the intended pharmacologic effect. The percentage of medication that circulates to other tissue sites will either exert no effect or will exert unwanted side effects (see **Figure 11-5**).

The protein to which many acidic and neutral medications bind is albumin. Some disease states can cause a decrease in the amount of albumin in the plasma. In this instance, medications that normally bind highly to albumin are unable to do so to the normal extent, and a greater proportion of those medications will be free and therefore active. Medications that are highly bound to albumin include phenytoin, an antiepileptic agent, and warfarin, an antithrombotic agent.

The blood levels of some medications can be measured, and the result can help guide appropriate therapy. Examples of medications whose levels are measured in the blood include many of the antiepileptics, such as phenytoin, carbamazepine, valproic acid, and phenobarbital; digoxin for atrial fibrillation; and some antibiotics, including aminoglycosides and vancomycin. Studies have been conducted in people to evaluate blood levels of these agents after certain doses are given. From these studies, researchers have been able to determine a normal, or *therapeutic*, level for these medications — the level at which most patients receive the desired effect with minimal side effects. Thus, blood levels of these medications can be checked, and it can be determined whether a change in therapy is needed or not on the basis of the laboratory results.

Volume of Distribution

The apparent volume of distribution describes the distribution characteristic of a particular medication throughout the body. Volume of distribution is defined as "the size of a compartment necessary to account for the total amount of drug in the body if it were present throughout the body at the same concentration found in the plasma."[11] It is not an actual body compartment; rather, it is a hypothetical compartment used to describe the size of the *pool* to which that drug is distributed. Some medications are distributed throughout the bloodstream and in many organs, fluids, and tissues (fat tissue or lean muscle tissue); other medications are not as widely distributed. In general, medications with a high volume of distribution will have a

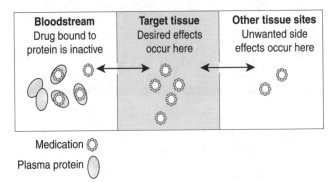

Figure 11-5. Medication distribution. This figure depicts the travel of medication from the bloodstream to the target tissue to other tissues. The double-headed arrows indicate that flow can occur in either direction. Medication bound to protein in the blood is inactive and cannot travel to other tissues, but the medication can dissociate or separate from the protein. Once separated, it can move about the body.

lower blood concentration, and medications with a low volume of distribution will have a higher blood concentration (see **Figure 11-6**). A simple way to think of this is to picture a swimming pool. A certain amount of confetti placed in a large swimming pool will be spread to all areas of the pool. The same amount of confetti placed in a swimming pool half the size of the first will also spread to all areas of the pool, but will look more colorful because the pool is smaller. The smaller pool will appear to contain twice the amount of confetti, when actually the same amount of confetti was used (see **Figure 11-7**).

Certain factors affect volume of distribution. Medications that have a low affinity (low attraction) to lipids or fat and medications that are highly bound to proteins in the bloodstream tend to have low volumes of distribution because they tend to stay in the bloodstream. Conversely, medications that have a high affinity to lipids and medications that are either bound to proteins in tissue or are not highly bound to plasma proteins tend to have high volumes of distribution—that is, they tend to be widely distributed throughout the body.

How does knowing the volume of distribution of a medication help? Knowing the volume of distribution of a certain medication can help to approximate the dose of medication needed to attain the desired level of drug in the body for it to be effective or to start working quickly. If a medication is widely distributed through the body

and the prescriber wants the medication to start working quickly, sometimes a loading dose of the medication (a larger first dose) will be given to more quickly achieve a higher drug concentration in the body. Examples of medications for which a loading dose is sometimes given include phenytoin, digoxin, and some antibiotics. As a general example, sometimes a prescription will be written as follows: "Take 2 tablets today, then take 1 tablet daily thereafter." Two tablets are used the first day as a loading dose, to help achieve a certain blood level of the medication to jump-start therapy. If a medication is not widely distributed through the body, a smaller loading dose or no loading dose will be needed. Most medications do not require a loading dose.

Metabolism

The metabolism of medication is the breakdown of medication in the body. Some organs in the body break down medications so they can be more easily eliminated from the body. The kidneys, lungs, and intestines can metabolize medications, but the major metabolic organ is the liver. It contains substances called *enzymes* that break down medication. Several different and specific metabolic processes can occur. Each medication has its own metabolic profile (the specific way in which it is metabolized).

Some medications are metabolized but some medications can *inhibit* the metabolism of other medications or can *induce*, or *potentiate*, the metabolism of other medications. Thus, knowing the metabolic profile of all medications dispensed to a patient can help determine if a drug interaction is likely to exist. For example, some antiepileptic medications are referred to as *enzyme inducers*, meaning they potentiate the metabolism of many other medications. Phentyoin, an antiepileptic, is an enzyme inducer, and it is known

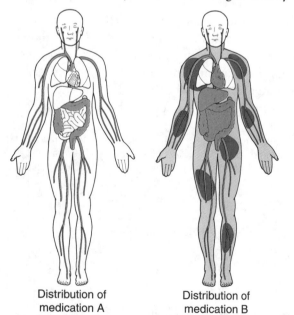

Distribution of medication A   Distribution of medication B

Figure 11-6. Volume of distribution. This schematic hypothetically and simplistically depicts drug distribution throughout the body. Medication A, shown on the left, appears to remain primarily in the bloodstream and is distributed to the target organ, the large intestines. Medication B, shown on the right, appears to be widely distributed throughout the body.

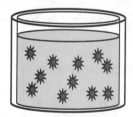

One 8 oz package of confetti   One 8 oz package of confetti

Figure 11-7. Volume of distribution. Although the same amount of confetti was used to fill each pool, it looks more abundant in the smaller pool. Likewise, the same amount of medication that is less widely distributed throughout the body will appear to be more abundant in the bloodstream, as evidenced by a higher blood plasma concentration.

to increase the metabolism of more than 100 other medications.[12] This can result in lessening of the activity of the other medication, because it is broken down and excreted from the body more quickly than normal. Conversely, some medications can inhibit the metabolism of other medications. For example, erythromycin, some antifungal medications, and cyclosporine (an immune suppressant used post-transplant) are all potent *enzyme inhibitors*, or medications that are known to inhibit the metabolism of many other medications. This can result in higher, more prolonged blood levels of these other medications, which may lead to prolonged duration of action of the other medications and the development of side effects.

Some medications are metabolized to an *active metabolite*, or another substance that is also pharmacologically active and able to exert a therapeutic or toxic effect. It is important to know that the active metabolite does not always act in the same manner as the parent drug, or the initial drug. An example of an active metabolite is seen with the drug fluoxetine, used primarily for depression. Fluoxetine is metabolized to norfluoxetine, which is active and exerts an antidepressant effect, but is longer acting than fluoxetine, so its effect lasts longer.[8,13] This prolonged effect can be perceived as good or bad, depending on the situation and specific patient characteristics. The good thing is that this long-acting metabolite allows convenient dosing of the medication once a day, or less frequently with the advent of a once-weekly formulation;[13] the bad thing is that this long-acting metabolite may remain in the system longer than wanted, so when side effects occur, they may occur for a prolonged period, especially in the elderly, who tend to eliminate the drug more slowly anyway.

Elimination/Clearance

Clearance is the elimination of medication from the blood and body. It is defined as "the intrinsic ability of the body or its organs of elimination to remove drug from the blood or plasma."[11] The kidneys and liver are the major organs that eliminate medications. Medications are cleared unchanged (not metabolized) from the body by the kidneys or via metabolism by the liver. Several factors can affect the clearance of medication from the body, including kidney function, hepatic function, cardiac output, and body weight. Patients with kidney or liver dysfunction may not eliminate some medications well. Patients with depressed cardiac output will have decreased blood flow to the kidneys and liver and therefore decreased elimination of

medications. Patients who are markedly overweight or underweight may have differing abilities to eliminate medications because kidney and liver size and blood flow are proportional to body weight.[11]

Changes in medication clearance affect drug dosing. If a medication is cleared less well because of kidney dysfunction, the dose will need to be reduced or the dosing interval increased to avoid potential side effects and prolonged effects. To determine if a lower dose is needed, an estimate of kidney function can be calculated mathematically. Mathematical estimates of kidney function often use a substance called creatinine as a marker of kidney function. Creatinine is a substance in the body that is normally present in the serum and is cleared from the body by the kidneys. A laboratory can easily measure serum creatinine from a blood sample. Because creatinine is excreted by the kidneys similarly to the way medications are excreted, it is possible to estimate medication clearance by measuring creatinine clearance. A common equation used to calculate creatinine clearance is the Cockroft–Gault equation:[14]

$$\text{Estimated CrCl (mL/min) in males} = \frac{(140 - \text{age})\,(\text{weight, in kilograms})}{(72)\,(\text{Scr})}$$

Scr = serum creatinine
CrCl = creatinine clearance

The result of this equation is multiplied by 85 percent for females.

A creatinine clearance for a young, healthy individual is approximately 120 mL/min. Medications that are excreted by the kidneys need to be dose adjusted for patients with depressed creatinine clearances, usually 60 mL/min or less. The manufacturer of each medication whose elimination is affected by kidney dysfunction determines at what creatinine clearance the dose needs to be adjusted and by how much. For instance, amantadine, a medication used for Parkinson's disease, requires varying degrees of close adjustment depending on the degree of kidney dysfunction, as shown in **Table 11-1**. **Table 11-2** provides a list of common medications that require dose adjustment when used in patients with renal dysfunction.[8]

Pharmacodynamics

Just as pharmacokinetics can be thought of as what the body does to the drug, pharmacodynamics can be thought of as what the drug does to the body. Pharmacodynamics is defined as "the study of the relationship between the concentration of a drug and the response

TABLE 11-1. RENAL DOSING OF AMANTADINE

Renal Function	Initial Dose of Amantadine
CrCl > 60 mL/min	100 mg po bid (monotherapy) 100 mg po daily (combination)
CrCl 50–60 mL/min	200 mg/daily alternating with 100 mg/daily
CrCl 40–50 mL/min	100 mg po daily
CrCl 30–40 mL/min	200 mg po twice weekly
20–30 mL/min	100 mg po three times weekly
CrCl 10–20 mL/min	200 mg load then 100 mg po weekly

TABLE 11-2. COMMON MEDICATIONS WITH A SIGNIFICANT RENAL COMPONENT TO ELIMINATION (TABLE NOT ALL-INCLUSIVE)

Allopurinol*	Enalapril*
Aminoglycosides	Famotidine
Atenolol	Lisinopril
Captopril	Methotrexate
Cimetidine	Procainamide*
Ciprofloxacin	Quinapril
Clonidine	Ranitidine
Digoxin	Triamterene
Disopyramide*	Vancomycin

*Drug has major active metabolite that is renally excreted.

Adapted from Chapron DJ. In: Therapeutics in the elderly. 3rd ed. Delafuente JC, Stewart RB, eds. Cincinnati, OH: Harvey Whitney Books Company; 2001.

obtained in a patient."[15] Examples of pharmacodynamic responses include an increase in bone mass with a bisphosphonate used for osteoporosis, a decrease in blood pressure with an antihypertensive agent, and a decrease in blood glucose with a sulfonylurea used in the management of diabetes.

For a pharmacological effect to occur, a drug needs to be absorbed into the systemic circulation and travel to its intended site of action, or target organ, as described earlier. Next, it needs to bind to a specific receptor like a lock and key. A receptor is defined as "a protein, which is embedded in a cell membrane that facilitates communication" between the outside and the inside of a membrane.[16] Endogenous ligands, or natural body substances, usually bind to the receptor and exert a normal bodily response. For example, when a substance called epinephrine binds to specific receptors called beta-receptors, the response is an increase in heart rate. Medications mimic these natural substances because medications are made to be chemically similar to these natural substances. This way, medications

can "fool" the receptor and can bind to it and exert a similar response. When a medication binds to the receptor, it physically blocks the endogenous substance from binding to the receptor. Only by binding to its receptor can a medication exert an effect (see **Figure 11-8**). After a medication binds to a receptor, the receptor helps to communicate specifics about the medication to the inside of the cell by generating a signal in the cell about the medication (see **Figure 11-9**).

By binding to the receptor, medications can either augment or block the signal normally brought about by binding of the endogenous substance to the receptor. Medications that augment or enhance a signal normally communicated in a cell are called *agonists*. Medications that block the transmission of a signal normally communicated in a cell are called *antagonists*. As mentioned before, natural beta agonists bind beta-receptors to increase heart rate. If a beta agonist medication binds to that receptor, the resultant effect would be an increase in heart rate, similar to the effect of a natural beta agonist binding to the receptor. Isoproterenol is a beta agonist that would do just that. Conversely, a beta antagonist, such as metoprolol, will antagonize the normal effects of a beta adrenergic substance bound to a beta receptor and thus would block an increase in heart rate.

The drug-receptor complex forms the basis of medication effects on the body. This drug-receptor interaction is what makes medications work—what makes the antacid the technician dispenses soothe the stomach, the antibiotic the technician prepares and dispenses help fight infection, and the pain medication the technician dispenses relieve pain.

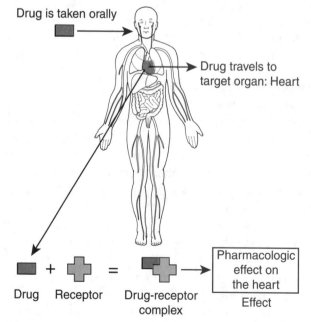

Figure 11- 8. Drug-receptor complex.

A. Endogenous ligand-receptor complex and associated physiologic response

Outside the heart cell

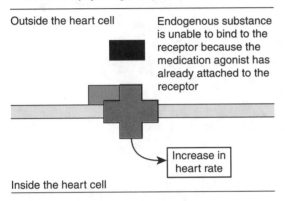

Increase in heart rate

Inside the heart cell

B. Medication agonist- receptor complex and associated physiologic response

Outside the heart cell

Endogenous substance is unable to bind to the receptor because the medication agonist has already attached to the receptor

Increase in heart rate

Inside the heart cell

C. Medication antagonist- receptor complex and associated physiologic response

Outside the heart cell

Endogenous substance is unable to bind to the receptor because the medication antagonist has already attached to the receptor

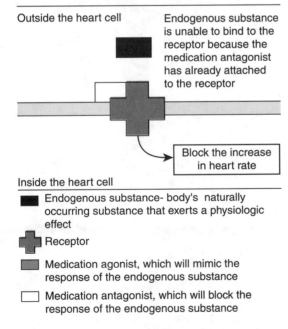

Block the increase in heart rate

Inside the heart cell

Endogenous substance- body's naturally occurring substance that exerts a physiologic effect

Receptor

Medication agonist, which will mimic the response of the endogenous substance

Medication antagonist, which will block the response of the endogenous substance

Figure 11-9. A closer look at drug-receptor complexes and pharmacologic response. Note that the medication agonist and antagonist are able to bind to the receptor because they look like the endogenous substance and fit the receptor well. By binding to the receptor as a key fits a lock, the medication prevents the endogenous substance from doing so and exerting its own effect.

Summary

Biopharmaceutics, pharmacokinetics, and pharmacodynamics collectively describe how medications are prepared and handled by the body, and affect the body. These studies correlate the physical and chemical properties of medications with their clinical effects. A pharmacy technician must become familiar with the basic principles of these studies to appreciate their contribution to the clinical effects of medication. When the technician is asked if a medication can be crushed, he or she will know why this seemingly simple question is a very important one with potentially problematic consequences if wrong directions are given. When the computer system alerts the technician to a drug interaction between an enzyme inducer and another medication, he or she will understand the mechanism of the interaction. And knowledge about loading doses will help the technician understand dosing and assist in recognizing when doses make sense and when they should be questioned.

Recommended Reading

Bimark Healthcare Communications. Alternative oral dosage forms for the geriatric patient. Novartis Pharmaceuticals Corporation; 1999.

Chapron DJ. Drug disposition and response. In: Therapeutics in the elderly, 3rd ed. Delafeunte JC, Stewart RB, eds. Cincinnati, OH: Harvey Whitney Books Company; 2001:257–88.

Shargel L, Yu ABC. Biopharmaceutic considerations in drug product design. In: Applied biopharmaceutics and pharmacokinetics. 3rd ed. Shargel L, Yu ABC, eds. East Norwalk, CT: Appleton and Lange; 1993.

Winters ME. Basic clinical pharmacokinetics. 3rd ed. Vancouver, WA: Applied Therapeutics, Inc.; 1994.

References

1. Lindly CM, Tully MP, Paramsothy V et al. Inappropriate medication is a major cause of adverse drug reactions in elderly patients. *Age Aging.* 1992; 21:294–300.

2. Hanlon JT, Gray SL, Schmader KE. Adverse drug reactions. In: Therapeutics in the elderly, 3rd ed. Delafeunte JC, Stewart RB, eds. Cincinnati, OH: Harvey Whitney Books Company; 2001:289–314.

3. Nolan L, O'Malley K. Prescribing for the elderly, part 1: sensitivity of the elderly to adverse drug reactions. *J Am Geriatr Soc.* 1988; 36:132–40.

4. Stewart RB, Cooper JW. Polypharmacy in the aged: practical solutions. *Drugs Aging.* 1994; 4:449–61.

5. Montamat SC, Cusack B. Overcoming problems with polypharmacy and drug misuse. *Clin Geriatr Med.* 1992; 8:143–58.

6. Shargel L, Yu ABC. Biopharmaceutic considerations in drug product design. In: Applied biopharmaceutics and pharmacokinetics. 3rd ed. Shargel L, Yu ABC, eds. East Norwalk, CT: Appleton and Lange; 1993.

7. Stedman CAM, Barclay ML. Comparison of the pharmacokinetics, acid suppression and efficacy of proton pump inhibitors. *Aliment Pharmacol Thera.* 2000; 14 (8):963–78.

8. Drug facts and comparisons updated monthly. St. Louis, MO: Facts and Comparisons: A Wolters Kluwer Company; 2002.

9. Eli Lilly and Company. Humalog prescribing information. Indianapolis, IN: Eli Lilly and Company; May 31, 2002.

10. Aventis. Lantus prescribing information. Kansas City, MO: Aventis; August 2002.

11. Winters ME. Basic principles. In: Basic clinical pharmacokinetics. 3rd ed. Koda- Kimble MA, Young LY, eds. Vancouver, WA: Applied Therapeutics, Inc.; 1994.

12. Hansten PD, Horn JR, eds. Drug interaction analysis and management. St. Louis, MO: Facts and Comparisons: A Wolters Kluwer Company; 2001.

13. Eli Lilly and Company. Prozac product information. Indianapolis, IN: Eli Lilly and Company; February 2001.

14. Cockroft DW, Gault MH. Prediction of creatinine clearance from serum creatinine. *Nephron.* 1976; 16: 31–41.

15. Bauer LA. Clinical pharmacokinetics and pharmacodynamics. In: Pharmacotherapy: a pathophysiologic approach. 5th ed. Dipiro JT, Talbert RL, Yee GC, eds. New York, NY: McGraw Hill Medical Publishing Division; 2002.

16. Brody TM, Garrison JC. Sites of action: receptors. In: Human pharmacology: molecular to clinical. 3rd ed. Brody TM, Larner J, Minneman KP eds. St. Louis, MO: Mosby; 1998.

17. Montamat SC, Cusack BJ, Vestal RE. Management of drug therapy in the elderly. *New Engl J Med.* 1989; 321(5): 303–9.

Self-Assessment Questions

1. Which of the following is the FIRST process that a solid dosage form must undergo to exert a pharmacologic effect?
   a. disintegration
   b. dissolution
   c. distribution
   d. demethylation

2. Which of the following dosage forms needs to be shaken before dispensing the medication?
   a. elixir
   b. solution
   c. syrup
   d. suspension

3. Which of the following pharmacokinetic processes is most impaired in the presence of renal disease?
   a. absorption
   b. distribution
   c. metabolism
   d. elimination

4. Which of the following routes ensures complete absorption into the systemic circulation?
   a. intravenous
   b. subcutaneous
   c. intramuscular
   d. intradermal

5. Which of the following product formulations may be crushed?
   a. timed-release capsule
   b. sustained-release tablet
   c. controlled-release caplet
   d. immediate-release tablet

6. If a patient has kidney disease, which of the following should be double-checked before dispensing?
   a. route of medication
   b. dose of medication
   c. formulation of medication
   d. number of concomitant medications

7. What does an enzyme inducer do?
   a. It increases the metabolism of other medications.
   b. It increases the absorption of other medications.
   c. It increases the distribution of other medications.
   d. It increases the bioavailability of other medications.

8. Why is it possible for a dose of an intravenous medication to be 2 mg, and the dose of the same medication given orally to be 4 mg?
   a. Metabolism of the medication by different routes is different.
   b. Bioavailability of the medication by different routes is different.
   c. Elimination of the medication by different routes is different.
   d. Distribution of the medication by different routes is different.

9. Which of the following studies the effects of medications at a target site?
   a. biopharmaceutics
   b. pharmacokinetics
   c. pharmacodynamics

10. To what does a medication have to bind to produce a clinical effect?
    a. a plasma protein
    b. a receptor
    c. an organ
    d. a blood cell

Self-Assessment Answers

1. a. Disintegration is the first of several processes that must occur before a medication can exert a pharmacological effect. Disintegration is the breakdown of the medication from the original solid formulation. The next step is dissolution, or the dissolving of drug into solution. Disintegration makes dissolution easier, as smaller particles are easier to dissolve than large particles.

2. d. Suspensions need to be shaken because particles in suspension do not remain suspended in solution. Rather, they aggregate at the bottom of the suspension. All the other options remain in the original mixed state and do not need to be resuspended.

3. d. The kidneys are responsible for excreting or eliminating many medications from the body. When kidney function is compromised, the elimination of renally excreted medications is hindered.

4. a. Intravenous medication administration is medication administration directly into the vein, and therefore into the bloodstream. Absorption of medications, by definition, is the absorption of medication into the bloodstream. The other routes administer medication outside the bloodstream, so medication administered by other routes needs to travel to the bloodstream from where the medication was administered.

5. d. Immediate-release medications can usually be crushed because altering the dosage form will not alter the rate of medication absorption and effect. Controlled-release, sustained-release, and timed-release medications are specially formulated to release medication over a prolonged period of time. Altering such dosage forms alters the special release mechanism and may cause all the medication to be released at once, like an immediate-release medication.

6. b. Because kidneys eliminate medication from the body, kidney disease may hinder the elimination of medication. Decreased elimination of medication may lead to accumulation of the drug in the body and may contribute to prolonged medication effects and side effects. For this reason, patients with kidney disease are often given lower doses of medications that are renally eliminated.

7. a. Enzyme inducers increase the metabolism of other medications that undergo the same type of metabolism as the inducer. For example, phenytoin is an enzyme inducer. It increases the metabolism of other medications, such as phenobarbital, carbamazepine, and valproic acid. Therefore, higher doses of these medications may be needed when given with phenytoin.

8. b. Bioavailability is the percentage of a medication dose that is absorbed into the bloodstream. Medications given intravenously are instantaneously and completely taken up by the bloodstream. Conversely, not all of an oral medication dose is taken up by the bloodstream. Therefore, the oral dose of a medication is often higher than the intravenous dose of the same medication.

9. c. The study of medication at its target site is the study of pharmacodynamics. Biopharmaceutics is the study of medication formulation and its effects on drug disposition. Pharmacokinetics is the study of medication absorption, distribution, metabolism, and excretion.

10. b. A medication needs to bind to a receptor to produce a clinical effect. Medications can bind to other proteins, such as albumin, but they are inactive when bound to a protein and therefore do not exert a clinical effect at that time. Medications may affect certain organs and can also affect the blood, but they do not affect them directly; they must bind to a receptor on that organ or to a receptor that will trigger a response to affect the blood.

Drug Classification and Pharmacologic Actions

12

SHERI STENSLAND

After completing this chapter, the technician should be able to

1. Identify the common drug names for each classification.

2. Describe the important actions or therapeutic uses for the major classes of drugs.

3. Describe the most common or most serious adverse effects for the major classes of drugs.

4. Describe special dispensing precautions for the major classes of drugs.

A drug can be defined as any substance that, when introduced into the body, alters the body's functions. An ideal drug would have several characteristics: (1) it would be effective for its therapeutic use, (2) it would be safe even if large quantities were ingested, and (3) it would not have any adverse effects. The ideal drug does not exist. All drugs have some adverse effects, and many drugs are toxic when more than the recommended dose is taken. Therefore, the decision to use any drug therapy is made after weighing the benefits of the drug against the risks involved with its use.

Drugs discussed in this chapter are arranged according to the body organ systems in which they have their major effects. Drugs often have actions in more than one part of the body and thus may be mentioned in several areas. This chapter covers the major actions or uses of drugs, their major adverse effects, and important characteristics of specific drugs, especially where these characteristics are important in dispensing activities. Many of the drugs discussed are listed in tables by both their generic and trade names. The United States Adopted Names Council (USAN) has approved stems for generic names that help to classify medications according to their mechanism of action. For example, a generic medication that has an *olol* ending is classified as a beta-blocking agent that is commonly used to treat hypertension or glaucoma. Learning to recognize these stems will help the technician identify the classifications for different medications. Besides the stems, many drug classes are identified by abbreviations. **Table 12-1** lists some commonly used drug and medical abbreviations. The drugs bolded in the tables in this chapter are the most commonly prescribed medications. This chapter presents only major drug classes. For readers who desire more in-depth information or information on less commonly used medications, a list of recommended reading is included at the end of the chapter.

TABLE 12-1. ABBREVIATIONS	
ACE —	Angiotensin converting enzyme
ADH —	Antidiuretic hormone
AIDS —	Acquired immunodeficiency syndrome
ARB —	Angiotensin receptor blocker
AQ —	Aqueous
BPH —	Benign prostatic hyperplasia
CMV —	Cytomegalovirus
COPD —	Chronic obstructive pulmonary disease
FDA —	Food and Drug Administration
GERD —	Gastroesophageal reflux disease
HDL —	High-density lipoprotein
HIV —	Human immunodeficiency virus
HMG-CoA —	Hydroxymethylglutaryl-Coenzyme A
LDL —	Low-density lipoprotein
MAOI —	Monoamine oxidase inhibitor
NSAID —	Nonsteroidal anti-inflammatory drug
PUD —	Peptic ulcer disease
RSV —	Respiratory syncytial virus
SSRI —	Selective Serotonin reuptake inhibitor
T_3 —	Triiodothyronine
T_4 —	Levothyroxine
TB —	Tuberculosis

Respiratory System

Some common diseases of the respiratory system are pneumonia, asthma, and chronic obstructive pulmonary disease (COPD). Pneumonia is a lung infection. Antibiotics for the treatment of pneumonia are discussed in the section on infectious disease. Asthma is characterized by a reversible narrowing of the air passages caused by overresponsiveness of the airways to various stimuli and inflammation of the airways. The stimuli that can cause inflammation and airway narrowing include viruses, cold air, exercise, pollens, dust, cigarette smoke, and animal dander. COPD is an irreversible chronic obstruction of airways. Emphysema and chronic bronchitis are examples of COPD. The symptoms of asthma and COPD are similar—wheezing, difficulty breathing, and coughing. These diseases differ in their cause, development, and reversibility. Similar drugs are used to treat both (see **Table 12-2**).

TABLE 12-2. AGENTS USED TO TREAT ASTHMA AND COPD

Generic Name	Brand Name	Common Side Effects
Short-Acting Bronchodilators		
Albuterol	**Proventil, Ventolin,**	Tremors, nervousness, fast heart rate
	Proventil HFA,	
	Ventolin HFA	
	Volmax	
Metaproterenol	Alupent	
Pirbuterol	Maxair	
Levalbuterol	Xopenex	
Long-acting Bronchodilators		
Salmeterol	**Serevent**	Tremors, nervousness, fast heart rate
Formeterol	Foradil	
Theophylline	various brands	Nausea, vomiting, fast heart rate, headache, insomnia
Inhaled Corticosteroids		
Triamcinolone	**Azmacort**	Thrush, hoarseness
Budesonide	Pulmicort	
Fluticasone	**Flovent**	
Flunisolide	Aerobid, Aerobid-M	
Beclomethasone	Beclovent, Vanceril, Q-Var	
Mast Cell Stabilizers		
Nedocromil	Tilade	Dizziness, headache, rash
Cromolyn sodium	Intal	
Anticholinergics		
Ipratropium	**Atrovent**	Flushing, dry mouth, constipation, confusion
Leukotriene Inhibitors		
Zafirlukast	Accolate	Headache, cough, abdominal pain
Montelukast	**Singulair**	
Zileuton	Zyflo	
Combination Agents		
Salmeterol/Fluticasone	**Advair**	
Ipratropium/Albuterol	**Combivent**	

Bronchodilators

Bronchodilators are drugs that open up, or dilate, the bronchioles. There are three types of bronchodilators: (1) Beta–2(β_2)-agonists, (2) xanthines, and (3) anticholinergics.

The β_2-agonists act on the nerves that control the smooth muscles in the bronchial airways. These agents are available in several dosage forms: metered-dose inhalers, solutions for inhalation via a nebulizer machine, oral tablets, oral liquids, and injections. Most patients use metered-dose inhalers. The proper use of inhalers is critical to the success of treatment with these drugs. Patient counseling should always include proper use of inhalers.

Common side effects of β_2-agonists are rapid heartbeat, tremors, anxiety, and nausea. Most of these side effects will disappear as the body adjusts to the medication. Rare, but more serious, side effects are chest pain, fast or irregular heartbeat, severe headache, dizziness, and severe nausea and vomiting. Overuse of β_2-agonists can result in decreased effectiveness of the agents. The beta-blockers used in cardiovascular diseases and glaucoma should not be used together with bronchodilators because the drugs have opposite effects.

β_2-agonists differ in how they work: short-acting β_2-agonists are used to stop an attack, whereas long-acting β_2-agonists are used on a daily basis to prevent attacks. Epinephrine and ephedrine are drugs that produce bronchodilation similarly to the β_2-agonists, but they act on more than just the lungs. This lack of selectivity increases the number of side effects these agents cause. Epinephrine and ephedrine are available in over-the-counter formulations, but they should not be used without medical supervision.

The xanthines are another class of bronchodilators. The exact mechanism of action of these drugs is not known, but it may be related to an anti-inflammatory effect. The xanthines most commonly used are aminophylline and theophylline. Aminophylline is a salt of theophylline. If theophylline is substituted for aminophylline, the dose should be 80 percent of the aminophylline dose.

Theophylline has a high incidence of side effects that often occur at therapeutic doses. Nausea and vomiting are common. Other side effects include irritability, restlessness, headache, insomnia, muscle twitching, and rapid heartbeat. Age, diet, smoking, other medications, and illnesses are all factors that can change the amount of theophylline a patient needs to achieve and maintain therapeutic theophylline blood concentrations. Blood levels are often measured periodically to ensure that patients achieve and maintain therapeutic concentrations. Xanthines are not used often, because of the need for monitoring and the side effect profile.

Anticholinergic drugs are the third class of bronchodilators. These drugs act on different nerves than the β_2-agonists but have the same result of relaxing the muscles in the airways. The anticholinergic drugs are more useful in COPD than in asthma. Combined use with β_2-agonists may increase the benefit. Anticho-

linergic agents are available in both oral and inhaled formulations. Because of the side effects associated with the oral formulations, such as atropine, the inhaled formulations (e.g., metered-dose inhalers and nebulization solutions) are commonly used. Common side effects of anticholinergic drugs include dizziness, headache, nausea, dry mouth, cough, hoarseness, or blurred vision.

Other Agents for Asthma and COPD

Because asthma is an inflammatory reaction, preventing or reducing the inflammation can eliminate or lessen the severity of acute asthma attacks. Mast cell stabilizers and corticosteroids are often used for this purpose.

Mast cell stabilizers are often used in patients with allergic asthma or exercise-induced asthma. In patients with these conditions, the release of histamine and other chemicals from the mast cells in the body causes the bronchioles to constrict. The mast cell stabilizers will hinder the release of these substances and prevent the constriction of the bronchioles. These agents are used to prevent asthma attacks, but they are not useful in resolving acute asthma attacks. Adverse reactions are rare and include irritation and dryness of the throat, cough, and bronchospasm (involuntary contracting/narrowing of the airways).

Corticosteroids are used to prevent asthma attacks and, in combination with bronchodilators, to interrupt acute attacks. The inhaled route of administration is useful in pulmonary diseases to prevent the numerous side effects these drugs can cause when given systemically (see Musculoskeletal System). Inhaled corticosteroids used to be avoided in children because of reports that they retard growth. More recent studies have disproved this theory, and current guidelines support the use of corticosteroids in children to control asthma. The most common side effects of inhaled corticosteroids are thrush (fungus of the throat and mouth) and hoarseness. Patients can prevent these effects by using a spacing device with the inhaler and rinsing the mouth with water after use. Some patients may require oral corticosteroids to control their symptoms.

The leukotriene inhibitors are a relatively new class of medications taken orally to treat asthma. This class of medications causes the muscles in the bronchioles to relax and tends to reduce inflammation. Leukotriene inhibitors are often used in patients who awaken at night with asthma symptoms. A key to recognizing the generic names of these agents is the -lukast stem on the names.

Patients with pulmonary diseases may use combinations of the drugs discussed above. Patients should be able to identify which inhalers are to prevent an attack (i.e., their *controllers*) and which are to abort an acute attack (i.e., their *quick-relief*). If both corticosteroid and bronchodilator inhalers are used, the bronchodilator should be used first to open up the airways to allow better penetration of the corticosteroid.

Antihistamines, Decongestants, Expectorants, and Antitussives

The common cold remains one of the most bothersome illnesses. More than 120 strains of viruses are responsible for causing the common cold. Most colds are self-limiting and can be self-treated. Treatment is aimed at reducing the symptoms: runny nose (rhinitis), sore throat (pharyngitis), and cough. These symptoms are produced by an inflammatory response of the lining of the nose, throat, and lungs to the viral invasion. Influenza (flu) viruses cause similar symptoms but may cause more damage to the lining of the respiratory tract. A lasting cough is common after the flu.

Many of the same symptoms occur with allergic rhinitis, a reaction of the nasal lining to allergic stimuli (called allergens). Similar products are used to treat symptoms of both diseases. Decongestants reduce the swelling of the lining of the nose. Antihistamines prevent the release of histamine, which is responsible for symptoms of allergic rhinitis. Antitussives reduce the frequency of cough. Expectorants decrease the thickness and ease expulsion of sputum from the lungs.

Decongestants can be used topically in the nose (see Intranasal Products) or taken orally. They constrict blood vessels in the nose, which decreases nasal swelling and congestion. Topical decongestants are often preferred because they reduce congestion better, last longer, and have fewer side effects than oral decongestants. Patients with hypertension, heart disease, overactive thyroid, diabetes mellitus, or an enlarged prostate gland should use caution if taking decongestants. The only oral decongestant currently available is pseudoephedrine. Side effects include tremors, nervousness, fast heart rate, and nausea. In 2000, the FDA recommended the removal of the oral decongestant phenylpropanolamine from the market because of its potential to cause strokes in women over the age of 50.

During the initial part of an allergic reaction, cells release histamine. Antihistamines block the body's response to histamine and thus reduce or prevent symptoms of allergic rhinitis, such as sneezing, nasal congestion, mucus secretion, and itching and tearing of the eyes. Reducing mucus secretion is a side effect of antihistamines. Antihistamines often help stop the runny nose associated with a common cold thanks to this side effect.

Antihistamines have many side effects. The one that concerns most people is drowsiness. This effect varies among antihistamines and is the reason they are sometimes used as sleep aids. The newer prescription antihistamines cause less sedation (see **Table 12-3**). In children and the elderly, a paradoxical reaction, excitation rather than drowsiness, is sometimes seen. Anticholinergic effects, such as dry mouth, blurred vision, difficulty urinating, and constipation, occur with many antihistamines. Patients with glaucoma, peptic ulcer, or an enlarged prostate gland should avoid most antihistamines. Many antihistamines are available over the counter and in combination with decongestants, expectorants, and antitussives.

A cough can be classified as productive or nonproductive depending on whether phlegm is expectorated with it.[4] A productive cough is helpful if it removes phlegm from the airways. This type of cough should be treated only if the coughing is frequent enough to disturb sleep or is unbearable to the patient. A nonproductive cough without chest congestion can be treated with an antitussive (cough suppressant). A nonproductive cough with chest congestion can be treated with an expectorant to facilitate the expectoration of phlegm. Persistent cough or any cough with chest congestion could indicate a serious condition, such as asthma or pneumonia.

TABLE 12-3. ANTIHISTAMINES		
Generic Name	**Brand Name**	**OTC or Rx**
First Generation Antihistamines		
Chlorpheniramine	Chlor-Trimeton	OTC
Clemastine	Tavist, Tavist-1	OTC
Diphenhydramine	Benadryl	OTC
Hydroxyzine	Atarax	Rx
Promethazine	Phenergan	Rx
Second Generation Antihistamines		
Cetirizine	Zyrtec	Rx
Loratadine	Claritin	OTC
Third Generation Antihistamines		
Desloratadine	Clarinex	Rx
Fexofenadine	Allegra	Rx

Antitussives are drugs that reduce the frequency of cough. Codeine, hydrocodone, dextromethorphan, and diphenhydramine suppress the cough center in the brain. Codeine and hydrocodone are narcotic drugs that can depress breathing and have addiction potential. Their most common side effects are nausea, drowsiness, lightheadedness, and constipation. Dextromethorphan is chemically related to codeine and has similar antitussive efficacy, although it does not have pain-relieving properties, cause respiratory depression, or have addictive potential when used as directed. Dextromethorphan is widely used in over-the-counter cough medicines. Drowsiness and gastrointestinal upset are the most common side effects. Diphenhydramine is an effective cough suppressant that is used in many over-the-counter cough and cold remedies. The sedative and anticholinergic side effects of this drug are discussed with the antihistamines.

Expectorants are controversial because there is little scientific evidence that they effectively decrease the thickness of phlegm and thus aid in its expectoration (which may indirectly treat a cough). Guaifenesin is the only expectorant recognized as safe and effective by the FDA.[2] Increased intake of fluids and humidification of air may also be effective in treating cough.

Guaifenesin is available in over-the-counter and prescription entities as a single drug or in combination with antihistamines, decongestants, and antitussives. It is available in liquid forms and as regular- and sustained-release capsules and tablets. There are no absolute contraindications to the use of guaifenesin. Nausea and vomiting, dizziness, headache, and rash are rare side effects.

Central Nervous System Disorders

Psychoactive Drugs

The true causes of most mental illnesses are unknown. The drugs used to treat these disorders work by altering the various chemicals, called neurotransmitters, found at the nerve junctions in the brain. Norepinephrine, epinephrine, serotonin, and dopamine are examples of neurotransmitters. The following types of drugs alter neurotransmitter activity: antidepressants, antipsychotics, anxiolytics, sedatives, and hypnotics.

Antidepressants

Depression is a common illness in the United States. Depression may be reactive (in response to a stimulus such as grief) or endogenous (a chemical disorder in the brain). Antidepressant medications can be used in either type of depression, but they are most often used for endogenous depression. Drugs can also cause depression, in which case, the suspected drug should be withdrawn. Symptoms of depression include depressed mood, inability to experience pleasure in activities, changes in sleep habits, loss of energy, changes in appetite, inability to concentrate, and thoughts of suicide.

Antidepressants (see **Table 12-4**) can be divided into several classes on the basis of their chemical structures and chemical actions in the brain. The most frequently used drugs are tricyclic antidepressants, monoamine oxidase inhibitors (MAOIs), and selective seratonin reuptake inhibitors (SSRIs). Several antidepressant drugs, such as bupropion, venlafaxine, nefazadone, trazodone, and mirtazapine, do not fit into these classifications. All the classes of antidepressants are effective treatments for depression. The adverse effects associated with a drug are a factor in the choice of a particular drug for a patient.

TABLE 12-4. ANTIDEPRESSANTS

Generic Name	Brand Name	Common Side Effects
Tricyclic antidepressants		
Amitriptyline	Elavil	Sedation, dry mouth, blurred vision, constipation, difficulty urinating, dizziness standing
Nortriptyline	Pamelor	
Protriptyline	Vivactil	
Imipramine	Tofranil, Tofranil-PM	
Desipramine	Norpramin	
Doxepin	Sinequan	
Clomipramine	Anafranil	
MAOIs		
Isocarboxazid	Marplan	Postural hypotension or hypertensive crisis
Phenelzine	Nardil	
Tranylcypromine	Parnate	
SSRIs		
Fluoxetine	Prozac	Nausea, diarrhea, anorexia
Paroxetine	Paxil	
Sertraline	Zoloft	
Citalopram	Celexa	
Escitalopram	Lexapro	
Fluvoxamine	Luvox	
Miscellaneous Agents		
Nefazodone	Serzone	Same as Tricyclics
Trazodone	Desyrel	
Venlafaxine	Effexor, Effexor-XR	
Bupropion	Wellbutrin, Wellbutrin-SR, Zyban	Seizures
Mirtazapine	Remeron	Agranulocytosis

Tricyclic antidepressants, the most widely used antidepressants for many years, have the stem *-triptyline* on their names. Their mechanism of action is unclear, but they are thought to enhance the action of norepinephrine and serotonin in the brain. These antidepressants are effective but have a large number of bothersome side effects, including dry mouth, blurred vision, constipation, difficulty urinating, dizziness upon standing, sedation, and sexual dysfunction. These side effects may cause patients to stop taking their medication. Overdose with these drugs can be lethal because of their effects on the heart and because they can cause convulsions. Because depressed patients often have suicidal tendencies, the overdose potential of these drugs is an important consideration when selecting a drug for treatment.

MAOIs are thought to work by preventing the natural breakdown of neurotransmitters. Until the availability of the SSRIs, the MAOIs were the most effective antidepressants. The distinguishing feature of the MAOIs has to do with the drug–diet interactions with tyramine-containing foods and the drug–drug interactions. Hypertensive crisis, an extreme elevation of blood pressure that can be fatal or produce organ damage, is a potential adverse reaction with MAOIs. This event most often occurs when certain foods or drugs are taken with the MAOI. Therefore, patients must be fully informed of the foods (e.g., aged cheeses, sausages, and red wine) and medications (e.g., pseudoephedrine in decongestants or diet pills) they should avoid. The most common side effect of MAOIs is postural hypotension, which is a drop in blood pressure upon arising (moving from a sitting or lying position to a standing position) that results in dizziness.

The SSRIs are the newest class of antidepressants. Tricyclics and MAOIs affect several neurotransmitters, but SSRIs affect only one neurotransmitter, serotonin. Many of the drugs in this class have approvals not only for depression but also for obsessive-compulsive disorders (OCD) and to treat the eating disorder bulimia. SSRIs gained quick acceptance because the side effect profile is more tolerable compared with the previous classes of antidepressants, and the SSRIs are less dangerous at normal or excessive doses. Their common side effects are nausea, anorexia, diarrhea, anxiety, nervousness, and insomnia. Sexual dysfunction does occur infrequently. Recently Prozac®, an SSRI, was the first antidepressant to gain approval for a once-weekly dosing. Patients must first be stabilized on the daily dosing and thereafter may be switched to the weekly dosing.

The category of antidepressants also includes miscellaneous agents. Nefazadone, trazodone, venlafaxine, bupropion, and mirtazapine do not fit into the usual classes of antidepressants. Nefazadone and trazodone share some of the adverse effects of the tricyclic antidepressants, such as sedation and postural hypotension, but they are less likely to cause heart rhythm disturbances or anticholinergic effects, such as dry mouth, blurred vision, constipation, and difficulty urinating. Like the tricyclic antidepressants, bupropion can cause constipation and dry mouth. The most serious adverse reaction of bupropion is seizures. Bupropion is unique in that it has gained approval to be used for smoking cessation. Venlafaxine's most common adverse effects are nausea, drowsiness, insomnia, dry mouth, dizziness, nervousness, sweating, and sexual dysfunction. An increase in blood pressure can occur in patients taking venlafaxine. Mirtazapine is not likely to cause heart rhythm disturbances or seizures, but it can cause agranulocytosis—a decreased production of all types of blood cells—and neutropenia—a decreased production of white blood cells.

Antidepressants are usually started at low doses and gradually increased. It may take 3 to 4 weeks before a patient will respond to them.[5] Patients must use caution when discontinuing one antidepressant and starting another to avoid adverse effects. Antidepressants should be discontinued over several weeks. During this time, the dose should be tapered gradually. Drug interactions are common with most antidepressants. Patients should be warned to check with their doctor or pharmacist before taking other prescription or nonprescription medications.

Antipsychotics

Psychosis is a mental disorder in which a person's capacity to recognize reality is distorted. Schizophrenia is one type of psychosis. Common symptoms of psychosis include hallucinations (hearing or seeing things that are not real), delusions (fixed beliefs that are false), and thought processes that are not logically connected.

The antipsychotics are classified as *conventional* or *atypical* agents (see **Table 12-5**). Although the precise mechanism of action is not known, conventional antipsychotics are thought to act by blocking the action of the neurotransmitter dopamine. The newer agents, marketed in the 1990s and classified as *atypical agents,* appear to block not only dopamine but also serotonin and have a more favorable side-effect profile. Many of

TABLE 12-5. ANTIPSYCHOTICS

Generic Name	Brand Name	Formulations
Conventional Antipsychotics		
Low-Potency		
Chlorpromazine	Thorazine	Tablets, concentrated liquid, suppositories, injection
Thioridazine	Mellaril	Tablets, suspension
Intermediate-Potency		
Perphenazine	Trilafon	Tablets, concentrated liquid
Loxapine	Loxitane	Capsules, concentrated liquid
High-Potency		
Trifluoperazine	Stelazine	Tablets, concentrated liquid
Fluphenazine	Prolixin	Tablets, decanoate injection, liquid, elixir
Thiothixene	Navane	Capsules
Haloperidol	Haldol	Tablets, concentrated liquid, injection, deconoate injection
Atypical Antipsychotics		
Clozapine	Clozaril	Tablets
Olanzepine	**Zyprexa**	Tablets
Risperidone	**Risperdal**	Tablets, solution
Quetiapine	Seroquel	Tablets
Ziprasidone	Geodon	Capsules
Aripiprazole	Abilify	Tablets

the antipsychotics are available as injections and oral tablets. Oral solutions, which should be diluted with liquids such as fruit juice, are available for patients who refuse tablets. Fluphenazine and haloperidol are available as long-acting injections for patients who may not be compliant with daily medication regimens. The effectiveness of haloperidol decanoate injections lasts 4 weeks. Long-acting fluphenazine is available as fluphenazine decanoate, which will last more than 4 weeks.

Adverse effects of the antipsychotics differ by classification and potency. The low-potency conventional agents tend to produce more sedation and anticholinergic effects, while the high-potency agents produce extrapyramidal effects. Extrapyramidal symptoms (EPS) include abnormal muscle contractions, some of which can be life threatening (such as when the throat muscles contract), and restlessness. Anticholinergic side effects include dry mouth, blurred vision, constipation, difficulty urinating, and increased heart rate. The atypical agents tend to cause postural hypotension. Clozapine has special monitoring parameters because of its ability to cause fatal agranulocytosis, and the distribution of this drug is tightly controlled to ensure proper monitoring.

Drugs for Bipolar Disorder

Bipolar disorder, also called manic-depressive disorder, is characterized by mood swings. Patients cycle between an agitated or overexcited and a depressed state. Manic episodes have traditionally been treated with lithium. Lithium is also taken as a maintenance drug to prevent episodes. Two other drugs now commonly used for bipolar disorder are carbamazepine and valproic acid. These drugs are both generally used to prevent seizures (i.e., they are anticonvulsants). They are discussed in more detail in the section on Drugs for Neurological Disorders.

The mechanism of action of lithium is unclear. Lithium affects many of the salts in the blood, leading to adverse effects, such as increased thirst and urination. Tremors, a common side effect of lithium, can be alleviated with propranolol. Lithium also decreases thyroid function in a high percentage of patients and causes kidney toxicity. The amount of lithium in the blood can be measured to ensure that the dose is high enough to be effective but low enough to avoid adverse effects.

Sedatives, Hypnotics, and Anxiolytics

Sedative-hypnotic drugs are used to treat anxiety and sleep disorders. Sedatives are used to reduce anxiety or produce a calming effect. Hypnotic drugs are used to produce sleep or drowsiness. Some drugs have sedative effects at lower doses and hypnotic effects at higher doses.

Drugs used for anxiety (anxiolytics) include the benzodiazepines (BZDs), barbiturates, and buspirone. Since the development of the BZDs, barbiturates are rarely used for anxiety. Barbiturates have a higher risk of adverse effects and toxicity than BZDs.

The characteristic ending to the benzodiazepines is *-azepam*. BZDs are the most commonly used drugs for anxiety and sleeplessness (see **Table 12-6**). Other indications for BZDs include depression, muscle tension, and convulsive disorders (see Anticonvulsants in the Drugs for Neurological Disorders section). Injectable forms of midazolam, and less frequently, diazepam, are used for sedation for surgical procedures or endoscopy.

TABLE 12-6. SEDATIVES AND HYPNOTICS

Generic Name	Brand Name	Comments
Benzodiazepines		
Alprazolam	Xanax	Used for anxiety, sedation
Chlordiazepoxide	Librium	Used for anxiety
Clorazepate	Tranxene	Used for anxiety, sedation
Diazepam	Valium	Used for anxiety, status epilepticus, muscle relaxant
Lorazepam	Ativan	Used for anxiety, status epilepticus, muscle relaxant
Midazolam	Versed	Used for sedation in surgical procedures
Oxazepam	Serax	Used for anxiety
Estazolam	Prosom	Used for sedation
Flurazepam	Dalmane	Used for sedation; longest acting hypnotic
Temazepam	Restoril	Used for sedation
Triazolam	Halcion	Used for sedation; shortest acting hypnotic
Quazepam	Doral	Used for sedation
Other Agents (nonbenzodiazepines)		
Buspirone	Buspar	Low abuse potential; less sedating; used for anxiety
Zolpidem	Ambien	Used for sedation
Zaleplon	Sonata	Used for sedation
Phenobarbital	Luminal	Used for sedation, anticonvulsant
Secobarbital	Seconal	Used for sedation
Choral Hydrate	Aquachloral	Used for procedure sedation

The most common side effects of BZDs are drowsiness and slowed reactions. These effects are enhanced when drugs such as alcohol or narcotics are used simultaneously with BZDs. All patients on BZDs or other medications that can cause sedation should be counseled about possible impairment of driving abilities, ability to operate machinery, and judgment. Amnesia, or memory loss, is often considered an adverse effect, but it is desirable when these drugs are used for sedation during painful medical procedures. Withdrawal symptoms may occur when patients who have taken these drugs for a long time abruptly stop therapy. When an overdose of BZDs occurs, a drug called *flumazenil* is available as an antidote to reverse some of the effects, such as sedation and respiratory depression.

Buspirone is chemically unlike the BZDs. Buspirone's advantage over BZDs is its lower likelihood of causing drowsiness and slowed reactions. It also has a low potential for abuse and no withdrawal symptoms.

Hypnotics may be used to treat a variety of sleep problems: difficulty in falling asleep, frequent awakening during the night, early morning awakening, and not feeling rested even after what should be an adequate amount of sleep. Nondrug therapies, such as establishing a regular bedtime and wake-up time and reducing the use of alcohol, caffeine, and nicotine, are usually tried first. General guidelines for the use of hypnotics include using the lowest effective dose for the shortest duration possible.

Like sedatives, hypnotic drugs include barbiturates; BZDs; and nonbarbiturate, nonbenzodiazepine drugs. Because of their potential for the development of tolerance, fatal overdose, dependence, withdrawal symptoms, and drug interactions, barbiturates have been used as hypnotics less often since the development of benzodiazepines.[5] Amobarbital, pentobarbital, and secobarbital are the barbiturates most often used as hypnotics.

The effects of some hypnotics carry over into the daytime. This carryover of drowsiness and decreased concentration, called a *hangover effect*, is an important consideration in the use of hypnotics. Elderly patients tend to metabolize drugs at a slower rate, tend to exhibit more confusion and disorientation upon waking, and are at greater risk for falls. Hypnotics with a hangover effect should be used with caution in these patients. BZDs that are metabolized and excreted rapidly are less likely to produce a hangover.[5] *Tolerance*, a loss of effectiveness over time, may occur with all BZDs.

Nonbenzodiazepine and nonbarbiturate hypnotics include several groups of drugs. A newer drug that is not chemically a BZD but has similar actions is zolpidem. Other drugs are used as hypnotics because drowsiness is one of their most common side effects. The antihistamine diphenhydramine is used this way because it frequently causes drowsiness. Many nonprescription sleep aids contain diphenhydramine. Antidepressants such as amitriptyline, doxepin, and trazodone are often used for patients who do not feel rested after adequate sleep or who should not take BZDs. Chloral hydrate has many of the same disadvantages as the barbiturates and is rarely used today as a hypnotic. Its place in therapy has been limited to sedation during procedures in certain patients.

Drugs for Neurological Disorders

Anticonvulsants

Epilepsy is a disorder of the central nervous system characterized by recurrent seizures. Seizures are brief episodes of brain dysfunction that result from abnormal firing of nerves in the brain. There are four main types of seizures: (1) generalized tonic-clonic seizures (grand mal), which involve sudden sharp muscle contractions followed by rigidity; (2) generalized absence seizures (petit mal), which consist of a sudden cessation of ongoing activities or a blank stare; (3) generalized myoclonic seizures, in which muscle contractions of isolated parts of the body, such as the face or arms, occur; and (4) partial seizures, which may precede a generalized seizure or involve other sensory components. Status epilepticus is an emergency situation in which seizures last for longer than 30 minutes or seizures have no period of consciousness in between them. Status epilepticus may result in brain injury or death if not treated immediately.

Anticonvulsant drugs, also called *antiepileptics*, are used to reduce the frequency of seizures. They do this by reducing the excitability of the nerve cells in the brain. All anticonvulsants have adverse effects, so their use is called for only when the probability of recurrent seizures is more worrisome than the adverse effects of the drugs.

The major drugs used to control seizures are phenytoin, carbamazepine, and valproic acid. Other drugs are listed in **Table 12-7**, along with the types of seizures they treat. Several of these agents have been available for only a few years.

Two BZDs are used for status epilepticus. Injectable forms of diazepam and lorazepam are commonly used initially to stop the repetitive seizure activity, and then long-acting drugs, such as phenytoin, are given to prevent the recurrence of seizures.

Phenytoin has been available for many years and effectively prevents many types of seizures. Dosing phenytoin is complicated, and blood levels are usually measured to ensure that enough phenytoin is present to prevent seizures but not so much as to cause side effects. This drug is known to have a narrow therapeutic index, which means small changes in the dose may result in large changes in effects. Side effects that are dose-related include double vision, loss of muscle coordination, and sedation. Common side effects that are not affected by decreasing the dose are overgrowth of the gums (gingival hypertrophy) and excessive body hair (hirsutism). Phenytoin also has many drug interactions. Patients should be warned not to take extra doses

TABLE 12-7. ANTICONVULSANTS

Generic Name	Trade Name	Seizure Indication
Phenytoin	Dilantin	Status epilepticus, tonic-clonic
Fosphenytoin	Cerebyx	Status epilepticus, tonic-clonic
Ethotoin	Peganone	Status epilepticus, tonic-clonic
Diazepam	Valium	Status epilepticus
Lorazepam	Ativan	Status epilepticus
Clonazepam	Klonopin	Absence, myoclonic
Valproic acid	Depakene	Absence
Divalproex Na	Depakote	Absence, partial
Ethosuximide	Zarontin	Absence
Carbamazepine	Tegretol, Tegretol-XR	Tonic-clonic, partial
Primidone	Mysoline	Tonic-clonic
Gabapentin	Neurontin	Tonic-clonic, partial
Oxcarbazepine	Trileptal	Partial
Lamotrigine	Lamictal	Partial
Felbamate	Felbatol	Partial
Levetiracetam	Keppra	Adjunctive to partial
Tiagabine	Gabitril	Adjunctive to partial
Zonisamide	Zonegran	Adjunctive to partial
Topiramate	Topamax	Adjunctive to tonic-clonic, partial

or other drugs without checking with their doctor or pharmacist. Phenytoin is available in capsule, tablet, oral suspension, and injectable form.

A new injectable drug, fosphenytoin, is converted to phenytoin in the body. Fosphenytoin, because of chemical properties that differ from phenytoin, has fewer administration-associated side effects but, once it is converted to phenytoin in the body, the two drugs have the same therapeutic effects.

Some anticonvulsant drugs have other therapeutic uses, such as for psychiatric disorders, for a painful facial nerve condition called trigeminal neuralgia, for other nerve pain conditions, and for restless leg syndrome. As with phenytoin, blood levels of many anticonvulsants are measured to ensure that the dose is producing therapeutic blood levels but not levels high enough to result in adverse effects. Liver function and red blood cell production must be monitored with several of the anticonvulant drugs. Carbamazepine can cause a rare, serious adverse effect called pancytopenia, which is a depression of the production of all types of blood cells (red cells, white cells, and platelets). Liver toxicity is the most serious side effect of valproic acid use, but it is reversible if the drug is stopped. Other side effects of valproic acid are nausea, vomiting, headache, weight gain, increased appetite, and hair loss. Phenobarbital is effective against fewer seizure types than some of the newer drugs. The adverse effects of phenobarbital, in particular excessive sedation, and the potential for dependence and withdrawal symptoms limit its usefulness. One agent, felbamate, was found after being marketed to have an unacceptable occurrence of serious blood reactions. It should not be used except for patients whose seizures cannot be controlled with other drugs.

Many of the newer antiepileptics have been studied more in combination with older drugs than alone. These agents are often called *adjunct therapy*, meaning they are used in addition to another agent to work effectively.

Antiparkinson Drugs

Parkinson's disease is a nervous system disorder characterized by movement abnormalities: tremor, extreme slowness in movement, and rigidity or stiffness of joints. Common movement abnormalities seen in these patients are *pill rolling* with the thumb and index finger, a cogwheel or ratcheting-appearing movement of the arms or legs, a stooped posture, and a blank stare caused by decreased blinking.

Although the cause of Parkinson's disease is unknown, the basis of drug therapy is to correct an imbalance of two chemicals in the brain, dopamine and acetylcholine. The available drug therapies control only symptoms; despite therapy, the disease will progress with increasing debilitation.

Levodopa is the major drug used in Parkinson's disease. It increases the amount of the chemical dopamine in the brain and other areas of the body. The increased amount of dopamine in the brain helps to reduce the symptoms of Parkinson's, but the increases in dopamine in the rest of the body can cause adverse reactions. Therefore, levodopa is usually given in combination with carbidopa. Carbidopa inhibits the conversion of levodopa to its active form outside the brain and thus reduces the adverse effects.

Levodopa can cause nausea and vomiting and effects on the heart rate and rhythm. These are not major problems when carbidopa is combined with levodopa (Sinemet®). However, certain movement disorders are more common in patients taking the combination product than in those taking levodopa alone. A variety of other side effects, including depression, anxiety, agitation, inability to sleep, confusion, and hallucinations, can occur with both. Levodopa should not be given to psychotic patients. Its actions are the opposite of the antipsychotic drugs, so it may worsen the symptoms of

psychosis, just as most antipsychotics may worsen the symptoms of Parkinson's disease.

Another set of drugs used as adjunctive therapy to levodopa is known as catechol-O-methyltransferase (COMT) inhibitors. COMT is an enzyme that breaks down levodopa. Inhibiting this enzyme leaves more levodopa available to be converted to dopamine. The two COMT inhibitor agents available are tolcapone (Tasmar®) and entacapone (Comtan®). Common side effects include GI (gastrointestinal) effects, such as abdominal pain, constipation, and diarrhea. Tolcapone has a high risk for liver toxicity (hepatotoxicity), so liver function should be tested periodically.

Other agents used in Parkinson's disease—amantadine, bromocriptine, pergolide, and selegiline—mimic or increase the actions of dopamine. These drugs are usually used in combination with levodopa, although they may be used alone. Their side effects are similar to those of levodopa: mental changes and movement disorders.

Anticholinergic drugs used in Parkinson's disease are benztropine, biperidin, procyclidine, trihexyphenidyl, ethopropazine, and diphenhydramine. Their mechanism of action is related not to dopamine but to the other chemical involved in Parkinson's disease, acetylcholine. Anticholinergics are more useful for patients with tremor and rigidity than those with slowed movement. These drugs have many side effects. Mental side effects include drowsiness, confusion, restlessness, and hallucinations. Common physical side effects are dry mouth, blurred vision, difficulty urinating, constipation, nausea and vomiting, and rapid heart rate.

Cardiovascular System

Antihyperlipidemic Agents

Heart attack and stroke are caused by blockage of blood vessels to the heart and brain. Hyperlipidemia—increased levels of cholesterol in the blood—is a risk factor in the development of these diseases. Lowering blood cholesterol has been shown to decrease the death rate from stroke and heart attack.

Cholesterol and triglycerides are the fats that contribute to heart disease. Cholesterol is measured as total cholesterol, which is a combination of low-density lipoprotein (LDL), the so-called "bad" cholesterol, and high-density lipoprotein (HDL), the "good" cholesterol. Drugs have differing effects on these various components of blood cholesterol and triglycerides. Drugs are selected on the basis of the type of fats that are elevated as well as the side-effect profiles of the drugs.

Initially, hyperlipidemia is treated with diet and exercise. If these methods fail, drugs may be added. The agents used today are bile acid sequestrants, hydroxymethylglutaryl coenzyme A (HMG-CoA) reductase inhibitors, fibrates, and nicotinic acid (see **Table 12-8**). These agents may be used alone or in combination to lower cholesterol. Because drug therapy always has unwanted side effects, the patient's risk factors for heart disease and degree of blood cholesterol elevation are considered before drug treatment is started.

Bile Acid Sequestrants

The liver and gallbladder secrete bile into the intestine to aid the absorption of fats from food in the intestines. The bile secreted into the intestine is reabsorbed into the blood. Bile acid sequestrants bind the bile in the intestines and prevent it from being reabsorbed. Instead, the bile is excreted in the feces. The loss of bile stimulates production of more bile, which requires cholesterol. Because the body uses cholesterol to make more bile, which is then bound and excreted, this cycle leads to a decrease in LDL and total cholesterol. The most common side effects with these drugs are constipation, aggravation of hemorrhoids, abdominal cramping, gas, nausea and vomiting, diarrhea, and heartburn. Tablet forms of these drugs are available, but for convenience these drugs are often given as a powder mixed in juice. If insufficient fluid is given with the bile acid sequestrants, they can form a solid mass in the esophagus or the intestines, blocking these parts of the digestive tract. In the same way that these drugs bind bile acids, they can also bind other medications. Other drugs should be taken 1 hour before, or 4 to 6 hours after, the bile acid sequestrants.

HMG-CoA Reductase Inhibitors

Much of the cholesterol in the body is not ingested as cholesterol but is made in the body from fats. The HMG-CoA reductase inhibitors, also known as the *statins*, prevent the formation of cholesterol from fats. They effectively increase the good cholesterol—HDL—and decrease the bad cholesterol—LDL—as well as decrease total cholesterol and triglycerides. The most common side effects are muscle and joint pain, headache, and gastrointestinal distress. The most serious effects include abnormalities of liver function tests, although liver damage does not usually occur. A more serious muscle disease, rhabdomyolysis, can occur, usually in patients taking these drugs in combination with the fibrates and possibly other drugs. HMG-CoA reductase inhibitors may cause increased sensitivity to sunlight, so sunscreen should be used when exposure to the sun cannot be avoided.

Fibrates

Clofibrate lowers LDL and total cholesterol but is more useful for its triglyceride-lowering effect. Gemfibrozil decreases triglycerides and raises HDL. The mechanism of action of fibrates is unknown. The most common side effects are nausea and other gastrointestinal symptoms, muscle and joint aches, skin rash, fatigue, taste disturbances, and weakness. More serious side effects are a possible increased risk of liver cancer, gallstones, and decreased white and/or red blood cells.

Other Lipid-Lowering Agents

Nicotinic acid (niacin) is a form of vitamin B that reduces serum cholesterol and triglycerides. Another form of this vitamin, nicotinamide (niacinamide), does not affect blood cholesterol levels. The most bothersome adverse effect of nicotinic acid is a flushing sensation, or a feeling of warmth, as well as itching, tingling, or headache. Taking an aspirin tablet 30 minutes before the niacin dose can alleviate this effect. GI upset can also occur. More serious effects include abnormal liver function tests. Liver damage is more likely to occur with sustained-release preparations. Decreased blood pressure can occur, causing dizziness, especially upon suddenly rising to a sitting or standing position. Larger doses are needed for treatment of high blood cholesterol than for vitamin supplementation.

TABLE 12-8. ANTIHYPERLIPIDEMICS

Generic Name	Trade Name	Common Side Effects
Bile Acid Sequestrants		
Cholestyramine	Questran	Constipation, nausea, gas, abdominal cramping
Colestipol	Colestid	
Colesevelam	Welchol	
HMG-CoA Reductase Inhibitors ("statins")		
Fluvastatin	**Lescol**	Headache, GI upset, muscle and joint pain, abnormal liver function tests
Lovastatin	Mevacor	
Atorvastatin	**Lipitor**	
Pravastatin	**Pravachol**	
Simvastatin	**Zocor**	
Rosuvastatin	**Crestor**	
Fibrates		
Gemfibrozil	**Lopid**	GI symptoms, dizziness, taste disturbances
Fenofibrate	**Tricor**	
Miscellaneous Agents		
Nicotinic acid	Niacin, Niaspan	Flushing, GI symptoms
Niacin/lovastatin	Advicor	
Ezetimibe	Zetia	GI symptoms, arthralgia

Antihypertensives

Other diseases or medications can cause high blood pressure, but 90 percent of high blood pressure is essential hypertension and is of unknown cause.[6] Hypertension usually has no symptoms, but is important to treat because it is a risk factor for heart attack and stroke. Untreated hypertension also can lead to blindness, kidney damage, and blood vessel diseases that affect the arms, hands, legs, and feet. Compliance with medication regimens is a problem in hypertension because patients usually have no symptoms of the disease. Patients may actually feel worse with medication, because they were never aware of their hypertension and now have side effects from the drugs. Patients who receive counseling about their disease and medication are more likely to be compliant with their drug and dietary regimens. Antihypertensive agents should not be discontinued abruptly. Patients should be screened for potential drug interactions as well as for drug–disease contraindications whenever a new medication is added to their regimen.

Like hyperlipidemia, the primary treatment for hypertension is lifestyle changes, such as changes in diet, weight loss (if overweight), and exercise. If these changes do not control blood pressure, then drug therapy may be needed.

Many classes of drugs are used to treat hypertension. Diuretics and beta-blockers have been shown in controlled studies to reduce the number of people who die from heart attacks and strokes.[6] Angiotensin converting enzyme inhibitors (ACE inhibitors), calcium channel blockers, and alpha-blockers have advantages in certain types of patients. Other agents used are central alpha-2-agonists, peripheral adrenergic antagonists, and direct vasodilators.

Diuretics

Diuretics decrease blood pressure by decreasing the blood volume. Commonly called water pills, diuretics work on the kidneys to increase urinary excretion of sodium, chloride, and water. Because all diuretics increase urination, they should be taken as early in the day as possible so the need to urinate does not interrupt the patient's sleep.

Three types of diuretics are used to treat hypertension (see **Table 12-9**): (1) thiazides, (2) loop diuretics, and (3) potassium-sparing diuretics. Thiazide diuretics in low doses are usually effective for hypertension. Loop diuretics are more effective in patients with mild kidney failure. Both thiazide and loop diuretics cause decreased

TABLE 12-9. DIURETICS		
Generic Name	**Brand Name**	**Comments**
Thiazide Diuretics		
Hydrochlorothiazide (HCTZ)	Hydrodiuril, Microzide	May cause loss of potassium, may alter blood glucose levels
Chlorothiazide	Diuril	
Indapamide	Lozol	
Chlorthalidone	Hygroton	
Metolazone	Zaroxolyn	
Loop diuretics		
Furosemide	Lasix	More potent than thiazides, may cause loss of potassium
Bumetanide	Bumex	
Torsemide	Demadex	
Ethacrynic acid	Edecrin	
Potassium-Sparing Diuretics		
Spironolactone	Aldactone	Potassium supplements usually not needed. Often these agents are used in combination with thiazides to increase potency
Triamterene	Dyrenium	
Combination Agents		
Triamterene/HCTZ	Dyazide, Maxzide	Diuretics
Spironolactone/HCTZ	Aldactazide	
Amiloride/HCTZ	Moduretic	
Losartan/HCTZ	Hyzaar	ARB/Diuretic
Lisinopril/HCTZ	Zestoretic	ACE-I/Diuretic
Bisoprolol/HCTZ	Zebeta	Beta-blocker/Diuretic
Valsartan/HCTZ	Diovan HCT	ARB/Diuretic

potassium in the body and may require potassium supplements to replace lost potassium. Potassium-sparing diuretics are weak diuretics that are sometimes added to other diuretics to prevent potassium loss.

Although the thiazide diuretics are well tolerated by patients, certain precautions should be noted. Thiazide diuretics may alter blood glucose control in diabetics. Patients who are taking thiazide diuretics may be more sensitive to sun, so they should be warned to avoid exposure or use sunscreen. Patients allergic to sulfonamides may also be allergic to thiazide diuretics.

Loop diuretics are more potent and may affect electrolytes, such as sodium, potassium, chloride, calcium, and magnesium, to a greater degree than the thiazides. Adverse effects similar to those of the thiazides may occur, including altered blood glucose control in diabetics, sun sensitivity, drug interactions, and allergic reactions in sulfonamide-allergic patients. Hearing loss and kidney damage have occurred in patients taking loop diuretics but are not considered common side effects.

Potassium-sparing diuretics used alone do not cause potassium loss like the other diuretics. Potassium-sparing diuretics are sometimes used with other diuretics to combine the greater potency of a loop or thiazide diuretic with their potassium-sparing effects. Combination drugs are Dyazide®, Maxzide®, Moduretic®, and Aldactazide®. Hydrochlorothiazide has also been combined with other types of antihypertensive drugs to make convenient dosage forms (see Table 12-9).

Beta-Blockers

Beta-blockers block the action of certain nerves in the cardiac muscle, the lungs, and the smooth muscles of the blood vessels. As a result, the heart rate decreases, heart muscle contraction is less forceful, the airways in the lungs constrict, and the dilation of blood vessels is blocked. The drugs lower blood pressure by decreasing the volume of blood pumped by each contraction of the heart. Beta-blockers are first-line drugs for treatment of hypertension and, like diuretics, have been shown to reduce the number of people who die from heart attack or stroke. They also have many other indications, including angina pectoris, cardiac rhythm disturbances, heart attack, migraine headache, tremor, and anxiety.

Beta-blockers are classified as *cardioselective* if they are more selective for the nerves in the heart (β_1) or *noncardioselective* (β_1 and β_2) (see **Table 12-10**). The selectivity is dose dependent, and they may act on the nerves in the lungs and blood vessels at higher doses.

Contraindications for the use of beta-blockers include conditions in which the heart rate is slow, the presence of asthma or COPD, and the presence of diseases in which the blood supply to the extremities (hands, feet, arms, and legs) is insufficient. Beta-blockers also block the symptoms of low blood sugar and should be used cautiously in patients with diabetes. Undesirable side effects include central nervous system effects, such as dizziness, tiredness, and depression. Some patients may develop tingling, loss of sensation, or intolerance to cold in the hands and feet. Increased cholesterol levels, weight gain or loss, and impotence are also possible.

ACE Inhibitors and Angiotensin Receptor Blockers

ACE inhibitors prevent the production of certain chemicals in the blood that cause the constriction of blood vessels and retention of sodium and water. By blocking blood vessel constriction and salt and water retention, these drugs can lower blood pressure. Like the beta-blockers, they have many other uses: ACE inhibitors may slow or prevent the development of

TABLE 12-10. BETA-BLOCKERS, ACE INHIBITORS, AND ARBS		
Generic Name	**Brand Name**	**Comments**
Beta-Blockers		
Atenolol	Tenormin	Note -*olol* ending.
Metoprolol	Lopressor, Toprol-XL	Contraindicated in patients
Nadolol	Corgard	with asthma and diabetes
Propranolol	Inderal, Inderal LA	
Timolol	Blocadren, Timoptic	
Carteolol	Cartrol	
Bisoprolol	Zebeta	
Pindolol	Visken	
Sotalol	Betapace	
Acebutolol	Sectral	
Carvedilol	Coreg	
Labetolol	Normodyne, Trandate	
ACE-Inhibitors (ACE-Is)		
Captopril	Capoten	Note -*pril* ending.
Benazepril	Lotensin	May cause dry cough, may
Enalapril	Vasotec	not require potassium
Fosinopril	Monopril	supplements. Patients with
Lisinopril	Prinivil, Zestril	diabetes may use for kidney
Quinapril	Accupril	protective qualities
Ramipril	Altace	
Tramdolapril	Mavik	
Perindopril	Aceon	
Moexipril	Univasc	
Angiotensin II Receptor Blockers (ARBs)		
Losartan	Cozaar	Note -*artan* ending.
Valsartan	Diovan	Does not cause dry cough,
Irbesartan	Avapro	effects similar to ACE-Is
Candesartan	Atacand	
Telmisartan	Micardis	
Eprosartan	Teveten	
Olmesartan	Benicar	

kidney disease in diabetic patients. They may increase survival, alleviate symptoms to some extent, and decrease hospitalization in patients with heart failure.

Adverse reactions to ACE inhibitors are uncommon and usually mild. A unique side effect of ACE inhibitors that may lead to discontinuation of the drug is a bothersome dry cough. Some patients experience temporary dizziness and fainting when they begin therapy. ACE inhibitors can also cause skin rashes, abnormal taste in the mouth, and potassium retention.

A new class of antihypertensive agents, the angiotensin receptor blockers (ARBs), was approved in 1995. This class works in the kidney to lower blood pressure in the kidney by inhibiting the angiotensin II receptors and blocking blood vessel constriction. The side effects are similar to those of the ACE inhibitors, except there is less incidence of the dry cough.

Calcium Channel Blockers

The movement of calcium in and out of cells is essential to nerve conduction and muscle contraction. Calcium channel blockers inhibit this movement. The result is a decreased force of contraction of the heart; blocked contraction of smooth muscle in the blood vessels, resulting in dilation of blood vessels; and slowed conduction of nerve impulses throughout the heart, resulting in a slowed heart rate. The drugs in this class vary in the selectivity of their actions on heart rate, blood vessel dilation, or heart contraction.

Calcium channel blockers are first-line agents for hypertension. They are also used for angina pectoris, heart rhythm disturbances, migraine headache, and diseases of the heart muscle. One drug, nimodipine, has a special indication for reducing nerve damage caused by bleeding in the brain, called subarachnoid hemorrhage.

The drugs in this class are grouped by their chemical structure, as shown in **Table 12-11**. In general, drugs with similar structure have similar uses and side effects. Patients who are taking beta-blockers or digoxin can experience problems taking verapamil or diltiazem because they may slow the heart too much. Drugs in the dihydropyridine group can increase the heart rate. Adverse effects of the calcium channel blockers include dizziness, headache, constipation, and, occasionally, swelling of the legs or feet.

The immediate-release formulations of this class are indicated for use in patients with angina pectoris. Many of these agents have sustained-release formulations available that are indicated for the treatment of hypertension, allowing for once- or twice-daily dosing, which may increase patient compliance.

TABLE 12-11. CALCIUM CHANNEL BLOCKERS

Generic Name	Brand Name	Comments
Dihydropyridines		
Amlodipine	Norvasc	Note the -*dipine* ending.
Nifedipine	Procardia XL, Adalat CC	Headache, flushing, and gum overgrowth are
Felodipine	Plendil	side effects
Isradipine	DynaCirc	
Nicardipine	Cardene SR	
Nisoldipine	Sular	
Nimodipine	Nimotop	
Nondihydropyridines		
Diltiazem	Cardizem (SR, CD), Tiazac, Dilacor XR	Nausea, headache are common
Verapamil	Calan SR, Verelan, Isoptin SR, Covera HS	

Miscellaneous Antihypertensives

The alpha-1 blockers, alpha-2 agonists, peripheral-acting adrenergics, and direct vasodilators are other classes of drugs used to treat hypertension. They act through various effects on nerve pathways to dilate the blood vessels and reduce blood pressure. Because these drugs block the ability of blood vessels to constrict, people who take them often get dizzy or feel faint when they stand up after sitting or sit up after lying down. This is called *postural hypotension*. Because of their high incidence of side effects and the discovery of more effective therapies, these agents are not often used, but may be seen as an adjunct in patients requiring multi-drug therapy to control their disease.

The alpha-1 blockers are doxazosin (Cardura®), prazosin (Minipres®), and terazosin (Hytrin®). In addition to postural hypotension, they can cause weakness, rapid heartbeat, and headache.

The alpha-2 agonists are clonidine, guanabenz, guanfacine, and methyldopa. Common side effects in addition to postural hypotension are drowsiness, sedation, dry mouth, and fatigue. Clonidine is available as a patch that is changed weekly. The Catapres-TTS® patch system consists of an active patch containing the drug and an inactive overlay; both patches must be dispensed. The patient must be taught to apply the patches properly, being sure to use both. Because the patches are only changed weekly, a patient would go a full week without medicine if the inactive overlay were applied alone.

The peripherally acting adrenergics are guanadrel, guanethidine, and reserpine. In addition to postural hypotension, guanadrel and guanethidine can cause diarrhea. Reserpine can cause lethargy, nasal congestion, and mental depression.

The direct vasodilators hydralazine and minoxidil can cause headache, rapid heartbeat, and fluid retention. Minoxidil was found to increase the growth of body hair in patients and is now available as a topical product (Rogaine®) for stimulating hair growth in people with balding or thinning hair.

Drugs Used for Angina Pectoris

Angina pectoris is chest pain of short duration caused by a lack of oxygen in the cardiac muscle cells. The pain subsides when the imbalance between the amount of oxygen the cells need and the amount of oxygen supplied to the cells is corrected. The pain of angina pectoris may not be limited to the chest. The pain is frequently felt in the arm or neck, usually on the left side of the body. An acute angina pectoris attack not relieved within 30 minutes by the use of two or three nitroglycerin tablets should receive medical attention for possible heart attack. Drugs used to treat angina pectoris include those used to abort an acute attack and those used on a daily basis to prevent attacks. Such drugs include nitrates, beta-blockers, and calcium channel blockers. The beta-blockers and calcium channel blockers are discussed in the antihypertensive section.

Nitrates

The nitrates are the most commonly used medicines for treating angina pectoris. Nitrates help resolve acute angina attacks by increasing the amount of oxygen delivered to the heart and by decreasing the oxygen needs of the heart. Nitrates work by dilating the arterial and venous blood vessels. Dilating the coronary arteries also allows more oxygen to flow to the heart.

Nitrates are available in many dosage forms. For acute attacks, sublingual tablets, inhalants, or translingual (on or under the tongue) sprays are used. In the hospital setting, nitroglycerin may be given as an intravenous infusion. For prophylaxis of angina, oral sustained-release tablets and capsules, topical ointment, and transdermal patches are used. The nitrates available are nitroglycerin, isosorbide dinitrate (Isordil®), and isosorbide mononitrate (Ismo®, Imdur®).

An important concern in choosing dosage forms and dosage regimens for nitrates is the development of tolerance. After 24 hours of continuous therapy, nitrates no longer work. Increasing the dose does not restore efficacy, but a nitrate-free period does. For this reason, nitrates are not usually dosed around the clock. Long-acting tablets and capsules may be given orally once daily or twice daily at 8 a.m. and 2 p.m. Isosorbide mononitrate regular release is frequently given as two doses 7 hours apart during the day. Nitroglycerin patches are often applied in the morning and removed at night. All these schedules provide a nitrate-free period at night.

Common side effects of nitrates include headaches, postural hypotension, dizziness, and flushing. Headache is so common, it is considered by some to be an indicator of the drug's activity. It can be treated with aspirin or acetaminophen.

Patients should be instructed on the use of the various dosage forms. They need to understand which products to use routinely and which to use for an acute attack. Patients also must understand the importance of the dosage schedule to prevent tolerance.

A drug commonly used in patients with angina is aspirin. Aspirin is prescribed in doses from 81 mg to 325 mg daily to prevent heart attacks. Heart attacks involve the formation of a clot in an already narrowed blood vessel supplying the heart. Aspirin inhibits the aggregation of certain blood cells, called *platelets*, preventing clot formation.

Cardiac Glycosides and Drugs Used for Heart Failure

In heart failure, the heart dose not function adequately as a pump. Symptoms of weakness and fatigue result from an inadequate oxygen supply to tissues. When the left side of the heart cannot pump all the blood that enters it, fluid backs up into the lungs, causing shortness of breath and cough. With reduced pumping of blood, less blood flows to the kidneys. The end result is retention of fluid and sodium, causing weight gain and swelling in the legs and feet. These symptoms may be mild to severe depending on how much the pumping ability of the heart is decreased.

As in many cardiac diseases, diet modification is part of the treatment. Fluid restriction and a low-sodium diet will be prescribed to reduce fluid retention. Drug therapy includes several types of drugs: ACE inhibitors, the combination of hydralazine and isosorbide dinitrate, diuretics, beta-blockers, and cardiac glycosides. The choice of drugs will be based on the severity of disease and the patient's symptoms. An ACE inhibitor is the first drug used in most patients. ACE inhibitors are useful for patients with mild to severe disease. ACE inhibitors, hydralazine, isosorbide dinitrate, and beta-blockers dilate the blood vessels, allowing for increased blood flow (see the Antihypertensive section for further information). Diuretics are used to reduce fluid retention in patients with fluid overload.

The role of cardiac glycosides is not well defined, but they have been shown to increase the force of heart muscle contraction in some patients.[5] Cardiac glycosides have been used for more than 200 years to treat heart failure and are still recommended for patients with symptomatic disease. The three currently available cardiac glycosides are digoxin (Lanoxin®), deslanoside, and digitoxin. Digitoxin and deslanoside are rarely used. Digitoxin differs from digoxin mainly in its onset, length of action, and route of elimination from the body. Its actions are otherwise similar to digoxin.

Digoxin acts on both the heart muscle and the nerve conduction system of the heart. It increases the rate and force of heart muscle contractions. The end result is improved pumping of blood and a slower heart rate. Digoxin is used to treat heart failure and rhythm disturbances of the heart.

Digoxin has a narrow therapeutic index and can have serious toxicities. Effects on nerve impulses in the heart can cause rhythm disturbances that can be fatal. Therefore, digoxin blood levels are monitored to help ensure safe dosing. Patients or caregivers should be aware of the early symptoms of toxicity: loss of appetite, nausea, vomiting, diarrhea, headache, weakness, confusion, and visual disturbances (particularly blurred vision, yellow or green vision, or a halo effect). An antidote, digoxin immune fab, is administered intravenously to treat life-threatening digoxin intoxication.

Digoxin is available as an injection, a tablet, an elixir, and a capsule. The amount absorbed from the different preparations varies, so the dose may need to be adjusted when dosage forms are switched. A loading dose may be given for more immediate effects, but loading doses increase the risk of toxicity.

Antiarrhythmics

Disturbances in the rate or rhythm of the heartbeat are called *arrhythmias*. Arrhythmias are often classified by where they occur in the heart. Common arrhythmias originating in the upper chambers of the heart, the atria, are *atrial fibrillation* and *atrial flutter*. Common arrhythmias occurring in the lower chambers of the heart, the ventricles, are *premature ventricular contractions, ventricular tachycardia, ventricular fibrillation*, and *torsades de pointes*. Arrhythmias may cause too rapid, too slow, or unsynchronized heart muscle contractions. The result is a decrease in the amount of blood pumped by the heart. Symptoms include dizziness, fatigue, and palpitation (forcible and rapid heartbeats that are usually noticed by the patient).

Antiarrhythmic drugs are classified according to their effects on the conduction of impulses through the heart and their mechanism of action. Drug therapy of arrhythmias is limited by the serious toxicities associated with the drugs. Many of the drugs used to treat arrhythmias can also cause arrhythmias. Drug therapy is used only when patients have life-threatening arrhythmias or intolerable symptoms. Common side effects of these drugs, which may be severe, are GI disturbances, such as nausea, vomiting, abdominal pain, and diarrhea.

Class IA antiarrythmic drugs—quinidine, procainamide, and disopyramide—are used for both atrial and ventricular arrhythmias. They all affect cardiac nerve conduction in a similar way as well as

treat arrhythmias. Procainamide can be given as an intravenous infusion or orally. Quinidine is given by intramuscular (IM) or intravenous (IV) injection or orally. Disopyramide is given orally. The milder side effects of procainamide include dizziness and mood changes. Procainamide has two serious side effects: lupus erythematosus and neutropenia. Lupus erythematosus is a syndrome of joint pain, rash, fever, and possible kidney dysfunction. Neutropenia is a decrease in white blood cells, resulting in a higher susceptibility to infection. Side effects of disopyramide include dry mouth, difficulty urinating, dizziness, constipation, and blurred vision. The most serious side effects are low blood pressure and heart failure.

Another subset of class I antiarrhythmics, class IB, includes lidocaine, tocainide, and mexilitine. The anticonvulsant phenytoin can also be used as an antiarrhythmic drug and has properties similar to these drugs. Class IB drugs are useful for ventricular arrhythmias. Like the IA drugs, they can cause as well as treat arrhythmias. Lidocaine is given intravenously. Its side effects are related to its effects on the central nervous system: dizziness, confusion, mood changes, hallucination, drowsiness, vision disturbances, muscle twitching, and seizures. The side effects of tocainide are similar to lidocaine, but tocainide can also cause blood disorders and lung disease. The side effects of mexilitine are also similar to lidocaine.

Flecainide and propafenone are class IC antiarrhythmics. Drugs in this class have been found to increase mortality in patients with asymptomatic, non-life-threatening arrhythmias. These drugs are now used only to treat life-threatening ventricular arrhythmias and some life-threatening atrial arrhythmias. Both of these drugs are available only as oral dosage forms and have mild side effects that are similar: dizziness, tremor, and blurred vision.

Several beta-blockers, such as propranolol, esmolol, and acebutolol, have antiarrhythmic properties and are used as class II antiarrhythmics. They are described in more detail in the Antihypertensives section of this chapter.

The class III antiarrhythmics are bretylium, amiodarone, and sotalol. They are used to treat ventricular arrhythmias. Bretylium is given intravenously. Low blood pressure is a common side effect.

Adverse reactions are common with amiodarone. A unique side effect with amiodarone is a blue-gray discoloration of the skin that is irreversible. Less serious side effects are visual disturbances, increased sensitivity to sunlight, fatigue, tremor, and changes in thyroid gland function. More serious side effects are microdeposits in the cornea of the eye that result in visual halos or blurred vision; lung toxicity; and liver toxicity. Amiodarone is given both orally and intravenously. Dosing of both forms involves a higher initial loading dose and a lower maintenance dose. Sotalol is a beta-blocking drug with antiarrhythmic properties similar to bretylium and amiodarone. Sotalol is only given orally.

The calcium channel blocker verapamil is used as an antiarrhythmic drug. It is discussed in the Antihypertensives section of this chapter. Also, digoxin is used for atrial arrhythmias. It is discussed in the Cardiac Glycosides section of this chapter.

Anticoagulants

Coagulation of blood (clot formation) is essential to prevent bleeding to death from cuts. But abnormal blood clot formation within blood vessels can cause heart attack, stroke, or pulmonary embolism (a blood clot in the lung), all potentially fatal conditions. Anticoagulants are used to prevent these potentially fatal clots from forming. Anticoagulants are commonly called *blood thinners*. Because anticoagulants slow clot formation, the main concern with anticoagulant therapy is excessive bleeding. Blood tests are used to monitor patients to maintain a level of anticoagulation that will prevent clot formation but not allow excessive bleeding. These tests are usually used for patients on warfarin or heparin therapy. Unfractionated heparin and low molecular weight heparins (LMWHs) are used to prevent or treat clot formation.

To treat clot formation, heparin is administered intravenously while LMWHs are administered subcutaneously. For prophylaxis, heparin and LMWHs are administered subcutaneously. A possible adverse reaction to heparin is a decrease in the number of platelets, a type of blood cell involved with clot formation. If the effects of heparin need to be reversed, protamine sulfate can be given.

The LMWHs enoxaparin (Lovenox®), dalteparin (Fragmin®), and Tinzaparin (Innohep®) are recent additions to anticoagulant therapy in the United States. These drugs are derived from heparin but have different actions on the clotting mechanism and more reliable activity by subcutaneous injection. They are currently used to prevent clot formation after orthopedic or abdominal surgeries. Enoxaparin is indicated for the treatment of deep vein thrombosis (DVT) and may be used on an outpatient basis. Advantages of using LMWHs are that excessive bleeding and reduction in platelets may be less common with these drugs, and blood tests are not needed for monitoring as with heparin.

Warfarin (Coumadin®) is the most commonly used oral anticoagulant. The maximal effect of warfarin takes 3 to 5 days to occur, so heparin is often given until warfarin takes effect. When the full effect of warfarin is present according to a blood test used to measure it, the heparin is discontinued. LMWHs can also be used until warfarin takes effect. As with other anticoagulants, bleeding is the most serious adverse effect. Nausea, diarrhea, skin rashes, mouth ulcers, and red-orange urine are other possible side effects. Many drug interactions, as well as changes in diet, can alter the effectiveness of warfarin. To avoid drug interactions, patients should always inform health professionals of all the drugs they take or have taken, including herbal supplements. Important counseling points for patients on warfarin should include the signs of abnormal bleeding and the importance of taking their medication at approximately the same time every day; avoiding major diet changes, especially with foods high in vitamin K (e.g., green leafy vegetables); and having blood tests taken as instructed. Consistency in diet is important because vitamin K counteracts the effects of warfarin.

Gastrointestinal System

The most common disorders of the gastrointestinal system are peptic ulcer disease (PUD), gastroesophageal reflux disease (GERD), nausea and vomiting, diarrhea, constipation, and inflammatory bowel disease. Drugs used to treat peptic ulcer disease, GERD, diarrhea, and constipation are discussed here. Drugs used to treat nausea and vomiting are discussed in the Oncology section.

Peptic ulcer disease and GERD are both related to the acid secretion of the stomach. Most gastrointestinal ulcer treatments work by reducing the acid content of the stomach. The most commonly used agents are antacids, histamine-2 receptor antagonists, proton pump inhibitors, a prostaglandin drug, and sucralfate.

Antacids

Antacids neutralize existing acid in the stomach. They do not reduce the secretion of acid. Sodium bicarbonate (baking soda) has been a household heartburn remedy for generations. It reacts with acid to create sodium chloride (ordinary table salt), water, and carbon dioxide, which reduces stomach acid but causes other problematic effects. The production of carbon dioxide, a gas, may result in flatulence and distention of the abdomen. The sodium, chloride, and bicarbonate are absorbed and can cause undesirable electrolyte changes in patients with such disorders as kidney disease, swelling of the ankles or feet, heart failure, liver failure, or hypertension.

Calcium carbonate (the ingredient in Tums®) similarly reacts with acid in the stomach to produce calcium chloride, water, and carbon dioxide. The calcium is not absorbed as well as sodium is, so systemic effects are less likely. Patients with renal failure may develop high blood levels of calcium. Calcium carbonate and other calcium salts are also used as nutritional supplements to provide calcium. Use of calcium antacids may result in the milk-alkali syndrome, which consists of high blood levels of calcium, a low blood acid content, irritability, headache, vertigo, nausea, vomiting, weakness, and muscle aches. Calcium salts may bind phosphates in food so they cannot be absorbed. Calcium salts are used for this purpose in patients with kidney failure to prevent the absorption of too much phosphate.

Aluminum hydroxide is a commonly used antacid. It reacts with acid to produce aluminum chloride and water. Although the aluminum chloride is poorly absorbed, it can cause problems in patients with kidney failure. If used in large amounts, the unabsorbed aluminum may prevent the absorption of phosphates. Aluminum hydroxide is used, as are the calcium salts, in patients with kidney failure for this purpose. Aluminum antacids commonly cause constipation.

Magnesium hydroxide may be used as an antacid. It reacts with stomach acid to form magnesium chloride and water. Little magnesium is absorbed, but, like the other salts, accumulation may occur in patients with kidney failure. Magnesium products commonly cause diarrhea. Therefore, combinations of aluminum and magnesium hydroxides are used to try to avoid either constipation or diarrhea. The diarrhea effect tends to predominate in these combinations.

Alginic acid is combined with the antacids sodium bicarbonate, aluminum hydroxide, and magnesium trisilicate in a product called Gaviscon®. This product is useful in GERD. The alginic acid does not neutralize acid but floats on the surface of the stomach contents as a thick solution. It may prevent reflux of the stomach acid or act as a barrier between the esophagus and the acid when reflux occurs.

Antacid preparations differ in potency (acid-neutralizing ability). They must be taken in adequate amounts to treat peptic ulcer disease or GERD. Timing of doses is important because the duration of effect of antacids is only 15 to 30 minutes. They are often taken before and after meals and at bedtime.

Antacids are implicated in many drug interactions. Antacids generally affect how well drugs are absorbed. They either react with the drug itself or cause changes in the acidity of the stomach that inhibit the absorption. Patients can reduce interactions by separating antacid doses from other medications by at least 2 hours.

Sucralfate is an aluminum salt that functions differently than the antacids. In an acid environment, sucralfate binds to an ulcer, forming a protective barrier between it and the acid environment. Adverse effects, drug interactions, and precautions are similar to those of other aluminim antacids.

Histamine-2 Receptor Antagonists

The histamine-2 receptor antagonists (H_2 antagonists) were a significant discovery in the treatment of peptic ulcer disease and GERD. These drugs block a different histamine receptor than the antihistamines used for allergic conditions. When histamine binds to the H_2 receptors on cells in the stomach, it stimulates the secretion of acid. H_2 antagonists reduce the output of acid from stomach cells by blocking this receptor.

The H_2 antagonists are similar in action and side effects. The agents currently available are cimetidine (Tagamet®), ranitidine (Zantac®), famotidine (Pepcid®), and nizatidine (Axid®). They are safe and well-tolerated drugs. The most common side effects are gastrointestinal disturbances. Central nervous system effects, such as drowsiness and headache, may occur. More severe central nervous system effects, such as confusion, agitation, and hallucinations, occur most often in severely ill patients.[9] All these drugs are available as oral or injectable formulations, except nizatidine, which is available only in capsules. All these products also are available over the counter as well as in prescription-only strengths. Because of its route of metabolism, cimetidine is most likely to cause drug interactions.

Proton Pump Inhibitors

Proton pump inhibitors (see **Table 12-12**) act within the stomach cells to prevent the production of acid. They can lower the stomach's acid output more than the H_2 antagonists. Adverse reactions are similar to those of the H_2 antagonists—chiefly nausea, diarrhea, and headache. The drugs administered as capsules contain enteric-coated pellets to protect them from the acid environment of the stomach. When they pass into the less acidic duodenum, the coating breaks down and the drug is absorbed. If a patient cannot swallow the whole capsule, then the pellets can be administered. However, if the capsules are crushed or put into an alkaline substance (such as antacids), then the coating will break down and the drug will be destroyed by the acid in the stomach. The generic names have a *-prazole* stem, allowing for easy recognition of the class.

Current findings suggest that a bacterium commonly found in the lining of the stomach, *Helicobacter pylori (H. pylori)*, causes peptic ulcer disease. This bacterium produces an enzyme that degrades the mucus barrier and allows acid to come in contact with the stomach lining. Treatment of peptic ulcer disease is now directed at elimination of this bacterium. Drug regimens directed at eradicating *H. pylori* include various combinations of antibiotics, such as amoxicillin, metronidazole, tetracycline, and clarithromycin, with histamine-2 receptor antagonists or proton pump inhibitors and bismuth subsalicylate (see Antidiarrheals).

Antidiarrheals

The frequency of normal bowel movements varies from one stool every 2 or more days to more than three stools per day. Diarrhea, therefore, is hard to define but is usually considered to be an increased frequency of loose, watery stools. Diarrhea can be acute or chronic and can be a symptom of another disease.

Diarrhea may result when the operation of the large intestine is disrupted. Decreased absorption of water, increased secretion of electrolytes into the intestinal contents, excessive amounts of mucus production, bleeding into the intestine, or alteration of the movements of the intestine can all result in diarrhea. Infection, toxins, drugs, diet, laxative abuse, or other diseases may cause these disruptions of intestinal function. Diarrhea accompanied by fever may have a bacterial cause. Persistent diarrhea should be referred to a physician.

Antiperistaltic drugs treat diarrhea by inhibiting the propulsive movements of the intestine. Slowing passage of the intestinal contents allows absorption of water and electrolytes, and cramping and stool frequency are reduced. Loperamide and diphenoxylate are antiperistaltic drugs. High doses of diphenoxylate have some narcotic effects, including euphoria. Atropine is added to diphenoxylate to discourage, through unpleasant side effects, the abuse of large doses of diphenoxylate. Antiperistaltic agents should not be used to treat diarrhea caused by bacteria, because doing so may prolong the diarrhea.

Adsorbent antidiarrheal drugs adsorb bacteria and toxins. They also adsorb nutrients, digestive enzymes, and drugs. Kaolin, pectin, attapulgite, and polycarbophil are adsorbent antidiarrheals. Polycarbophil adsorbs water and treats both diarrhea and constipation. The other adsorbent drugs do not have proven efficacy.

Bismuth subsalicylate has been used for indigestion, for nausea, for diarrhea, and as adjunct treatment in *H. pylori* infections previously discussed. Bismuth appears to have an antisecretory action that blocks the copious fluid flow in diarrhea. It has been used to treat infectious diarrhea, including diarrhea common in travelers to foreign countries. Bismuth subsalicylate does contain salicylate, so patients taking aspirin, which also contains salicylate, should be warned so they do not inadvertently take too much salicylate. The signs of high levels of salicylate are ringing in the ears, nausea, and vomiting. Salicylate is also contraindicated in children because of the possibility of causing Reye's syndrome.

Laxatives

As mentioned previously, the frequency of bowel movements varies. The common misconception that daily bowel movements are necessary for good health may lead to the misuse of laxatives and worsen bowel problems. A wide range of diseases, as well as drugs and diet, may cause constipation. Laxatives should be used only after causative diseases have been identified, causative drugs have been discontinued, and dietary adjustments have been tried.

TABLE 12-12. PROTON PUMP INHIBITORS		
Generic Name	**Brand Name**	**Formulations**
Omeprazole	Prilosec	Capsules
Pantoprazole	Protonix	Tablets, injection
Lansoprazole	Prevacid	Capsules, suspension
Rabeprazole	Aciphex	Tablets
Esomeprazole	Nexium	Capsules

Laxatives are used to increase patient comfort and also to prevent complications. Hemorrhoids may be aggravated by constipation. In some cases of constipation, the bowel may become so distended with fecal content that perforation of the bowel or loss of blood supply to the bowel may occur. Laxatives are also commonly used to empty the bowel before various diagnostic procedures.

Bulk-forming laxatives dissolve or swell as they mix with the fluid in the intestine. The increased bulk in the intestine stimulates the movement of the intestine. Because this is a natural method of stimulating bowel movement, these laxatives are usually the first choice. Bulk laxatives do not act quickly. They take 12 to 24 hours or longer to act. They must be given with adequate water to prevent them from forming an obstruction in the esophagus or intestine. Examples of bulk-forming laxatives are polycarbophil, methylcellulose, and psyllium.

Emollient laxatives are also known as *stool-softeners*. They facilitate the mixing of fatty and watery substances in the intestine to soften the fecal contents. These drugs are better suited to preventing constipation than treating it. They are not fast acting in treating constipation; they may take up to 5 days to act. As with bulk laxatives, fluid intake should be increased with emollient laxatives. These drugs are commonly used in patients who should avoid straining with stool passage. Examples of emollient laxatives are docusate sodium, docusate calcium, and docusate potassium.

Saline laxatives contain salts that are not absorbed. These salts draw water into the intestines. The increased pressure in the intestine from this water stimulates movement in the intestine. These drugs are indicated for acute evacuation of the bowel. Examples of saline laxatives are milk of magnesia, magnesium citrate, and sodium phosphates. These drugs act within 30 minutes to several hours.

Hyperosmotic laxatives draw water into the intestine. The (the time they take to work) is within 30 minutes. Glycerin suppositories are a hyperosmotic laxative. Their effect may be enhanced by the irritant effect of sodium stearate in the suppository.

Stimulant laxatives irritate the lining of the intestine or the nerves in the wall of the intestine, which causes the intestines to evacuate their contents. They also may act by increasing the amount of water and electrolytes the body secretes into the intestine. These drugs produce thorough evacuation of contents within hours of administration. They also may cause cramping,

colic, mucus secretion, and excessive loss of fluid. Their chronic abuse may result in a poorly functioning colon. Examples of stimulant laxatives are senna, castor oil, and bisacodyl. Bisacodyl tablets are coated to prevent action in the stomach. Administering these tablets with antacids or milk of magnesia may cause the coating to dissolve, which may result in vomiting.

Gastrointestinal Stimulants

Drugs that increase gastrointestinal tract motility have a number of therapeutic uses. In patients with GERD, these drugs appear to increase the tone of the muscle separating the stomach and esophagus so that reflux is prevented. Gastrointestinal stimulants are also used in a complication of diabetes called *gastroparesis*. Gastroparesis is a reduced motility of the stomach that results in delayed emptying of the stomach contents into the intestine. Symptoms of gastroparesis are nausea, vomiting, and abdominal distention.

Metoclopramide (Reglan®) is a gastrointestinal stimulant. Metoclopramide has other effects that not only make it useful as an antiemetic drug but also account for some side effects. Metoclopramide can cause drowsiness, nervousness, fatigue, dizziness, weakness, depression, diarrhea, and rash. Uncommon possible reactions are extrapyramidal symptoms and movement disorders that are common with antipsychotic drugs (see Central Nervous System).

Musculoskeletal System

Many diseases of the musculoskeletal system cause pain or inflammation of the muscles or joints. Agents used to treat these conditions are discussed in this section.

Anti-inflammatory and Antipyretic Agents

Inflammation is the body's response to infection or trauma. The blood vessels send fluid, dissolved substances, and cells into areas of tissue injury or death. This reaction protects and aids in the healing of tissue. However, a prolonged or unneeded response produces unnecessary pain or discomfort.

The signs of inflammation include redness, heat, pain, swelling, and altered function of the involved tissue. These signs of inflammation are common symptoms of such inflammatory diseases as rheumatoid arthritis, lupus erythematosis, tendonitis, bursitis, and gout. Anti-inflammatory agents do not cure these diseases; they just relieve the symptoms.

The nonsteroidal anti-inflammatory drugs are a large class of agents commonly abbreviated as *NSAIDs*.

The term *nonsteroidal* is used to differentiate these agents from corticosteroid hormones, which also have anti-inflammatory properties and are discussed later in this chapter. NSAIDs also have analgesic (pain-relieving) and antipyretic (fever-reducing) properties. Aspirin is the oldest of this class of drugs; for other drugs in this category, see **Table 12-13**.

All NSAIDs can cause serious bleeding and ulcers in the stomach. Many of the drugs used to treat ulcers (see section on Gastrointestinal System) can be given to prevent damage to the stomach lining. One drug specific to treating ulcers caused by NSAIDs is misoprostol. Although misoprostol is effective in preventing NSAID-induced ulceration, patients often cannot tolerate it because of the abdominal pain and diarrhea it causes. Other side effects of misoprostol are nausea, flatulence, headache, vomiting, and constipation. Misoprostol can stimulate uterine contractions, so female patients must be sure they are not pregnant and will not become pregnant while taking this drug. One agent—Arthrotec®—is available that combine a NSAID and misoprostol.

NSAIDs have also been shown to cause kidney dysfunction. Because they inhibit platelet formation, NSAIDs also have blood-thinning properties. Aspirin has a longer acting effect on platelets than the other NSAIDs and should be used cautiously in patients on anticoagulant therapy.

In 1998 a new class of anti-inflammatory agents was approved called the *cycloxygenase-2 (COX-2) inhibitors*. They have the same indications as the NSAIDs and most of the same side effects. The benefit of the COX-2 inhibitors was thought to be less GI disturbances and less incidence of ulcer development. Recent studies have not shown the GI problems to be significantly different than with the NSAIDs. Another benefit of the COX-2 inhibitors is a longer duration of action that allows once- or twice-daily dosing. These agents are also listed in Table 12-13.

Because of the potential harm associated with the use of aspirin in children, two special cautions are mentioned here. The first is the occurrence of Reye's syndrome. This syndrome can cause liver disease and central nervous system damage when aspirin is used to treat fever in children with viral infections, such as chicken pox and influenza. The second caution is the frequency with which aspirin is a cause of poisoning in children. The similarity of chewable aspirin tablets in taste and appearance to candy probably contributes to its potential as a poison.

Analgesics

Control of pain (analgesia) is an important part of medicine. Analgesics are drugs that relieve pain by altering the way the brain receives and interprets the sensation of pain from the nerves. Effectively controlling pain puts patients at ease and promotes recovery.

Opioid analgesics (also called narcotic analgesics) all act on the same types of receptors in the brain to control pain. These drugs do not reduce inflammation or lower fever but do have other therapeutically useful properties, such as the suppression of cough. A large number of opioid analgesics are available, most in injectable and oral forms. Butorphanol is available as a nasal spray. Morphine, hydromorphone, meperidine, and fentanyl are some of the most potent opioid analgesics. Some less potent agents are codeine, oxycodone, hydrocodone propoxyphene, nalbuphine, butorphanol, buprenorphine, dezocine, and tramadol (Ultram®). The choice of drug depends on factors such as the site, duration, and severity of the pain.

All opioid analgesics have similar adverse effects. Depression of the breathing reflex is the most important adverse effect. Overdose of opiod analgesics may result in death. Combining analgesic with other drugs, such as alcohol, that also depress breathing may have additive effects. Opioid analgesics also produce drowsiness, so patients must be warned about driving and other activities that require them to be alert. Nausea and constipation are other common side

TABLE 12-13. NONSTEROIDAL ANTI-INFLAMMATORY AGENTS

Generic Name	Brand Name	Comments
Ibuprofen	**Motrin, Advil**	Note -*profen* ending
Ketoprofen	Orudis, Oruvail	
Flurbiprofen	Ansaid	
Diclofenac	**Voltaren**	
Sulindac	Clinoril	
Etodolac	Lodine	
Ketoralac	Toradol	Indicated for short-term use only
Naproxen	**Naprosyn, Naprelan**	
Mecloxicam	Mobic	
Piroxicam	Feldene	
Oxaprozin	Daypro	
Indomethacin	**Indocin**	Used to treat gout
Nabumetone	Relafen	
Cox-2 Inhibitors		
Celecoxib	**Celebrex**	Note -*coxib* ending
Rofecoxib	**Vioxx**	
Valdecoxib	Bextra	

effects. Patients on several days of therapy may need to take a stool softener to prevent constipation.

The most popular nonopioid analgesic is acetaminophen. This drug is similar to aspirin in its ability to relieve pain and reduce fever, but it has no anti-inflammatory properties. Acetaminophen is a useful alternative to aspirin in children with chicken pox or other viral illnesses, in patients with stomach or intestinal ulcers, in patients with conditions likely to cause bleeding, and in patients with aspirin allergies. In usual doses, acetaminophen rarely causes side effects, but in larger doses, it can cause liver damage. Acetaminophen is available without prescription and is widely used in oral and rectal dosage forms. It is often combined with stronger opioid analgesics. For example, acetaminophen with codeine, hydrocodone with acetaminophen (Vicodin®, Norco®), and propoxyphene with acetaminophen (Darvocet-N®) are all narcotic analgesics with acetaminophen added.

Skeletal Muscle Relaxants

Two main groups of drugs have skeletal muscle relaxant effects: (1) those given intravenously and (2) those given orally. Intravenous drugs are used to relax muscles during medical procedures. Oral drugs include those used for painful muscle conditions, such as sprains or strains, and those used mainly for muscle spasms.

The intravenous drugs are called *neuromuscular blocking agents*. They block the nerve impulse at the point where it is transmitted from the nerve to the muscle. Neuromuscular blocking agents prevent muscles from moving when movement would interfere with the medical treatment or procedure. These drugs have no effect on pain or level of consciousness, so other agents must be used to control pain and anesthetize the patient. Neuromuscular blocking agents include succinylcholine, tubocurarine, mivacurium, rocuronium, pancuronium, atracurium, vecuronium, and doxacurium. Drugs are chosen for different types of procedures according to how quickly they start to act and how long their effects last. At the end of a procedure, the actions of these drugs are commonly reversed with such drugs as neostigmine, pyridostigmine, or edrophonium. Adverse effects of neuromuscular blocking agents are usually extensions of their action: slow recovery of breathing and muscle weakness.

Another group of skeletal muscle relaxants is used orally for painful muscle conditions, such as sprains and strains. It is not known whether these drugs

actually relax muscles or relieve pain as a result of their sedative properties. Drugs in this group include carisoprodol (Soma®), chlorzoxazone, cyclobenzaprine (Flexeril®), metaxalone (Skelaxin®), methocarbamol (Robaxin®), and orphenadrine. Drowsiness is a shared adverse effect. These drugs are commonly given with pain relievers, which may add to the drowsiness. Patients should be warned about driving or other activities that require them to be alert.

Diazepam and baclofen are used mainly for muscle spasticity, which is seen in such diseases as cerebral palsy and multiple sclerosis and following stroke. Diazepam is a sedative-hypnotic drug used for its muscle relaxant properties in these diseases. Baclofen is also used in these diseases and has the advantage of producing less sedation than diazepam.

Systemic Corticosteroids

Corticosteroids are hormones secreted by the adrenal gland, a part of the endocrine system. These drugs are discussed under this section because they are commonly used to suppress inflammation and the immune response. They are useful in a wide spectrum of diseases, including rheumatoid arthritis, bursitis, asthma, allergic reactions, lupus erythematosis, inflammatory bowel disease, ulcerative colitis, psoriasis, and organ transplantation.

Other names for the corticosteroids are adrenocorticosteroids, glucocorticosteroids, and, simply, steroids. Drugs available include hydrocortisone, prednisone, prednisolone, methylprednisolone, triamcinolone, dexamethasone, betamethasone, and flunisolide. Dosage forms available are topical creams, ointments, and lotions; eye drops; injectable products for intramuscular, intravenous, and intra-articular (into the joint) injections; enemas; oral inhalers; nasal sprays; and tablets.

While short-term use of corticosteroids carries little risk of adverse effects, long-term use is indicated only when the benefits outweigh the risks. Long-term oral corticosteroid use can lead to Cushing's syndrome, which is characterized by a rounded, puffy face; thinning of the skin; osteoporosis (bone weakening); muscle loss; and high blood glucose. Therapeutic use of corticosteroids suppresses natural adrenal gland function, which is essential to the body in times of physical stress. The dose of corticosteroids must be tapered when they are to be discontinued so that the adrenal gland can recover and begin to secrete natural hormones. Another method of dosing is to use alternate-day therapy (alternating days with and without drug) to allow the natural adrenal function to recover on the drug-free days.

Endocrine System

Endocrine drugs can be either natural or synthetic. Endocrine drugs are used to compensate for a deficiency or excess of a specific hormone, to block the production or effects of a hormone, or to treat a nonendocrine disease. Examples of the latter include corticosteroid therapy for asthma or the use of vasopressin to minimize bleeding in the esophagus of alcoholics. The indications for endocrine drugs discussed here are diabetes mellitus, thyroid diseases, oral contraception, fertility agents, osteoporosis, benign prostatic hypertrophy, and pituitary functions.

Diabetes

Diabetes mellitus is the most common endocrine disease. There are two types of diabetes mellitus: (1) Type 1 (also called insulin-dependent diabetes mellitus) and (2) Type 2 (also called noninsulin-dependent diabetes mellitus). Type 1 diabetes is characterized by a lack of insulin production from the pancreas and must be treated with insulin. This type of diabetes is the less common of the two and is more often diagnosed in children and adolescents than in adults. Type 2 may be characterized by either decreased production of insulin or normal amounts of insulin with abnormal sensitivity of the tissues to the insulin that is present. This type of diabetes may be treated with diet alone, with oral hypoglycemic agents, with insulin, or with a combination of these agents. Type 2 diabetes is the more prevalent type and is more often diagnosed in adulthood, although recent statistics indicate an increase in diagnosis of Type 2 diabetes in children.

Insulin is one of the two treatments for diabetes mellitus. Insulin can be given only by injection, either subcutaneous or intravenous. There are many types of insulin (see **Table 12-14**), but only regular insulin can be given intravenously. The types of insulin differ in their onset of action and duration of action. Human insulin is now used because it causes fewer side effects than animal-source insulin. Insulin doses are measured in units. Special insulin syringes should be used to measure the dose properly.

Oral hypoglycemics (see **Table 12-15**) are used to lower blood sugar in Type 2 diabetes. There are several

TABLE 12-14. INSULIN		
Insulin Type	**Onset of Action**	**Duration of Action**
Rapid-Acting Lispro Aspart	5–15 min	3–4 hr
Short-Acting Regular	30–60 min	4–6 hr
Intermediate-Acting NPH Lente	2–4 hr 3–4 hr	10–16 hr 12–18 hr
Long-Acting Ultralente Glargine	6–10 hr 4 hr	18–20 hr 24 hr (no peak)

classes of oral hypoglycemics, and each has a different mechanism of action. The *sulfonylureas* are the oldest agents available. They work by increasing the secretion of insulin from the pancreas. The sulfonylureas are further classified into first and second generations, with the first generation agents having more side effects. The most common side effect is low blood sugar (hypoglycemia). Other side effects include weight gain, GI upset, and skin rash. Another class of agents, the *secretogogues*, works similarly to the sulfonylureas but appear to have a lower incidence of hypoglycemia.

The *biguanides* lower blood sugar by decreasing the amount of sugar produced by the liver, and they may increase the sensitivity of insulin receptors, allowing for more sugar to be used by the body. The biguanides may cause weight loss, which is a benefit to many patients with diabetes who need to lose weight. This class also does not cause hypoglycemia. Nausea, vomiting, and diarrhea are the common side effects. Patients with renal problems should not use the biguanides.

The *thiazolidinediones*, also known as the *glitazones*, improve insulin sensitivity, allowing the muscle and fat to use glucose. These agents should be used only as adjunct therapy to one of the previously described agents. Edema (fluid retention) and weight gain are common with these agents. The first agent in this class was withdrawn from the market because of liver toxicities, but the newer agents do not appear to have this problem, although liver function should be monitored.

The last class is the *alpha-glucosidase inhibitors*. These agents lower blood sugar levels by delaying the breakdown of sugar and carbohydrates in the intestine, thus slowing their absorption. Abdominal cramping and gas are common with these agents and limits their use.

TABLE 12-15. ORAL HYPOGLYCEMICS

Generic name	Brand Name	Comments
Sulfonylureas		
First Generation		
Chlorpropamide	Diabinese	Long-acting agent
Tolbutamide	Orinase	
Second Generation		
Glyburide	Micronase, Diabeta, Glynase	May be used as monotherapy or in combinations
Glipizide	Glucotrol, Glucotrol XL	
Glimepiride	Amaryl	
Meglitinides (secretogogues)		
Repaglinide	Prandin	May be used as monotherapy or with metformin
Nateglinide	Starlix	
Biguanides		
Metformin	Glucophage, Glucophage XR	Once-daily formulation helps with GI discomfort
Thiazolidinediones (Glitazones)		
Rosiglitazone	Avandia	Monitor liver enzymes
Pioglitazone	Actos	
Alpha-Glucosidase Inhibitors		
Acarbose	Precose	Take with meal
Miglitol	Glyset	
Combination Agents		
Glyburide/ metformin	Glucovance	New combinations developed to increase patient compliance
Glipizide/metformin	Metoglip	
Rosiglitazone/ metformin	Avandamet	

These agents need to be taken before each meal, requiring multiple doses daily.

Thyroid Diseases

The thyroid gland influences the rate of metabolism and the development of the body from youth to maturity. Diseases of the thyroid gland include hypothyroidism, which is an underproduction of thyroid hormone, and hyperthyroidism, which is an overproduction of thyroid hormone.

Autoimmune disease (the immune system attacking the body's own cells), radiation or surgical treatment of hyperthyroidism, iodine deficiency, and pituitary disease all can cause hypothyroidism. Goiter, an enlargement of the thyroid gland causing a lump in the neck, may occur with hypothyroidism. Symptoms of hypothyroidism are related to decreased metabolism.

These symptoms include fatigue, hoarseness; cold intolerance; decreased sweating; cool, dry skin; facial puffiness; and slow movement.

Hypothyroidism is treated by the administration of thyroid hormone. Naturally produced thyroid hormone actually consists of several substances, including triiodothyroxine (T_3) and levothyroxine (T_4). Levothyroxine (Synthroid®) is the most commonly prescribed drug for hypothyroidism. Thyroid USP is dried animal thyroid gland that contains both T_3 and T_4. Thyroid USP is often prescribed in grains; all the other preparations are prescribed in milligrams or micrograms. Liotrix® is a combination of T_3 and T_4. All these drugs are usually given once daily. Liothyronine must be given more frequently, so it is used more often for thyroid function tests than for treatment.

Adverse effects related to thyroid hormone replacement include increased heart rate, which can be dangerous in patients with heart disease. Therefore, older patients or those with heart disease should begin therapy with low doses. Other adverse effects include nervousness, heat intolerance, heart palpitation, and weight loss. Patients with these effects usually should have a blood test to evaluate the appropriateness of the dose.

Hyperthyroidism is most often caused by an immune system disorder, such as Graves' disease. Symptoms of hyperthyroidism are usually the opposite of hypothyroidism. Heat intolerance, weight loss, increased sweating, palpitations, swelling of the feet, diarrhea, tremor, and nervousness are common symptoms. Hyperthyroidism is most often treated with nondrug therapies—surgery or radioactive iodine—to remove the gland. Often hypothyroidism will occur after removal of the gland, and thyroid hormone replacement will be necessary.

Antithyroid drugs block the synthesis of thyroid hormones. They are used most often in children and young adults who do not need permanent removal of the gland. Methimazole and propylthiouracil (PTU) are the primary antithyroid drugs. The most common adverse effect of these drugs is a raised, itchy rash. A rare but serious side effect is agranulocytosis, which is a pronounced decrease in blood cells. This effect is usually reversible if the drug is discontinued. Antithyroid drug therapy, like surgery and radioactive iodine, can cause hypothyroidism.

Iodides were the major antithyroid drugs many years ago, but today they are infrequently used to inhibit thyroid hormone release. Forms of iodine used include Lugol's solution, containing 8 mg of iodide per drop, and saturated solution of potassium iodide (SSKI®), containing 50 mg of iodide per drop. Both these products are dosed in drops, not teaspoonfuls, and diluted in juice or another liquid. Pharmacy personnel must alert patients and caregivers to the proper dose to avoid overdose.

Oral Contraceptives and Fertility Agents

A woman's menstrual cycle is controlled by hormones released in sequence that cause ovulation and prepare the uterus for implantation of a fertilized egg. Manipulating the levels of these hormones can prevent pregnancy (contraception) or make pregnancy more likely. Oral contraceptives are used to prevent pregnancy. This is the most common use of these agents; other uses include regulating menstruation or treating endometriosis, polycystic ovary syndrome, and even acne vulgaris.

Oral contraceptives include two types of preparations: estrogen and progestin combinations and progestin-only preparations. Too many of these agents are available to list in this chapter, so the reader should refer to any drug listing for individual agents. The combination pills work largely by inhibiting ovulation. They also change the lining of the uterus, slow the movement of the egg through the fallopian tubes to the uterus, and thicken the cervical mucus so that it is more difficult for sperm to penetrate it. These effects make fertilization of the egg and implantation of the fertilized egg less likely should ovulation occur. The combination pills have failure rates of 0 to 6 percent overall. These agents contain the lowest doses of hormones considered effective. The progestin-only pills do not inhibit ovulation as reliably and are more reliant on the other mechanisms to prevent pregnancy.

Three types of combination oral contraceptives are in use: (1) monophasic, (2) biphasic, and (3) triphasic. Monophasic pills contain the same amounts of estrogen and progestin in each of the 21 pills taken per cycle. Biphasic pills contain a different ratio of estrogen to progestin for the first 10 days and the last 11 days of the cycle. Triphasic pills vary the amount of hormones three times during the 21 days. The biphasic and triphasic pills mimic normal hormonal changes more closely and therefore have fewer side effects. Progestin-only oral contraceptives contain the same amount of progestin (norethindrone or norgestrel) in each pill.

The risks associated with these pills occur rarely and are higher for women who smoke or take higher-dose preparations. The greatest risk in smokers is the occurrence of blood clots. The low-dose combinations available have been found not to increase the risk of developing other conditions, such as gallbladder disease, strokes, and heart attacks. Researchers are not sure if oral contraceptive use can result in an increased risk of breast or cervical cancer.

Side effects that are less serious but bothersome include irregular vaginal bleeding or spotting, headache, and breast tenderness. Progestin-only pills have a higher incidence of abnormal bleeding but do not have the risk of blood clots associated with estrogen. Other side effects of oral contraceptives include nausea and vomiting.

Other formulations of hormonal contraceptives are used as long-acting contraceptives. A once-monthly injection with estradiol cypionate and medroxyprogesterone is available. Medroxyprogesterone acetate is given as an injection every 3 months. Levonorgestrel is available as an implant under the skin in the upper arm and as an intrauterine device (IUD) providing protection for 5 years. A transdermal patch containing ethinyl estradiol and norelgestromin (Ortho-Evra®) can be worn for 7 days. The advantage of these forms is that patients do not have to take a pill every day.

Fertility agents are used to increase the likelihood of pregnancy in patients having difficulty conceiving. They stimulate the pituitary hormones that release the egg from the ovary (ovulation). Clomiphene, urofollitropin, and menotropins are the drugs used to stimulate ovulation. An injection of human chorionic gonadotropin (HCG) is given after a cycle of urofollitropin and menotropins. Timing the doses of these drugs to coincide with the woman's cycle is important to success in inducing ovulation. Therefore, pharmacy personnel must ensure that HCG will be available when the patient needs it. Women should see their physicians frequently while taking fertility agents so that adverse effects are noticed early. Multiple births occur more commonly in women who have taken fertility agents. Other adverse effects are not common.

Osteoporosis

Osteoporosis, a disease characterized by the loss of bone, occurs when more calcium and phosphorus salts are absorbed into the blood from bone than are deposited back into the bone. Osteoporosis can result in misshapen bones, such as curvature of the backbone seen in the elderly, or in easily broken bones. In general, bones are constantly being remodeled during our lifetime. This remodeling occurs by resorption, in which a cavity is formed in the bone, and formation, in which new bone is generated. During osteoporosis, the process of resorption outweighs the formation of new bone.

Drugs used to treat osteoporosis can be grouped into those that decrease the reabsorption of calcium and phosphorus into the blood and those that increase the deposition of calcium and phosphorus. Drugs that decrease reabsorption of calcium and phosphorus are estrogens, calcium, calcitonin, vitamin D, and biphosphonates. A drug that stimulates bone formation (deposition) is sodium fluoride, but it is not approved for this use in the United States.

Estrogens are used both to prevent and to treat osteoporosis. Ethinyl estradiol and conjugated estrogens (Premarin®) are the drugs most commonly used for this purpose. For prevention, they are taken at the time of menopause—either natural menopause or menopause caused by removal of the ovaries. Progesterone is also commonly given to postmenopausal patients who have not had a hysterectomy to decrease the risk of cervical cancer. When estrogens are used alone, they are given for 21 to 25 days a month. When estrogens are given with progesterone, the progesterone may be added for 5 to 10 days of the cycle or given all 25 days with the estrogen. Estrogens are available as pills and patches. Combination estrogen and progesterone tablets (Prempro®) are now available to ease compliance.

Adequate calcium intake is essential to prevent and treat osteoporosis. The various calcium salts provide different amounts of elemental calcium, the active part of the salt. Calcium carbonate, calcium lactate, calcium phosphate, calcium chloride, and calcium acetate are commonly given orally. Calcium carbonate has a high calcium content and a low cost. Taking calcium salts between meals may increase calcium absorption.[5] Constipation is the most common side effect of calcium salts.

Calcitonin is a hormone that inhibits bone resorption. Human-source calcitonin is available as an injection. Calcitonin from salmon is available as an injection and as a nasal spray (Miacalcin®). Development of antibodies (neutralizing substances produced by the body) to salmon calcitonin limits its effectiveness. Antibody development is less likely when salmon calcitonin is used in low doses, intermittently or intranasally.

Bisphosphonates are drugs that inhibit bone resorption by becoming part of the bone structure, thus allowing the formation of new bone. Alendronate (Fosamax®) and risedronate (Actonel®) are more potent inhibitors of bone resorption than etidronate or pamidronate. Both alendronate and risedronate are administered orally, and recently both have been marketed as once-weekly dosing tablets to aid patient compliance. To prevent damage to the esophagus and to promote absorption, alendronate and risedronate should be taken with a full glass of water immediately upon arising from sleep. Patients should remain upright and not eat for at least 30 minutes after taking either of these agents.

Benign Prostatic Hypertrophy

Benign prostatic hypertrophy (BPH) is a noncancerous enlargement of the prostate gland that develops in older men. Because the prostate gland encircles the urethra and urine leaves the body through the urethra, enlargement of the prostate can cause difficulties in urinating.

Surgery has been the main treatment for BPH, but alpha-adrenergic blocking drugs and finasteride are useful alternatives. The alpha-adrenergic blocking drugs prazosin, doxazosin, and terazosin are used to relieve the urinary symptoms of BPH but do not effect the growth of the prostate tissue. These drugs are discussed in more detail in the section on Antihypertensives.

Finasteride reduces the size of the prostate by inhibiting production of the hormone that causes enlargement of the prostate gland. Finasteride does not work in all patients and may take up to 6 months to produce a noticeable effect. The adverse effects of finasteride include impotence, decreased sex drive, and headache. Finasteride may cause abnormalities in a male fetus. Therefore, women who are or may become pregnant should not be exposed to this drug, including contact with crushed tablets or contact with semen from a sexual partner taking finasteride. Whole tablets are film coated to protect against contact with the drug.

Pituitary Hormones

The pituitary gland controls some of the body's functions by producing hormones that control the production of other hormones. For example, the production of thyroid, adrenocortical, and reproductive hormones are controlled by other hormones produced in the pituitary gland. The pituitary gland also regulates growth in children, water retention by the kidneys, and uterine contraction. The pituitary hormones available as pharmacological agents are oxytocin, vasopressin, and adrenocorticotropin.

Oxytocin is used to induce or augment labor and to control bleeding after giving birth. Two synthetic versions of oxytocin, ergonovine and methylergonovine, are used to control uterine bleeding after giving birth. Oxytocin is also administered as a nasal spray to help milk flow in nursing mothers.

Vasopressin, also called antidiuretic hormone (ADH), has an important role in regulating blood pressure. This hormone increases water reabsorption by the kidneys. A lack of vasopressin results in diabetes insipidus, a disease that is different from, and much less common than, diabetes mellitus. In diabetes insipidus, too much water and sodium are lost in the urine. Vasopressin and a synthetic agent, desmopressin acetate (DDAVP), are used to treat diabetes insipidus. Because vasopressin also constricts blood vessels, it is used to stop bleeding from blood vessels in the esophagus and stomach in alcoholic liver disease. DDAVP has also been useful to treat bedwetting in children and to prevent blood clotting in certain blood disorders. DDAVP can be given by injection or by nasal spray.

Adrenocorticotropin (ACTH) stimulates the release of hormones from the adrenal gland. ACTH and a synthetic version, cosyntropin, are used most often to diagnose diseases of the adrenal gland. Because ACTH causes the release of cortisol, a corticosteroid, from the adrenal gland, it can be used to treat asthma, rheumatoid arthritis, inflammatory bowel disease, and neurological diseases. However, using corticosteroids is usually preferred in these diseases. ACTH is sometimes used for flare-ups of multiple sclerosis.

Infectious Diseases

The term *infection* refers to the invasion of tissue by a foreign substance, such as a microorganism. In response, the body sends white blood cells to destroy the microorganisms. Invading microorganisms include bacteria, viruses, fungi, protozoa, and parasites such as amoebas, flukes, and worms. Tissue damage can occur directly from the invading organisms or from the white blood cells sent to fight the organisms. The body can also increase its temperature to help kill the invaders. Therefore, common symptoms of infection are similar to those of inflammation: fever, pain, heat, redness, and swelling. The emphasis of this section is on drugs used to treat bacteria, with some discussion of antivirals and antifungals.

Organisms from the environment invade the body every day. Some of these organisms are not harmful and some are even helpful, such as the bacteria that normally live in the gastrointestinal tract. When too many organisms are encountered or when the body's defenses cannot overcome the organism, signs of the infection may occur. Antibiotics are used when the body's defenses need help fighting an infection or if the infection may cause serious long-term effects. Many of the infective organisms acquired by patients in hospitals or long-term care facilities are more difficult to kill than those acquired by patients at home.

Antibiotics are used three different ways: (1) empirically, (2) definitively, and (3) prophylactically. The selection of an antibiotic depends on how it will be used and the type of infection. Patients in hospitals may receive prophylactic, empirical, and definitive antibiotic therapies within a short period.

Empirical antibiotic therapy is used when the organism causing the infection is unknown. The choice of drug is based on the organisms usually found at the site of infection (e.g., urinary tract, sinus, lungs). Samples of fluid or tissue from the site of infection are grown (cultured) in the laboratory to try to identify the infecting organism.

When cultures have identified the organism, definitive therapy is started. Drugs used for definitive therapy are those known to be effective against the organism. When cultures are done, various antibiotics may also be tested to see which ones kill the organism (sensitivities). Antibiotic therapy can then be based on these sensitivities.

In prophylactic, or preventive, use, antibiotics are used to prevent infection from occurring in such situations as surgery. In surgery, cutting tissues open may expose them to bacteria from the skin or the environment. Antibiotics are given before surgery to prevent the few organisms that enter the body from multiplying and causing an infection. Patients with weakened immune systems, such as cancer patients and patients with acquired immunodeficiency syndrome (AIDS), may receive antibiotics to prevent infections that are common in these populations. Patients planning to travel to areas with diseases, such as malaria, that are not prevalent in the United States may take antibiotics to prevent contracting such diseases.

Antibiotics are divided into classes on the basis of their chemical structures. Antibiotics may differ between classes and within classes in several ways:

- The bacteria against which they are effective
- Whether they actually kill bacteria (bactericidal) or just prevent the multiplication of bacteria (bacteriostatic)
- Their adverse effects
- The sites of infection in which they are most effective (e.g., skin, lungs, kidneys, bone)
- How they are removed from the body
- Routes by which they are given (oral, IV, IM)

The infection, characteristics of the antibiotic, and characteristics of the patient are all considered when an antibiotic is selected.

Beta-lactam Antibiotics

Beta-lactam antibiotics have a common chemical structure but vary widely in the organisms against which they are effective (broad-spectrum) and in how easily organisms develop resistance to them. The beta-lactam drugs have relatively few adverse effects and are distributed well into many body tissues. Beta-lactam antibiotics are further broken down into *penicillins*, *cephalosporins*, *carbapenems*, and *monobactams*.

Penicillin

Penicillins were one of the first antibiotics developed and can be identified by the *-cillin* ending on the agent name. The original penicillin G was effective against limited organisms. Since penicillin G was introduced, many bacteria have developed enzymes that destroy the drug. Therefore, penicillin G is of limited use now. The next group of penicillins developed, ampicillin and amoxicillin, are effective against more organisms but can also be destroyed by the enzymes some bacteria produce. Oxacillin, dicloxacillin, nafcillin, and methicillin were developed to be stable against the enzymes produced by *Staphylococcus aureus*, a common organism. These antibiotics are used when this organism is suspected. The newest penicillins are broad spectrum, meaning they are effective against many types of bacteria. Broad-spectrum antibiotics include carbenicillin, mezlocillin, ticarcillin, piperacillin, and azlocillin. Some of these penicillins are also combined with a beta-lactamase inhibitor, a substance that inactivates the enzymes bacteria produce and prevents the destruction of the antibiotic. An example is amoxicillin with clavulanic acid (Augmentin®).

Penicillin allergies are estimated to occur in 5 to 8 percent of the population and can be fatal.[10] All patients should be carefully questioned about their allergy histories before they are given any drug of this class. Allergies, including the type and severity of the reaction, should be documented accurately on the patient medication profile.

Cephalosporins

Cephalosporins are another group of beta-lactam antibiotics. These drugs are resistant to some of the bacterial enzymes that destroy penicillins. Some patients who are allergic to penicillin can also be allergic to cephalosporins. This condition is called cross-sensitivity.

Cephalosporins are divided into generations on the basis of their spectrum of activity (i.e., how many different types of bacteria they are effective against; see Table 12-16). First generation cephalosporins have the most limited activity but are effective against many bacteria that cause skin infections and urinary tract infections. Second generation cephalosporins have broader activity than first generation cephalosporins. Third generation cephalosporins have the broadest spectrum of activity. Some of them are used to treat serious hospital-acquired infections.

Carbapenems and Monobactams

The two other types of beta-lactam antibiotics are carbapenems and monobactams. Imipenem-cilastatin and meropenem are carbapenems with activity against many bacteria that have developed resistance to other antibiotics. Some patients who are allergic to penicillin will also be allergic to imipenem-cilastatin and

TABLE 12-16. CEPHALOSPORIN

Generic Name	Brand Name	Route of Administration
First Generation Agents		
Cefadroxil	Duricef	Oral
Cephalexin	**Keflex, Keftab**	Oral
Cefazolin	Ancef, Kefzol	IV, IM
Second Generation Agents		
Cefaclor	Ceclor	Oral
Loracarbef	Lorabid	Oral
Cefoxitin	Mefoxin	IV
Cefuroxime	**Zinacef, Ceftin**	IV, IM, oral
Cefprozil	**Cefzil**	Oral
Third Generation Agents		
Cefixime	Suprax	Oral
Ceftriaxone	Rocephin	IM, IV
Cefdinir	Omnicef	Oral
Cefpodoxime	Vantin	Oral
Cefotaxime	Claforan	IV, IM

meropenem. Aztreonam is a monobactam with good activity against some of the hospital-acquired organisms but not as many as the third generation cephalosporins and carbapenems. Patients who are allergic to penicillin can usually take aztreonam without a reaction.

Macrolides

Macrolides are antibiotics that are especially useful against several organisms that cause respiratory infections. Patients who are allergic to penicillin can usually take any of the macrolides. Erythromycin, the oldest drug in this group, frequently causes diarrhea and gastrointestinal cramping. The newer drugs in this group, clarithromycin (Biaxin®) and azithromycin (Zithromax®), are effective against more bacteria and cause less diarrhea. These agents have gained favor in recent years because once- and twice-daily dosing increases compliance. In addition, azithromycin has a shorter duration of therapy, often only 5 days.

Sulfonamides

Sulfonamides are effective against many bacteria that cause respiratory, urinary tract, and ear infections. The most frequently used sulfonamide is a combination of the sulfonamide sulfamethoxazole and trimethoprim. This combination is often abbreviated as *TMP/SMX*. Because the two drugs act in different ways to inhibit bacteria, the development of resistance is less likely than with a single drug. Sulfisoxazole is another available sulfonamide.

Allergic reactions to sulfonamides are common but usually not fatal. A serious skin reaction occurs only rarely. Patients with penicillin allergies can usually take sulfonamides. Sulfonamides can precipitate in the urinary tract, so patients should be told to drink plenty of water while taking them. Also, a patient may sunburn more easily when taking sulfonamides. Patients should be told to avoid sun exposure, use sunscreens, and not use artificial tanning lamps.

Tetracyclines

Tetracyclines have a broad spectrum of activity, but they only inhibit the reproduction of organisms (bacteriostatic). Despite their broad spectrum, their inability to kill organisms limits their usefulness to mild infections. Tetracyclines are useful against some of the organisms involved in sexually transmitted diseases, mild respiratory infections, and acne. The most commonly used are tetracycline hydrochloride, doxycycline, and minocycline.

Because tetracyclines combine with such metals as iron, aluminum, calcium, and magnesium, they should not be given with iron tablets, antacids, or milk products. The large molecule formed when they combine with these metals prevents their absorption and renders the drug ineffective. Because tetracyclines react with calcium, they can be deposited in newly formed bone and teeth. The complex they form with calcium can be weaker than normal tooth and bone and discolor tooth enamel. Because this reaction is of more concern in children or developing fetuses, who are actively forming bone and teeth, these drugs should not be given to children or pregnant women.

Allergies to tetracyclines are uncommon, and these drugs can be given to people with penicillin allergies. However, sun sensitivity may occur as with sulfonamides, and the same precautions should be urged.

Aminoglycosides

Aminoglycosides can kill many organisms, including most of the hospital-acquired organisms. These drugs include gentamicin, tobramycin, amikacin, netilmicin, streptomycin, kanamycin, and neomycin. The first four of these drugs are almost always given intravenously, although gentamicin and tobramycin are found in topical medications (see the Ophthalmic section). These four drugs are commonly used for serious infections and in combination with other antibiotics, both to broaden the spectrum of bacteria that will be killed and to lessen the development of resistance in bacteria. None of the aminoglycosides is absorbed well when given orally. This poor absorption and resulting high gastrointestinal concentration makes neomycin a useful agent for cleansing the gastrointestinal tract before intestinal surgery. Neomycin and erythromycin are often used together for this purpose.

Allergies to aminoglycosides are uncommon, and these drugs can be used in patients with penicillin allergies. Damage to the ear nerves and the kidneys are serious side effects that can be avoided by careful dosing. Many hospitals have pharmacokinetics programs to help improve the dosing of aminoglycosides and prevent side effects.

Fluoroquinolones

Fluoroquinolones act by a different mechanism than beta-lactam or aminoglycoside antibiotics and may be useful against bacteria that have developed resistance to other antibiotics. Fluoroquinolones may also be useful in penicillin-allergic patients. Currently available fluoroquinolones are norfloxacin (Noroxin®), ofloxacin

(Floxin®), ciprofloxacin (Cipro®), levofloxacin (Levaquin®), and moxifloxacin (Avelox®). Note the *-floxacin* ending to each of the generic names, which helps to classify these agents. Ciprofloxacin, levofloxacin, ofloxacin, and moxifloxacin are available as oral and intravenous preparations. They attain similar blood levels by either route, which allows them to be used orally for some serious infections that are usually treated with intravenous antibiotics. Fluoroquinolones are particularly useful for prostate gland infections because they penetrate this tissue better than most antibiotics. Fluoroquinolones are also used to treat urinary tract infections, respiratory infections, and gastrointestinal infections and as single-dose therapy for some sexually transmitted diseases.

Common side effects of fluoroquinolones are nausea and vomiting, skin rashes, headache, and photosensitivity (increased sensitivity to the sun). In large doses or when drug accumulation occurs because of renal failure, seizures can occur. Pregnant women and children should not take fluoroquinolones because of possible effects on bone growth. Patients should be cautioned to avoid excessive sun exposure while taking these agents.

Miscellaneous Antibiotics

Clindamycin

Clindamycin (Cleocin®) is effective against many organisms found on the skin and in the mouth. Because of its activity against mouth organisms, it is used in pneumonias that occur in patients who inhale their mouth secretions because of poor swallowing reflexes. It is also used in combination with other antibiotics for some abdominal infections. There is no cross-sensitivity in penicillin-allergic patients. Diarrhea is a common side effect.

Metronidazole

Metronidazole (Flagyl®) is the most effective antibiotic against anaerobic bacteria (bacteria that grow without oxygen). Anaerobic bacteria cause infections primarily in the abdomen and vagina. To cure vaginal infections, both the woman and the sexual partner must be treated. Metronidazole is also used to treat an anaerobic bacterium that frequently causes diarrhea. Metronidazole is not effective against other bacteria, so it is often given in combination with other antibiotics. To prevent a severe drug reaction, patients taking metronidazole must avoid alcohol.

Vancomycin

Vancomycin is effective against certain bacteria, methicillin-resistant *Staph aureus* for example, that are resistant to most of the penicillins. It is also useful for treating infections in patients who are allergic to penicillin. Infections acquired in a nursing home or the hospital are more likely to be caused by bacteria that are resistant to penicillins than are infections acquired at home. Patients who have long-term intravenous lines, such as cancer patients, also are likely to develop infections that are resistant to penicillins. Vancomycin is often used in these situations and to treat infections of the heart or heart valves.

Vancomycin is usually given intravenously. It should be well diluted and given slowly. A reaction, referred to as *Red Man Syndrome*, may occur if the drug is given too rapidly. This syndrome is characterized by low blood pressure (hypotension) with or without a rash on the upper trunk, face, and arms. Older preparations of vancomycin were impure and damaged hearing and kidney function. Preparations available today are purified and rarely cause this damage unless combined with other drugs that are toxic. To prevent these toxicities, blood levels of vancomycin have been measured and pharmacokinetics programs have been established to promote dosing regimens unlikely to result in toxicity. Because these toxicities are less common with the improved preparations, many hospitals are no longer checking blood levels for vancomycin in all patients. Oral vancomycin is not absorbed well enough to treat systemic infections, but is used to treat pseudomembranous colitis.

Antitubercular Drugs

Tuberculosis (TB) was a common and dreaded disease before the development of effective diagnosis and treatment practices in the 1940s and 1950s. Currently in the United States, certain groups, such as drug addicts, patients with end-stage renal disease, homeless shelter residents, nursing home residents, and patients with AIDS, are more likely to acquire active TB.[11]

Antitubercular drugs are used to prevent and treat TB. Preventive therapy is used for people with a positive skin test for TB or for people exposed to patients with active cases of TB. Treatment is given to patients with active TB. Because therapy with just one drug often leads to the development of bacterial resistance, TB treatment regimens consist of multiple drugs that are effective against tuberculosis. The use of two or more drugs simultaneously minimizes the development of resistance to all of the drugs.

The Centers for Disease Control and Prevention, an agency of the U.S. government, has published guidelines for the prevention and treatment of TB. The major drugs included in these guidelines are isoniazid, rifampin, pyrazinamide, ethambutol, and streptomycin.

Isoniazid is the mainstay of preventive therapy and is one of the drugs used in treatment when drug resistance is not suspected. Patients receiving isoniazid may also receive vitamin B$_6$ (pyridoxine) to prevent side effects, such as numbness or tingling in the hands or feet. Liver failure is the most dangerous adverse effect, but it rarely occurs.

Rifampin and pyrazinamide are the other drugs recommended to treat tuberculosis and are also given for prevention if isoniazid resistance is suspected. Rifampin has also been added to antibiotic therapy of other infections to prevent the development of resistance. Rifampin imparts a harmless orange color to urine, sweat, and tears and can stain contact lenses orange. Patients should be forewarned of this possibility. Rifampin also has many significant drug interactions. Pyrazinamide can cause hypersensitivity reactions, such as rash, fever, and joint pain. Like isoniazid, its most serious adverse effect is liver damage.

Combination tablets of isoniazid with rifampin as well as isoniazid with rifampin and pyrazinamide, are now available. These combinations are intended to make compliance with long-term therapy easier for some patients. Because tuberculosis drugs must be taken for at least 6 months and resistance is more likely to develop if patients take medication erratically, directly observed therapy is recommended. Directly observed therapy means that the patient comes to an office or clinic and takes the medicine in front of the health care worker.

Addition of a fourth drug to the treatment regimen is now recommended by the Centers for Disease Control. The fourth drug improves the likelihood that a resistant strain will be covered and thus enhances the effectiveness of the regimen. This increased effectiveness also allows the patient to take the medication twice a week instead of daily, which is more convenient for directly observed therapy. The fourth drug is usually ethambutol, although streptomycin is used sometimes. The disadvantages of streptomycin are that it must be given intramuscularly and that it can damage the nerves involved with hearing and balance.

When patients cannot tolerate one or more of the drugs used in the regimens described here, or when different types of tuberculosis occur, regimens that include capreomycin, kanamycin, amikacin, cycloserine, ethionamide, ciprofloxacin, ofloxacin, or clofazimine can be used instead.

Antivirals

Until the 1980s, many drugs were available that were effective against bacteria, but few were effective against viruses. The emergence of viral diseases, such as AIDS and genital herpes, and the increased severity of common viral infections, such as chicken pox, in patients with weakened immune systems spurred the development of many new antiviral drugs.

Herpes simplex virus is the cause of fever blisters (cold sores). Another strain of the herpes simplex virus causes genital herpes, characterized by painful lesions on the genitalia that are spread by sexual contact. Several drugs—acyclovir (Zovirax®), famciclovir (Famvir®), and valaciclovir (Valtrex®)—can decrease the symptoms caused by these viruses and other human immunodeficiency virus (HIV)-related infections. These drugs are also used to reduce the severity of the symptoms caused by herpes zoster virus. Herpes zoster causes the very painful symptoms of shingles and the potentially serious cases of chicken pox in children with weakened immune systems (e.g., children with leukemia).

Amantadine and rimantidine have limited usefulness against the influenza virus. These drugs are reserved to prevent infection after exposure to influenza or to reduce symptoms in some patients who develop infection. There are several types of influenza viruses, but amantadine and rimantidine are effective only against Influenza A. The side effects associated with amantadine are hallucinations, blurred vision, and difficulty urinating. Rimantadine has fewer side effects. Amantadine also has some effects that rimantadine does not, which has made it useful in Parkinson's disease (see Central Nervous System Disorders section).

Ribavirin is an antiviral drug used for a respiratory virus that is common in infants and small children called *respiratory syncytial virus* (RSV). This drug can also be used for Influenza A and B infections. Ribavirin is administered as an aerosol in an oxygen hood or tent. Ribavirin can harm a fetus, so women who are or who may become pregnant should avoid contact. Nursing or respiratory care personnel, as well as visitors, who are in the patient room where the drug is being aerosolized should be made aware of this precaution.

TABLE 12-17. HIV AGENTS

Generic Name	Brand Name	Comments
Reverse Transcriptase Inhibitors		
Nucleoside Reverse Transcriptase Inhibitors (NRTIs)		
Zidovudine	AZT, ZDV, Retrovir	May cause severe anemia, lactic acidosis, and enlarged liver
Didanosine	ddI, Videx	Take on empty stomach. May cause lactic acidosis and enlarged liver
Zalcitabine	ddC, Hivid	May cause peripheral neuropathies, lactic acidosis, and enlarged liver
Stavudine	d4T, Zerit	May cause lactic acidosis
Lamivudine	3TC, Epivir	and enlarged liver
Abacavir	ABC, Ziagen	
Nucleotide Reverse Transcriptase Inhibitors		
Tenofovir	TFV, Viread	May cause lactic acidosis and enlarged liver
Non-Nucleoside Reverse Transcriptase Inhibitors (NNRTIs)		
Nevirapine	NVP, Viramune	Severe hepatotoxicity
Efavirenz	EFV, Sustiva	Dizziness, headaches
Protease Inhibitors (PIs)		
Indinavir	IDV, Crixivan	Take on empty stomach
Ritonavir	RTV, Norvir	Take with food, refrigerate. Capsules, not solution
Nelfinavir	NFV, Viracept	Diarrhea and hyperglycemia
Saquinavir	Invirase, Fortovase	are common side effects
Amprenavir	APV, Agenerase	Large quantities of propylene glycol in solution may cause toxicities

The anti-HIV antivirals (see **Table 12-17**) work on different enzymes involved with replication of the virus. Because they work on different enzymes, a combination of drugs from different classes enhances their effectiveness and delays the emergence of resistant strains of HIV. Scientists continue to develop more effective agents or more effective ways to use these agents to treat AIDS.

Zidovudine, a nucleoside reverse transcriptase inhibitor, was the first drug available with activity against HIV. Currently, zidovudine is used alone or in combination with other drugs to treat patients with AIDS, to treat patients with HIV infection but no symptoms, and to decrease the likelihood of transmission of the HIV virus from mother to fetus. The major side effect of zidovudine is decreased white blood cell count, which increases the likelihood of infection.

The protease inhibitors are the most potent anti-HIV drugs available. All the drugs in this class have many drug interactions. Indinavir can cause nausea,

abdominal pain, and elevated liver function tests. To avoid the formation of kidney stones, patients should drink six glasses of water daily.

Nevirapine, the only non-nucleoside reverse transcriptase inhibitor, should always be used in combination with other antiviral drugs. The most common adverse effects of nevirapine are rash, fever, nausea, headache, and abnormal liver function tests. The rashes associated with nevirapine can be severe and life threatening. Nevirapine can be taken with or without food.

Opportunistic infections occur in patients with abnormally weak immune systems (immunocompromised), such as patients with AIDS or leukemia.

Ganciclovir and foscarnet are antivirals used to treat another virus, cytomegalovirus (CMV), which can cause infections in the eye, colon, lungs, and liver. CMV usually occurs in immune-compromised patients. These drugs can also be used to treat or prevent the same infections in patients who have had a kidney or liver transplant. Ganciclovir may decrease white blood cell count. Foscarnet's major adverse effect is kidney toxicity. Because foscarnet does not affect white blood cells, it can be useful for treating AIDS patients who have decreased white blood cells. Ganciclovir causes less kidney toxicity than foscarnet, which makes it useful for kidney transplant patients. Because ganciclovir can cause tumors and changes in cellular chromosomes, it is advisable to handle and dispose of ganciclovir according to guidelines for cancer chemotherapy drugs.

Antifungals
Antifungals are often used for skin, nail, or vaginal infections. This section focuses on antifungal agents used for internal fungal infections.

Like many other types of infections, fungal infections have increased in recent years because of the increased number of patients whose immune systems are not able to control the growth of fungi (e.g., AIDS, cancer, and transplant patients). Additionally, the widespread use of antibiotics kills the bacteria that normally control the growth of fungi.

Amphotericin B remains the "gold standard" antifungal drug. It can be given by intravenous injection and as a bladder irrigation for fungal bladder infections. Although amphotericin B is effective against most of the fungi that cause disease in humans, its usefulness is limited by its adverse effects, which include fever, chills, vomiting, and headache. These reactions can be limited by the administration of acetaminophen, diphenhydramine, methylprednisolone, or meperidine. More serious reactions include kidney toxicity, decreased red blood cell count, and changes in the salts normally found in the blood.

The search for effective agents without the side effects of amphotericin B led to the development of ketoconazole, fluconazole, and itraconazole. These drugs can be used to treat both topical and internal infections.

Ketoconazole is available as an oral agent. It is an inexpensive, effective agent for thrush, a fungal infection of the mouth and throat. Thrush is common in cancer patients treated with drug therapy or radiation. An acidic environment is necessary for the absorption of ketoconazole, so antacids or histamine-2 blockers, such as ranitidine and cimetidine, that decrease stomach acidity should not be given with ketoconazole.

Fluconazole (Diflucan®) is an antifungal that can be given orally or intravenously. It is just as effective orally as intravenously, so IV use is necessary only in patients who cannot take the oral formulation or absorb the oral form reliably. Like ketoconazole, fluconazole is useful for thrush and esophageal infections, but it is more effective than ketoconazole for fungal infections in the lungs, blood, abdomen, and urinary bladder. A single dose of fluconazole can be used to treat vaginal yeast infections. Some patients may prefer a single oral dose to the use of topical creams. Fluconazole is well absorbed even in a nonacidic stomach. It has fewer side effects than amphotericin B, but amphotericin B is more effective for some infections. Serious side effects are rare with fluconazole, but it can cause liver damage and severe skin disorders.

Itraconazole is the newest antifungal agent. It is indicated for the treatment of onychomycosis (nail fungus) and other types of infections that fluconazole cannot treat. The Sporanox® Pulsepak became popular in treating nail fungus with a 1-week-per-month therapy pack for 3 months. Like fluconazole, itraconazole can cause liver damage. For optimal absorption, itraconazole should be taken with a full meal or with a cola beverage.

Oncology

Cancer can occur in any tissue of the body. It is not a single disease but rather a set of more than 100 disorders occurring in different tissues.[5] Cells are constantly dividing to replace cells that have died. In cancer, a change occurs in some cells that causes them to disregard the normal controls that stop cellular growth after a certain number of cells have developed. Therefore, cells multiply out of control and are generally nonfunctional. They can form a large mass called a tumor, which compresses healthy cells around it and steals nutrition from the healthy cells. This results in a decrease in the number of cells that are functional. Cancerous cells can also break off from the primary site and migrate through blood or the lymphatic system to other tissues. This process is called *metastasis*. The ability of cancer to spread is the reason early detection is so important. Treating cancer in one area is much easier than treating cancer that has spread throughout the body.

Three types of treatment—or combinations of these treatments—are used for cancer: (1) surgery, (2) radiation, and (3) chemotherapy (drug therapy). Combinations tailored to specific cancers allow for more successful elimination of cancerous cells and less damage to normal tissue. Chemotherapy is administered to kill cells in large tumors as well as cancer cells that remain after the bulk of the tumor is removed by surgery or killed by radiation therapy.

Several factors contribute to the success of chemotherapy regimens. These factors include the growth cycle of the cancerous cells during therapy, the mechanism by which chemotherapeutic agents kill cancer cells, the combination of agents used for therapy, and the severity of the adverse effects the agents cause. Because chemotherapy is more effective against rapidly dividing cells, it is given in cycles that allow rest periods during which the normal tissue is allowed to recover and tumor cells are allowed to re-enter a rapid division phase for the next cycle of therapy. The risk-benefit ratio of chemotherapy must be favorable. In other words, the benefits of therapy must outweigh the harm caused by the adverse effects.

Chemotherapeutic agents are divided into classes on the basis of how they kill cells. Common chemotherapeutic agents are listed below. The toxic effects of these agents on healthy cells can be the limiting factor in the effectiveness of chemotherapy. Many chemotherapy drugs have several commonly used names and abbreviations, which can lead to confusion and medication errors. Because these drugs have so many dose-related adverse effects, mistakes with chemotherapy (e.g., giving the wrong drug or dose) are often fatal.

Common Chemotherapeutic Agents

Alkylating Agents

> Mechlorethamine, Chlorambucil, Streptozocin, Dacarbazine
>
> Cyclophosphamide, Lomustine, Carmustine,
>
> Busulfan, Cisplatin, Carboplatin, Ifosfamide, Melphalan

Antimetabolites

> Methotrexate, Fluorouracil, Floxuridine, Gemcitabine
>
> Cytarabine, Mercaptopurine, Cladribine, Fludarabine

Hormones

> Megestrol Acetate, Medroxyprogesterone, Diethystilbestrol, Estramustine, Tamoxifen, Leuprolide, Letrozole, Flutamide

Antibiotics

> Bleomycin, Doxorubicin, Daunorubicin, Mitoxantrone, Mitomycin, Dactinomycin, Idarubicin

Mitotic Inhibitors

> Etoposide, Vincristine, Paclitaxel
>
> Vinblastine, Vinorelbine, Docetaxel

Miscellaneous

> Hydroxyurea, Procarbazine, Dacarbazine, Interferon alpha 2a and 2b, Asparaginase, Paclitaxel

Combinations of chemotherapeutic agents usually lead to higher response rates and a longer period of remission than therapy with a single agent. The selection of drugs for combination is based on different mechanisms of action, responsiveness to dosage schedules, and the toxicity of the agents. Combination therapy often allows decreased doses of each drug, which may decrease the incidence and severity of toxicity. Chemotherapy combinations are called *regimens,* and they are abbreviated with the initials of the drug names. The initials stand for trade and generic names, and the same letters do not always stand for the same drugs in different regimens. Orders without the drug names can be confusing. An example of a chemotherapy regimen is *MAC*, used for ovarian cancer. MAC stands for mitomycin, Adriamycin® (doxorubicin), and cyclophosphamide. In the MOPP regimen for Hodgkin's disease, the *M* stands for mechlorethamine, the *O* stands for vincristine (Oncovin®), and the *P*s stand for Procarbazine and Prednisone. As shown here, *M* in one abbreviation is not the same as *M* in another abbreviation. Using abbreviations is dangerous and should be avoided. Mistakes with chemotherapy can be fatal.

Chemotherapeutic agents cause many severe adverse effects. The bone marrow, where new blood cells are produced, is inhibited by many chemotherapeutic agents. This leads to decreased numbers of white blood cells (neutropenia), which makes the patient vulnerable to infection. Filgrastim and sargramostim can be used to stimulate the production of white blood cells and minimize the risk of infection caused by low white blood cell counts. Decreased numbers of platelets in the blood can result in bruising or bleeding. Other common side effects of chemotherapy are hair loss, kidney damage, nerve damage, lung damage, heart damage, inflammation of the bladder, diarrhea, and nausea and vomiting.

Antiemetics

Nausea and vomiting is one of the major adverse reactions to chemotherapy. Patients can lose so much fluid through vomiting that they must be admitted to the hospital to receive intravenous fluids. Additionally, many cancer patients cannot maintain adequate nutrition because of nausea. This lack of nutrition is especially devastating because cancer cells are stealing nutrition from healthy cells. Perhaps most important, nausea and vomiting adversely affect the patient's quality of life. Drug therapy to control vomiting is therefore an important part of chemotherapy.

Antiemetics prevent nausea and vomiting. The antiemetic drug used will depend on how common and how severe nausea and vomiting are with the chemotherapy regimen the patient is to receive. Combinations of antiemetics are used to increase effectiveness. Granisetron (Kytril®) and ondansetron (Zofran®) are given either orally or intravenously with chemotherapeutic agents that cause the most severe emesis (vomiting). Dexamethasone and lorazepam are often given in combination. Other drugs used to control chemotherapy-induced nausea and vomiting include metoclopramide, droperidol, haloperidol, dronabinol, prochlorperazine, trimethobenzamide, and diphenhydramine.

Topical Medications

Ophthalmic Medications

Diseases of the surface or near the surface of the eye can often be treated with topical medications. The most common ophthalmic diseases are conjunctivitis, glaucoma, and dryness of the eyes. **Table 12-18** lists the

TABLE 12-18. OPHTHALMIC AGENTS

Generic name	Brand name	Formulations
Antibiotic Agents		
Gentamicin		Solution, ointment
Tobramycin	Tobrex	Solution, ointment
Na sulfacetamide	Sulf-10	Solution, ointment
Ciprofloxacin	Ciloxan	Solution
Ofloxacin	Ocuflox	Solution
Levofloxacin	Quixin	Solution
Norfloxacin	Chibroxin	Solution
Combination Agents		
Neomycin/Polymixin/ Hydrcortisone	Cortisporin	Solution, ointment
Neomycin/Polymixin/ Dexamethasone	Maxitrol	Solution, ointment
Tobramycin/ Dexamethasone	Tobradex	Solution, ointment
Antiviral Agents		
Vidarabine	Vira-A	Ointment
Trifluridine	Viroptic	Solution
Ganciclovir	Vitrasert	Implant
Idoxuridine	Herplex	Solution
Antihistamine/Decongestant Agents		
Lodoxamide	Alomide	Solution
Levocabastine	Livostin	Solution
Ketotifen	Zaditor	Solution
Olopatadine	Patanol	Solution
Emedastine	Emadine	Solution
Azelastine	Optivar	Solution
Antiglaucoma Agents		
Beta-blockers		
Betaxolol	Betoptic, Betoptic-S	Solution, suspension
Carteolol	Ocupress	Solution
Levobunolol	Betagan	Solution
Timolol	Timoptic, Timoptic-XE	Solution
Carbonic anhydrase inhibitors		
Dorzolamide	Trusopt	Solution
Brinzolamide	Azopt	Solution
Prostaglandin analog		
Lotanoprost	Xalatan	Solution

drugs used to treat these conditions. Topical treatment of eye diseases is advantageous because the side effects that might occur with systemic medication can be avoided.

Eye drops and ointments must be used properly to obtain the desired benefit. Drops and ointment should be placed in the lower lid pouch. Ophthalmic solutions and suspensions tend to cause a burning or stinging sensation upon initial use. If eye products are not used correctly, the drug can drain out of the eye without producing the desired effect. Ointments allow the medication longer contact with the eye, but they tend to cause blurry vision. To alleviate complaints of blurred vision, ointments are often recommended for use at night. If too much drug is used, systemic side effects can result. The external coat of the eye is resistant to infection. Once this surface is broken, the eye is very susceptible to infection. For this reason, ophthalmic products must be made and kept sterile. Ophthalmic preparations should be labeled "For the eye."

Medications for Conjunctivitis

Conjunctivitis is the most common eye disease in the Western hemisphere.[1] Conjunctivitis is an inflammation of the conjunctiva. It can be caused by bacterial infection, allergy, chemical irritation, or other diseases. The signs and symptoms of conjunctivitis include redness, tearing, secretions, drooping of the eyelid, itching, a scratchy or burning sensation, sensitivity to light, and the sensation that a foreign body is present in the eye. The treatment of conjunctivitis depends on the cause and the symptoms.

Conjunctivitis that is caused by infection can be treated with antibiotics or antiviral eye drops. Antibiotics harm or kill invading bacteria. Newborn infants are routinely given erythromycin ophthalmic ointment to prevent conjunctivitis caused by bacteria that might have entered the eye during birth. Patients who have intense itching and inflammation in addition to an infection may benefit from combination agents. Combination agents have antibiotics combined with steroids to fight the infection as well as to provide an anti-inflammatory action. Antiviral ophthalmic preparations are effective against herpes simplex viruses and CMV. CMV infections occur in patients whose immune systems have been compromised by drugs used to prevent transplant organ rejection or by AIDS. The antiviral drug ganciclovir is used specifically to treat CMV; the other antiviral agents listed in Table 12-18 are used to treat herpes simplex viruses.

Agents used to treat allergic conjunctivitis depend on the symptoms. Artificial tears may soothe itchy, watery, red eyes. If artificial tears do not work, an antihistamine may be used. Antihistamines stop the release of histamine that causes an allergic response and will help alleviate itchy, watery eyes. Another set of agents act as both antihistamines and mast cell stabilizers, making them more potent allergy agents. Mast cell stabilizers work differently than antihistamines. They keep the mast cell walls from bursting and releasing not only histamine but also other chemicals that can lead to allergic reactions.

Medications for Glaucoma

Glaucoma is a disease caused by increased pressure within the eye. Untreated glaucoma can damage the optic nerve, resulting in partial to total loss of sight. Many drugs are used to treat glaucoma by lowering the pressure. Sympathomimetic drugs lower pressure by increasing the fluid drainage from the eye. Beta-blocking drugs decrease the production of aqueous humor in the eye. These agents are often considered first-line therapy for glaucoma because of their efficacy and favorable side-effect profile. Although these drugs have low systemic absorption, they have caused bronchoconstriction and slowed heart rate in some patients (see Antihypertensives section). Because of these effects, these drugs should be used cautiously in patients with lung disease, heart failure, and diabetes. A newer class of agents, which also work by decreasing the production of aqueous humor, are the carbonic anhydrase inhibitors. The first of the two agents, dorzolamide, was approved in 1994. Miotic drugs, such as carbachol, pilocarpine, physostigmine, demecarium, echothiophate iodide, and isoflurophate, constrict the pupil size, thus increasing the fluid drainage. These agents were the first available to treat patients with glaucoma, but they are no longer considered first-line agents. Pilocarpine is available in a controlled-release unit that is placed under the lower eyelid and releases medication for 1 week. The antiglaucoma drug echothiophate is available as a powder that must be reconstituted and labeled with an expiration date before dispensing.

The most common adverse effects of all of these drugs are discomfort, stinging or burning, and blurred vision upon administration. The miotic agents, which constrict the pupil, can cause poor night vision. The drug dorzolamide is a sulfonamide and should be avoided in patients with a sulfonamide allergy because it can cause severe allergic reactions.

Medications for Dryness

A large number of ophthalmic preparations are available as artificial tear solutions for the relief of dry eyes. These products contain salts in the same concentrations as found in the tissues and fluids of the eye. They also contain buffers to maintain the same acidity as the eye tissues and thickening agents to prolong the time they stay on the surface of the eye. All these products are available over the counter. A prescription-only insert, Lacrisert®, is available that provides relief from dryness with once-daily insertion as opposed to application of drops several times daily.

Ophthalmic vasoconstrictors are commonly used to reduce redness in the eyes from minor irritations. Several products are available over the counter for this purpose. These products are also used to dilate the pupil for eye examinations and surgery. The over-the-counter products should not be used for more than 72 hours without consulting a physician. Products include phenylephrine, oxymetazoline, naphazoline, and tetrahydrozoline. Some of these drugs are available in combination with antihistamines or with zinc sulfate as an antiseptic for minor eye irritations.

Corticosteroids are available in topical ophthalmic preparations and are indicated for inflammatory conditions, such as allergic conjunctivitis, selected infections of the eye, chemical and other burns, and penetration of foreign bodies. Prednisolone and dexamethasone are available as single drugs and in combination with many different anti-infective agents. Other agents available in ophthalmic formulations are NSAIDs, which are indicated for inflammatory conditions.

Otic Medications

Topical otic medications are effective for treating conditions of the external ear. Conditions involving the middle or inner ear require systemic treatment. Topical ear treatments are most commonly used for impacted earwax and minor infections or irritation of the auditory canal. Several products have names similar to ophthalmic products, and care should be taken to avoid confusion and mistakes. Otic preparations should be labeled "For the ear." Topical otic products should not be used if the eardrum is perforated.

The antibiotic chloramphenicol is available as an otic preparation for infections of the auditory canal. Antibiotic combinations of neomycin and polymyxin B with the corticosteroid hydrocortisone are also used to treat these infections. Acetic acid, M-cresyl acetate, boric acid, benzalkonium chloride, benzethonium chloride, ciprofloxacin, and aluminum acetate are antibacterial or antifungal ingredients in ear drops, and they may also be combined with corticosteroids. Treatments for some infections involving the middle ear may combine an oral antibiotic with one of the agents listed above. These infections tend to be painful.

One combination contains antipyrene and benzocaine (Auralgan®) and is used solely as a pain reliever.

Otic preparations that contain carbamide peroxide and glycerin are used to soften and disperse earwax. After these agents have been instilled, the wax is removed by irrigating the ear with a syringe. A physician should remove any wax not responding to these drugs after 4 days.

Intranasal Products

The major ailment of the nose that is treated with topical products is rhinitis. Rhinitis may also be treated with oral drugs. Rhinitis is a hyper-reactivity of the lining of the nose to stimuli. The stimuli may include seasonal allergens such as pollen, perennial allergens such as animal dander, or nonallergic stimuli such as stress, temperature changes, and other environmental factors. Rhinitis also occurs during infections such as the common cold or the flu. Symptoms of rhinitis may include nasal congestion, runny nose, postnasal drainage, sneezing, itching, redness of the membrane lining the nose, watery eyes, dark circles under the eyes, and inability to breathe through one's nose.

Intranasal corticosteroids are used for rhinitis and other allergic or inflammatory conditions of the nose. Intranasal corticosteroids are considered long-term treatment for conditions and should not be used for immediate resolution of symptoms. With doses that exceed the recommended range, and occasionally with recommended doses, systemic effects may occur. The mechanism of action of corticosteroids is discussed under the Anti-inflammatory and Antipyretic Agents section. Several of these agents, listed in **Table 12-19**, are also available as oral inhalers, so care must be taken to dispense the product for the correct route of administration. Some aqueous (AQ) preparations sting less than other preparations and are longer acting, allowing for fewer daily administrations.

Decongestant drugs are available in intranasal sprays, drops, or inhalers. These drugs act on the nerves of the blood vessels in the nose. They cause the blood vessels to constrict, which decreases swelling and stuffiness in the nose. Topical agents are associated with rebound congestion when used for more than 3 to 5 days. Essentially, the nasal lining becomes more congested as the effect of the drug wears off. This increased stuffiness may cause the patient to increase the use of the decongestant, creating a cycle that is difficult to break.

TABLE 12-19. INTRANASAL FORMULATIONS

Generic Name	Brand Name	Onset of Action
Antihistamines		
Azelastine	Astelin	Immediate
Corticosteroids		
Beclomethasone diproprionate	Beconase, Vancenase, Beconase AQ, Vancenase AQ	Few days to 2 weeks
Budesonide	Rhinocort, Rhinocort AQ	24 hours
Flunisolide	Nasalide, Nasarel	Few days to 2 weeks
Fluticasone	**Flonase**	Few days
Mometasone	**Nasonex**	2 days
Triamcinolone acetonide	**Nasacort, Nasacort AQ**	12 hrs to a few days
Mast Cell Stabilizers		
Cromolyn sodium	Nasalcrom	1 to 2 weeks
Topical decongestants		
Oxymetazoline	Neo-Synephrine 12-hour Duration Afrin 12-hour Dristan 12-hour Nostrilla 12-hour	Immediate
Xylometazoline	Otrivin Natru-Vent	Immediate
Naphazoline	Privine	Immediate

Naphazoline, oxymetazoline, and xylometazoline are topical decongestants. Xylometazoline and oxymetazoline are long acting and can be used every 8 to 10 hours and every 12 hours, respectively. Reactions such as stinging, burning, and sneezing may occur. Patients with hypertension or other cardiovascular disease, overactive thyroid, diabetes mellitus, or an enlarged prostate gland should not use these products because of possible detrimental effects.

Dermatological Agents

Dermatitis and hypersensitivity reactions are common diseases of the skin. Contact dermatitis can be an acute or chronic reaction to irritants or allergens. Symptoms of contact dermatitis are redness, oozing, hives, swelling, and scaling. Poison ivy rash is an example of contact dermatitis. Sunburn is a dermatitis that results from overexposure to the sun. Normal exposure to the sun can also result in sunburn in patients who are taking drugs that sensitize the skin. Drug reactions and hives caused by foods and inhalants are other forms of dermatitis. Psoriasis is a noninfectious, chronic dermatitis that is characterized by white scale over red patches of skin, most commonly on the elbows, knees, scalp, lower back, genitalia, and feet. The cause of psoriasis is unknown. Generally, psoriasis may improve and then relapse.

Coal tar and salicylic acid have been used for many years to treat psoriasis. These products are available as ointments, creams, lotions, shampoos, and bath additives. They have an unpleasant odor and can stain clothing and hair. They should not be applied to broken skin. Salicylic acid is also used to remove warts, calluses, and corns. Some newer drugs for treating psoriasis include anthralin and calcipotriene. Anthralin can stain clothing and hair.

Corticosteroid creams, ointments, and lotions can be used for psoriasis. Other uses for corticosteroid topical products include other skin conditions involving itching and inflammation, such as contact dermatitis, reactions to insect and spider bites, burns and sunburns, diaper rash, and inflammation associated with fungal infections of the skin. Corticosteroids vary in potency and available strengths and formulations, as shown in **Table 12-20.** When topical steroids are being dispensed, the correct formulation (ointment, cream, or lotion) and strength must be carefully selected. Hydrocortisone and hydrocortisone acetate are available over the counter in 0.5 and 1 percent strengths. Many combinations with antifungals, antibiotics, and antibacterial agents are available. Such products should be applied sparingly. Systemic effects can occur if a significant amount of the corticosteroid is absorbed through the skin. Significant absorption of corticosteroids is more likely to occur when patients use more potent steroids, apply them to large surface areas, use them for prolonged periods, and apply occlusive dressings over the steroid.[2]

Numerous organisms may infect skin. Parasites, such as lice and mites, can cause rashes and itching by biting or laying eggs in the skin. Fungal and yeast infections are most common in skin folds, such as under the breasts and in the groin areas. Fungal infections can also occur on the feet (athlete's foot), on the scalp or body (ringworm), around the nails, or in the mouth. Viral infections that involve the skin include warts, cold sores, sexually transmitted herpes simplex, and herpes zoster rash (shingles). Bacterial infections that involve the skin include impetigo, a honey-colored crust commonly seen around the mouth and nose in children, and various sexually transmitted diseases.

Many topical anti-infective agents are available. Mupirocin, tetracycline, chloramphenicol, erythromycin, gentamicin, bacitracin, neomycin, and combina-

TABLE 12-20. TOPICAL AGENTS

Generic Name	Trade Name	Formulations
Low Potency Corticosteroids		
Desonide	DesOwen	Cream, ointment, gel, spray
Hydrocortisone	Various brands	Cream, ointment, gel, spray, solution, lotion
Medium Potency Corticosteroids		
Hydrocortisone valerate	Westcort	Cream, ointment
Mometasone	**Elocon**	Cream, ointment, lotion
High Potency Corticosteroids		
Betamethasone diproprionate	Diprosone	Cream, ointment, lotion
Betamethasone valerate		Ointment
Desoximetasone	Topicort	Cream, ointment, gel
Fluocinolone	Synalar	Cream, ointment
Fluocinonide	Lidex	Cream, ointment, gel
Halcinonide	Halog	Cream, ointment
Triamcinolone	Aristocort	Cream, ointment, lotion
Very High Potency Corticosteroids		
Clobetasol	Temovate, Embeline, Cormax	Cream, ointment
Diflorasone	Psorcon-E	Cream, ointment (emollient)
Halobetasol	Ultravate	Cream, ointment
Augmented betamethasone diproprionate	Diprolene	Cream, ointment
Topical Antifungals		
Clotrimazole	Lotrimin AF, Mycelex	Cream, lotion, solution
Miconazole	Micatin, Desenex	Cream, powder, spray
Terbinafine	Lamisil AT	Cream
Tolnaftate	Tinactin, Aftate	Cream, solution, powder, aerosol
Ketoconazole	Nizoral	Cream, shampoo
Naftifine	Naftin	Cream, gel
Econazole	Spectazole	Cream

tions of polymyxin B, neomycin, and bacitracin are examples of topical anti-infective agents. Many of the antifungal agents are listed in Table 12-20 and are marketed for athlete's foot and jock itch. These agents should not be used alone to treat onychomycosis (nail fungal infections)—an oral antifungal agent must be used in this condition. Acyclovir is available as an antiviral ointment.

Acne is a chronic condition in which lesions, called *comedones,* appear on the skin. Comedones are commonly called *whiteheads* and *blackheads.* Acne is most common in teenage years. Hormones, friction, sweating, and stress can all cause and increase the severity of acne.[4]

A large number of topical products are available for treating acne. Most acne products work to prevent breakouts by one of four mechanisms: (1) increasing the rate of turnover of skin cells, (2) killing bacteria on the skin, (3) inhibiting inflammation, and (4) decreasing the production by the skin of oily substances.[5] Tretinoin, benzoyl peroxide, azelaic acid, and sulfur are examples of topical preparations. Combinations of sulfur drugs, salicylic acid, and resorcinol are also available. Antibiotics such as tetracycline, meclocycline, erythromycin, and clindamycin are available to treat acne topically (see the Infectious Diseases section). In more severe cases of acne, systemic treatment with antibiotics or isotretinoin can be used. In some cases, both topical and systemic therapies are used.

Nutritional Products

Vitamins

Vitamins are compounds involved in the cellular chemical reactions that are essential to normal tissue growth, maintenance, and function. The body can synthesize vitamin D on exposure to sunlight, but the rest of the essential vitamins must be supplied by the diet. The recommended dietary allowance (RDA) is the daily level of intake needed to meet the nutritional needs of most healthy people.

Vitamins are classified as *fat-soluble* or *water-soluble*. The fat-soluble vitamins are vitamins A, D, E, and K. These vitamins are absorbed with fats in the diet, so very low-fat diets and conditions that impair fat absorption may decrease amounts of these vitamins in the body. Excessive use of mineral oil as a laxative may cause decreased absorption of the fat-soluble vitamins. These vitamins are stored in fats in the body when excess amounts are ingested. Toxic effects may occur when large amounts are taken. The water-soluble vitamins are vitamin C, folic acid, and the B vitamins. With normal kidney function, excess of these vitamins is excreted in the urine and toxic levels do not accumulate.

Many vitamins have more than one name. Knowing the alternate names may be helpful for dispensing the correct product. Listed below are some duplicate names:

Vitamin A = Retinol

Vitamin E = Tocopherol

Vitamin B_1 = Thiamine

Vitamin B_2 = Riboflavin

Vitamin B_3 = Niacin = Nicotinic Acid

Vitamin B_5 = Pantothenic Acid

Vitamin B_6 = Pyridoxine

Vitamin B_{12} = Cyanocobalamin

Several forms of vitamin D are available but are not interchangeable in all patients. These forms include cholecalciferol, 25-hydroxycholecalciferol, 1,25-dihydroxycholecalciferol, and ergocalciferol.

Vitamins are used therapeutically in some situations. Vitamin A may be used for certain skin disorders. Vitamin D is used for patients with bone malformation caused by kidney disease. Vitamin K may be given to reverse the effects of the blood thinner warfarin. Niacin (vitamin B_3) is used to treat high blood cholesterol.

Vitamins are also given as supplements. Supplements are indicated when a patient's diet is poor, such as with some elderly patients and alcoholics. Vitamin supplements also may be given during periods of increased metabolic requirements, such as pregnancy, major surgery, or cancer. Poor absorption is another indication for vitamin supplementation. Some patients lack a substance necessary for the absorption of vitamin B_{12} and must receive B_{12} by injection. Some drugs may affect the absorption of, or requirements for, some vitamins. Patients taking the antituberculosis drug isoniazid may have an increased need for pyridoxine (vitamin B_6) to avoid adverse effects on nerves.

Minerals

Minerals are parts of enzymes, hormones, and vitamins and are essential to processes such as muscle contraction, nerve conduction, and water and acid balance. The minerals present in the body in relatively large amounts are calcium, phosphorus, potassium, chloride, magnesium, and sulfur. The minerals present in small amounts (trace elements) include iron, zinc, iodine, chromium, selenium, fluoride, copper, and manganese.

Diets may vary in their mineral content to a greater extent than vitamin content. Plants take up minerals from soil, so the mineral content of the soil where they grow influences the amount of minerals present in foods. Deficiencies of certain food groups in the diet may cause deficiencies in certain minerals. For instance, dairy products are the most important source of calcium. Patients who are intolerant of dairy products or are strict vegetarians may require calcium supplements to get enough calcium.

Minerals, like vitamins, may be given individually when only one is needed. For instance, to prevent the bone disease osteoporosis, postmenopausal women are frequently given calcium supplements. The four minerals that are most commonly administered as single entities are calcium, iron, potassium, and magnesium. Minerals, especially iron, are also added to many multivitamin preparations.

Calcium is available as many different salt forms that vary in the amount of calcium provided. Calcium is also available as injectable salts for intravenous use.

Iron deficiency anemia can result from poor absorption of iron, inadequate intake of iron, or iron loss secondary to bleeding. Iron is administered as many different salts that contain varying amounts of iron. Iron is also available in an injectable preparation for intramuscular or intravenous use.

Potassium is the primary mineral found inside cells. Potassium imbalance adversely affects cellular metabolism and nerve and muscle function. Potassium salts are available as tablets and liquids for oral use. The amount of potassium present is normally expressed as milli-equivalents (mEq) rather than milligrams (mg). Potassium chloride is the salt most commonly prescribed. Liquid forms tend to have an unpleasant taste, but they may be preferred by patients who are unable to swallow the large tablets or capsules. One tablet form of potassium chloride, K-Dur®, is a tablet of pressed pellets that can be suspended in liquid to provide a tasteless liquid form. Effervescent potassium tablets are also available to be dissolved in water or juice. Potassium salts are irritating to the stomach, so they are usually given as wax or polymer forms that minimize irritation by slowly releasing potassium in the gut. Potassium chloride and potassium phosphate are also available for intravenous use. Overly concentrated intravenous potassium solutions are irritating to veins. Intravenous solutions must be administered slowly to avoid heart rhythm disturbances.

Magnesium is the second most abundant mineral found inside cells. It is important to many of the body's enzymes, nerves, and muscles. Magnesium may be administered as oral tablets, liquids, or by injection. As with the other minerals, the amount of magnesium in different salts varies. The amount may be expressed as *mEq*. Magnesium sulfate is the salt used for intravenous administration. Various salts are used for oral replacement. Diarrhea is a common side effect of oral formulations.

Recommended Reading

USP DI, Volume II, Advice for the patient. Rockville, MD: United States Pharmacopeia Convention, Inc; 2003.

USP DI, Volume I, Drug information for the health care professional. Rockville, MD: United States Pharmacopeia Convention, Inc.; 2003.

Facts and comparisons. St. Louis, MO: Facts and Comparisons, Inc.

DiPiro JT. Pharmacotherapy: a pathophysiologic approach, 5th ed. McGraw-Hill Companies, Inc. 2002:1396.

References

1. Principles of management of common ocular disorders In: Vaughan D, Asbury T, eds. General ophthalmology, 11th ed. Los Altos, CA: Lange Medical Publications; 1986:54–65.

2. Facts and comparisons. St. Louis, MO: Facts and Comparisons, Inc.; 2003.

3. The skin: assessment. Syntex Laboratories, Inc.; 1986.

4. Covington T, et al., eds. Handbook of nonprescription drugs, 13th ed. Washington, DC: American Pharmaceutical Association; 2002.

5. DiPiro JT, e.a., Pharmacotherapy: a pathophysiologic approach, 5th ed. 2002:1396. McGraw-Hill Companies, Inc.

6. The Fifth Report of the Joint National Committee on Detection, Evaluation and Treatment of High Blood Pressure (JNC V). *Arch Intern Med.* 1993; 153:154–83.

7. Immediate-release nifedipine labeling will warn against off-label uses, FDA indicates following calcium channel blocker advisory committee review. F-D-C Reports 1996; 58(5):3–5.

8. McEvoy G, et al., eds. AHFS drug information 2002. Bethesda, MD: American Society of Health-System Pharmacists.

9. Katzung B, ed. Basic and clinical pharmacology, 6th ed. Norwalk, CT: Appleton & Lange; 1995.

10. Des Prez RM, Heim CR. Mycobacterium tuberculosis. In: Mandell GL, Douglas RG, Bennett JE, eds. Principles and practice of infectious diseases. New York: Churchill Livingstone, Inc; 1990:1877–82.

1. Which of the following antibiotics can be prescribed for a patient who is allergic to penicillin?
   a. ticarcillin
   b. erythromycin
   c. amoxicillin
   d. dicloxacillin

2. Which of the following drugs is used in the treatment of Parkinson's disease?
   a. dobutamine
   b. oxytocin
   c. levodopa/carbidopa
   d. ciprofloxacin

3. Insulin *cannot* be given by which of the following routes?
   a. oral
   b. intravenous
   c. subcutaneous
   d. intravenous drip

4. Several of the most commonly prescribed drugs are used for depression. Which of the following is *not* an antidepressant?
   a. fluoxetine
   b. sertraline
   c. amitriptyline
   d. diazepam

5. Which of the following is *not* an action of ibuprofen?
   a. anti-inflammatory
   b. fever reduction (antipyretic)
   c. pain relief (analgesic)
   d. nausea relief (antiemetic)

6. Which of the following statements is true about chemotherapy agents (drugs used for cancer)?
   a. The naming of chemotherapy regimens (such as MAC, MOPP, CHOP) has been standardized so that the same letter always stands for the same drug.
   b. Chemotherapy drugs frequently have similar-sounding names that can be easily confused.
   c. Chemotherapy drugs are very safe and have few adverse effects.
   d. Chemotherapy drugs are the only treatment available for cancer.

7. Which drug inhibits ovulation and is used in birth control pills?
   a. conjugated estrogens
   b. ethinyl estradiol
   c. clomiphene
   d. oxytocin

8. Corticosteroids may be used to treat all but which of the following diseases?
   a. rheumatoid arthritis
   b. asthma
   c. allergic reactions
   d. peptic ulcer disease

9. When corticosteroids are no longer needed, how should the drug be discontinued?
   a. The drug should be stopped immediately and all extra tablets washed down the sink.
   b. The drug should be gradually stopped by reducing the dose over days to weeks.
   c. The drug should never be discontinued.
   d. The oral form should be changed to injectable.

10. Which of the following drugs is to treat AIDS (acquired immunodeficiency syndrome)?
    a. glyburide
    b. enalapril
    c. zidovudine
    d. albuterol

11. Conjunctivitis (inflammation of the eye) can be treated with all of the following *except*:
    a. corticosteroid eye drops
    b. antiallergy agents
    c. antibiotic eye drops
    d. beta-blocker eye drops

12. Bronchodilators for asthma
    a. are often used as oral metered-dose inhalers.
    b. are obsolete since the introduction of nedocromil.
    c. include theophylline, β_2 agonists, and corticosteroids.
    d. are ineffective by the inhaled route.

13. Lovastatin
    a. lowers blood pressure in patients with angina pectoris.
    b. lowers the bad cholesterol and raises the good cholesterol.
    c. prevents the absorption of fat in food.
    d. commonly causes a dry cough.

14. Drugs used to treat hypertension include all of the following *except*:
    a. verapamil

b. hydrochlorothiazide

c. atenolol

d. digoxin

15. Effects of warfarin include all *except*:

a. decreasing the formation of blood clots

b. nose bleeds

c. red-orange urine

d. ringing in the ears

16. If a patient has a feeding tube into the stomach and is taking omeprazole,

a. empty the capsule, crush the pellets, and dissolve them in Maalox® to flush down the tube.

b. consult the pharmacist for the correct action to take.

c. give omeprazole in the intravenous fluid.

d. tell the nurse to discontinue the drug.

17. The minerals calcium and iron

a. are needed by the body in trace amounts.

b. may interfere with the absorption of tetracycline.

c. are only available in vitamin/mineral combinations.

d. must be given as supplements because they are not found in food.

18. Levothyroxine and thyroid USP are used to replace natural thyroid hormone in hypothyroidism.

a. True

b. False

19. Ciprofloxacin and tetracycline are good drugs for pediatric infections because they are available in liquid forms.

a. True

b. False

20. Acetaminophen is preferred to aspirin to lower fever in children with chicken pox.

a. True

b. False

21. Prescriptions for opioid analgesics should have a label affixed to the bottle to warn patients against the use of alcohol with these drugs.

a. True

b. False

22. Intranasal beclomethasone is used to treat asthma.

a. True

b. False

23. If relief of the common cold does not occur with an intranasal decongestant, increase the dose and use the drug more often.

a. True

b. False

24. Nitrates are effective only if they are used every day, around the clock.

a. True

b. False

25. Emollient laxatives (stool softeners) are effective drugs for preventing constipation.

a. True

b. False

26. Large doses of vitamins might not help you, but they won't hurt you.

a. True

b. False

27. Match the trade name with the appropriate generic name.

Trade Name	Generic Name
1.___Premarin	A. Alprazolam
2.___Lanoxin	B. Captopril
3.___Prozac	C. Phenytoin
4.___Zantac	D. Albuterol
5.___Mevacor	E. Conjugated estrogens
6.___Capoten	F. Ranitidine
7.___Ceclor	G. Digoxin
8.___Xanax	H. Fluoxetine
9.___Proventil	I. Lovastatin
10.___Dilantin	J. Cefaclor

Self-Assessment Answers

1. b. Erythromycin. All of the other answers are penicillins and would cause a similar allergic response. Erythromycin is safe to use in penicillin-allergic patients. Cephalosporins should be used with caution, as cross-sensitivity does occur.

2. c. Levodopa/carbidopa. Levodopa/carbidopa is the mainstay of therapy of Parkinson's disease. Dobutamine is used for cardiac conditions and shock. Oxytocin is a hormone that causes uterine contractions and milk flow. Ciprofloxacin is an antibiotic.

3. a. Oral. Insulin is destroyed in the stomach when given orally. Regular insulin can be given intravenously either as a bolus injection or a drip. Other forms of insulin are given subcutaneously.

4. d. Diazepam. Diazepam is a sedative-hypnotic that is also used sometimes as an antispasmolytic and as an antiepileptic. Fluoxetine, sertraline, and amitriptyline are all antidepressants.

5. d. Nausea relief. Ibuprofen may have nausea as an adverse effect. Ibuprofen is a nonsteroidal anti-inflammatory agent, so it provides all three of the other actions: anti-inflammatory, antipyretic, and analgesic.

6. b. Chemotherapy drugs frequently have similar-sounding names that can be easily confused. Vinblastine and vincristine sound so much alike that they have been the source of fatal drug errors. The letters in chemotherapy regimens do not always stand for the same drug, so confusion is likely. Chemotherapy drugs have many serious adverse effects. Chemotherapy is one of three medical treatments for cancer. Radiation and surgery are other treatments.

7. b. Ethinyl estradiol. Ethinyl estradiol is found in many combination birth control pills. Conjugated estrogens are a type of estrogen, but they are used only for postmenopausal estrogen replacement and osteoporosis prevention and treatment. Clomiphene is used to stimulate ovulation to enhance fertility. Oxytocin is a hormone that stimulates uterine contraction during and after labor and stimulates milk flow.

8. d. Peptic ulcer disease. Corticosteroids suppress inflammation and suppress the immune system. They are useful for diseases characterized by inflammation, such as rheumatoid arthritis, asthma, and allergic reactions. Corticosteroids have no role in the treatment of peptic ulcer disease.

9. b. The drug should be gradually stopped by reducing the dose over days to weeks. Gradually reducing the dose allows the adrenal gland to recover its important function. Corticosteroids can be stopped immediately only if a very low dose has been taken for a short time. The answer c is incorrect because corticosteroids should only be taken as long as the benefit outweighs the risks. The oral form would not be changed to injectable. Usually the opposite is done—injectable drug is given for greater effect and then changed to oral, and finally oral drug is gradually discontinued.

10. c. Zidovudine. Zidovudine is an antiviral drug with activity against HIV, which is the cause of AIDS. Glyburide is an oral hypoglycemic agent for Type 2 diabetes mellitus. Enalapril is an angiotensin converting enzyme (ACE) inhibitor used for high blood pressure. Albuterol is a drug used to relax the lungs in asthma and other breathing disorders.

11. d. Beta-blocker eye drops are used to treat glaucoma but have no role in the treatment of conjunctivitis.

12. a. Nedocromil is not a bronchodilator and plays a different role in asthma treatment than the bronchodilators. Corticosteroids are not bronchodilators. Bronchodilators other than theophylline are used by the inhaled route.

13. b. Lovastatin has no effect on blood pressure and does not prevent absorption of fat. It prevents the formation of cholesterol from fats after they are absorbed. ACE inhibitors are the drugs associated with dry cough.

14. d. Digoxin is used to treat heart failure and atrial fibrillation but has no role in the treatment of hypertension. Verapamil, hydrochlorothiazide, and atenolol are all used to treat hypertension.

15. d. Decreasing the formation of blood clots is the therapeutic effect of warfarin. Nosebleeds and red-orange urine are side effects of

warfarin. Ringing in the ears is associated with aspirin, salicylates, quinine, and quinidine, but not with warfarin.

16. b. The pharmacist will need to assess how to give the drug and whether there are any drug-nutrient interactions. Crushing the pellets and mixing with Maalox will destroy the coating and expose the drug to the acid in the stomach. Omeprazole is destroyed by acid. Omeprazole does not have an injectable dosage form. Telling the nurse to discontinue the drug would be inappropriate for a technician. The pharmacist or nurse could consult the physician about alternative therapies.

17. b. Iron is a trace element, but calcium is needed in larger amounts. Calcium and iron are available in single-ingredient tablets, as well as in some combination products. A normal diet provides adequate amounts of these minerals in most people.

18. a. Hypothyroidism is the underproduction of thyroid hormone. It is treated with replacement hormone such as levothyroxine or thyroid, USP.

19. b. Ciprofloxacin and tetracycline should not be used in children because of adverse effects.

20. a. Aspirin should not be used in children with chicken pox or viral illnesses, because they are at increased risk of developing Reye's syndrome.

21. a. Alcohol can add to the sedative effect and depression of breathing that can occur with opioid analgesics.

22. b. Orally inhaled beclomethasone is used to treat asthma. Intranasal beclomethasone is used to treat allergic rhinitis.

23. b. Overuse of intranasal decongestants can lead to rebound congestion.

24. b. Tolerance to nitrates develops. A daily "nitrate-free" period improves their effectiveness.

25. a. Stool softeners are preferred for preventing rather than treating constipation.

26. b. Water-soluble vitamins in large doses are excreted by the kidney in healthy people. But fat-soluble vitamins, even in healthy people, accumulate in body fat and may cause toxic effects.

27. Answers: 1-E; 2-G; 3-H; 4-F; 5-I; 6-B; 7-J; 8-A; 9-D; 10-C

Footnote

[*] See Chapter 7 for more information about medication references.

Nonsterile Compounding and Repackaging

DOUGLAS C. HIGGINS

After completing this chapter, the technician should be able to

1. Understand the concept of compounding medications from individual chemicals.

2. Understand and name several compounded dosage forms.

3. Understand the concept of, and reasons for, repackaging medications.

4. Understand the importance of record keeping for compounding and repackaging.

For many years, compounding was disappearing. Chemicals were difficult to obtain. Technical support was sparse. Knowledge was spread primarily among older pharmacists. In the past two decades, however, companies that support compounding pharmacists have spurred a renewed interest in meeting patient needs through compounding. Several thousand pharmacies have thriving practices in human and veterinary compounding—some are compounding-only pharmacies. The expertise of a compounding pharmacist in using medications for a wide variety of conditions offers a unique clinical experience and close patient contact through the patient-physician-pharmacist triad.

Opportunities abound for compounding. Commercial medications typically come in just a few strengths and dosage forms. Compounding offers opportunities to meet patient needs by preparing medication in the proper strength and dosage form. Some possible areas of practice include the following:

- Discontinued medications
- Flavors
- Veterinary medications
- Hospice and palliative care
- Hormone replacement therapy
- Pain control
- Wound care
- Dermatology

Proper packaging of compounded and commercially available medications provides stable preparations with a maximum shelf life. Many commercial medications are available in unit-of-use packaging; however, there is still a need to repackage many medications to meet patient or institutional needs.

As pharmacists are evaluating patient needs, counseling patients, developing formulations, and performing other clinically oriented activities, technicians perform much of the actual dosage form preparation through compounding and repackaging medications.

Good Compounding Practices

Chemicals for compounding are approved by the Food and Drug Administration (FDA); however, the practice of compounding is controlled by individual state boards of pharmacy. Until 1997, certain aspects of compounding and the role of the FDA were not clearly defined in federal law. In response, in 1997, the Food and Drug Administration Modernization Act (FDAMA) was passed. This legislation clearly defined the roles of both compounding pharmacies and the FDA. In the summer of 2002, however, the legislation was declared unconstitutional because of advertising restrictions. The guidelines of the 1997 FDAMA still offer a structure for compounding pharmacists to follow until future legislation addresses the issue again.

The *United States Pharmacopeia (USP 27)* offers guidelines for compounding. The following chapters review specific areas of compounding:

Chapter 795, Pharmaceutical Compounding—Nonsterile Preparations

Chapter 797, Pharmaceutical Compounding—Sterile Preparations

Chapter 1075, Good Compounding Practices

Chapter 1160, Pharmaceutical Calculations in Prescription Compounding

This chapter will focus primarily on Chapter 795 and to a lesser extent on Chapter 1075.

The following are the key areas that will be covered in this chapter:

1. Responsibility of the compounder
2. Compounding environment
3. Stability of compounded preparations
4. Ingredient selection
5. Compounded preparations
6. Compounding process
7. Compounding records and documents
8. Material Safety Data Sheet (MSDS) file
9. Quality control
10. Patient counseling

Responsibility of the Compounder

The compounder is responsible for all aspects of the compounding process, including, but not limited to, appropriately trained personnel and the key areas of chapter 795 of *USP 27* that follow.

Compounding Environment

The compounding area should have adequate space for equipment and support materials. Controlled temperature and lighting are needed for chemicals and finished medications. The area must be kept clean for sanitary reasons and to prevent cross-contamination. A sink with hot and cold running water is essential for hand washing and equipment cleaning.

Stability of Compounded Preparations

Stability is defined in *USP 27* as "the extent to which a preparation retains, within specified limits, and throughout its period of storage and use, the same properties and characteristics that is possessed at the time of compounding."[1]

Primary packaging of the finished medication is of utmost importance. The choice of the proper container is guided by the physical and chemical characteristics of the finished medication. Whether the medication is light sensitive or binds to the container are examples of considerations in maximizing stability.

Beyond-use labeling should be included on all medications. (Expiration dates apply to manufactured products.) Examples of considerations for determining beyond-use dates include whether the medication is aqueous or nonaqueous, the expiration dates of the ingredients used, the storage temperature, and the references documenting the stability of the finished medication.

Ingredient Selection

Sources of ingredients vary widely. USP or National Formulary (NF) chemicals are the preferred chemicals for compounding. Other sources may be used, but the compounder has a responsibility to be certain the chemical meets purity and safety standards. Manufactured medications are another acceptable source of ingredients. It would be inappropriate to use any chemical withdrawn from use by the FDA.

Compounded Preparations

Preparations should contain at least 90 percent, but not more than 110 percent, of the labeled active ingredient, unless more restrictive laws apply. Compounding guidelines in *USP 27* specifically address the following:

- Capsules, powders, lozenges, and tablets
- Emulsions, solutions, and suspensions
- Suppositories
- Creams, topical gels, ointments, and pastes

Compounding Processes

The goal of the compounding process is to "minimize error and maximize the prescriber's intent."[2] A sampling of areas to consider in the compounding process follows:

- Evaluation of the appropriateness of the prescription
- Calculations of the amount of ingredients
- Identification of equipment needed to compound the prescription properly
- Proper hand cleaning and gowning
- Evaluation of the final medication for weight variation, proper mixing, and consistency
- Proper notations in the compounding log
- Appropriate labeling of the final medication

Compounding Records and Documents

The goal of record keeping is to allow another compounder to reproduce the same formulation at a later date. Two parts of the records and documentation are the formula (or formulation record) and the batch log (or compounding record).

The formulation record is a file of compounded preparations, much like a recipe. It includes chemicals in the formula, equipment needed to prepare the formula, and mixing instructions for preparing the formula.

The compounding record is the log (or record) of an actual batch being prepared. It includes manufacturers and lot numbers of chemicals used, the date of preparation, an internal identification number (commonly called lot number), a beyond-use date, and any other pertinent information regarding the preparation.

Material Data Safety Sheets (MSDS) File

MSDS on each chemical should be readily accessible to all employees.

Quality Control

Quality control is a final check on the preparation to ensure its safety and quality. The compounder must evaluate the finished preparation both physically and by

reviewing the compounding procedure to be certain the preparation is accurate. Discrepancies should be noted and evaluated to determine if the preparation is acceptable.

Patient Counseling

As with any prescription, the patient should be counseled on the correct use of the medication. Compounded medications are often different in method of use or the type of dispensing container, so special care should be taken to be certain the patient thoroughly understands the proper use of the medication.

Nonsterile Compounding

Compounding is simply using one or more active or inactive chemicals to produce a final medication. The compounder must follow a strict procedure to achieve the proper strength and consistency of medication. A logical progression is to use chemicals to create formulas and formulas to create batches. Chemical lot numbers, manufacturers, and beyond-use dates are recorded in a log each time a formula is compounded. See **Figure 13-1** on the next page for an example of a log.

Equipment

Compounding requires specialized equipment. An electronic balance is commonly used for speed and accuracy of measurement (see **Figure 13-2**). The balance must be maintained and calibrated regularly. Balances commonly come enclosed to minimize inaccuracy in measurement caused by air currents or inadvertent bumping. The surface on which the balance rests must be stable and solid.

Mortars and pestles are used to crush, grind, and blend various medicinal ingredients. The mortar is a deep bowl, and the pestle is a club-shaped tool that, when stamped or pounded vertically into the well of the mortar, pulverizes the contents of the mortar (see

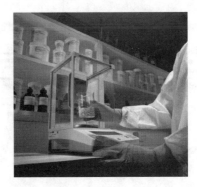

Figure 13-2. Electronic balance.

Logged Formula Worksheet
03/25/2004 4:50:45 PM
Page 1

DOUG'S PHARMACY
239 N. TAFT ST.
SUITE 1
PAXTON, IL 60957 ph. 217-379-3684

DIETHYLSTILBESTEROL 1MG CAP
0

| | PCCA ID: | | Schedule: - 393 | Active ☑ |
| Description: | | | Formula ID: 393 |

Pricing calculations from the log

Quantity made: 100 CAPS
Date made: 03/24/2004
Lot number: 20040324@6
Discard after: September 20, 2004 _____ Time to make: 30
Pharmacist: DOUGLAS C. HIGGINS
Technician: - NONE   NDC1: 393
Packaging:
Equipment needed:
Labeling: 393
Stability information:
Log note:

Chemicals		Sch.	Quantity used	QS	(Balance)
1 DIETHYLSTILBESTROL, USP POWDER		L	0.1 GM	☐	
Lot #: 88743	Mfg: PCCA		Exp. date:		Whsr. PROFESSIONAL COMPOUN
Balance Qty used calcs 0.1 = 0.1 / 100 * 100					Each CAPS contains 0.001 GM or 0.1%
2 LACTOSE HYDROUS NF POWDER		O	22.4 GM	☐	
Lot #: C103266	Mfg: PCCA		Exp. date:		Whsr. PROFESSIONAL COMPOUN
Balance Qty used calcs 22.4 = 22.4 / 100 * 100					Each CAPS contains 0.224 GM or 22.4%
3 FOOD COLOR, YELLOW POWDER		O	0.05 GM	☐	
Lot #: C104470	Mfg: PCCA		Exp. date:		Whsr. PROFESSIONAL COMPOUN
Balance Qty used calcs 0.05 = 0.05 / 100 * 100					Each CAPS contains 0.0005 GM or 0.05%
4 MAGNESIUM STEARATE N.F. POWDER		.	0.25 GM	☐	
Lot #: C102299	Mfg: PCCA		Exp. date: 4/18/2004		Whsr. PROFESSIONAL COMPOUN
Balance Qty used calcs 0.25 = 0.25 / 100 * 100					Each CAPS contains 0.0025 GM or 0.25%
5 CAPSULE P-LOK #3 CLEAR CAPSULE			100 CAP	☐	
Lot #: PH03012902	Mfg: B&B		Exp. date:		Whsr. RAWKINS CHEMICAL, IN
Balance Qty used calcs 100 = 100 / 100 * 100					Each CAPS contains 1 CAP or 100%

(Added all GM & GMS: 22.80)

Mixing directions

1. WEIGH ALL POWDERS
2. MIX IN MORTAR
3. ENCAPSULATE USING STANDARD TECHNIQUE

| Sterile item: ☐ Sterility checked: ☐ Date checked: | Checked by: |
| Method used: | |

Date entered: 03/24/2004 11:35:47 AM   Last modified: 03/25/2004 4:46:41 PM   by: Current pharmacist

Figure 13-1. Department of Pharmacy Services Repackaging Production Worksheet.

Figure 13-3). Mixing is usually achieved by moving the pestle in a circular motion in the mortar. Mortars are available in a variety of materials and sizes. Glass, porcelain, ceramic, and Wedgwood™ are commonly used. Wedgwood™ offers a rough surface to allow grinding and reduction of particle size, but it is very difficult to clean to prevent cross-contamination of preparations. Glass and porcelain offer smooth, easy-to-clean surfaces.

Ointment mills are commonly found in compounding pharmacies (see **Figure 13-4**). Most have three rollers with small, adjustable spaces between the rollers. When preparations pass through the rollers, particle size is reduced.

Depending on the needs of the pharmacy, spatulas, beakers, graduated cylinders, tube sealers, blenders, vacuum pumps, weigh boats, syringes, suppository molds, jet pipettes, and funnels may be found in the compounding pharmacy (see **Figure 13-5**).

Inactive Ingredients

In addition to the active, or therapeutic, ingredient(s), medications may contain a number of inactive, or nontherapeutic, ingredients that function as diluents, binders, colors, glidants, lubricants, flavoring, sweeteners, or suspending agents, to name a few. The term *inert* is often used to describe these ingredients.

Commonly Compounded Products

Transdermals

One exciting newer area of compounding involves transdermal (across the skin) medications. Many chemicals cross the skin readily with the aid of penetrating bases. The bases most commonly use lecithin as the carrier. Typically, the lecithin is dissolved as minute droplets (known as micelles) in water-based gels. Medications for both local and systemic use are common. Therapeutic agents include, but are not limited to, nonsteroidal anti-inflammatory medications, neuropathic pain medications, circulation enhancers, antinauseants, and local anesthetics.

Use of transdermal medications may replace less desirable administration routes, such as rectal suppositories. Patients unable or unwilling to swallow often benefit from transdermal administration of medications. In veterinary use, applying a small therapeutic dose to the inside of the animal's ear is common.

Ointments and Creams

Numerous varieties of ointments and creams are available, from petrolatum-based products to emollient and vanishing creams. When mixing the active ingredients into the base, an ointment mill or power mortar and pestle with rotating blades offer two methods of dispersing and reducing particle size to allow the final product to be of optimal effectiveness and cosmetic appeal. A few examples of medications incorporated into ointments and creams include corticosteroids, antifungals, antibiotics, prostaglandins, and hormones.

Preparations may be for topical, rectal, or vaginal use. The choice of base depends on the type of condition being treated. For instance, a vaginal medication would commonly use an emollient or vanishing cream. Ointments may be used for occlusive preparations. Compounding pharmacies commonly use plastic or metal tubes or collapsible ointment jars for dispensing ointments or creams.

In the past, ointments and creams were prepared on a glass plate or paper pad. Today, specialized mixers with blades offer very uniform mixes. Use of an ointment mill will also offer a uniform mix with the advantage of reducing the particle size of powders

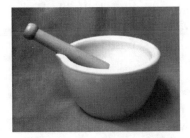

Figure 13-3. Mortar and pestle.

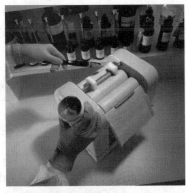

Figure 13-4. Ointment mill.

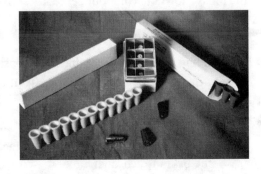

Figure 13-5. Suppositories and molds.

being incorporated into the final product. Milling a preparation enhances the final product and removes any graininess, which often is felt in ointments and creams prepared without milling.

Solutions and Suspensions

Solutions and suspensions may be oil based but are more commonly water based. Solutions and suspensions are generally easy to compound and offer wide flexibility of dosing. Dosing can be individualized to the patient by varying the concentration of the medication. Whenever possible, it is preferable to obtain the pure chemical to compound the solution or suspension. When the pure chemical is unavailable, tablets or capsules may be used to compound the medication.

Flavoring and sweetening the preparations is almost always necessary. A wide variety of sweeteners, including sucrose, stevia, acetylsulfame, aspartame, and saccharin, are available. Flavors range from traditional raspberry, cherry, marshmallow, mint, and chocolate to newer flavors such as piña colada, green apple, and tutti frutti. Some flavorings are available in both water- and oil-soluble forms. For veterinary use, flavors include fish, chicken, beef, and liver.

Suppositories

Suppositories are made using molds. The molds are made of brass, aluminum, rubber, or, most commonly today, disposable plastic. When using the plastic molds, the suppository may be sealed and dispensed in the mold. A variety of sizes are available, depending on the amount of active ingredient. One mold uses a shape similar to a golf tee for a suppository that remains in the rectal sphincter to release the active ingredient slowly to the local area.

In making a suppository, the first step is to determine the type of base to be used. Common bases include fatty acid and polyethylene glycol. Calibrating the mold allows the compounder to know the quantity of base in each suppository.

The mold is calibrated as follows:

- Using the desired base, fill 10 suppositories.
- After the base solidifies, weigh all 10 suppositories.
- Divide the weight of all 10 suppositories by 10.
- The resulting weight equals the average weight of the base in each cavity.
- If 10 suppositories weighed 13 gm, the average weight would be 1.3 gm.

A suspending agent should also be used in the mixture to minimize settling of the active ingredient while the suppository hardens. The most common suspending agent for this purpose is silica gel powder. While the base is melting on a heat source, usually a hot plate with magnetic stirring rod, the silica gel powder and active ingredient are mixed in a mortar. After the base is melted, the powder is added to the base with rapid stirring and mixed thoroughly. The base is poured into the mold, allowed to solidify at room temperature, and then refrigerated.

Capsules

Compounding pharmacists prepare a wide variety of capsules. Numerous capsule sizes and colors are available. Capsules may be *immediate release* or *slow release*. Using a percentage method, the amount of each ingredient to be used is calculated. For example, if the active ingredient occupies 50 percent of the capsule volume, inactive ingredients will occupy the other 50 percent of the capsule. Food color is often used to aid in the uniform mixing of the powders. Powders are commonly mixed in a mortar, plastic bag, or specialized blender.

In the past, capsules were packed by hand, but most compounding pharmacists now use a capsule-filling machine. After the capsules are loaded into the machine, the lids are removed, the capsules drop even with the plate, the powder is dispensed into the capsules, and the lids are replaced. Many capsules can be filled in a short time using this method.

Rapid-Dissolve Tablets

Rapid-dissolve tablets are a relatively new dosage form. The active ingredient(s) are mixed in a flavored base. The mixture is loaded into a mold and baked. The final product dissolves in approximately 15 seconds on the tongue. Some absorption occurs through the tissues in the mouth and some occurs through the gastrointestinal tract as the dissolved tablet is swallowed. Rapid-dissolve tablets offer an alternative dosage form for children, patients with trouble swallowing, prison inmates, and others.

Lollipops

Lollipops are becoming more popular for dosing medications. Drugs such as local anesthetics or healing agents may be added to the lollipop for local effect. Other drugs may be used for systemic administration through either the oral mucosa or gastrointestinal tract.

Troches

Troches are small, medicated squares resembling candy. A troche is dissolved between the cheek and gum. Troches offer an alternative to oral medications. Troches allow medications to be absorbed through the oral mucosa. The molds are commonly plastic, 24- or 30-place molds. After the base is melted, the active ingredient(s), flavoring(s), and inactive ingredients are stirred in. The mixture is thoroughly mixed, then poured into the mold and allowed to cool and solidify.

Powders

Powders are a dosage form that is valuable for specialized uses. Used in folds of creases in the skin, powders offer a drying or lubricating effect. An active ingredient may be mixed in the powder. The powder is sprinkled or sprayed on the area, often using a collapsible plastic container with a small, long-tip opening.

A polyox bandage powder can be used to form a gelatin layer over a wound or skin area. Active ingredients are incorporated into the powder. The powder is applied in sandwich-like layers, wetting each successive layer. Typically, about three layers of powder form a good gel layer. A polyox bandage powder is especially useful for oral lesions and sores to coat the mucosa. It is also often used for skin ulcers.

Tablet Triturates

Tablet triturates resemble nitroglycerin tablets. A paste containing the active and inactive ingredients is pressed into a mold, allowed to dry, and then removed from the mold.

Record Keeping

With specialized pharmacy practices such as compounding comes the need for complete record keeping. Tracking chemicals, building formulas from the chemicals, and batching formula preparation into logs requires meticulous record keeping, tying each step together.

Record keeping may be done manually, with formulas and logs of individual lots kept on paper. A more practical approach is using software designed to integrate the process of tracking each step, from chemicals to final product. Such software is available from several vendors.

Each container with a final preparation should be properly labeled with the name of the preparation, lot number, and beyond-use date. Beyond-use dates are calculated on the basis of the stability of the ingredients in the preparation. Consulting with the pharmacist or other resources, such as compounding consultants, will assist in determining the appropriate beyond-use date. The length of time until the beyond-use date is most commonly noted in the formula.

Repackaging

As pharmaceutical manufacturers prepare, package, and distribute more and more of the commonly prescribed medications, the role of the pharmacy has changed from formulator, compounder, and packager to repackager of commercially available products. Pharmacies repackage medications from bulk containers into patient-specific containers, including unit-of-use, single-unit, and single-dose packaging.

Unit-of-Use Packaging

Unit-of-use packaging is characterized by a vial, an envelope, or a plastic bag containing several doses of the same medication. Before dispensing, a prescription label with the patient's name and administration directions is affixed to the package. Unit-of-use packaging is suitable for inpatient or outpatient dispensing. Medications are packaged this way in advance of requests.

As the benefits of unit-of-use packaging became known, further modifications gave rise to the unit-dose concept. Unit-dose packaging includes single-unit and single-dose packages.

Single-Unit Packaging

Single-unit packaging contains a single-dosage form, for example, one tablet or capsule, or one teaspoonful (5 milliliters [ml]) of an oral liquid.

Single-Dose Package

The single-dose package is often confused with the single-unit package. The important difference is that the single-dose package always contains one dose of the drug for a given patient. A single-dose package, for example, contains two tablets when a given patient's dose is two tablets, whereas a single-unit package contains only one tablet. (A glossary of terms can be found at the end of this book.)

The availability of single-unit and single-dose packages from manufacturers has reduced the need for pharmacy personnel to repackage. However, repackaging is still performed because not all medications are available in unit-of-use packages, especially oral liquid medications for pediatric patients and a number of the less commonly prescribed oral solids.

Extemporaneous Versus Batch Repackaging

Extemporaneous repackaging is repackaging quantities of medications that will be used within a short period of time. *Batch* repackaging is the periodic repackaging of large quantities of medications in unit-dose or single-dose packages.

Extemporaneous repackaging is done on an as-needed basis. The quantities repackaged are based on the anticipated immediate need. Usually these medications have limited or unknown stability or are prescribed infrequently.

Batch repackaging is done for medications that have extended stability and are prescribed frequently. Batch repackaging is also thought to save time, materials, and money. Good manufacturing practices are used with batch repackaging programs to prevent errors.

Containers and Repackaging Materials

Repackaging materials and the package itself must protect the drug from harmful external elements, such as light, heat, moisture, air, and (in the case of sterile products) microbial contaminants. The material must not deteriorate during the shelf life of the drug. Packages should be lightweight and made of materials that do not interact with the dosage form. Repackaging materials should not absorb, be absorbed by, or chemically interact with the drug. Materials that are recyclable or biodegradable are preferred over those that are not.

Packages should be constructed so they do not deteriorate with normal handling. They should be easy to open and use and should not require any additional training or experience to use. Packages should allow for the contents to be inspected by the person administering the medication, unless the pharmaceutical properties of the drug preclude its being exposed to light. *USP XXII* defines containers and closures on the basis of the degree to which the contents are protected. These degrees of protection are defined as follows:

1. *Light-resistant containers* protect the drug from the effects of incident light by virtue of specific properties of which they are composed, including any coating applied. If protection from light is required, a clear and colorless or a translucent container may be made light-resistant by means of an opaque enclosure.

2. *Well-closed containers* protect the contents from extraneous solids and from loss of the drug under ordinary handling, shipment, storage, and distribution conditions.

3. *Tightly sealed containers* protect their contents from contamination by extraneous liquids, solids, or vapors; from loss of the drug; and from effervescence, deliquescence, or evaporation under ordinary handling, shipment, storage, and distribution conditions.

4. *Hermetic containers* are impervious to air or any other gas under ordinary or customary conditions of handling, shipment, storage, and distribution.[2]

The classification set forth by *USP XXII* designates package types as class A, least amount of moisture permeation; class B, more moisture permeation; class C, more moisture than class B; and class D, highest amount of moisture permeation. Manufacturers of repackaging materials and repackaging equipment describe their products on the basis of the type of package that is achievable—class A, B, C, or D—with class A being the best and class D being the worst. It is generally accepted that class A or class B packages are needed to extend the stability of a repackaged product beyond a few days following repackaging.

Repackaging Equipment

Repackaging equipment can be manual, semi-automated, or fully automated. These systems are reviewed as they pertain to repackaging of oral solids, oral liquids, and injectables. The more manual the system, the more variability is introduced in the package quality and the less chance the package has of attaining a class A or class B rating. More repackaging systems are available for oral solids than for any other dosage form, because most doses dispensed in institutions are oral solids.

Oral Solid Systems

Blister and Pouch Systems

Oral solids may be packaged in blister packages or in pouch packages. Blister packages are composed of an opaque and nonreflective backing that is usually used for printing or labeling. The backing, generally composed of paper or a paper-foil laminate, should be easy to peel from the blister portion of the package. Backing that is made entirely of paper may range in thickness from light (about the thickness of construction paper) to heavy (about the thickness of light cardboard).

The blister portion is composed of a flat-bottomed dome or bubble of transparent plastic. The plastic may be either high-density or low-density polyethylene or a combination of polyethylene densities and polypropylenes. Polyvinylchloride (PVC) has also been used as a blister package plastic.

Blister packages are more rigid than pouch packages and therefore may protect the contents better, but they do not lend themselves to the automated repackaging systems found in institutional practice. Automated blister packaging is generally confined to the pharmaceutical industry, but blister packages are used with some manually operated repackaging programs in institutional practice.

Pouch packages have one or both sides composed of an opaque, nonreflective surface intended for printing. This surface is generally a paper-foil laminate. The opposite side of the pouch can be made of the same paper-foil laminate, a paper-foil-polyethylene laminate, or a transparent polyethylene-coated cellophane.

The pouch package is probably the most common type for batch repackaging. The pouch package lends itself to relatively inexpensive automated machinery applications in institutional practice.

Manual Systems

Manually operated oral solid repackaging systems use either pouch packages or blister packages. Both pouch packages and blister packages use either heat sealing or adhesive sealing. As a rule, adhesive sealing systems produce class B, C, or D packages and heat-sealing systems produce class A, B, C, or D packages.

Pouch Systems

Manual pouch repackaging systems use clear or light-resistant plastic bags (usually PVC). The tablet or capsule is dropped into the bag, and the bag opening is sealed with an adhesive. This system provides a class D package. Manual pouch systems can also be heat sealed by a hot knife blade sealing the end of the plastic bag. Although heat sealing provides a better seal than adhesive, the package is usually class D because of the packaging material. A label is typed directly on the package before the product is added or on a regular

stock label and affixed to the package after it is sealed. This system is generally reserved for extemporaneous packaging.

Blister Systems

Manual blister repackaging systems use a plastic blister package made of a clear PVC or a laminate of PVC and low-density polyethylene plastic. The blisters or bubbles come in various sizes, depending on the type and size of the product being repackaged. The blisters can be filled on a tabletop or placed in specially designed holders to cradle the package. The blisters are filled with the drug, and then a paper, paper-foil, or vinyl-paper-foil backing is attached to the blister by removing a protective covering from an adhesive strip on the backing material and applying pressure to the blister and backing material. Blister packages are heat sealed in a heat seal press, which resembles a waffle iron. The heat seal applies heat and pressure to the backing material, while the blisters remain protected by the well-like device that holds them.

The adhesive blister package can create a class B, C, or D package. The heat seal blister system can create a class A, B, C, or D package.

Automated Systems

Automated oral solid repackaging systems, or unit-dose strip packaging machines, operate in basically the same fashion as blister packing machines. They all produce a pouch package made of two polyethylene-paper-foil laminates or a polyethylene-paper-foil laminate and a polyethylene-cellulose laminate. Tablets or capsules are manually fed into a wheel that drops the dose into a pouch formed by two heated wheels, and the package is sealed. A serrated knife blade that perforates the strip of pouches as it passes out of the machine separates individual packages. The labeling information is printed on the laminate by means of a stencil-and-ink system (wet or hot stamp) or a computer-generated printing system that interfaces with the packaging machine. The printing process occurs before the dose is dropped into the pouch.

Automated repackaging machines can package 60 to 120 doses of a single drug per minute. A device can be attached to the top of the automated strip packaging machine to eliminate the need for an operator to feed tablets and capsules into the wheel.

To prevent contamination of oral solid packaging equipment, only nonpenicillin and nononcolytic drugs should be repackaged.

Oral Liquid Systems

Manual Systems

Manual repackaging systems for oral liquids can be divided into those that use a glass or plastic vial as the reservoir for the liquid medication and those that use a glass or plastic syringe. Manual repackaging systems that require vials have three different closure systems: screw cap vials, vials with permanently affixed tops and small fill holes for medication, and vials that require the addition of a cap that must be crimped. An operator uses syringes, burettes, pipettes, or graduates to measure and transfer the liquid into the vial.

Manual systems for repackaging oral liquids into syringes use either of two methods of repackaging. The first method relies on the operator transferring the liquid to a suitable vessel (such as a beaker) and withdrawing the liquid into the syringe. An ordinary syringe can be used for this process if the number of dosage units is relatively small. Many pharmacies use a reusable glass or disposable plastic Cornwall-type syringe (often referred to as a magic syringe or a spring-loaded syringe) to speed the filling process. The Cornwall syringe method also offers greater reliability in fill volume, because the syringe is preset with the appropriate volume to dispense. Some systems use a burette instead of a syringe. With the burette method, the operator attaches a specially designed cap to the bulk bottle that allows a syringe to be introduced into the bottle; the contents are then withdrawn via the syringe by inverting the bottle.

Semiautomated Systems

Semiautomated systems are manual systems that use some piece of automated equipment as part of the filling or sealing process. Semiautomated filling pumps are either volumetric or peristaltic in design and can be used with either oral syringes or vials.

Volumetric pumps operate on the same principle as do Cornwall syringes. The volume to be dispensed into the container is preset on the basis of the draw-back setting and the type of reservoir selected for the pump.

Peristaltic pumps get their name from the form of pumping action they employ in delivering fluid. Peristaltic action is created by a series of roller wheels being pulled across a length of tubing. As each wheel passes over the tubing, the tubing is crimped and a small volume of fluid is forced down the tubing. Peristaltic pumps offer some advantages over volumetric pumps, including a faster rate of delivery for larger volumes (10 ml and above) and the ability to deliver fairly viscous liquids.

When many units are to be produced, a peristaltic pump usually requires frequent recalibration. Volumetric pumps need less recalibrating than peristaltic pumps and are more accurate and reliable for delivering fluid volumes of less than 10 ml.

Like most mechanical devices, these pumps offer several convenience factors. Most pumps display the volume of fluid being dispensed and the number of dispensing cycles (number of units filled); allow fill cycle times to be set automatically with rest periods established between each fill; and are equipped with alarms to alert the operator to an empty container. Pumps also are furnished with foot-pedal actuators that allow the operator to control the delivery and rest cycle of the fill.

Automated Systems

Automated liquid repackaging machines are available that fill, seal, and label the medication. Plastic cups are used as the fluid reservoir, and the sealing system is a PVC-paper-foil overseal. The overseal acts as the label stock, and the labeling is printed directly on the seal as the machine fills and seals the product in much the same way automated oral solid packaging machines do. A peristaltic pump delivers a predetermined amount of fluid into each cup as the cups pass by the filling orifice. The overseal is attached by applying heat and pressure until a strong bond is made between the cup and the PVC-paper-foil seal. The individual finished packages are separated when the machine cuts the overseal paper between cups. Machines are equipped with a variety of sensors that detect and signal problems associated with the fill cups, sealing foil, printing tape, and general machine failure. These machines, capable of producing 20 to 32 units per minute, are used in packaging liquids with volumes of 15 ml, 30 ml, or 45 ml. The packages these machines produce can attain a class A rating.

Commonly Repackaged Products

Oral Liquids

Oral liquids are usually repackaged in glass or plastic oral vials or oral syringes. Glass containers were commonly used in the past because of their properties of inertness, visibility of contents, stability, and FDA acceptance.

Plastics began to be used for repackaging pharmaceuticals in the 1980s. The acceptance of plastics was slow at first because of some of the early materials used. They have become more popular because newer products are inert, are cheaper to produce and ship, weigh less than glass, and are usually unbreakable.

Glass or plastic vials are the most frequently used containers for oral liquids. They are composed of the reservoir and a closure system, generally a rubber stopper or a plastic or metal screw cap. The rubber stopper is frequently made of butyl rubber with an aluminum or plastic overseal to hold the stopper in place. The screw cap is generally lined with a paper-vinyl inner cap. Some plastic and glass vials use a paper-lined aluminum foil cap as a closure system; this cap is affixed to the vial by crimping the top over a lip in the vial. Other systems contain a preaffixed rubber seal that accepts a blunt cannula for semiautomated filling. After filling, a tamper-evident seal is applied to the self-sealing closure to help ensure product integrity.

Another oral liquid container system is a plastic vial with a unique closure system. A plastic ball fits into a small filling hole in the bottom of the vial. The ball provides a friction fit to prevent liquid from escaping from the container. The top of the vial has a paper-foil laminate pull-off tab that allows for labeling or just serves as a tear-off seal.

Oral syringes are similar to injectable syringes, except they are not sterile and a hypodermic needle cannot be connected to the syringe, which prevents the injection of oral products parenterally. Oral syringes are composed of either a glass barrel and a plunger made of plastic and rubber or a plastic barrel and a plastic plunger. Many oral syringe systems have caps for the syringe hub to help maintain the integrity of the liquid in the syringe. A tamper-evident seal can be applied over the cap and barrel of the syringe. Caregivers who use the oral syringe system should be cautioned to ensure that the syringe caps are kept out of reach of small children to prevent the children from accidentally swallowing a cap. These caps should not be placed on syringes intended for outpatient use.

Topical Medications

Topical medication in an ointment or cream vehicle can be repackaged into glass or plastic jars or tubes. Topical creams and gels intended for administration into the vagina may be repackaged into vaginal syringes specifically designed for this purpose. These syringes can be purchased with a tube adapter to fit almost any size tube of ointment or cream.

Beyond-Use Dating, Labeling, and Record Keeping

Labeling is the responsibility of the dispenser, who should take into account the nature of the drug repackaged, the characteristics of the containers, and the storage conditions to which the article may be subjected in order to determine a beyond-use date for the label. *USP 27* offers standards for determining an appropriate expiration date in the absence of published stability data.[3]

Considerable technical advances have occurred in the area of labeling, partly as a result of using computers in institutional practice. In particular, personal computers have greatly improved the quality and efficiency of the label production process. Current federal labeling requirements are described in the *ASHP Technical Assistance Bulletin on Single Unit and Unit Dose Packages of Drugs.* The technical bulletin states that the control number or the lot number should appear on the package. The lot number, which is the number assigned by the repackager to the dosage form being repackaged, is often generated from the date the product is repackaged, and another number or letter is added to designate the order in which the dosage form was repackaged that day. For example,

Lot Number: A111502

was the first product repackaged on November 15, 2002. The second product repackaged on that date would be

Lot Number: B111502.

The repackaging date may also be displayed backwards, as follows:

Lot Number: A021511.

The lot numbering system should be simple to use. The more complicated the system, the greater the likelihood for errors to occur in assigning and interpreting the lot number.

Most labels are applied manually to the finished product, but labeling guns similar to those used in retailing for affixing price labels to goods are available, which make labeling semi-automated.

Standards of practice and government regulation require maintaining accurate and complete records of the repackaging process. Accurate records help in managing inventory and monitoring the efficiency of the repackaging process. Such records can provide a focal point for a quality assurance program and maximize the technician's role in repackaging.

Like labeling systems, most record-keeping systems are now computerized. Although computerized record-keeping programs provide more flexibility in the quantity and type of information that can be gathered, hard copies of certain records, such as sample labels and production sheets, are still needed. The types of repackaging records that should be kept include formulation records, prepackaging records, and daily repackaging logs.

Formulation records give the repackaging technician pertinent information about container type, labeling information, stability, processing equipment, and hazardous materials on a drug-by-drug basis. For example, the following information would be kept on file and referred to each time tamoxifen citrate 10 milligram (mg) tablets are repackaged.

Drug: Tamoxifen citrate

Strength: 10 mg

Dosage form: Oral tablet

Packaging material: Poly-foil to poly-foil

Equipment: MPL strip packager

Precautions: The operator should use gloves and mask during production.

Beyond-use dating: Use FDA guidelines

Repackaging records contain actual information about the drug being repackaged, as in the following example:

Drug: Tamoxifen citrate

Strength: 10 mg

Dosage Form: Oral tablet

Date of repackaging: 11/15/02

Manufacturer's data

Name: XYZ

Lot number: 9AJB57

Beyond-use date: 6/04

Repackager's data

Lot number assigned: A111502-1

Beyond-use date assigned: 05/15/03

Expected yield:_____

Quantity repackaged:_____

Signatures

Person packaging: JG

Person checking: DF

Repackaging records are organized by drug so that several batches can be entered in the same record and contain information on all the repackaging runs of the drug. See Figure 13-1 for an example of a repackaging control record form. Note that because the formulation and repackaging records contain overlapping information, they can be combined into a single record for a given drug. Finally, the repackaging record should have a label, such as the following, affixed:

Tamoxifen citrate: (XYZ)

10 mg oral tablet

Beyond-use date: 051503

Lot number: A111502-1

Anytown Hospital, Anycity

The production worksheet shown in Figure 13-1 lists daily repackaging activity and is used to track production records for a given shift or person. It should contain the following information:

Date

Drug, strength, and form repackaged

Lot number assigned

Quality packaged

Extemporaneous or batch

Name of repackager

This record is not a necessity, but many pharmacies find it helpful in tracking productivity. It can serve an important function in recording lot numbers if lot numbers are determined by the date and order in which products are repackaged.

Quality Control

A well-defined quality control program is essential to ensure the continuous production of high-quality repackaged medications. Because several technicians and pharmacists may deal with many products when repackaging medications, strict adherence to the principles of good manufacturing practices is essential to quality control.

Quality control of repackaging involved in-process controls such as written procedures and end-product testing. In-process controls include written procedures, formal training of the operators of the system, maintenance of equipment, and checkpoints during the process.

Personnel Training and Competency

Formal training programs are important because they promote consistency and standardization. Over time, training programs can pay for themselves by preventing the loss of medication, supplies, and personnel time associated with improper repackaging. Training can extend the life of equipment by teaching proper operating procedures, cleaning and maintenance, and adjustment and repair of malfunctioning machinery. Teaching aids, such as programmed texts and video presentations, are available through professional organizations.

Written Procedures

Technicians should be familiar with the pharmacy's procedures for repackaging. Most procedures will include expectations regarding cleanliness; labeling format; assignment of beyond-use dates; container size in relation to the size or volume of the drug being repackaged; operational procedures for the setup, operation, and cleanup of equipment; the type and detail of records; and quality assurance and testing procedures. Because procedures are usually reviewed and updated annually, it is a good idea to review the procedures with the staff after each update.

Maintenance of Equipment

Most equipment that is used in the repackaging process requires maintenance. Maintenance can be part of the daily operation of the equipment or can be done on a set schedule. Regularly scheduled preventive maintenance can extend the life of equipment, which decreases overhead in the repackaging operation. Preventive maintenance reduces equipment failures and ensures that equipment is operating to the manufacturer's specifications.

Checkpoints

Checkpoints are the steps in the repackaging process that are crucial to ensuring a high-quality package. It is important to double-check each step. Checkpoints include the following:

1. Double-checking to ensure that the drug and dosage form being repackaged are the ones that are supposed to be repackaged. It is also important to ensure that the bulk product has not expired.

2. Double-checking the fill volumes to ensure that the amount of liquid delivered is proper for the dose and the container selected.

3. Double-checking any calculations that may be needed for reconstituting a product to arrive at a given dosage.

4. Double-checking the information (e.g., spelling) on a label, stencil, or computer screen to ensure that the label is complete and accurate.

End-Product Testing

End-product testing is the type of quality control most industries practice. End-product testing requires sampling the final product and determining whether it meets all the standards it met before being repackaged. Examples of end-product testing include testing a sterile product for sterility and testing a package of a solid or liquid oral dosage for moisture impermeability. The uniformity and potency of a product can be tested by a number of chemical analyses. End-product testing is not generally performed for basic repackaging processes, but it may be used more commonly in institutional practice to validate certain types of sterile compounding.

Conclusion

Compounding offers a unique clinical experience in meeting patient needs. Patients benefit from the customized medication and the care of the pharmacist in meeting their needs with dosage forms, routes of administration, or strengths of medication not commercially available. The demand for compounded medications is increasing as more pharmacies offer this service. With the superb technical support provided by compounding support services, compounding pharmacists and technicians offer a new level of patient care. When commercial medications are available but not in the packaging best suited to the needs of the patient or staff, repackaging offers a convenient, cost-effective method of providing medications to the patient.

References

1. USPC. *The United States Pharmacopeia*, 27th rev., and the *National Formulary*, 22nd ed. Rockville, MD: The United States Pharmacopeial Convention; 2003:2346.

2. USPC. *The United States Pharmacopeia*, 22nd rev., and the *National Formulary*, 17th ed. Rockville, MD: The United States Pharmacopeial Convention; 1989.

3. USPC. *The United States Pharmacopeia*, 27th rev., and the *National Formulary*, 22nd ed. Rockville, MD: The United States Pharmacopeial Convention; 2003:2347.

Self-Assessment Questions

1. When preparing compounded medications, what should the compounder avoid?
   a. using gloves to protect hands from chemical contact
   b. using a mask to prevent inhalation of chemical powders
   c. having food or beverages in the preparation area
   d. use of hazardous chemicals

2. Which of the following would not typically be recorded when preparing a compound medication log?
   a. the chemical expiration date
   b. the name or initials of the person preparing the compound
   c. the number of times the preparation has been compounded
   d. the manufacturer of the chemical

3. Which of the following is an example of equipment *not* typically found in a compounding pharmacy?
   a. an ointment mill
   b. mortars and pestles
   c. a capsule-filling machine
   d. a tablet press

4. When choosing repackaging materials, what should one refer to?
   a. *USP* standards
   b. Food and Drug Administration standards
   c. state pharmacy board standards
   d. local health department standards

5. Dispensing units of repackaged medications would *not* commonly include which of the following?
   a. unit-of-use packaging
   b. single-dose packaging
   c. liquid medications
   d. reusable containers

6. Compounded medications would *not* include which of the following?
   a. preparations discontinued by manufacturers
   b. veterinary preparations
   c. unique routes of delivery, such as transdermal administration
   d. medications prepared by a manufacturer

7. Inactive ingredients in compounded medications
   a. never affect the absorption of the medication.
   b. can be used for flavoring.
   c. should not be used as suspending agents.
   d. is never referred to as inert.

8. A compounded medication
   a. does not contain more than one active ingredient.
   b. can contain more than one inactive ingredient.
   c. never mixes chemical powders and liquids.
   d. does not include powder dosage forms.

9. Repackaging records may
   a. be destroyed when the medication supply has been dispensed.
   b. be useful for quality control purposes.
   c. not be used to evaluate whether or not the medication was correctly packaged.
   d. not be inaccurate.

10. Considerations for repackaging materials include
    a. the day of the week to repackage.
    b. the type of packaging material and medication to be repackaged.
    c. the sensitivity of the repackaging person to light.
    d. the time of day when repackaging.

Self-Assessment Answers

1. c. Food or beverages may contaminate the preparation(s) and also may be contaminated by the chemicals in the compounding area.
2. c. Knowing the number of times the preparation has been compounded is not essential to the process, although the other choices are essential.
3. d. Tablets are most commonly prepared in manufacturing.
4. a. *USP* standards are the published standards for repackaging.
5. d. Reusable containers would be difficult to use due to sanitary reasons.
6. d. Compounding, by definition, is not manufacturing.
7. b. Flavorings are commonly used in medications, but are not active ingredients.
8. b. Many compounded medications contain more than one inactive ingredient, such as flavoring and suspending agents.
9. b. Knowing details from repackaging records can be useful in many quality control areas, such as knowing expiration dates, knowing the person who did the repackaging, and so on.
10. b. The repackaged medication may have stability needs, such as light sensitivity, to be met by the materials.

Aseptic Technique, Sterile Compounding, and Intravenous Admixture Programs

14

SCOTT M. MARK

Aseptic technique, along with its application to different dispensing and administration systems and dosage types, is the primary focus of this chapter. Potential risks of parenteral therapy are addressed in the second section of the chapter to emphasize the importance of using the proper techniques and appropriate caution when preparing these products. Nurses are often referred to as the primary caregivers involved in administering the products described in this chapter; however, in some hospitals or home care settings the primary caregiver may be another health care professional, the patient, or the patient's family members. The training and skills of the caregiver, or caregivers, should be taken into consideration when products are prepared and dispensed, because this may influence the intravenous (IV) delivery system chosen for the patient.

The purpose of this chapter is to help the pharmacy technician develop a basic understanding of sterile products and the methods used to prepare them. This chapter should be mastered in sequence with the rest of the *Manual for Pharmacy Technicians*, especially chapters that have related information, including Pharmacy Calculations (Chapter 5), Medication Orders (Chapter 9), and Home Care (Chapter 4). It is also suggested that this chapter be used in conjunction with the ASHP videotapes *Aseptic Preparation of Parenteral Products* and *Safe Handling of Cytotoxic and Hazardous Drugs.*˙ More detailed information is also available in the *ASHP Guidelines on Quality Assurance for Pharmacy-Prepared Sterile Products* (Appendix) and in the book *Compounding Sterile Preparations, 2nd edition*.

Many small hospitals prepare and administer hundreds of sterile products daily, and larger hospitals may prepare thousands. In addition, many patients now receive IV drug therapy in the home. The correct procedures must be followed when preparing IV drug therapy to ensure that the final product is safe and effective. For example, a structured IV admixture program is needed to ensure the stability, sterility, and appropriate

Learning Objectives

After completing this chapter, the technician should be able to

1. Describe the basics of IV drug therapy.

2. Describe the key elements of working in a laminar airflow hood.

3. Perform basic manipulations needed to prepare a sterile product by using aseptic technique.

4. Prepare products for the IV systems most commonly used for IV administration of drugs and fluids.

5. Describe the risks of handling cytotoxic and hazardous drugs.

6. List the steps in drug preparation and handling that are unique to cytotoxic and hazardous drugs.

7. List the typical ingredients of a total parenteral nutrition solution.

8. Describe the manual and automated means of preparing total parenteral nutrition solutions.

9. Describe the benefits of a formal IV admixture program.

labeling of IV products. Technicians and pharmacists work as a team in the IV preparation environment, each with his or her own role and expertise, to ensure that the patient receives the right drug in the right amount.

Drugs are given parenterally if patients cannot take oral medications, if patients have difficulty absorbing medications, if a more rapid onset of action is desired (as in an emergency situation), or if the drug is not available in a suitable oral dosage form. Although the parenteral route of drug administration offers many advantages, it also has some unique preparation requirements that must be followed to ensure that patients are not harmed.

Since the drug or solution is being injected directly into the body, it bypasses the body's barriers to infection.[1] Therefore, it is extremely important that the solution be sterile, that is, free from bacteria or other living organisms. If a contaminated drug or solution is inadvertently injected into a patient, the adverse effects can be fatal. *Aseptic technique* is the term used for all procedures and techniques used to keep a sterile product from becoming contaminated.

Parenteral Drug Administration

Medications can be administered to patients in numerous ways. Medications not given to patients by mouth (enterally) are referred to as being *parenterally* administered. Parenteral administration includes intravenous (IV), intramuscular (IM), intrathecal (IT), epidural, intraarticular, intraarterial, intraocular, intraperitoneal, and subcutaneous (SQ, SC, SubQ) routes of administration. IV solutions are commonly administered to patients to replace body fluids and introduce drugs into the body. Medications do not benefit the patient until they reach the blood and are distributed to the body. IV medications are introduced directly into the blood and therefore have the most rapid onset of action. This route has many benefits over oral medications, which have to be absorbed from the gastrointestinal tract, or IM medications, which have to be absorbed from the muscle mass. IV medications are also beneficial in that they can be given to patients who are unconscious, uncooperative, nauseated, vomiting, or otherwise unable to take oral medications. Direct administration of IV medications

into the blood also provides a predictable rate of administration. Some medications are simply not suitable for IV administration because of their stability or adsorptive properties. IV medications also have disadvantages, such as the risk of infection, the pain of the injection, and the immediate effect of the administration in the event of an error.

Special training is required for all personnel who prepare and administer sterile IV solutions. As mentioned, the process of preparing IV products using predetermined steps to ensure a sterile final product is known as *aseptic technique*. Basic aseptic technique should be used when handling parenteral dosage forms, as well as irrigations and ophthalmics (see Chapter 7, Routes of Administration). This chapter will address the IV route of administration since it is the most common route through which parenteral doses are administered in health systems today.

Risks of IV Therapy

IV therapy offers a rapid, direct means of administering many lifesaving drugs and fluids. A high percentage of IV therapy is administered without any problems, but there are some risks. Many of the issues addressed in this training manual are aimed at teaching proper technique and therefore minimizing the potential for these risks. The following are some reported complications of IV therapy that may increase the risk to patients.[2]

Infection—Infections can result if a product contaminated with microorganisms or pathogens is infused into a patient. Since the IV route bypasses the body's normal barrier system, microorganisms reach the bloodstream directly. These microorganisms may be introduced into products during preparation, administration, or production or through improper storage. The rate of infection or sepsis from contaminated infusions has steadily decreased since health care practitioners and product manufacturers have implemented training, good manufacturing practices (GMPs), and quality assurance programs. Despite these efforts, human touch contamination continues to be the most common source of IV-related contamination.

Air embolus—The incidence of an air embolus is low because many solutions are administered using air-in-line alarms, which are infusion pumps equipped with an alarm that sounds when air is in the IV line. Solutions infused by gravity do not need alarms, because the infusion automatically stops when there is no more fluid for gravity to push through the IV line. Even when a bag runs dry, large amounts of air are not infused. In adults, it takes 15 to 20 milliliters (mL) of air given quickly to result in harm. Infants and pediatric patients are adversely affected by much lower amounts of air.[3] Air-eliminating filters, which also stop air bubbles and add another measure of safety, are available on some IV sets.

Bleeding—IV therapy may or may not cause bleeding. When the IV catheter is removed, bleeding may occur around the catheter site. Also, if the patient has a condition that results in prolonged bleeding time or is receiving an anticoagulant medication, extra care and caution should be used, especially when removing the catheter.

Allergic reaction—When a patient has an allergic reaction to a substance given parenterally, the reaction is usually more severe than if the same substance were given by another route (e.g., by mouth, topically, or rectally). One reason for this is that substances given parenterally cannot be retrieved like substances given by other routes. For example, substances administered topically can often be washed off, those given orally can be retrieved by inducing vomiting or by pumping the stomach, and those given rectally can be flushed out using an enema. When a drug that has caused allergic reactions in a large number of patients is given intravenously, therefore, the patient should be monitored closely. If the likelihood of an allergic reaction is especially high, a test dose (a small amount of the drug) may be given to see how the patient reacts before administering the full dose of the medication.

Incompatibilities—Some drugs are incompatible with other drugs, containers, or solutions. If an incompatibility exists, the drug may precipitate, be inactivated, or adhere to the container. These outcomes are undesirable and may be difficult to detect with the naked eye. A visual inspection of the final product should always be performed to observe any cloudiness or signs of irregularity. Solutions with known or detectable incompatibilities should not be administered to patients.

Extravasation—Extravasation occurs when the IV catheter punctures and exits the vein under the skin, causing drugs to infuse, or infiltrate, into the tissue. Extravasation may take place when the catheter is being inserted or after it is in place if the extremity with the IV catheter is moved or flexed too much. Using a stiff-arm board to prevent excessive movement near the catheter site may help maintain regular flow and prevent extravasation and infiltration, both of which can be painful and usually require that the IV be restarted in a different location. Some drugs, such as certain chemotherapy agents, may cause severe damage

if they infiltrate the tissue. Medications can alleviate some of the effects of the drug and hot and cold compresses can arrest progression, but in some cases the tissue damage can be so severe that it requires surgery or even loss of the limb.

Particulate matter—Particulate matter refers to unwanted particles present in parenteral products that can cause adverse effects to the patient if injected into the bloodstream. Some examples of particulate matter are microscopic glass fragments, hair, lint or cotton fibers, cardboard fragments, undissolved drug particles, and fragments of rubber stoppers, known as cores. Improvements in manufacturing processes have greatly reduced the presence of particulates in commercially available products. Similar care must be taken in the pharmacy to prevent particulate matter from contaminating compounded products. All products should be visually inspected for particulate matter before dispensing. Some institutions use inline filters to help minimize the amount of particulate that reaches the patient.

Pyrogens—Pyrogens, the by-products or remnants of bacteria, can cause reactions (e.g., fever and chills) if injected in large enough amounts. Because a pyrogen can be present even after a solution has been sterilized, great care must be taken to ensure that these substances are not present in quantities that would harm the patient. If the pyrogen is smaller than the filter being used it may be introduced into the bloodstream.

Phlebitis—Phlebitis, or irritation of the vein, may be caused by the IV catheter, the drug being administered (because of its chemical properties or its concentration), the location of the IV site, a fast rate of administration, or the presence of particulate matter. The patient usually feels pain or discomfort, often severe, along the path of the vein. Red streaking may also occur. If phlebitis is caused by a particular drug, it may be helpful to further dilute the drug, give it more slowly, or give it via an IV catheter placed in a larger vein with a higher, faster-moving blood volume.

Types of IV Administration

Medications can be administered intravenously through several different systems or processes. An IV injection is generally a small volume of solution administered directly from a syringe into the vein. When given over a short period of time, an IV injection is referred to as an *IV push*. Solutions that are administered over a longer period of time are known as *IV infusions*. While IV infusions are commonly larger-volume solutions, they may not be in the case of pediatric doses. Infusions can be given either continuously or intermittently. Continuous infusions are given over extended periods of time, while intermittent infusions generally are given over a short period of time, usually to administer medications. In most IV solutions, one or more drugs are added to prepare the final sterile product. The drug is referred to as the *additive* and the final product is referred to as the *admixture*.

Basic Continuous IV Therapy

In the basic setup, the IV fluid is a large-volume parenteral (LVP), usually more than 100 mL, which is hung on an IV pole or other device approximately 36 inches higher than the patient's bed or head. This allows the flow of IV solution to be maintained by gravity (see **Figure 14-1**).[2] Attached to the LVP is a set of sterile tubing that is usually referred to as a primary IV set. The primary IV set extends down from the LVP to a catheter that has been placed in the patient's vein. IV solution setups may differ because of the infusion device or the patient's special needs.

The LVP is usually a simple solution of dilute dextrose, sodium chloride, or both. It may contain additives, such as potassium, if the patient's clinical condition warrants it. The solution is infused continuously to keep blood from clotting in the catheter and plugging it up. The fluid is also used to deliver drugs and to help prevent or reverse dehydration.

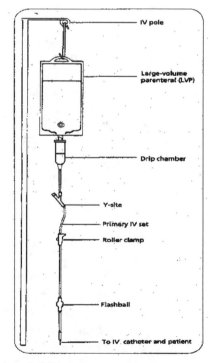

Figure 14-1. A LVP hanging on an IV pole, showing the primary IV set, including drip chamber, Y-site and flashball injection sites, and roller clamp, which can be used to control the flow of fluid.

Administration Systems for Parenteral Products

As mentioned, patients receiving IV therapy usually have either a basic IV setup that includes an LVP solution or a catheter specifically designed for periodic injections (heparin lock, butterfly, etc.). On the basis of the setup, IV drug administration systems are typically classified as either *continuous infusions* or *intermittent injections*.

Continuous Infusions

Some drugs are administered as a continuous infusion because they are more effective and less toxic than when given intermittently. Continuous infusions include basic fluid and electrolyte therapy, blood products, and drugs that require tight administration control to minimize adverse effects.

Intermittent Injections

Intermittent injection systems are used to administer medications that work better when infused at defined time intervals rather than when infused continuously, possibly because periodic administration of the drug increases efficacy or reduces toxicity. Examples of drugs commonly given intermittently are antibiotics and drugs used to treat or prevent gastrointestinal ulcers.

Several types of systems are available for intermittent injections. Each system has advantages and disadvantages related to cost, flexibility, waste rates, and so on. This section addresses how to prepare products for use with each system. Institutional policies dictate specific labeling, expiration dating, and storage conditions, and so they are not addressed here.

Large-Volume Parenterals

LVPs are IV solutions greater than 100 mL in volume. LVPs are usually solutions of dilute dextrose or sodium chloride with or without drug additives and are usually given as continuous infusions, although they may be used for intermittent infusions as well. These preparations may be used in their commercially available form or may have drug additives added in the pharmacy.

Commercially Available

LVPs with additives manufactured in standard concentrations are stable in solution for long periods of time and are available in a variety of sizes (250 mL, 500 mL, 1000 mL) and containers (glass or plastic) depending on the product and its use. Examples include lidocaine, potassium, nitroglycerin, dopamine, bretylium, and aminophylline. Ready-to-use products are advantageous because they reduce handling by the pharmacy and, therefore, the potential for contamination. In some cases these agents are used for emergency situations and may be stocked in the patient care area for immediate access. Standard concentrations of IV medications can decrease potential medication errors in compounding and administration.

Pharmacy Prepared

Some solutions are made in the pharmacy to meet the specific needs of patients. Solutions are prepared in different volumes (250 mL, 500 mL, or 1000 mL) and different containers (glass or plastic, bag or syringe) depending on the drug and its intended use. The preparation of LVPs in the pharmacy should follow the techniques described later in this chapter in the section titled Aseptic Preparation of Parenteral Products.

Syringe Systems

The most common drug delivery systems that use syringes are syringe pumps, volume control chambers, gravity feed, and IV push systems. Syringe systems require that the pharmacy fill syringes with drugs and label them. Drug stability in syringes may differ from the stability of the same drug in other dosage forms because of concentration differences.

Syringe Pumps

Syringes can be used to administer drugs by means of a specially designed syringe pump and tubing set. The pump is adjusted to administer the desired volume from the syringe over a given period of time. Pumps are operated by either a battery or a compressed spring and can administer a single dose per setup or a 12- or 24-hour supply at preprogrammed intervals. Most of these setups require a special small-bore tubing set that determines the rate at which the drug is administered. The pharmacy must supply doses in standard syringe

sizes and concentrations. This procedure allows safer administration to patients, because many syringe pumps are preprogrammed to deliver volumes that are based on standard concentrations.

Volume Control Chambers (Buretrol or Volutrol)

Syringes can be used to administer drugs through a volume control, or volumetric chamber (see **Figure 14-2**). The drug is injected through a port on top of the chamber and solution is added from the primary LVP. This system can use minimal amounts of fluid per dose, a method that may be beneficial in fluid-restricted or pediatric patients. This setup allows for controlled administration of fluids since the nurse can clamp off the solution after the volume in the chamber has infused. Since multiple drugs might be in the chamber at the same time, potential for incompatibilities and unpredictable rates of administration exist. For this reason, it is important that each medication be followed by an IV flush with normal saline. A disadvantage to this system is the increased potential for infection because multiple manipulations may occur.

Gravity Feed

Syringes can be used to administer drugs directly by gravity if a specially designed tubing set is used (see **Figure 14-3**). The set has a vent through which air enters the syringe as fluid is pulled out by gravity. The

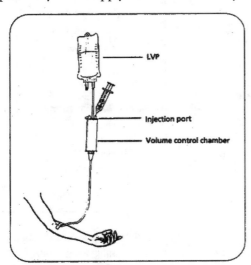

Figure 14-2. A volume control setup.

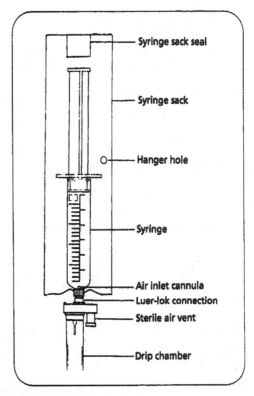

Figure 14-3. A gravity-feed syringe.

syringe is prepared in the pharmacy, labeled, and sent to the nurse for administration. The system is relatively inexpensive and requires no other special equipment.

IV Push

Drugs given by IV push are injected directly into the IV tubing and pushed into the patient quickly (see **Figure 14-4**). The drug is injected into an injection port, a Y-site on the IV tubing, or an injection flashball. The primary IV set usually is clamped off just above the injection port so the drug is delivered to the patient directly, resulting in the rapid onset of the drug's effects.

This system is used in emergencies as well as more routine situations. Disadvantages of the IV push method are that the rate of drug delivery with a syringe is difficult to control and many drugs cause adverse effects when given too quickly.

Small Volume Parenterals ("Piggyback" Systems)

A common method of preparing drugs is adding the drug solution to a small volume parenteral, or piggyback (any IV solution of less than or equal to 100 mL), and labeling it. The nurse simply attaches tubing to the piggyback and connects this secondary IV set to the primary IV set at the proximal Y-site (see **Figure 14-5**). Piggybacking offers the benefits of flexibility and ease of administration.

The piggyback is placed higher than the primary IV (usually an LVP) so that gravity causes the drug solution to run into the patient's vein

before the primary fluid. The back-check valve at the proximal Y-site closes while the piggyback is being administered, thus preventing the piggyback solution from entering the primary IV. Once the piggyback solution has infused, the primary IV resumes flowing. A number of systems are variations of the basic piggyback concept.

Many drugs and doses are available in premixed form. If premixed products are not stable for long periods of time at room temperature, they are often sold frozen and thawed by the pharmacy shortly (hours or days) before being administered. Adding drugs to these solutions is generally not recommended, and most containers do not have an injection port. These solutions are administered and handled by the nurse in the same manner as other piggyback setups.

Add-Vantage®

The Add-Vantage® system (see **Figure 14-6**) uses a specially designed bag and vial that contains drug for reconstitution. The vial is screwed into a special receptacle on the top of the bag. To reconstitute the drug, the vial's stopper is removed from outside of the bag and the stopper remains in the bag. The IV solution then flows from the bag into the vial and dissolves or dilutes the drug. The bag is inverted several times to mix the drug and the IV solution. The bag is then administered to the patient in a fashion similar to the traditional piggyback setup.

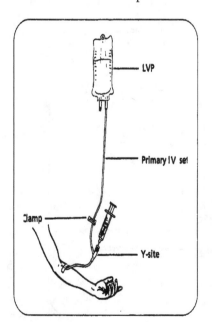

Figure 14-4. IV push setup using a Y-site.

Figure 14-5. A small volume parenteral, or piggyback setup. Note that the piggyback hangs higher than the primary IV.

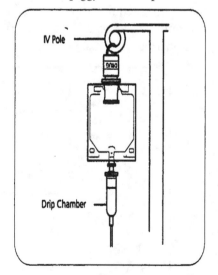

Figure 14-6. The ADD-Vantage® system setup is shown here. Note the special port at the top of the bag, which holds the medication vial.

The act of screwing the vial onto the bag receptacle should be performed in a laminar airflow hood (LAH). The actual vial top and receptacle are sterile and shielded by a protective cover until used. The pharmacy technician removes the cover at the time the vial is screwed on.

The bag's expiration date is usually 30 days after the date the vial is attached and changes to the drug expiration date when the stopper is pulled and the drug is mixed, or activated. For that reason, the pharmacy usually leaves the stopper in place and the nurse pulls it before administering the dose. That way, changes in the drug order do not result in wasted doses.

Vial Spike Systems

The Add-a-Vial® and Mini-Bag Plus® systems are similar in concept to the Add-Vantage® system. The drug-containing vial is attached to the bag in the pharmacy, but it is not activated or mixed until just before administration. The Add-a-Vial® system uses a vial adapter, which has a spike at each end; one spike is inserted into the drug vial and the other is inserted into the injection port of the bag. The Mini-Bag Plus® system (see **Figure 14-7**) uses a special container that has a vial adapter and a breakaway seal. The pharmacy is responsible for attaching the drug-containing vial to the bag.

The Add-a-Vial® spike that is inserted into the bag is snapped off, or the Mini-Bag Plus® breakaway seal is

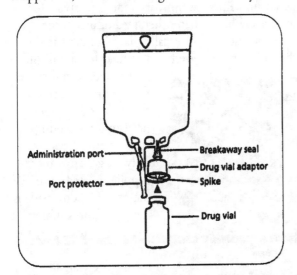

Figure 14-7. The Mini-Bag Plus® system has a special manufacturer's bag equipped with a drug vial adapter. The adapter is pushed down on the vial and snapped into place. The Add-a-Vial® system operates on a similar principle except the drug vial adapter is separate from the bag and is spiked on both ends. It is attached to the drug vial first, then assembled with the bag. With both systems, the assembled product is sent to the nursing unit, where, just prior to administration, the breakaway seal is broken and the solution is mixed with the drug.

broken just before administration, allowing solution from the bag to enter the drug vial and be mixed. The system does not require special vials because the adapters are designed to fit commonly used vial sizes. Add-a-Vial® can be used with various manufacturers' bags. Mini-Bag Plus® requires that the manufacturer's bag be used because the drug vial adapter is attached. With each of these systems, it is important to ensure that the product is activated so that the patient receives the dose of medication.

Premixed Solutions

Bags/bottles containing powder for reconstitution. Some drugs are available in powdered form in final containers of plastic or glass. This system requires that the pharmacy add 20 to 100 mL of sterile diluting fluid, such as 0.9 percent sodium chloride or sterile water for injection, to reconstitute the drug. Once reconstituted and labeled by the pharmacy, these products are administered via piggyback systems. These systems are also referred to as *drug manufacturer piggyback bottles*, or DMPBs.

Controlled-release infusion system.® A method of intermittent drug delivery somewhat different from syringe and piggyback systems is the controlled-release infusion system (CRIS®; see **Figure 14-8**). The CRIS® delivers medication directly from the vial when it is attached to a special adapter that is aligned with the primary IV solution. The drug-containing vial is sent from the pharmacy in ready-to-use form (powders are reconstituted before being dispensed). The nurse attaches the drug vial to the special adapter and turns a dial to direct solution flow through the drug vial and down the tubing. This system presents a labeling

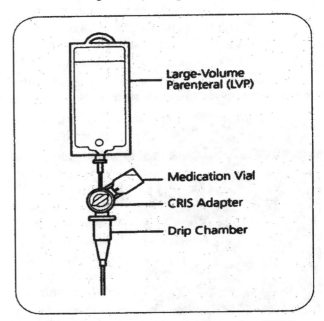

Figure 14-8. The controlled-release infusion system (CRIS®).

challenge to the pharmacy since ready-to-use vials have limited space for patient-specific labels and expiration date stickers. The CRIS® requires a special primary IV set onto which a reconstituted vial of drug fits. The vial is spiked onto the set, and the CRIS® adapter is turned so fluid from the primary IV enters the spiked vial to deliver drug to the patient.

Patient-Controlled Analgesia

A method of drug administration used for injectable pain medications is patient controlled analgesia, or PCA (see **Figure 14-9**), which is very effective in managing pain. Two advantages of PCAs are that they eliminate the need for painful intramuscular injections and they reduce patients' anxiety about controlling their pain. The goal of PCA therapy is to relieve pain as soon as the patient recognizes a need for it. PCA may also reduce nursing time associated with the administration of pain medications. Patients generally are given a basal dose (or constant rate) of drug and can supplement this with a bolus (or immediate dose) of medication as needed.

PCA is usually administered by using either a stationary or portable pump that infuses analgesics directly into an IV line. When the patient pushes a button, the pump releases a programmed amount of the pain medication into the IV tubing. The amount of pain medication is specific for that patient's weight and condition. The pump is also programmed to limit how often the patient will receive pain medication after pushing the button. For example, the pump may be programmed to allow a patient to receive a maximum of 1 mg of morphine sulfate every 15 minutes. When the patient pushes the button, the pump injects 1 mg. If the patient pushes the button again in 10 minutes, the pump does not release drug. If the patient pushes the button at least 5 minutes later (15 minutes since the last injection), the pump again administers 1 mg. This is often referred to as a *15-minute lockout period*.

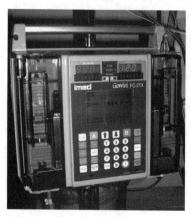

Figure 14-9. A PCA Pump.

PCA preparations may be available commercially or prepared in the pharmacy. Preparation of these products involves the same techniques as other parenteral products. They differ from most other products in two regards. First, if the patient does not have other means of pain control, there may be an urgency to initiate therapy; much of this urgency can be avoided with preplanning among the physician, the nurse, and the pharmacy. Second, these doses usually contain enough medication to last at least 8 hours and often up to 24 hours or more. The result is usually a very large amount of narcotic in one container, necessitating awareness of security issues to prevent diversion or theft.

PCA solutions are sometimes administered subcutaneously. As with IV infusions, PCAs should never be administered without an infusion pump to protect against inadvertent overdosage.

For infusions containing controlled substances, it is common for the final product to be hung in an *IV locking box* (see **Figure 14-10**), which is a plastic box that encases the IV to discourage potential drug diversion.

Unique Infusion Devices and Containers

The delivery systems described thus far meet the needs of typical hospitalized patients. A number of new types of infusion devices and containers have been developed in the past 20 years to meet patient needs not met by the traditional systems. Many of these products are designed to deliver drugs through a compact system that allows the patient to receive therapy outside of the hospital. The system may be drug or therapy specific, such as an implanted pump with a drug reservoir for continuous low-dose chemotherapy administration. This type of system is surgically placed under the skin and the catheter is inserted in a vein. It has a built in

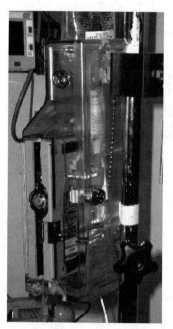

Figure 14-10. IV Lock Box.

power source and space for the drug solution, so the patient does not need to carry a pump, start a new IV periodically, or get any other supplies related to the IV therapy. The downside is that it requires surgery and can be used only for drug therapies administered in very small amounts over long periods of time.

Another type of system uses an elastomeric infusion device (EID) that acts as its own pump, not requiring gravity or a power source. EIDs are similar in concept to a water balloon inside a plastic bottle. The balloon is filled with drug solution and the pressure of the container forces it through the tubing, eliminating the need for a separate pump. These systems, whether used for hospitalized or home care patients, present unique challenges in filling technique, drug stability, and administration methods. Personnel preparing drugs for use in these systems should become familiar with the devices themselves to prevent errors and complications. Some of the commercially available EIDs are the Intermate®, Home Pump®, and Eclipse®. Each device is labeled with a flow rate in mL/hour. The duration of the infusion depends on the volume of drug solution added by the pharmacy.

Administration Sets

Primary IV Set
The primary IV set attached to the LVP can be one of several varieties, but the IV sets that flow by the force of gravity have several common features. The tubing has a drip chamber that is used to estimate the administration rate by counting drops as they fall through the chamber. Drip chambers typically are classified as *macrodrip* or *minidrip* on the basis of the size of the drop that is formed in the drip chamber. Each set of tubing is labeled according to the number of drops it produces from one mL of solution. This number is used to determine how many drops should fall in a minute for the desired volume of mL per hour. Macrodrip sets deliver 10 to 20 drops per mL, and minidrip sets deliver 60 drops per mL.

The rate of flow through the tubing is set by use of a roller clamp rate-controlling device or an electronic infusion device. The roller clamp crimps the IV tubing as it is adjusted to control the flow of fluid. Electronic infusion devices, typically categorized as either pumps or controllers, are used to increase the precision and accuracy of administration. Electronic infusion devices usually are used in fluid-restricted patients or when the IV solution contains a drug that must be administered at a precise rate that cannot be ensured by using the gravity method.

The tubing may have injection ports, either Y-sites or flashballs. Drugs or other solutions can be injected through the injection ports so they can be administered with the main IV solution. The systems used to give drugs through this means vary in setup.

Secondary IV Sets
Drugs that are routinely given through the same basic IV setup usually are attached to a *secondary IV set* that is connected to the primary set (see Figure 14-5).

Venous Access Devices

Peripheral Venous Catheters
Peripheral venous catheters are inserted into a peripheral vein (that is, a vein of the arm, leg, hand, foot, or scalp) or a central vein (that is, in the chest near the heart). The location of the catheter depends, in part, on the contents of the IV solution. Peripheral insertion is more common than central insertion. With peripheral catheters, there are limitations on what can be infused and at what rate. The central catheter is more complicated and riskier to insert and maintain, but it has fewer restrictions on the concentration of drug, rate of administration, and time the venous access can remain in place.

There are several types of peripheral catheters. The most common is plastic because it is flexible and can bend as the vein flexes or moves and is therefore the most comfortable for the patient. Another type is a steel needle with a short end of tubing. This type is referred to commonly as a *scalp vein* or *butterfly* because of its appearance. This type of catheter may be left in the patient's vein even without a running IV if it is periodically flushed (rinsed) with a solution to prevent it from being blocked by blood clots. It is usually used in patients that require IV therapy but are otherwise able to eat and drink, do not require supplemental fluids, and may even be ambulatory.

Central catheters can be temporary, meaning they are used for days or weeks (such as during a hospital stay), or permanent, meaning they can be used for months or years (such as with home care patients or cancer patients who require frequent infusions). The physician inserts temporary central catheters via a minor surgical procedure in the patient's room, which involves a small incision and insertion of the catheter into a vein near the heart. Permanent placement of central catheters also involves minor surgery, but it must be done in an operating room. The central catheter gives direct access into a vein that has a high flow of blood; therefore, solutions that might be irritating or damaging to peripheral blood vessels, which have a lower blood flow, are given centrally.

Two commonly used permanent catheters are the Hickman® and the Broviac®. Each of these is a tunnel catheter, which remains outside the body to provide readily available access for patients receiving multiple injections. Port-a-cath® catheters are another form of central injection port that is located below the skin. Another type of catheter that offers some of the benefits of both central and peripheral catheters is called a peripherally inserted central catheter (PICC). The PICC line, as its name implies, is inserted peripherally, but it is a long flexible catheter that is threaded through the venous system and its tip ends near the heart, where there is a high volume of blood flow. Caution needs to be exercised when manipulating all catheters, as they can become seeded or colonized with bacteria and become a source of infection. (For additional information on central lines, see Chapter 4, Home Care Pharmacy Practice.)

Heparin Lock

Heparin locks (see **Figure 14-11**) are used to maintain catheter access to a vein without having to run a continuous drip to keep the vein open. Heparin locks have an IV catheter or needle on one end and a resealable rubber diaphragm on the other end. The main purpose of a Heparin lock is to provide a port through which medications can be administered intermittently. The concentration of heparin used in heparin locks is usually 10 units or 100 units per mL.

Needleless Systems

Needleless systems are becoming a cost-effective alternative to traditional needle systems. They reduce the risks of needle sticks and, subsequently, the potential risk of disease transmission to health care workers who regularly draw blood or administer medications to patients. Some states and some health care systems require needleless systems by law. Needleless systems contain specially designed components, which may include a *cannula* (see **Figure 14-12**), or positive pressure cap, that may be directly connected to a syringe tip and a needleless injection site. Cannulas function like a needle, but contain a blunt tip. The injection site must have the ability to accept the cannula.

Final Filters

Final filters are inline filters located in the tubing used for drug administration. Final filters can be used to remove particles that may be present in the IV solution but are not visible to the naked eye. These particles, although small, can be harmful to patients if they become trapped in small capillaries or accumulate in the body. Final filters should be used with drugs prepared from ampules and any drug where particulate matter is commonly found in the final solution.

Aseptic Preparation of Parenteral Products

As the use of parenteral therapy continues to expand, the need for well-controlled admixture preparation has also grown. Recognizing this need, many pharmacy departments have devoted increased resources to programs that ensure the aseptic preparation of sterile products. These programs focus on the following main elements:[4,5]

- development and maintenance of good aseptic technique in the personnel who prepare and administer sterile products

- development and maintenance of a sterile compounding area, complete with sterilized equipment and supplies

- development and maintenance of the skills needed to properly use an LAH

Aseptic Technique

Aseptic technique is a means of manipulating sterile products without compromising their sterility. Proper use of the LAH and strict aseptic technique are the most important factors in preventing the contamination of sterile products. Thorough training in the proper use of the LAH and strict aseptic technique, followed by the development of conscientious work habits, is therefore of utmost importance to any sterile products program.

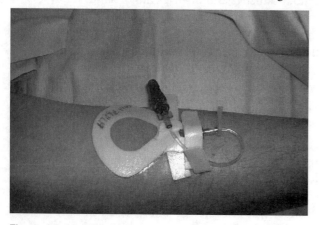

Figure 14-11. Heparin Lock.

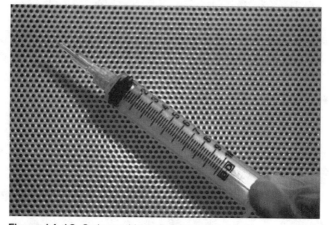

Figure 14-12. Syringe with cannula.

Sterile Compounding Area (Clean Room)

Sterile parenteral solutions must be free of living microorganisms, pyrogens, and visible particles. Room air typically contains thousands of suspended particles per cubic foot, most of which are too small to be seen with the naked eye. These contaminants include dust, pollen, smoke, and bacteria. Reducing the number of particles in the air improves the environment in which sterile products are prepared. These particles can be reduced by following several practices to maintain the sterile compounding area.

A sterile compounding area should be cleaned daily and segregated from normal pharmacy operations, patient specimens, nonessential equipment, and other materials that produce particles. For example, the introduction of cardboard into the clean environment should be avoided; traffic flow into a clean area should be minimized; floors should be disinfected periodically; and trash should be removed frequently and regularly. In addition, care should be taken to take the trashcans outside of the IV room before removing the trash from the container. This will minimize the creation of particulate matter or the risk of spills in the IV room. Other, more sophisticated aspects of clean-room design include special filtration or treatment systems for incoming air (see **Figure 14-13**), ultraviolet irradiation, air-lock entry portals, sticky mats to remove particulate matter from shoes, and positive room air pressure to reduce contaminant entry from adjacent rooms or hallways. Clean rooms are often adjoined by an *anteroom* that is used for nonaseptic activities related to the clean-room operation, such as order processing, gowning, and handling of stock.

Sterile products should be prepared in Class 100 environments, which means they contain no more than 100 particles per cubic foot that are 0.5 micron or larger in size. LAHs are frequently used to achieve a Class 100 environment.

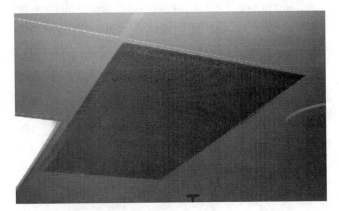

Figure 14-13. Ceiling HEPA Filter.

Laminar Airflow Hoods

The underlying principle of LAHs is that twice-filtered laminar layers of aseptic air continuously sweep the work area inside the hood to prevent the entry of contaminated room air. There are two common types of laminar flow hoods: horizontal flow and vertical flow.

Horizontal LAHs sweep filtered air from the back of the hood to the front (see **Figure 14-14**). Horizontal flow hoods use an electrical blower to draw contaminated room air through a prefilter. The prefilter, which is similar to a furnace filter, removes only gross contaminants and should be cleaned or replaced on a regular basis. The prefiltered air is then pressurized to ensure that a consistent distribution of airflow is presented to the final filtering apparatus. The final filter constitutes the entire back portion of the hood's work area. This *high efficiency particulate air*, or HEPA, filter removes 99.97 percent of particles that are 0.3 micron or larger, thereby eliminating airborne microorganisms, which are usually 0.5 microns or larger.

Vertical LAHs have a vertical flow of filtered air. In vertical LAHs, HEPA-filtered air emerges from the top and passes downward through the work area (Figure 14-14). Because exposure to some antineoplastic (anticancer) drugs may be harmful, these drugs should

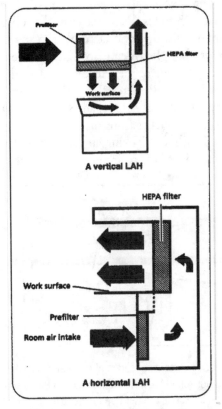

Figure 14-14. Horizontal and vertical laminar flow hoods with the basic components labeled.

be prepared only in vertical LAHs to minimize the risk of exposure to airborne drug particulates. The types of vertical LAHs used for the preparation of anti-neoplastics contain airflow within the hood and are referred to as biological safety cabinets (BSCs). BSCs and the preparation of antineoplastics and cytotoxic medications are covered later in this chapter.

The critical principle of using LAHs is that nothing should interrupt the flow of air between the HEPA filter and the sterile object. The space between the HEPA filter and the sterile object is known as the *critical area*. The introduction of a foreign object between a sterile object and the HEPA filter increases wind turbulence in the critical area, and contaminants from the foreign object may be carried onto the sterile work surface and thereby contaminate the injection port, needle, or syringe. To maintain sterility, nothing should pass behind a sterile object in a horizontal LAH or above a sterile object in a vertical LAH.

All materials placed within the LAH disturb the patterned flow of air blowing from the HEPA filter. This *zone of turbulence* created behind an object could potentially extend outside the hood, pulling or allowing contaminated room air into the aseptic working area (see **Figure 14-15**). When laminar airflow is moving on all sides of an object, the zone of turbulence extends approximately 3 times the diameter of that object. When laminar airflow is not accessible to an object on all sides (for example, when placed adjacent to a vertical wall), a zone of turbulence is created that may extend 6 times the diameter of the object (see Figure 14-15). For these reasons, it is advisable to work with objects at least 6 inches from the sides and front edge of the hood without blocking air vents; that way, unobstructed airflow is maintained between the HEPA

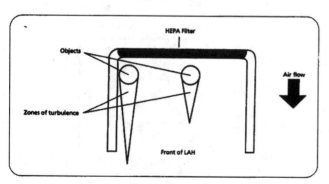

Figure 14-15. Examples of zones of turbulence created behind objects in a horizontal LAH. Notice that the zone of turbulence of the object on the left is greater due to the object's proximity to the side of the hood, and has extended outside of the LAH. (Note: figure is not drawn to scale.)

filter and sterile objects. The hands should also be positioned so airflow in the critical area between the HEPA filter and sterile objects is not blocked.

The following are general principles for operating LAHs properly:

- An LAH should be positioned away from excess traffic, doors, air vents, or anything that could produce air currents capable of introducing contaminants into the hood.

- If the LAH is turned off, nonfiltered, nonsterile air will occupy the LAH work area. Therefore, when it is turned back on, it should be allowed to run for 15 to 30 minutes before it is used. (Manufacturer's recommendations should be consulted for each hood.) This allows the LAH to blow the nonsterile air out of the LAH work area. Then the LAH can be cleaned for use.

- Before use, all interior working surfaces of the LAH should be cleaned with 70 percent isopropyl alcohol or another appropriate disinfecting agent and a clean, lint-free cloth. Cleaning should be performed from the HEPA filter in a side-to-side motion beginning in the rear of the hood toward the front of the LAH (in a horizontal LAH), so contaminants are moved out of the hood. The hood should be cleaned often throughout the compounding period and when the work surface becomes dirty. Some materials are not soluble in alcohol and may initially require water to be removed. After the water is applied and wiped off, the surface should be cleaned with alcohol. In addition, Plexiglas sides, found on some types of LAHs, should be cleaned with warm, soapy water rather than alcohol. Spray bottles of alcohol should not be used in the hood because they do not allow for the physical action of cleaning the hood, they can accidentally damage the HEPA filter, and they do not ensure that alcohol is applied to all areas of the surface to be cleaned. Once applied, alcohol should also be allowed to air dry, which will increase its effectiveness as a disinfectant.

- Nothing should be permitted to come in contact with the HEPA filter. This includes cleaning solution, aspirate from syringes, and glass from ampules. Ampules should not be opened directly toward the filter.

- Only objects essential to product preparation should be placed in the LAH. Do not put paper, pens, labels, or trays into the hood.

- Jewelry should not be worn on the hands or wrists when working in the LAH because it may introduce bacteria or particles into the clean work area.

- Actions such as talking and coughing should be directed away from the LAH working area, and any unnecessary motion within the hood should be avoided to minimize the turbulence of airflow.

- Smoking, eating, and drinking are prohibited in the aseptic environment.

- All aseptic manipulations should be performed at least 6 inches from the sides and front edge of the hood to prevent the possibility of potential contamination caused by the closeness of the worker's body and backwash contamination resulting from turbulent air patterns developing where LAH air meets room air.

- LAHs should be tested by qualified personnel every 6 months, whenever the hood is moved, or if filter damage is suspected. Specific tests are used to certify airflow velocity and HEPA filter integrity.

Although the LAH provides an aseptic environment that is safe for the manipulation of sterile products, it is essential that strict aseptic technique be used in conjunction with proper hood operation. The technician must remember that the use of the LAH alone, without the observance of aseptic technique, cannot ensure product sterility.

Personal Attire

The first component of good aseptic technique is proper personal attire. Clean garments, which are relatively particulate free, should be worn when preparing sterile products. Clean-room attire will depend on institutional policies and often are related to the type of product being prepared (see Appendix). Many facilities provide clean scrub suits or gowns for this purpose. Scrub suits should not be worn home to ensure that no contaminants are transported home and that the process of cleaning the clothing does not introduce lint onto the low-lint clothing. In addition, suits should be covered up when leaving the pharmacy to minimize the contamination from other areas, such as the cafeteria. Hair covers and shoe covers help reduce particulate or bacterial contamination, and the use of surgical masks and gloves is warranted as well. Nail polish and artificial nails should not be worn. Many facilities also require that all facial hair be covered.

Handwashing

Touching sterile products while compounding is the most common source of contamination of pharmacy-prepared sterile products. The fingers harbor countless bacterial contaminants, so proper hand washing is extremely important. The technician should scrub hands, nails, wrists, and forearms thoroughly for at least 30 seconds with a brush, warm water, and appropriate bactericidal soap before performing aseptic manipulations. Hands should be washed frequently and every time workers re-enter the sterile compounding area. Although many institutions require the use of sterile gloves to reduce touch contamination, the technician should be careful to avoid a false sense of security. Sterile gloves are sterile only until they touch something unsterile or until they are torn and allow bacteria from the hands to enter the work area. For example, if it becomes necessary to scratch or touch the face while wearing gloves, the gloves will need to be changed or disinfected with a foam hand sanitizer. For these reasons, washing bare hands thoroughly before unwrapping and putting on the gloves is necessary. Occasionally workers develop allergies to latex as a result of repeated use of latex gloves. As a result, many institutions have now turned to using only nonlatex gloves. Workers who have open sores on their hands or have an upper respiratory tract infection should inform their supervisor or consult their institution's quality assurance procedures. Often such procedures will require that they be removed from the work environment or employ additional precautions while working in the sterile compounding area.

Equipment and Supplies

In addition to hand washing, the correct use of appropriate sterile equipment and supplies, including syringes and needles, is another important factor in aseptic preparation of sterile products.

Syringes

Syringes are made of either glass or plastic. Most drugs are more stable in glass, so glass syringes are most often used when medication is to be stored in the syringe for an extended period. Some medications may react with the plastics in the syringe, which would alter the potency or stability of the final product. Disposable plastic syringes are most frequently used in preparing sterile products because they are inexpensive, durable, and are in contact with substances only for a short time, which minimizes the potential for incompatibility with the plastic itself.

Syringes are composed of a barrel and plunger (see **Figure 14-16**). The plunger, which fits inside the barrel, has a flat disk or lip at one end and a rubber piston at the other. The top collar of the barrel prevents the syringe from slipping during manipulation; the tip is where the needle attaches. To maintain sterility of the product, the technician should not touch the syringe tip or the plunger. Many syringes have a locking mechanism at the tip, such as the Luer lock, which secures the needle within a threaded ring. Some syringes, such as slip-tip syringes, do not have a locking mechanism. In that case, friction holds the needle on the syringe.

Syringes are available in numerous sizes, ranging from 0.5 to 60 mL. Calibration marks on syringes represent different increments of capacity, depending on the size of the syringe. Usually, the larger the syringe capacity, the larger the interval between calibration lines. For example, each line on the 10 mL syringes represents 0.2 mL, but each line on the 30 mL syringes represents 1 mL.

To maximize accuracy, the smallest syringe that can hold a desired amount of solution should be used. Syringes are accurate to one-half of the smallest increment marking on the barrel. For example, a 10 mL syringe with 0.2 mL markings is accurate to 0.1 mL and can be used to measure 3.1 mL accurately. A 30 mL syringe with 1 mL markings, however, is only accurate to 0.5 mL and should not be used to measure a volume of 3.1 mL. Ideally, the volume of solution should take up only one-half to two-thirds of the syringe capacity, which avoids inadvertent touch contamination caused when the syringe plunger is pulled all the way back.

When measuring with a syringe, the final edge (closest to the tip of the syringe) of the plunger piston, which comes in contact with the syringe barrel, should be lined up to the calibration mark on the barrel, which corresponds to the volume desired (see **Figure 14-17**).

Syringes are sent from the manufacturer assembled and individually packaged in paper overwraps or plastic covers. The sterility of the contents is guaranteed as long as the outer package remains intact; therefore, packages should be inspected, and any that are damaged should be discarded. The syringe package should be opened within the LAH to maintain sterility. The wrapper should be peeled apart and not ripped or torn. To minimize particulate contamination, the discarded packaging or unopened syringes should not be placed on the LAH work surface.

Syringes may come from the manufacturer with a needle attached or with a protective cover over the syringe tip. The syringe tip protector should be left in place until it is time to attach the needle. For attaching needles to Luer lock-type syringes, a quarter-turn is usually sufficient to secure the needle to the syringe.

Needles

Like syringes, needles are commercially available in many sizes. Two numbers, gauge and length, describe the needle size. The gauge of the needle corresponds to the diameter of its bore, which is the diameter of the inside of the shaft. The larger the gauge, the smaller the needle bore. For example, the smallest needles have a gauge of 27, while the largest needles have a gauge of 13. The length of a needle shaft is measured in inches and usually ranges from 3/8 to 3 1/2 inches.

The components of a simple needle are the shaft and the hub (see **Figure 14-18**). The hub attaches the needle to the syringe and is often color-coded to correspond to a specific gauge. The tip of the needle shaft is slanted to form a point. The slant is called the *bevel*, and the point is called the *bevel tip*. The opposite end of the slant is termed the *bevel heel*.

Needles are sent from the manufacturer individually packaged in paper and plastic overwraps with a protective cover over the needle shaft. This guarantees the sterility as long as the package remains intact. Therefore, packages that are damaged should be discarded.

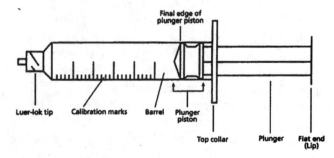

Figure 14-16. A syringe with the basic components labeled.

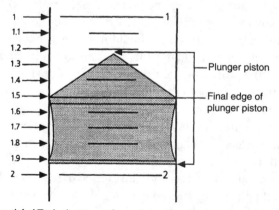

Figure 14-17. A close-up of a syringe showing how to measure 1.5 mL. Note that the final edge of the plunger piston is used to make the measurement.

No part of the needle should be touched. Needles should be manipulated by their overwrap and protective covers only. The protective cover should be left in place until the needle or syringe is ready to be used. A needle shaft is usually metal and is lubricated with a sterile silicone coating so that latex vial tops can be penetrated smoothly and easily. For this reason, needles should never be swabbed with alcohol.

Some needles are designed for special purposes and therefore have unique characteristics. For example, needles designed for batch filling have built-in vents (vented needles) to avoid the need to release pressure that might form in the vial. Another example is needles with built-in filters, which are intended for use with products requiring frequent filtering, such as drugs removed from a glass ampule.

When dealing with small volumes, it is important to account for the volume of solution left in the hub of the needle. As much as 0.3 mL may be present in the hub of the needle, which could represent a significant amount of the dose for a pediatric patient. When drawing up solutions using a needle, this volume remains in the hub of the needle. Thus, when removing the needle and replacing it with a cannula, this volume is discarded and the patient does not receive the correct amount of medication. It may be necessary to dilute the product to increase the volume or provide overfill in the syringe to account for this. The technician should consult his or her institution's policies and procedures for guidance.

Drug Additive Containers

Injectable medications may be supplied in an ampule, vial, or prefilled syringe. Each requires a different technique to withdraw medication and place it in the final dosage form.

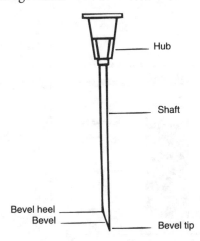

Figure 14-18. A needle with the basic components labeled.

Vials

Medication vials are glass or plastic containers with a rubber stopper secured to the top, usually by an aluminum cover. Vials differ from ampules in that they are used to hold both powders and liquids. A flip-top cap or aluminum cover usually protects the rubber stopper.

Protective covers do not guarantee sterility of the rubber stopper. Therefore, before the stopper is penetrated, it must be swabbed with 70 percent isopropyl alcohol and allowed to dry. The correct swabbing technique is to make several firm strokes in the same direction over the rubber closure, always using a clean swab. Swabbing helps achieve sterility in two ways: First, the alcohol acts as a disinfecting agent, and second, the physical act of swabbing in one direction removes particles.

When piercing vials with needles, the technician should avoid coring fragments out of the rubber stopper with the needle. A core is carved out of the rubber stopper when the bevel tip and the bevel heel do not penetrate the stopper at the same point. To prevent core formation, the stopper should first be pierced with the bevel tip and then pressed downward and toward the bevel as the needle is inserted (see **Figure 14-19**).

Vials are closed-system containers, because air or fluid cannot pass freely in or out of them. In most cases, air pressure inside the vial is similar to that of room air. To prevent the formation of a vacuum inside the vial (less pressure inside the vial than in the room), the user should normalize pressure by first injecting into the vial a volume of air equal to the volume of fluid that is going to be withdrawn. This step should not be done with drugs that produce gas when they are reconstituted, such as ceftazidime, or with cytotoxic medications.

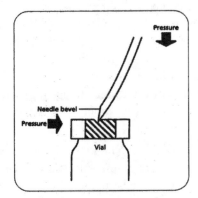

Figure 14-19. A non-coring technique of piercing a vial with a needle. Note that the needle is held on an angle—the bevel tip will pierce the vial first. As downward pressure is applied, there is a slight bend in the needle, and the bevel heel will enter through the opening made by the bevel tip.

If the drug within a vial is in powdered form, it has to be reconstituted. The technician should inject the desired volume of sterile diluting solution (the *diluent*), such as sterile water for injection, into the vial containing the powdered drug. An equal volume of air must be removed to prevent positive pressure from developing inside the vial. This is particularly important when dealing with medications that can be harmful if expelled into the air. The air should be allowed to flow into the syringe before the needle is removed from the vial, or a vented needle should be used, which allows displaced air to escape the vial through a vent in the needle. Care must be taken to ensure that the drug is completely dissolved before proceeding. Usually, gentle shaking adequately dissolves the drug contents. Some agents cannot be shaken because this will degrade the active ingredient (e.g., some biologic products, some investigational agents). As always, if the user is not familiar with preparation methods for the product, he or she should consult the package information or a supervisor.

Vials with drugs in solution are classified as *multiple-dose* (also called *multiple-use* or *multi-dose*). Multiple-dose vials contain a small amount of a preservative agent, added to retard the growth of bacteria or other organisms that may inadvertently contaminate a product. The presence of these substances does not make the solution self-sterilizing, and the use of strict aseptic technique is still required. Preservatives are included in "bacteriostatic water for injection" and any multiple-dose product. Common substances used as preservatives include benzyl alcohol, parabens, phenol, and benzalkonium chloride. The manufacturer typically adds these substances in small quantities that are not harmful when the product is dosed appropriately. Therefore, if a preparation calls for large amounts of drug solution that contains a preservative or a diluent with a preservative, the technician should consult the pharmacist to verify that the total amount of preservative to be administered will not be toxic. Because of their toxicity, solutions with preservatives should not be used for epidural or intrathecal dosage forms and should only be used with caution in pediatric or neonatal preparations.

Single-dose vials have no preservative and are intended to be used one time only. Once a vial is entered with a needle, whether in a patient care area or an LAH, it should be discarded.

Ampules

Ampules are composed entirely of glass and, once broken (i.e., opened), become open-system containers.

Since air or fluid may now pass freely in and out of the container, it is not necessary to replace the volume of fluid to be withdrawn with air.

Before an ampule is opened, any solution visible in the top portion (*head*) should be moved to the bottom (*body*) by swirling the ampule in an upright position, tapping the ampule with one's finger, or inverting the ampule and then quickly swinging it into an upright position (see **Figure 14-20**).

To open an ampule, the head must be broken from the body. To make the break properly, the ampule neck is cleansed with an alcohol swab. The swab should be left in place because it can prevent accidental cuts to the fingers as well as shattering of glass particles and aerosolized drug. The head of the ampule should be held between the thumb and index finger of one hand, and the body should be held with the thumb and index finger of the other hand. Pressure should be exerted on both thumbs, pushing away from oneself in a quick motion to snap open the ampule. Ampules should not be opened toward the HEPA filter of the LAH or toward other sterile products within the hood. Extreme pressure may result in crushing of the head between the thumb and index finger. Therefore, if the ampule does not open easily, it should be rotated so that pressure on the neck is at a different point. Some ampules are scored or have designated pressure points to facilitate opening. Reusable plastic openers are available in various sizes to open ampules. They provide greater protection but must be kept clean.

To withdraw medication from an ampule, the ampule should be tilted and the bevel of the needle placed in the corner space (or *shoulder*) near the opening. Surface tension should keep the solution from spilling out of the tilted ampule. The syringe plunger is then pulled back to withdraw the solution.

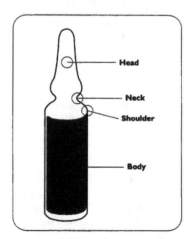

Figure 14-20. An ampule with the basic components labeled.

The use of a filter needle (e.g., a needle with a 5-micron filter in the hub) keeps glass or paint chips that may have fallen into the solution from being drawn into the syringe. To withdraw the solution, either use a filter needle and change to a regular needle before expelling the contents or start with a regular needle and change to a filter needle before expelling the contents. Either way, the filter needle must not be used for both withdrawing from the ampule and expelling from the syringe because doing so would nullify the filtering effect. Usually the medication is withdrawn from the ampule with a regular needle and then the needle is changed to a filter needle before pushing the drug out of the syringe. If the syringe is used as a final container for dispensing, a filter needle should be used to withdraw the solution. Sometimes, a medication (e.g., a suspension) may need to be withdrawn from an ampule with a regular needle so the active ingredient is not filtered out in the process.

Another device that can be used for withdrawing solutions from an ampule is the filter straw. The filter straw differs from the filter needle in that it is made out of plastic tubing rather than metal and it is longer, making it easier to reach the bottom of an ampule. The filter straw also reduces the risk of needle sticks during the manipulation because it does not have a sharp tip. Once the solution is withdrawn with a filter straw, however, a regular needle must be attached to the syringe to inject the solution into its final container.

Prefilled Syringes

Manufacturers produce a number of products that are packaged in ready-to-inject syringes. Drugs commonly given IM, IV, or SC are packaged this way to make them convenient for the health care provider. This packaging is also used if the drug is commonly used in emergency situations, because a prefilled syringe saves time. Prefilled syringes often have calibrations on the syringe barrel and are labeled with the concentration and total volume. These products may be used in the pharmacy to prepare sterile products but are more likely to be kept in patient care areas.

Preparation of IV Admixtures

The usual process for preparing an admixture is that an order is received in the pharmacy and reviewed by the pharmacist. If the order is deemed reasonable and appropriate, the pharmacist will input the information into the pharmacy records (usually by entering it into a pharmacy computer system) to document the preparation and generate a label. The pharmacist then assigns the preparation of the product to support personnel. The following sequence describes the common steps technicians follow to prepare IV admixtures. However, keep in mind that the final IV admixture may be prepared in a variety of containers, including flexible plastic bags, glass bottles, and semirigid plastic containers.

Before compounding, the technician assembles all materials and visually inspects vials, ampules, and IV solution containers for signs of cloudiness, particulate matter, cracks and punctures, expiration dates, and anything else that may indicate the product is defective. It is also important to ensure that an appropriate supply of all materials is available to complete the tasks. The technician places only materials that are necessary to prepare the product in the LAH.

Next, the technician will disinfect all injection surfaces and allow them to dry. The drug fluid is withdrawn from its container and measured, using the syringe size closest to the volume to be withdrawn. To obtain as accurate a measurement as possible, the technician should remove air bubbles from the syringe by first pulling back slightly on the plunger to draw any fluid trapped in the needle into the syringe barrel, then tap the barrel and slightly depress the plunger.

Flexible Plastic Bags

Flexible plastic bags made of polyvinyl chloride (PVC) are used frequently. They are easier to store, are less breakable than glass bottles, and eliminate the need to vent the container when removing fluid.

PVC bags are available in several sizes and contain a variety of solutions. They are packaged in plastic overwraps designed to limit fluid loss. The protective overwrap should not be removed from a PVC bag until it is ready to be used. To minimize air turbulence in the critical area, the injection port of a PVC bag, which is covered by an outside latex tip diaphragm, should be positioned toward the HEPA filter when preparing an IV admixture.

To add a drug to a PVC bag, a needle is inserted into the injection port and the appropriate volume of drug fluid is injected. A needle longer than 3/8 inch should be used because the injection port of the PVC bag has two diaphragms that must be pierced (see **Figure 14-21**). The outside diaphragm is the outside latex tip; the inside diaphragm, which is plastic, is about 3/8 inch inside the injection portal. (Note: Individual manufacturer's products may differ in appearance, but the design concept is the same.)

Glass Containers

To add a drug to a glass infusion container, the technician first removes the protective cap from the IV bottle, then swabs the rubber stopper or latex diaphragm with alcohol, lets it dry, and injects the drug fluid. To insert needles through rubber stoppers, the previously described noncoring technique should be used (see Figure 14-19). After admixing, a protective seal should be placed over the stopper of the glass container before it is removed from the LAH.

Semirigid Containers

When using a polyolefin, semirigid container for admixture preparation, the technician should remove the protective screw cap and add drugs through the designated injection portal. Disinfecting the portal and replacing the protective cap are not necessary.

Disposal of Supplies

Syringes and uncapped needles should be discarded according to institutional policy. In some institutions they are discarded in puncture-resistant, sealable containers, often called *sharps* containers. If the pharmacist needs the syringe to verify the amount of drug added to the admixture, institutions may allow needles used in compounding to be recapped for removal and disposal. When a syringe is used to verify the amount of drug added, the plunger is drawn back to the calibration mark to indicate the amount. Then the syringe and the drug vial are placed next to the completed and labeled product for the pharmacist to verify. It should be noted that recapping needles is generally considered to be an unsafe practice. Most institutions have policies against recapping needles, as required by OSHA and the CDC, to decrease the risk of needle-stick injuries with contaminated needles. Contaminated, uncapped needles and syringes must be disposed of in puncture-resistant containers. If recapping of needles is required, a one-handed scoop method should be used. For worker safety, two-handed recapping is never an acceptable practice.

Luer Locks

When the final product being dispensed is not intended for injection (such as an aerosol) a Luer lock tip (see **Figure 14-22**) may be placed on it to maintain sterility. These are attached either by friction or threaded grooves. Luer locks may also be used on syringes prepared for use with needleless systems.

Seals and Closures

Once a port has been penetrated with a needle, it will need to be properly sealed to reduce the risk of contamination from bacteria. The most common seals used are IV additive (IVA) seals, which are placed over the sterile port of a vial or a final product. These seals are made from aluminum and have a sterile pad in the center that maintains contact with the port to ensure the sterility. Other closures may include tamperproof caps that are placed on bottles or IV bags to prevent tampering. Tamperproof caps are commonly used on IV preparations containing controlled substances to discourage drug diversion once the product has left the pharmacy. Injection ports on IV bags are often sealed with metallic adhesive seals in the LAH after an admixture is made.

Automated Syringe Filling Equipment

Traditional syringe filling equipment involves the use of a portable minipump, which can be preprogrammed to dispense preset volumes into syringes. New technology has produced equipment that prepares and labels IV syringes ready for dispensing. These automated syringe filling cabinets receive data from the pharmacy computer system instructing them to prepare the appropriate patient doses. They then pull from a selection of drug vials that are preloaded into the cabinet, using

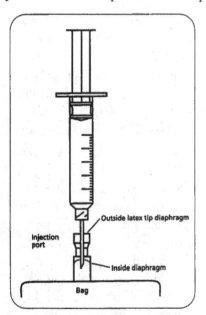

Figure 14-21. A syringe penetrating the injection port of a PVC bag. The needle must be long enough (greater than 3/8 inch) to penetrate the inside diaphragm. (Note: figure is not drawn to scale.)

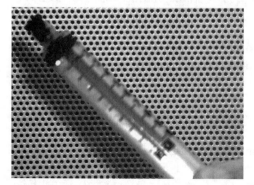

Figure 14-22. Luer Tip.

bar-code verification. The vial is swabbed and reconstituted, and the appropriate amount of final product is removed and labeled for dispensing.

Labeling

Once an IV admixture or other sterile product is compounded, it should be properly labeled with the following information:

1. Patient name, identification number, and room number (if inpatient)

2. Bottle or bag sequence number, when appropriate

3. Name and amount of drug(s) added

4. Name and volume of admixture solution

5. Approximate final total volume of the admixture, when applicable

6. Prescribed flow rate (in mL per hour)

7. Date and time of scheduled administration

8. Date and time of preparation

9. Expiration date

10. Initials of person who prepared and person who checked the IV admixture

11. Auxiliary labeling—supplemental instructions and precautions.

Many labels now also contain a bar code that contains information on the medication, the patient, and the anticipated administration. The pharmacy computer generates these bar codes to reduce the frequency of medication administration errors, and to facilitate charge and credit capture.

After the admixture is properly labeled, it is given a final inspection for cores and particulates. The pharmacist should check all drug and IV solution containers used in preparing the admixture to verify that the technician added the proper amount of the correct drug to the correct IV solution. A registered pharmacist must validate the label and final sterile product against the order for accuracy and completeness before dispensing it for patient use.

Each product should also include an expiration date beyond which it should not be used. This date might include a time 24 hours after preparation so that unused preparations are returned for potential reuse or it might reflect the actual time that the product is considered stable. Typically drugs are considered stable as long as they are within 10 percent of their labeled potency. Sterility concerns also factor into the assignment of expiration times. The pharmacist should assign the expiration time.

Methods for assigning those times, for both standard and nonstandard preparations, should be reflected in policies and procedures and substantiated by references, literature, or reasonable professional judgment.

Preparation and Handling of Cytotoxic and Hazardous Drugs

Some medications can be hazardous to those who touch or inhale them. Because hazardous drugs initially involved drugs used in treating cancer, the terms *antineoplastic* and *chemotherapeutic* were used to describe them. The term *cytotoxic*, or *cell killer*, was later used to refer to any agent that may be genotoxic, oncogenic, mutagenic, teratogenic, or hazardous in any way. Exposure to antineoplastics, as well as immunosuppressants, antiviral agents, and biological response modifiers, may pose some of these risks. Hazardous agents require special handling procedures to minimize the potential for accidental exposure.

Contact with hazardous drugs can cause immediate problems, such as dermatitis, dizziness, nausea, and headache.[7] Studies also suggest that repeated exposure to small amounts of the drugs may cause organ or chromosome damage, impaired fertility, and even cancer.[7]

Preparation of these agents requires special procedures for labeling, storage, and transport. Use of protective clothing, BSCs, and special handling of spills and wastage are also important. Special techniques related to the actual administration of these products to patients are not covered in this chapter. Additional information is available from ASHP in the *Technical Assistance Bulletin on Handling of Cytotoxic and Hazardous Drugs*.

Protective Apparel

There is no substitute for good technique, but protective apparel is another fundamental element in protecting personnel who handle or prepare hazardous drugs. Protective garments, such as disposable coveralls or gowns, gloves, and shoe and hair covers, should be used to shield personnel from exposure.

Most procedures require the use of disposable coveralls or a solid-front gown. These garments should be made of low-permeability, lint-free fabric. They must have long sleeves and tight-fitting elastic or knit cuffs. They should not be worn outside the work area and should be changed immediately if contaminated. Shoe and hair covers may also be required, depending on the institution's policies.

Wearing gloves is essential when working with hazardous drugs. Workers should wash hands thoroughly before putting on the gloves and after removing them, and they should use good quality, disposable, powder-free latex gloves, such as surgical latex. These gloves are preferred because of their fit, elasticity, and tactile sensation. If only powdered gloves are available, the powder should be washed off before beginning to work.

Depending on the procedure, one or two pairs of gloves may be required. If two pairs are needed, one pair should be tucked under the cuffs of the gown and the second pair placed over the cuff. If an outer glove becomes contaminated, change it immediately. Change both the inner and the outer gloves immediately if the outer glove becomes torn, punctured, or heavily contaminated. If only one pair is worn, tuck the glove under or over the gown cuff so the skin is not exposed.

Every work area in which hazardous drugs are prepared should have an eyewash fountain or sink and appropriate first aid equipment. If skin or eye contact occurs, established first aid procedures should be followed, medical attention should be obtained without delay, and the injury should be documented.

Biological Safety Cabinets

One of the most important pieces of equipment for handling hazardous drugs safely is the BSC. A BSC is a type of vertical LAH that is designed to protect workers from exposure as well as to help maintain product sterility during preparation. BSCs must meet standards set by the National Sanitation Foundation (NSF Standard 49).

Horizontal LAHs should not be used to prepare hazardous drugs because they blow contaminants

directly at the preparer. If possible, the technician should prepare sterile hazardous drugs in a Class II BSC. The front air barrier of the BSC protects the handler from contact with hazardous drug dusts and aerosols that are generated in the work zone. Room air is pulled into the front intake grill and filtered through a HEPA filter. The air then passes vertically, that is, downward, through the work zone. The air that has passed through the work zone goes through front intake and rear exhaust grilles, passes through a HEPA filter, and is recirculated through the work zone or exhausted to the outside. Placing objects on or near the front intake or rear exhaust grilles may obstruct the airflow and reduce the effectiveness of the cabinet.

There are several types of Class II BSCs. Type A BSCs pump about 30 percent of the air out the hood exhaust after it passes through a HEPA filter (see **Figure 14-23**). This air is then circulated to the room or exhausted to the outside depending on how the hood is vented. Workers must be sure not to block airflow from the exhaust filters. Type B BSCs send air from the work zone through a HEPA filter and then to the outside of the building through an auxiliary exhaust system (see **Figure 14-24**). Type B BSCs offer greater protection because filtered air is sent outside the building and they have a faster inward flow of air. It is preferable to have the BSC exhausted directly to the outside through dedicated venting rather than venting into the general hospital circulation.

BSCs must be operated continuously, 24 hours per day, and they should be inspected and certified by qualified personnel every 6 months. The manufacturer's recommendations for proper operation and mainte-

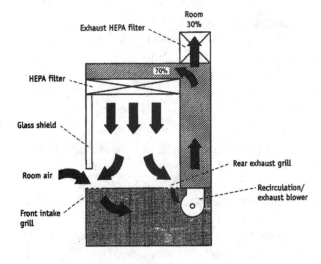

Figure 14-23. Class II Type A biological safety cabinet.

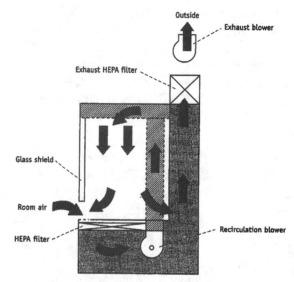

Figure 14-24. Class II Type B biological safety cabinet.

nance, particularly for replacement of HEPA filters, should be followed.

Workers should clean and disinfect the BSC regularly. The work surface and back and side walls should be cleaned with water or a cleaner recommended by the cabinet manufacturer. Aerosol cleaners should not be used; they could damage the HEPA filters and cabinet and allow contaminants to escape.

Before performing sterile manipulations, the work surface should be disinfected with 70 percent isopropyl alcohol or another suitable disinfectant and allowed to dry. Alcohol is a disinfectant and may remove some substances in the hood that water does not. The technician should be careful not to use excessive amounts of alcohol because vapors may build up in the BSC. Dispose of any gauze and gloves used to clean the BSC in sealable containers with other hazardous waste; they are contaminated.

Extensive decontamination should be performed, preferably on a weekly basis and immediately after a large spill. While cleaning and disinfecting the hood, technicians should wear a gown, latex gloves, a respirator, hair cover, and eye protection, because the front shield may need to be raised. The technician should keep the blower on and clean from the top, where contamination is least, to the bottom, where contamination is greatest, and use heavy toweling or gauze with cleaner and distilled deionized water. The HEPA filter cover should be removed and the inside of the BSC cleaned. The work tray should be lifted and propped against the back wall to clean underneath, and the drain spillage trough should be scrubbed thoroughly. Workers should change torn gloves immediately. The cleaner, water containers, protective apparel, and cleaning materials all must be handled and discarded as contaminated waste.

Preparing Hazardous Drugs

Before technicians handle a cytotoxic or other hazardous drug, they must demonstrate proper manipulative technique and use of protective equipment and materials.

Before preparing sterile hazardous drugs in a BSC, the technician should wash the hands and put on a gown and one or two pairs of latex gloves and then disinfect the work surface with alcohol. The technician should stand so the front shield protects his or her eyes and face. Some institutions place a plastic-backed liner on the work surface. Though this liner may introduce particles into the work zone, it will absorb any small spills.

The technician should assemble sufficient materials for the entire preparation process to avoid leaving and

re-entering the work zone. Only items necessary to the preparation process should be placed in the work zone, and these objects should not block the downward flow of air; for example, IV bags or bottles should not be hung above sterile objects. Sterile objects should be handled well inside the BSC so they are not contaminated by unfiltered air at the front air barrier. Air quality is lowest at the sides of the work zone, so the technician should work at least 3 inches away from each side wall.

If possible, IV sets should be attached to containers and primed before adding the drug. Syringes and IV sets with locking fittings should be used; they are less likely to separate than friction fittings. Needles are secured to these Luer lock fittings with a quarter turn.

When working with drugs in vials, pressure can build up inside the vial and cause the drug to spray out around the needle. The technician should maintain a slight negative pressure inside the vial to prevent this. Too much negative pressure, however, can cause leakage from the needle when it is withdrawn from the vial. Another way of preventing pressure buildup is to use a chemotherapy dispensing pin. This disposable device is attached at one end to the Luer lock fitting of the syringe, and a pin on the opposite end is inserted into the drug vial. The device also has a venting unit that allows for constant pressure equalization, therefore eliminating any problems due to pressure imbalances.

When reconstituting a drug in a vial, a syringe that can hold twice as much diluent as will be drawn into the syringe barrel should be used. This ensures that the plunger will not be pulled out of the barrel when the diluent is being drawn into the syringe. After drawing the diluent into a syringe, the technician should insert the needle into the vial top and draw the plunger back to draw air into the syringe and create a slight negative pressure inside the vial. Small amounts of diluent should be injected slowly and equal volumes of air drawn out of the vial. The technician should keep the needle in the vial and swirl the contents carefully until they dissolve completely. With the vial inverted, the proper amount of drug solution should be gradually withdrawn while equal volumes of air are exchanged for drug solution. Excess drug should remain in the vial. With the vial in the upright position, a small amount of air should be drawn from the vial into the needle and hub, and then the needle should be withdrawn from the vial.

If there is a need to transfer a hazardous drug to an IV bag, the technician should be careful not to puncture the bag. He or she should wipe the IV container and set with moist gauze and put a warning label on the

IV bag, then place the IV in a sealable bag so any leakage will be contained.

When withdrawing cytotoxic or hazardous drugs from an ampule, the technician should gently tap the contents down from the neck and top portion. The ampule neck should be sprayed or wiped with alcohol. The technician should then attach a 5-micron filter needle or filter straw to a syringe that is large enough to hold the ampule's contents, and draw the fluid through the filter needle, clearing it from the needle and hub. The filter needle should then be exchanged for a regular needle of similar gauge and length, and any air and excess drug should be ejected into a sterile vial, leaving the desired volume in the syringe. The technician should be careful not to create aerosols. The drug may then be transferred to an IV bag or bottle. If the dose is to be dispensed in the syringe, the plunger should be drawn back to clear fluid from the needle and hub, and the needle should be replaced with a locking cap. The syringe should be wiped with moistened gauze and labeled appropriately. In some institutions, the pharmacy is responsible for priming the line with the chemotherapeutic agent. Additional precautions will need to be taken if this is the case.

Good technique does not end with drug preparation. There are special requirements for waste disposal and cleanup. Any glass fragments and needles should be placed in a puncture- and leak-resistant container. Needles should not be clipped before disposal. All other materials should be placed in sealable plastic bags along with the outer pair of gloves. All waste containers should be sealed before removing them from the BSC, and they should be disposed of in designated, labeled containers. Next, the gown should be removed and disposed of, and, last, the inner pair of gloves should be removed and disposed of. When removing the gloves, the technician should be careful not to touch the fingertips of the gloves to the skin or the inside of the gloves. Finally, the technician should wash his or her hands.

Labeling, Storage, and Transport

Safe and effective labeling, storage, and transportation

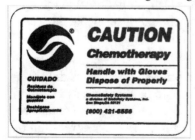

Figure 14-25. Example of a suitable warning label for cytotoxic and hazardous drugs. Other labels also may be suitable.

practices are essential to prevent accidental exposure to hazardous drugs. Following the appropriate guidelines with respect to these processes should begin the moment hazardous drugs enter the facility. Hazardous drugs should be identified by distinctive labels indicating that the product requires special handling (see **Figure 14-25**). Labels should be attached to drug packages and their storage shelves, bins, and areas. All hazardous drug storage areas should be marked clearly as containing hazardous drugs. Access to these areas should be limited to authorized personnel who have been trained in handling hazardous drugs.

Storage equipment should be designed to minimize breakage. For example, shelves should have front barriers and carts should have rims. Hazardous drugs should be kept at eye level or lower and stored in bins. Refrigerated hazardous drugs should be stored in bins that are separated from nonhazardous drugs.

Transporting hazardous drugs requires special precautions to prevent container leakage or breakage. For example, pneumatic tube systems cause mechanical stress to containers and should never be used for transporting hazardous drugs. Carts used to transport hazardous materials should have rims to prevent the containers from falling off the cart and breaking. Hazardous drug containers must be securely capped or sealed and properly packaged to protect against leakage or breakage during transport. If leakage or breakage occurs, the procedures described later in this section should be followed.

Waste Disposal and Spill Cleanup

The technician should review his or her institution's policies and procedures for identifying, containing, collecting, segregating, and disposing of hazardous waste. Hazardous waste should be disposed of in separate containers. Regular trash should not be placed in hazardous waste containers. Handle the outside of hazardous waste containers with uncontaminated gloves only.

Everyone who handles hazardous drugs should be familiar with the techniques and procedures for handling spills. In the event of a hazardous drug spill, the technician should use a spill kit, and the cleanup should follow established procedures. It is essential that the technician be familiar with the location and the use of the spill kit prior to requiring its use. Spill kits contain all the materials needed to clean up hazardous drug spills and protect health care workers and patients. Spill kits contain protective gear, eye protection, a respirator, utility and latex gloves, a disposable gown or coveralls, and shoe covers. They also contain the equipment needed to clean up the spill: a disposable scoop, a puncture and leak-resistant plastic container for disposing of glass fragments, absorbent spill pads, gauze and disposable toweling, absorbent powder, and sealable, thick plastic waste disposal bags. Hazardous waste must be stored in leak-resistant containers until it is disposed of in accordance with government and institution policy.

In the event of a spill, the technician should put up a warning sign to alert other people in the area of the hazard. All the protective equipment, including latex gloves covered by utility gloves, should be worn. Broken glass should be put in the puncture- and leak-resistant plastic container, and liquids should be absorbed with disposable towels or spill pads. Powders should be removed with dampened towels or gauze. The contaminated surface should be rinsed with water, washed with detergent, and then rinsed again. Cleaning should start at the outside of the spill and work toward the center. All the contaminated materials should be placed in sealable plastic disposal bags. In all cases, it is important that the circumstances and the handling of the spill be documented in writing (including completion of an incident report) and kept on file.

If the area is carpeted, the technician should refer to institutional policies and procedures for handling spills in carpeted areas. Absorbent powder and "hazardous drug only" vacuum cleaners are often used to clean up spills in these areas.

If a large spill occurs in a BSC, additional steps must be taken. The technician should use the spill kit described above and be sure to seal all contaminated materials in hazardous waste containers while the materials are still inside the BSC. He or she should use utility gloves when handling any broken glass. The drain spillage trough should be thoroughly cleaned and the BSC decontaminated if necessary. The waste containers should then be transferred to leak-resistant containers.

Total Parenteral Nutrition Solutions

Total parenteral nutrition (TPN), once known as hyperalimentation, refers to the IV administration of nutrients needed to sustain life. TPN contains carbohydrates, protein, fats, water, electrolytes, vitamins, and trace elements, hence the designation *total*.

TPN therapy is indicated for patients who cannot meet their nutritional needs from oral or other gastrointestinal means. TPN may be used for patients who cannot eat (e.g., after head and neck surgery, if comatose, or before or after surgery), who will not eat (e.g., patients with chronic diseases or psychologic disorders or geriatric patients), who should not eat (e.g., patients with esophageal obstruction or inflammatory bowel disease), or who cannot eat or absorb enough to sustain their nutritional needs (e.g., patients with cancer, burns, or trauma). Whenever the patient has a functional gastrointestinal system, it should be used preferentially over TPN, unless there is a medical contraindication.

Components of Parenteral Nutrition Solutions

TPN solutions contain base components and additives. Base components are usually mixed first and make up much of the volume of the TPN. They are composed of dextrose (carbohydrates) and amino acids (protein) and may also include fat and water. Additives are usually mixed with the base component and include life-sustaining nutrients, electrolytes, vitamins, and trace elements and may also include such drugs as heparin, insulin, and H_2 antagonists.

Carbohydrates are usually administered in the form of dextrose because of its low cost and easy availability. The commercially available concentrations of dextrose vary from 5 to 70 percent. Usually a 50 or 70 percent solution is used in TPN preparation, and the final dextrose concentration in the TPN is usually around 25 percent for solutions administered via a central vein. The dextrose concentration is significantly less—usually a maximum of 10 to 12.5 percent—for infusions intended for peripheral administration.

Protein is required for tissue synthesis and repair, transport of body nutrients and waste, and maintenance of immune function. Protein is usually given as commercially available synthetic crystalline amino acid formulations. These solutions are available in concentrated forms, such as 8.5 percent, 10 percent, or 15 percent and diluted during the compounding process. A number of special formulations are available for pediatric patients and patients who have kidney or liver disease or are in a high stress situation (e.g., intensive care patients).

Fats (or lipids) are usually administered as fat emulsions. Emulsions are needed because fat is insoluble in water. Administering fat emulsions not only prevents essential fatty acid deficiency but also provides a source of calories. Fat emulsions are commercially available as 10 or 20 percent emulsions that may be dispensed in a separate container that can be given through a peripheral IV line. Alternatively, fats can be added to the TPN solution. In this type of TPN, called a *3-in-1 solution* or *total nutrient admixture*, the fat emulsion is considered a third base component along with dextrose and amino acids. The 3-in-1 technique offers several nutritional advantages but has certain mixing, stability, and compounding disadvantages (see the Preparation of TPN Solutions section). Thirty percent fat emulsions are available for compounding admixtures only and should not be given as a separate IV infusion.

Water is in all preparations and is usually derived from the components used in the preparation. Sterile water for injection may be added to obtain the desired final concentration or volume. The purpose of adding water is to offset normal bodily losses and prevent dehydration. In addition to the TPN solution, separate fluids may be given for fluid replacement or for administration of medications.

Electrolytes are needed to meet daily metabolic needs and correct deficiencies. The electrolytes usually included in TPNs are sodium, potassium, chloride, acetate, phosphate, magnesium, and calcium. Electrolytes usually are administered as a specific salt of the product. For example, sodium may be admixed as sodium chloride, sodium acetate, sodium phosphate, or sodium lactate. Potassium can be given as potassium chloride, potassium acetate, or potassium phosphate. The patient's clinical condition and blood chemistries determine the amount and form of electrolytes required.

Vitamins usually are administered in a standard formulation of fat and water-soluble vitamins and are often abbreviated as *MVI* for *multiple vitamin infusion*. Commercial formulations include vitamins A, D, C, E, B_1, B_2, B_6, and B_{12}, folic acid, pantothenic acid, biotin, and niacin. When vitamin K (phytonadione) is needed, it is usually given separately as an IM injection. However, some clinicians add vitamin K to the TPN or use vitamin preparations that contain vitamin K. Pediatric formulations of MVI and vitamin K are also available.

Trace elements are required for proper enzymatic reactions and for use of energy sources in the body. Typical elements administered are copper, zinc, chromium, manganese, selenium, iron, and iodine. Commercial products are available that include combinations of trace elements and allow administration of a few milliliters to meet the daily requirements. It is extremely important to note that there are many trace element products and concentrations, so care must be taken to prevent incorrect dosing due to selection of the inappropriate product.

Other additives may be added to TPN preparations for consistency and ease of administration. These include, but are not limited to, octreotide, heparin, insulin, H_2 blockers (such as ranitidine), and iron. As with any additive, stability references should be checked before any admixture is prepared.

Orders for TPN Solutions

Procedures for ordering and dispensing TPN solutions vary and are specific to each institution. Many institutions use a standardized TPN ordering form to make the orders straightforward and consistent, yet patient-specific (see **Figure 14-26**). Often a cutoff time for order changes or new orders is used to maximize efficiency and minimize wastage. Since setting up to make just one TPN can be costly, this approach saves time and money by allowing multiple bags to be prepared consecutively.

TPN solutions are ordered specifically to meet a patient's metabolic and nutritional needs. These solutions usually are administered by means of a pump to maximize safety.

An order for central TPN solution might look like this:

Dextrose	250 g
Amino acids	42.5 g
Sodium chloride	60 mEq
Potassium chloride	40 mEq
Potassium phosphate	20 mEq
Calcium gluconate	1 g
Magnesium sulfate	1 g
Trace elements	2 mL
MVI-12	10 mL
Total volume	1000 mL

Infuse at 100 ml per hour.

Also give: Vitamin K 10 mg intramuscularly (IM) every week, 10% fat emulsion 500 ml intravenously 3 times per week.

Here is an example of an order for 3-in-1 central TPN solution:

Dextrose	250 g
Amino acids	85 g
Fat emulsion	50 g
Sodium chloride	80 mEq

ADULT TPN/PPN PHYSICIAN ORDERS

NOTE: All TPN orders (formula and rate) must be received in the Central Pharmacy by 12 Noon to be activated the same day. Orders received after 12 Noon will be activated the following day. A bag containing 24 hours of TPN will be sent. The adult hang time is 9 p.m.

DO NOT THIN FROM CURRENT CHART

Time Processed

Clerk's Initials

1. SELECT ONE:

	REGULAR FORMULA	LOW K FORMULA	NO K FORMULA	LOW ACET HIGH Cl	LOW Na FORMULA	PERIPHERAL FORMULA	SPECIAL FORMULA
AMINO ACIDS	☐ 6%	☐ 6%	☐ 6%	☐ 6%	☐ 6%	3%	☐ *
DEXTROSE	☐ 15% ☐ 25%	☐ 15% ☐ 25%	☐ 15% ☐ 25%	☐ 15% ☐ 25%	☐ 15% ☐ 25%	10%	+
SODIUM -mEq/L	45	45	45	45	20	45	
POTASSIUM-mEq/L	40.5	20	0	40	40.5	40.5	
CHLORIDE -mEq/L	57.5	59	69	89	44	57.5	XXX
ACETATE -mEq/L	92.8	81.7	52.2	52.2	72.6	66.8	XXX
CALCIUM - mEq/L	5	4.5	5	5	5	5	
MAGNESIUM - mEq/L	8	5	0	8	8	8	
PHOSPHORUS -mM/L	15	7.5	0	15	15	15	

* Other Amino Acid Concentrations Available -- 3% (Renal), 4.25%   + Other Dextrose Concentration Available -- 35%

2. RATE: 25 ml/hour for 8 hours, then 50 ml/hour for 8 hours, then _____ ml/hour for 8 hours, to a final rate of _____ ml/hour.
   Note: All solutions containing > 3% amino acids or > 10% dextrose must be given through a central line.
3. Vitamins (10 ml) and trace elements (5 ml) are added to TPN daily, unless otherwise ordered.
4. Vitamin K 10 mg is added to TPN every Monday, unless otherwise ordered.
5. (optional) Regular Insulin Human _____ units/liter of TPN.
6. (optional) Cimetidine _____ mg/bag of TPN.
7. FAT EMULSION: Infuse over 12 hours.

☐ 20% 250 ml.   ☐ Every day
☐ 20% 500 ml.   ☐ Every _____

ORDERS

1. STAT portable chest x-ray to verify central line placement, if not previously obtained. Infuse D5W at 20 cc/hr through central line until placement verified.
2. Label TPN catheter. On multi-lumen catheters, white port is designated for TPN. Do not draw blood, take CVP readings, or administer other fluid or drugs through TPN catheter/port.
3. Strict I&O's every 8 hours. Weigh ICU patients three times a week and floor patients weekly.
4. Hang fat emulsion at 0900; hang TPN at 2100. Discard unused portion of TPN.
5. Notify primary service, before hanging first bag of TPN, if blood sugar is >250 mg/dl or if phosphorus is<2.0 mM/dl.
6. Once TPN is hung, do not increase rate if blood sugar is >250 mg/dl.
7. Change TPN and fat emulsion administration sets every 24 hours.
8. Change central line dressing for TPN catheter every 96 hours or as needed per nursing policy (NS-21).
9. LABS: a. Astra-9, Magnesium, Hitachi, Ionized Ca, PT/PTT, CBC with diff with initiation of TPN, then every Monday and Thursday.
   b. Fasting triglyceride before first bottle of fat emulsion hung, then every Monday. (Draw at least 6 hours after fat emulsion infusion completed.)
   c. Obtain 24 hour urine for urea nitrogen (UNU) and creatinine (UCr) on first day of TPN, then every Monday (from 0600 - 0600).
10. Indirect Calorimetry per Nutrition Support Service
11. Finger stick for glucose every 6 hours. Follow designated sliding scale using regular insulin subcutaneously.

   A. 200-249 mg% - 5 u   B. 200-249 mg% - _____ u
   250-299 mg% - 10 u   OR   250-299 mg% - _____ u
   300-349 mg% - 15 u   300-349 mg% - _____ u
   350-399 mg% - 20 u   350-399 mg% - _____ u
   400 mg%- Call MD   400 mg% - Call MD

Supervising Physician Signature: _____

Physician Signature : _____   Physician Name Printed:_____

Beeper #:_____ Date: _____ Time: _____
WHITE-Chart   CANARY-Pharmacy   PINK-Nursing

Figure 14-26. Example of a TPN order form.

Potassium chloride	60 mEq
Potassium phosphate	60 mEq
Calcium gluconate	1 g
Magnesium sulfate	1 g
Trace elements	2 mL
MVI-12	5 mL
Total volume	2000 mL

Infuse over 24 hours. Give vitamin K 10 mg IM every week.

Preparation of TPN Solutions

Preparation of TPN solutions has changed considerably in the past 10 to 15 years. In the past, many of the components required preparation from nonsterile powders. Today, most TPN ingredients are available as sterile solutions, reducing the need for extemporaneous preparation. Most TPNs are made by gravity fill or by means of an automated compounding device.[8]

Gravity Fill

Gravity fill involves equipment that is normally part of an IV program. As the name implies, gravity is used to transfer the base components (dextrose and amino acids plus IV fat emulsion in a 3-in-1 solution) into the final container. The disadvantages of this method are that it limits flexibility in the volumes of base components used, it takes longer than automated methods, and volumes cannot usually be measured accurately. There are two gravity methods of filling bags: the empty bag method and the underfill method.

The *empty bag method* involves starting with an empty sterile bag that will be used as the final container. Commercially available bags have leads that can be connected to bottles or bags of the base components. The desired amounts flow into the empty bag by gravity. This method can be used for either traditional or 3-in-1 preparations.

The *underfill method* uses commercially available underfilled bags, which are partially filled with concentrated dextrose solution. A bottle of amino acids is connected to the underfilled bag by a tubing set and infused into the partially filled bag to make the final mixture.

With either method, other components are added by drawing each up into a syringe and injecting them through an injection port into the final container. This is usually the final step before labeling and dispensing. Great care must be taken both in technique and accuracy, since the potential for errors is high and their ramifications are serious. Each additive must be added in the correct amount; if even one is incorrect, the entire solution for that patient must be remade, and the solution made in error is likely to be wasted. The pharmacist must check each step. To prevent waste, some institutions require that the pharmacist check the calculations and amounts of additives in syringes before they are added to the bag.

Automated Compounding

Automated compounding involves the use of specialized equipment to prepare the TPN solution. Two primary versions of TPN compounders are available. One version provides a separate compounder for the base solutions and for the electrolytes, while the other version uses one compounder to infuse all the compounded ingredients (bases and electrolytes). In the former, three primary pieces of equipment are used, sometimes together and sometimes individually. An automated compounder prepares the base components dextrose, amino acids, and possibly fat emulsion and water; a second automated compounder adds most or all of the additives or other components; and a computer with software maintains the orders for the ingredients and controls the two compounders (see **Figure 14-27**).

The base compounder uses special tubing that can withstand the pumping action of the machine in allocating large volumes of solutions. It accounts for the specific gravity of the solutions being used and actually weighs the amount pumped into the final container. Some compounders also weigh the original container from which solutions are pumped. It stops pumping when the selected amount has been added. The base compounder can be used with the computer, or it can

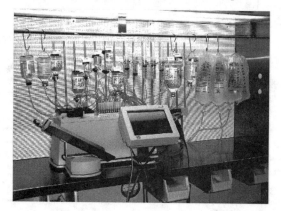

Figure 14-27. Example of the components of an automated TPN preparation device. The devices are (from L to R): The base nutrient compounder control and pump modules, micronutrient compounder, and computer for programming both compounders.

be used alone. When the base compounder is used alone, the operator enters the desired volume and specific gravity of the base solution components. The device weighs the correct amounts as described above.

The additives compounder also uses special tubing that delivers exact amounts of the solutions in very small quantities. It weighs the solutions to ensure proper volumes and flushes the line between injections to avoid incompatibility problems. The additives compounder must be used with the computer and cannot be programmed alone.

The computer software controls the system and offers many safeguards. It performs many of the calculations that would otherwise be done by hand and thus prone to human error, it allows the user to enter maximum safe quantities for different components, and it alerts the user to potential entry errors and inappropriate orders. Alarms are available to detect free-flowing ingredients and air bubbles in the line. The final products are checked subsequently by comparing the anticipated weight of the product against the actual weight of the product. Variances of more than +/- 3 percent are not accepted.

The accuracy provided by the automated compounders cannot totally substitute for all checks and balances in ensuring the quality of the product. Checks and balances must be built into each step of the TPN ordering, preparation, and administration process. Calculations should be verified and double-checked, and solutions and their ingredients should be checked and double-checked, regardless of the system used. The many additives that go into a TPN solution make it complicated with respect to compatibility and stability. For example, certain concentrations of electrolytes (e.g., calcium and phosphate) will precipitate when combined and warrant that all solutions be inspected carefully before they are dispensed. For this reason, software programs are designed to analyze key components of the order for potential incompatibilities. Admixture references should also be used before a solution is mixed. Special care must be taken when inspecting 3-in-1 solutions since the lipids may obscure the presence of white particulates and precipitates.

Automated compounders are used inside the LAH and must be cleaned daily according to the manufacturer's instructions. These systems require routine maintenance and calibration to ensure accurate compounding. To minimize the potential for errors, the compounders should be observed during operation. Quality control procedures may be implemented to

verify final contents of the product. These systems are occasionally used for compounding other solutions. Great care should be taken to avoid compounding errors.

Administration

Most TPN solutions are made for administration through a central line (see Basic Intravenous Therapy section). This route is used because it results in immediate dilution of the solution being administered, and therefore a very concentrated solution can be administered. Administering a concentrated solution often allows the medical team to completely meet an adult patient's daily nutritional needs with 2000 to 3000 mL of TPN solution.

Occasionally, parenteral nutrition is administered through a peripheral IV line. Peripheral parenteral nutrition (PPN) can contain many of the same components as TPN. However, to be administered peripherally, the PPN admixture may not be as concentrated (or have as high an osmolarity) as TPN. Since these solutions are more dilute, they may not meet all the patient's nutritional needs, that is, they are not "total" nutrition. Consequently, they are often used either as a nutritional supplement or for short-term nutritional intake.

Pediatric Parenteral Drug Administration

Pediatric patients receive many of the same products as adults, including intermittent medications, continuous infusions, chemotherapy, TPN, and analgesics. The unique aspect of this group of patients, of course, is that doses and solutions are much more individualized to meet their specific needs. Standardization of doses is not as common in pediatric patients as it is in adults. Doses are usually calculated on the basis of body weight, resulting in much smaller doses than most adults receive. The volume of solution is also limited since their blood volume is considerably less than that of an adult.

Intermittent doses are usually given by syringe through a volume control chamber or by using a syringe pump. These systems are used to maximize the accuracy of administration and minimize the amount of fluid given along with the dose of medication. Calculations should be checked and double-checked for these dilutions. A decimal point error could result in a 10-fold overdose or underdose of the drug, which could be significant, especially in a pediatric patient.

Epidural Administration

Epidural administration of drugs involves placing a special catheter into the epidural space of the spine. Some anesthetics and analgesics are injected into the epidural space to act on the nerve endings and provide the patient with pain relief. The placement of the catheter is a very delicate procedure and typically is performed by an anesthesiologist or a neurosurgeon. Because the drug is injected at the nerve ending, the dose needed for pain relief is greatly reduced as are many of the side effects (e.g., respiratory depression).[9]

Preparing parenterals for epidural administration requires the same aseptic technique as for other parenteral products. Good technique is of utmost importance with these products because an infection in the epidural space could rapidly become life threatening. Most epidurals must be prepared by the pharmacy and dispensed in syringes or special reservoirs designed to be used with special pumps. All solutions given epidurally must be free of preservatives to prevent toxicity in the spinal column. Dosage calculations should be checked and double-checked. The doses needed are very small, and an error resulting in an inadvertent overdose could have severe consequences.

Patient Controlled

The most common use of epidural analgesia is the administration of a loading dose to initiate pain control, followed by subsequent doses as needed and administered via a PCA pump. This method is very effective in attaining the benefits of both epidural analgesia and PCA. Pump programming is similar to that for IV PCA, with doses appropriate for the epidural route.

Continuous Infusions

Continuous infusions of epidural analgesics are given with a device that delivers solution at a known per-hour rate through the epidural catheter.

Bolus Injections

Bolus epidural injections of analgesics often are used to initiate therapy or when short-term therapy is required. Bolus dosing may be sufficient to control pain without the use of a pump or continuous infusion device.

Admixture Programs

Many of the practices described in this chapter are elements of an overall pharmacy-coordinated IV admixture program. The need for such well-developed programs is reinforced whenever there is a report of a patient who is harmed by an improperly prepared parenteral product. In almost all the cases reported, the proper equipment was not used, the ingredients were not correct, personnel preparing the product were not properly trained, or some other preventable reason led to the unfortunate outcome. Although an admixture program does not guarantee that problems will not occur, it does minimize risk to the patient by considering all factors that could potentially cause problems. The true benefit of a formal IV admixture program is that if it is well designed and managed, the whole will be greater than the sum of the parts. That is, each element alone will improve the quality of the products prepared, but with all the components working in concert, the improvement in quality will be even greater. This provides for the best possible outcome for the patient.

All IV admixture programs should comply with OSHA regulations of safe practice and USP Standards for Sterile Compounding, as well as ASHP Technical Assistance Bulletins.

Components of a Program

The basic components of a formal IV admixture program are listed below. The need for some components will depend on the scope of services provided and the type of patients served. For example, the structure of a program meeting the needs of a 100-bed hospital will differ from that of a home care pharmacy or a large teaching hospital. Each basic component is described below, along with an explanation of how its inclusion contributes to a system that is superior to one that does not use a formal program. Additional details and recommended practices are available and can be used to tailor your own program.[10]

Policies and Procedures

Written policies and procedures that are detailed and comprehensive serve as an important part of the foundation for an IV admixture program.[11,12] The *policy* portion of the document serves as a basis for decision-making, while the *procedure* portion serves as a description of how the task or function should be carried out.

Space

A coordinated program ideally has a space appropriate for the preparation of sterile products. Standards developed by ASHP and the United States Pharmacopeia (USP) describe the desirable room layout; wall, floor, and ceiling surfaces; air quality; cleanliness; maintenance; housekeeping; and processing areas needed as part of a formal program.[13] In many cases, an admixture service is operated from a room that is smaller than ideal, so the space must be well planned for movement of people, LAH requirements, and flow of patient orders.[4] The heating and cooling requirements of the room need to be properly assessed. The combination of people in the room and the heat generated by the LAHs can result in an uncomfortably warm environment. If possible, the room should be on its own cooling unit rather than part of a zone in the building. This will allow the room to be cooled without affecting other areas unnecessarily. The area should be well lit and located in a low traffic area. The floors, walls, and ceiling should have smooth surfaces that cannot easily harbor bacteria and can readily be cleaned and disinfected. Such items as cardboard boxes can produce particulates when handled and therefore should not be brought into the IV preparation area. Easily cleaned, moveable supply carts that can be removed from the room for restocking are ideal. A room that is clean, organized, and structured within these guidelines will be the safest and most efficient for preparation of sterile products within the hospital.

Training

Pharmacists and technicians who work with sterile products and prepare them on a daily basis should be knowledgeable about the process.[14] Pharmacy technicians who work with these products should be trained to understand basic aseptic technique (including handling supplies, hand washing, garb, etc.), sources of contamination, how to work within an LAH, how to prepare standard types of parenteral products, and how to prepare nonstandard types of preparations as needed. Technicians should demonstrate competency after learning from written training materials, videotapes, and hands-on demonstrations. They should not only demonstrate proper technique but also have a sample product tested for sterility and accuracy.

Equipment

Selection and maintenance of proper equipment is important in any function, but especially when relied on to provide a clean work environment for sterile product preparation (such as with an LAH). LAHs should be cleaned before use, and HEPA filters should be inspected every 6 months and have their prefilters changed regularly. Compounding equipment (such as syringe pumps used in compounding and automated TPN compounders) should be inspected, calibrated, and maintained according to manufacturers' recommendations. Temperature control equipment, such as refrigerators and freezers, should be monitored for temperature and equipped with an alarm that sounds when the temperature is outside USP guidelines. All equipment (including tables, chairs, etc.) should be made of materials that are easily cleaned and disinfected (e.g., laminate or stainless steel). All equipment maintenance should be performed on a schedule and documented.[15] Older recommendations stated that printers be located outside the IV room because of the dust generated from the impact printing mechanism. With new thermal and laser printers, however, that is less absolute. It is recommended that sinks not be located in the IV room because of the microbial growth that they create.

Computers often are used for a number of functions related to TPN production, including maintaining patient profiles, generating labels, screening for incompatibilities and duplicate orders, accessing patient information (e.g., labs or diagnosis), charging patients, and maintaining records.[4]

Standard and Nonstandard Preparations

An IV admixture program makes many different types of products, both standard (routine) and nonstandard. Using the expertise of those who work in such an environment can ensure that both types receive the same attention and care needed. Nonstandard preparations present challenges and, since they are often unusual, may result in errors when made by persons not familiar with them. The use of a coordinated program, references, procedures, and general knowledge will reduce the likelihood of one of these products being prepared incorrectly. Such a program also promotes consistency in preparation and labeling.

Labeling

Countless medication errors can be attributed to poor labeling of medications. An important benefit of a pharmacy IV admixture program is that it allows for consistent, complete labeling of products prepared.[16] The labeling formats must be clear and consistent.

Handling

Order flow and delivery are standardized in a formal IV program. This allows for proper storage (e.g., temperature control, etc.), retrieval of unused preparations (for potential reuse), and delivery of products. This effort improves the product integrity and reduces waste by promoting use of products before they pass their expiration date.[16]

Quality Assurance

Having all sterile products prepared in one department (and often in one area) aids in the development of a coordinated, meaningful quality assurance program. In large institutions that require compounding of sterile products at satellite sites, a standardized quality assurance program is recommended. Attempting to monitor and evaluate the quality of sterile products that are being prepared in numerous locations throughout a hospital or other setting would be difficult and inefficient without the use of common guidelines.

All IV admixture programs should have a *quality assurance program* to ensure that products and services are of desired quality. ASHP's *Guidelines on Quality Assurance for Pharmacy-Prepared Sterile Products* (Appendix) provides recommendations for preparation, expiration dating, labeling, facilities, equipment, personnel education, training, evaluation, and end-product testing. Some common methods of ensuring quality include air sample testing in the IV room, sampling of end products by the lab using pyrogen testing, flame testing, or tests for microbial contamination.

Revisions to the USP introduced in 2003 provide detailed recommendations for the development and implementation of quality assurance programs in IV admixture programs. The technician should refer to USP Chapter 797, "Pharmaceutical Compounding—Sterile Preparations," for a full description of recommendations and regulations regarding IV admixture programs.

The ASHP guideline describes three different levels of risk for products. Products are classified on the basis of how they are prepared, how long they can be stored, whether they are prepared for a single patient or as part of a batch, and whether they are from a sterile or nonsterile source. The characteristics of the different risk levels are listed below.

Risk Level 1

- Sterile products without preservatives for individual patients or are batch prepared with preservatives for multiple patients.

- Sterile products transferred into a sterile container (e.g., syringe, IV bag, or bottle).

- Storage time for these products, including administration time, should not exceed 28 hours at room temperature, 7 days under refrigeration, or 30 days if frozen.

Risk Level 2

- These products are batch-prepared without preservatives for multiple patients.

- These include products that require multiple sterile ingredients that are combined in a sterile container through a closed-system transfer that are then subdivided into multiple parts.

- Storage time for these products, including administration time, can exceed 28 hours at room temperature, 7 days under refrigeration, or 30 days frozen.

Risk Level 3

- These products are compounded from nonsterile ingredients, containers, or equipment or prepared from sterile or nonsterile ingredients in an open system.

Most hospital pharmacies are in Risk Level 1. Home care pharmacies may be in Risk Level 1 or 2. Risk Level 3 pharmacies are not very common.

Pharmacists are likely to be held responsible for ensuring compliance with the guidelines and other standards of practice, but technicians' work habits and activities will be affected as well. Areas of the document that affect the technician include training, policies and procedures, garb, aseptic technique, process validation, and end-product evaluation. The first four areas are covered in other sections of this chapter, but process validation and end-product evaluation require further explanation.

Process validation means that procedures that ensure that the processes used in sterile product preparation consistently result in sterile products of acceptable quality. For most aseptic processes, validation is actually a method for evaluating the aseptic technique of personnel. Validation may be accomplished through *process simulation*. Process simulation is carried out just like a normal sterile product preparation process except that a microbial growth medium is substituted for the products that would normally be used. Once the sterile product is prepared, the growth medium is incubated and evaluated for microbial growth over a period of time. No microbial growth indicates that the person performing the preparation did not contaminate the product. Individuals should complete a process validation program before being allowed to prepare sterile products, and technique should be re-evaluated regularly.

End-product evaluation is the final inspection made by the pharmacist before the product is allowed to leave the pharmacy. It includes an inspection for leaks, cloudiness, particulate matter, color, solution volume, and container integrity. In some instances, the growth medium fill procedure, described above, should be supplemented with a program of end-product sterility testing, and a method of recalling products not meeting specifications should be in place. The pharmacist also verifies compounding accuracy with respect to the correct ingredients and quantities. This check of the technician's work is an important step in ensuring that only quality products are sent for patient use.

Recommended Reading

Achusim LE et al. Comparison of automated and manual methods of syringe filling. *Am J Hosp Pharm.* 1990; 47:2492–5.

Buchanan EC, Schneider PJ. Compounding sterile preparations, 2nd ed. Bethesda, MD: American Society of Health-System Pharmacists; 2005.

American Society of Hospital Pharmacists. Compounding sterile preparations video training program (VHS and DVD: companion workbook). Bethesda, MD: American Society of Health-System Pharmacists; 2005.

American Society of Hospital Pharmacists. Safe handling of cytotoxic and hazardous drugs. (Videotape and study guide.) Bethesda, MD: American Society of Hospital Pharmacists; 1990. American Society of Parenteral and Enteral Nutrition. Safe practices for parenteral nutrition formulations. *JPEN.* 1998; 22:49–66.

Brier KL. Evaluating aseptic technique of pharmacy personnel. *Am J Hosp Pharm.* 1983; 40:400–3.

Cohen MR. Proper technique for handling parenteral products. *Am J Hosp Pharm.* 1986; 21:1106.

Hasegawa GR, ed. Caring about stability and compatibility. *Am J Hosp Pharm.* 1994; 51:1533–4.

Leff RD, Roberts RJ. Practical aspects of intravenous drug administration. 2nd ed. Bethesda, MD: American Society of Hospital Pharmacists; 1992.

McDiarmid MA. Medical surveillance for antineoplastic drug handlers. *Am J Hosp Pharm.* 1990; 47:1061–6.

United States Pharmacopeia. Pharmaceutical compounding—sterile preparations, chap. 797. Rockville, MD: United States Pharmacopeia; 2003.

References

1. Plumer AL. Principles and practice of intravenous therapy. Boston: Little, Brown and Co.; 1982.

2. Lindley CM, Deloatch KH. Infusion technology manual: a self-instructional approach and videotape. Bethesda, MD: American Society of Hospital Pharmacists; 1993.

3. Turco S, King RE. Sterile dosage forms, their preparation and clinical application. 4th ed. Philadelphia: Lea & Febiger; 1994.

4. Hunt ML. Training manual for intravenous admixture personnel. 5th ed. Chicago: Pluribus Press; 1995.

5. American Society of Hospital Pharmacists. Aseptic preparation of parenteral products. (Videotape and study guide.) Bethesda, MD: American Society of Hospital Pharmacists; 1985.

6. Trissel LA. Handbook on injectable drugs. 7th ed. Bethesda, MD: American Society of Hospital Pharmacists; 1992.

7. American Society of Hospital Pharmacists. Technical assistance bulletin on handling cytotoxic and hazardous drugs. *Am J Hosp Pharm.* 1990; 47:1033–49.

8. Abramowitz PW, Hunt ML Jr. Principles and advantages of automated compounding: a pharmacy education guide. Deerfield, IL: Clintec Nutrition; 1992.

9. Littrell, RA. Epidural infusions. *Am J Hosp Pharm.* 1991; 48:2460–74.

10. Buchanan EC, Schneider PJ. Compounding sterile preparations, 2nd ed. Bethesda, MD: American Society of Health-System Pharmacists; 2005.

11. Hethcox JM. The policy and procedure manual. In: Handbook of institutional pharmacy practice. 3rd ed. Brown TR, ed. Bethesda, MD: American Society of Hospital Pharmacists; 1992:53–62.

12. Buchanan EC. Policies and procedures for compounding sterile preparations. In: Compounding sterile preparations, 2nd ed. Buchanan EC, Schneider PJ, eds. Bethesda, MD: American Society of Health-System Pharmacists; 2005:235–42.

13. Buchanan EC. Sterile preparation facilities and equipment. In: Compounding sterile preparations, 2nd ed. Buchanan EC, Schneider PJ, eds. Bethesda, MD: American Society of Health-System Pharmacists; 2005:169–92.

14. Buchanan EC. Pharmacy technician education, certification, training, evaluation, and regulation. In: Compounding sterile preparations, 2nd ed. Buchanan EC, Schneider PJ, eds. Bethesda, MD: American Society of Health-System Pharmacists; 2005:159–68.

15. Schneider PJ. Equipment for compounding sterile preparations. In: Compounding sterile preparations, 2nd ed. Buchanan EC, Schneider, PJ, eds. Bethesda, MD: American Society of Health-System Pharmacists; 2005:27–34.

16. Buchanan EC. Handling of sterile products and preparations within the pharmacy. In: Compounding sterile preparations, 2nd ed. Buchanan EC, Schneider, PJ, eds. Bethesda, MD: American Society of Health-System Pharmacists; 2005:111–8.

Self-Assessment Questions

1. When is intravenous drug therapy used?
   a. when the patient is unable to take needed medications by mouth
   b. when a drug is needed in an emergency
   c. when a drug is not absorbed from the stomach
   d. all of the above

2. Parenteral drug products should be which of the following?
   a. free of particulate matter
   b. sterile
   c. free of pyrogens
   d. all of the above

3. In the typical IV setup, an LVP is attached to a primary set that is then attached to the catheter and inserted into the patient. How are drugs given intermittently usually administered?
   a. through another IV line (not through the one used for the LVP)
   b. through a Y-site injection port or flashball on the primary set
   c. by adding them to the LVP solution
   d. none of the above

4. IV tubing used as a primary set includes which of the following?
   a. macrodrip tubing (delivering 10 drops per minute)
   b. microdrip tubing (delivering 60 drops per minute)
   c. all purpose tubing (delivering 100 drops per minute)
   d. a and b

5. How are LVP solution containers with potent drugs that need to be infused with a high degree of accuracy and precision usually administered?
   a. with the aid of a roller clamp
   b. with the aid of an electronic infusion device
   c. these solutions are not given IV
   d. LAH

6. Sterile products should be prepared in a "class 100" environment. How is that accomplished in most pharmacies?
   a. with a room air filter
   b. with an LAH
   c. with a fume hood
   d. with a fan cycling air 100 times per hour
   e. none of the above

7. What is the term for the space between the HEPA filter and the sterile product being prepared?
   a. hot spot
   b. backwash zone
   c. zone of turbulence
   d. critical area
   e. none of the above

8. All manipulations inside an LAH should be performed at least _____ inches inside the hood to prevent _____ .
   a. 12 inches; smoke
   b. 6 inches; backwash
   c. 10 inches; contamination
   d. 2 inches; breakage from falling on the floor

9. What should the technician do before working in the LAH?
   a. wipe interior surfaces with 70 percent isopropyl alcohol
   b. operate the hood for at least 15 to 30 minutes
   c. wash hands with bactericidal soap
   d. all of the above

10. Items inside an LAH should be placed away from other objects and the walls of the hood to prevent what?
    a. zones of turbulence
    b. dead spaces
    c. windows of contamination
    d. laminar air

11. It is permissible to touch any part of the syringe while making sterile products as long as the technician is wearing sterile gloves.
    a. True
    b. False

12. A 30 mL syringe with 1 mL calibrations on its barrel can be used to accurately measure 15.5 mL of a solution for injection.
    a. True
    b. False

13. What should the user do to ensure sterility of a new needle?
    a. make sure the package was intact and not damaged
    b. wipe the needle with 70 percent isopropyl to disinfect it
    c. apply additional silicone so the needle self-sterilizes on insertion into a vial
    d. two of the above are correct

14. What should be done to prevent core formation when entering a vial diaphragm?
    a. use only small needles
    b. insert needles quickly before a core is formed
    c. insert the needle with the bevel tip first, then press downward and toward the bevel so the bevel tip and heel enter at the same point
    d. insert the needle straight into the vial diaphragm

15. How do ampules differ from vials?
    a. They are closed systems.
    b. They require the use of a filter needle.
    c. They can be opened without risk of breakage.
    d. They do not differ from vials.

16. Prior to compounding a product for parenteral administration, one should do all of the following *except*?
    a. Gather all needed supplies.
    b. Gather supplies anticipated for the entire shift and place them into the LAH.
    c. Inspect all materials for signs that they might be defective.
    d. Disinfect injection sites before entry.

17. Which of the following is(are) true regarding labels for IV products?
    a. They should be handwritten to show a personal touch.
    b. They should not include anything but the drug name and the patient's name, so the patient doesn't become alarmed when reading the label.
    c. They should be in a format that is consistent and easily understood.
    d. all of the above

18. Which is true of preservatives in parenteral products?
    a. They kill organisms and therefore eliminate the need for aseptic technique and LAHs.
    b. They are harmless and nontoxic in any amount.
    c. They are present in multidose vials.
    d. They should be used in epidural dosage forms to ensure sterility.

19. What is the name of an IV system that uses a threaded drug vial that is screwed into a corresponding receptacle on an IV bag?
    a. Drug-o-matic
    b. piggyback vial
    c. Add-Vantage®
    d. LVP
    e. cytotoxic

20. What is Buretrol a common name for?
    a. piggyback system
    b. Add-Vantage®
    c. Volume Control Chamber
    d. CRIS®

21. What can contact with cytotoxic drugs cause?
    a. dermatitis
    b. dizziness
    c. nausea
    d. possible chromosome damage, impaired fertility, or cancer
    e. all of the above

22. Cytotoxic agents can be which of the following?
    a. cell killers
    b. oncogenic
    c. mutagenic
    d. teratogenic
    e. any of the above

23. What does protective apparel for those preparing cytotoxic or hazardous injections in a BSC include?
    a. a low permeability, solid-front gown with tight-fitting elastic cuffs
    b. latex gloves
    c. a self-contained respirator
    d. two of the above

24. What are vertical LAHs that are Class II BSCs and exhaust 100 percent of their air outside of the building called?
    a. Type A
    b. Type B
    c. horizontal LAHs
    d. none of the above

25. How should a cytotoxic agent be transported after it is prepared in the pharmacy?
    a. immediately
    b. in a way that minimizes breakage
    c. expedited with systems such as pneumatic tubes
    d. by making the transporter aware of what they are carrying and what the procedure would be in the event of a spill
    e. two of the above

26. Contents of a "Chemo Spill Kit" include each of the following *except?*
    a. gloves
    b. goggles
    c. a respirator
    d. a disposable gown
    e. a loudspeaker

27. Electrolytes are added to TPN solutions to meet metabolic needs and correct deficiencies. What is(are) an example(s)?
    a. amino acids
    b. potassium chloride
    c. vitamin D
    d. lipid emulsions
    e. all of the above

28. Lipid or fat emulsions typically are administered by all of the following methods *except* which one?
    a. as a 10 percent emulsion given IV through a peripheral line
    b. as a 20 percent emulsion given IV through a peripheral line
    c. as part of a 3-in-1 TPN solution
    d. as an IV push

29. Dextrose is the base component of TPN solutions most commonly given as a source of carbohydrates. Which of the following statements is(are) true?
    a. It is available as a 5 percent solution that is commonly used in TPN solutions.
    b. It is available in a concentrated form (50 percent or more) that is diluted in the final TPN solution to approximately 25 percent.
    c. It is available as a 70 percent solution that is commonly given as a separate infusion for calories and energy.
    d. all of the above

30. Which of the following is *false* concerning the gravity fill method of preparing TPN solutions?
    a. The final solution can be either the traditional formulation (amino acids and dextrose as the base) or the 3-in-1 solution (with amino acids, dextrose, and fats as the base).
    b. It involves using an empty bag/bottle or using an underfilled container as the final container.
    c. It involves pumping ingredients into the final container; "gravity" really refers to the

administration process for these solutions.
    d. It involves numerous checks in the system since so many additives are being measured and injected, leaving greater potential for error.

31. What may automated compounding of TPN solutions use?
    a. a compounding device to pump base ingredients into the final container
    b. a device that accurately measures small quantities of electrolytes and injects them into the final container
    c. a computer and software to run the compounding device
    d. aseptic technique that should be done in an LAH
    e. all of the above

32. How are TPN solutions typically given?
    a. through a central IV line
    b. through a peripheral IV line
    c. through a pump
    d. through a syringe
    e. two of the above

33. Policies and procedures for a formal IV program typically include all of the following *except*
    a. personnel training guidelines
    b. quality assurance for the area
    c. environmental monitoring procedures
    d. names of staff working in the area

34. Which of the following is true of space and facilities used for sterile product preparation?
    a. They should be set up to meet recommendations of ASHP and USP.
    b. They can be anywhere within the pharmacy.
    c. They should be carpeted to minimize noise disturbances.
    d. They should have a good breeze to keep workers cool.

Self-Assessment Answers

1. d. IV drug therapy offers some benefits in drug delivery because it provides rapid blood levels of the medication, and many drugs are not stable or absorbed in the stomach. On the other hand, there are risks associated with parenteral therapy since it is being injected directly into the body. Parenteral therapy is more expensive than oral therapy because of the need for sterility and special equipment. Therefore, the oral route should be attempted first, but if this is not feasible, the parenteral route may be used.

2. d. A basic premise of the safe administration of any parenteral drug is that it be sterile (free of living microorganisms), free of particulate matter (undesirable particles), and free of pyrogens (by-products of organisms that cause fever, chills, and could lower blood pressure). Many aspects of a good IV admixture program are aimed at producing a product that meets these criteria. Products that do not meet these criteria should not be administered to the patient.

3. b. Intermittent drugs (e.g., antibiotics, antiulcer drugs) are often given every 6 or 8 hours through a designated location on the primary set. These locations include Y-sites (shaped like a "Y") or flashball injection sites. The only reasons another site might be required for the administration of these types of drugs would be if they were incompatible with the LVP solution or if the LVP contained a critical drug that could not be interrupted by the intermittent drug.

4. d. Caregivers can manually control the flow rate of LVPs by counting drops in the drip chamber and adjusting the roller clamp to obtain the desired rate. The sets have a drip chamber that is calibrated to different drop sizes so that the caregiver can visually count drops and calculate the rate of delivery. Usually the macrodrip tubing (delivering 10 drops per minute) is used when a solution is being given at a fast rate, while the microdrip tubing (delivering 60 drops per minute) is used when a slower rate is needed.

5. b. Potent drugs that are adjusted for their effect on the patient must be carefully controlled by the caregiver. Only the use of an electronic infusion device allows this type of control. A roller clamp does control the rate of flow, but only at an approximate level, and the rate of flow can easily be affected by the movement of the patient.

6. b. Class 100 is defined as an environment that contains no more than 100 particles per cubic foot that are larger than 0.5 microns in size. An LAH provides a class 100 environment that can be placed in a relatively small space and is comparatively low in cost. The hood uses a blower to push air through a HEPA filter and blow it across a work surface. Although some very sophisticated settings are able to filter and control air quality in an entire room and make it a class 100 environment, these are very expensive and probably more than is needed for preparation of routine sterile products.

7. d. A key principle in the use of an LAH is that nothing passes between the HEPA filter, which is blowing highly purified air, and the product being prepared. This area has been termed the *critical area* because of its importance.

8. b. Care must be taken so that manipulations are done well inside the hood (at least 6 inches) to prevent backwash (i.e., unfiltered room air entering the work surface). Air movement is minimal by the time it reaches the outside of the hood, and any movement or draft could allow room air to move into the hood. By working well inside the hood, this occurrence is minimized. Some users have a tendency to work on the outside edge because it is quieter than working well within the hood, but this obviously eliminates the benefits of using the hood.

9. d. The hood should be operated for a period of time so that room air is purged from the work area. The interior surfaces of the hood should be wiped down with 70 percent isopropyl alcohol to disinfect them. Hands should be washed in bactericidal soap so that bacteria on the hands are minimized.

10. a. Materials placed within the LAH disturb the patterned flow of air blowing from the HEPA filter. This zone of turbulence created behind

Self-Assessment Answers

an object could potentially extend outside the hood, pulling or allowing contaminated room air into the aseptic working area (see Figure 9-3). When laminar airflow is moving on all sides of an object, the zone of turbulence extends approximately 3 times the diameter of that object. When laminar airflow is not accessible to an object that is placed adjacent to a vertical wall, a zone of turbulence is created that may extend 6 times the diameter of the object.

11. b. The barrel of the syringe can be touched and handled, but the syringe tip and plunger should never be touched. Wearing sterile gloves while preparing sterile products does not guarantee sterility, because the gloves are no longer sterile once they have touched a nonsterile container or surface.

12. a. Syringes are accurate to one-half of the calibrated markings. In this example, that would be one-half of one mL. Since the needed volume is at that mark, it would be accurate.

13. a. Needles are sterile from the manufacturer as long as the protective overwrap is not damaged. Needles have a silicone lubricant that allows easier penetration into vials. Needles should not be wiped off, since it will remove this silicone coating.

14. c. Answer c best describes the special technique that should be used to prevent a core. The other answers describe techniques that could potentially lead to a core.

15. b. Ampules are made of glass and become an open system (air can pass freely) when they are opened. Glass fragments may end up in the solution, requiring the use of a filter needle, and the fragments can cut the finger of the user if they are not handled carefully. Vials are closed systems. They do not break on opening, so there is no risk of glass fragments and no need for a filter needle.

16. b. Only items needed for the preparation itself should be in the hood. Other items will introduce particulate matter unnecessarily into the work area and will create zones of turbulence disrupting the effectiveness of the LAH.

17. c. The label can play a big role in preventing medication errors. As much information as possible should be included on the label, including drug name, strength, hang time, solution, volume, patient name, room number, infusion instructions, frequency of administration, storage requirements, and so on. This information should be typed or computer generated so that it is readable and should be consistent in format.

18. c. Preservatives are added to retard the growth of microorganisms in multiple dose vials. The presence of these substances should not give a false sense of security that the solution is self-sterilizing, because it is not. Strict aseptic technique is still needed. Also, if doses of drugs are significantly higher than those originally intended, larger volumes of the drug solution are given, which results in larger amounts of the preservative being present, which might be toxic. Therefore, if preparations involve large amounts of drug solution that contain a preservative or a diluent with a preservative, the pharmacist should be consulted to verify that the total amount of preservative to be administered to the patient will not be toxic. Solutions with preservatives should not be used in preparations for neonates, or in epidural or intrathecal dosage forms because of their toxicity.

19. c. See text for description of available systems.

20. c. See text for description of available systems.

21. e. Cytotoxic agents require special handling and attention because of their potentially toxic effects. All handlers should be familiar with these special techniques and should be aware of the consequences of improper handling. All of the choices are potential effects of direct exposure to one of these agents.

22. e. Handlers should be aware of what types of agents are classified as *cytotoxic* and therefore require special handling. Typically, antineoplastics, immunosuppressants, and some antivirals are included in this category. Package inserts, material safety data sheets, or other references should be checked if a product's status is in question.

Self-Assessment Answers

23. d. Protective apparel is doubly important with cytotoxic agents because of not only protecting the product from contamination but also protecting the preparer from exposure. Those handling cytotoxics should wear a nonpermeable gown that ties in the back and has some type of tight fitting cuffs. They should also wear latex gloves that are nonpowdered. If the gloves have powder on them from the manufacturer, they should be wiped clean with 70 percent isopropyl alcohol before use, which will prevent the powder from becoming a particulate contaminant. Use of a respirator is not needed when preparing products in a BSC, because the hood filters and recycles the air.

24. b. One of the most important pieces of equipment for handling hazardous drugs safely is the BSC. A BSC is a type of vertical LAH that is designed to protect workers from exposure as well as to help maintain sterility during preparation. There are several types of Class II BSCs. Type A BSCs pump about 30 percent of the air back into the room after it passes through a HEPA filter. The technician should be sure not to block airflow from the exhaust filters. Type B BSCs send air from the work zone through a HEPA filter and then to the outside of the building through an auxiliary exhaust system. Type B BSCs offer greater protection because filtered air is sent outside the building and because they have a faster inward flow of air. Horizontal LAHs should not be used to prepare hazardous drugs because they blow contaminants directly at the preparer.

25. e. Delivery of cytotoxic agents does not have to occur immediately. Once prepared, the product can receive an expiration date like any other sterile product, with consideration for sterility and stability. Special handling and packaging should be used to prevent the container from breaking or leaking while in transit. Mechanical devices, such as pneumatic tubes, should not be used since they often jar the product, and any leakage or a spill inside a tube system would be very difficult to decontaminate.

26. e. Chemo spill kits are available commercially or can be compiled from the existing pharmacy stock. Spill kits should be assembled containing all the materials needed to clean up hazardous drug spills and protect health care workers and patients. Spill kits should contain the following protective gear: eye protection, a respirator, utility and latex gloves, a disposable gown or coveralls, and shoe covers. They should also contain the equipment needed to clean up the spill: a disposable scoop and a puncture and leak-resistant plastic container for disposing of glass fragments; absorbent spill pads; gauze and disposable toweling; absorbent powder; and sealable, thick plastic waste disposal bags.

27. b. The electrolytes usually include sodium, potassium, chloride, acetate, phosphate, magnesium, and calcium. Electrolytes usually are administered (and calculated) by using a specific salt of the product. For example, sodium is frequently given as sodium chloride. Potassium can be given as potassium chloride, potassium acetate, or potassium phosphate. The patient's clinical condition and laboratory values usually determine the amount and form of electrolytes. The other components listed are commonly in TPN solutions but are not electrolytes.

28. d. Fat emulsions are administered to prevent essential fatty acid deficiency and to provide a source of calories. They are commercially available as 10 or 20 percent emulsions and are isoosmolar and can be given through a peripheral IV line. Alternatively, fats can be added to the TPN solution. In this case, the fat emulsion is considered a third base component along with dextrose and amino acids, and the TPN is called a 3-in-1 solution or a total nutrient admixture. The 3-in-1 technique offers several nutritional advantages but has certain mixing, stability, and compounding disadvantages.

29. b. Commercially available concentrations vary from 5 to 70 percent. Usually a 50 or 70 percent solution is used for TPNs, and the final dextrose concentration in the TPN is

usually around 25 percent for solutions administered via a central vein. The dextrose concentration is significantly lower for infusions intended for peripheral administration.

30. c. All of the answers are true except for c. Gravity is used to transfer base solutions into the final container. This process can be slow since the dextrose is very thick in its concentrated form.

31. e. Automated compounding involves the use of specialized equipment to prepare the TPN solution. Three primary pieces of equipment are used, sometimes together and sometimes individually: (1) an automated compounder that prepares the base components, (2) a second automated compounder that adds most or all of the additives or other components, and (3) a computer with software that maintains the orders and controls the two compounders. The base compounder pumps the base components into the final container. The additives compounder also uses special tubing that delivers exact amounts of the solutions in very small quantities. It weighs the solutions to ensure proper volumes and flushes the line between injections to avoid incompatibility problems. The additives compounder must be used with the computer and cannot be programmed alone. The computer and software control the system and offer many safeguards because they perform many of the calculations that would otherwise be done by hand and be prone to human error. They also allow the user to enter maximum safe quantities for different components and alert the user to potential entry errors and inappropriate orders. The automated compounders are used inside the LAH and must be cleaned daily according to the manufacturer's instructions.

32. e. Most TPN solutions are made for administration through a central line. This route is used because it results in immediate dilution of the solution being administered, and therefore a very concentrated solution can be administered. This route

also allows the medical team to completely meet the adult patient's nutritional needs each day with 2000 to 3000 mL of TPN solution, depending on the weight and needs of the patient. Concerns over the adverse effects of a TPN solution that infuses too quickly require that a pump or other electronic infusion device be used to control its rate of administration.

33. d. Policies and procedures for IV programs typically include sections on personnel training and evaluation, acquisition, storage and handling of supplies, maintenance of the facility and equipment, personnel conduct and dress, product preparation methods, environmental monitoring, process validation, expiration dating practices, labeling guidelines, end-product evaluation, housekeeping procedures, quality assurance, and documentation records. Any specific information on individuals would not fall within the purpose of these documents.

34. a. A coordinated program ideally has an appropriate space for the preparation of sterile products. Standards developed by the ASHP and USP describe the desirable room layout, wall/floor/ceiling surfaces, air quality, cleanliness, maintenance, housekeeping, and process areas needed as part of a formal program. While ideal space and facilities are still not available in some institutions, the presence of such a program will serve to show the need for such facilities. In most hospitals, there is no better place to prepare these types of products.

APPENDIX

ASHP Guidelines on Quality Assurance for Pharmacy-Prepared Sterile Products

Patient morbidity and mortality have resulted from incorrectly prepared or contaminated pharmacy-prepared products.[1–7] Pharmacists seldom know that inaccurate or contaminated products are dispensed when pharmacy quality monitors are inadequate.[8–10] In contemporary health care organizations, more patients are receiving compounded sterile products that are stored for extended periods before use (allowing the growth of a pathological bioload of microorganisms[11]), more patients are seriously ill, and more patients are immunocompromised than ever before.

These ASHP guidelines are intended to help pharmacists and pharmacy technicians prepare sterile products of high quality.[a] The pharmacist is responsible for compounding and dispensing sterile products of correct ingredient identity, purity (freedom from physical contaminants, such as precipitates,[12] and chemical contaminants), strength (including stability[13] and compatibility), and sterility and for dispensing them in appropriate containers, labeled accurately and appropriately for the end user.

Other professional organizations have published useful guidelines on compounding and dispensing sterile products. The United States Pharmacopeia (USP) publishes the official compendium *The United States Pharmacopeia and The National Formulary (USP)* and its supplements, all of which may have legal implications for pharmacists.[14,15] The reader would especially benefit from studying the *USP* general information chapter on sterile drug products for home use,[13] which is referred to often in this ASHP guideline. The National Association of Boards of Pharmacy (NABP) has published less detailed model regulations for use by state boards of pharmacy.[16,17] The American Society for Parenteral and Enteral Nutrition (A.S.P.E.N.) recently published a special report on safe practices for parenteral nutrition formulations.[18]

Other governmental and accreditation sources are more general. The Joint Commission on Accreditation of Healthcare Organizations (JCAHO) publishes at least four sets of standards that mention pharmacy compounding. The hospital accreditation standards simply state that the organization adheres to laws, professional licensure, and practice standards governing the safe operation of pharmaceutical services.[19] The JCAHO home care standards require that medications be safely prepared, including "using appropriate techniques for preparing sterile and nonsterile medications and products." For example, the home care standards state that "appropriate quality-control techniques are used to check for preparation accuracy and absence of microbial contamination. Techniques for preparing sterile products follow guidelines established by the American Society of Health-System Pharmacists."[20] The JCAHO standards for long-term-care pharmacies list important conditions for product preparation, such as separate areas for sterile product preparation, use of a laminar-airflow workbench or class 100 cleanroom, and quality control systems to ensure the accuracy and sterility of final products.[21] The JCAHO standard for ambulatory care infusion centers states, among other things, several facility-related standards, for example the use of biological safety cabinets to protect personnel preparing cytotoxic or hazardous medications; work surfaces free of equipment, supplies, records, and labels unrelated to the medication being prepared; and a separate area for preparing sterile products that is constructed to minimize opportunities for particulate and microbial contamination.[22]

The Food and Drug Administration (FDA) publishes regulations on current good manufacturing practices that apply to sterile products made by pharmaceutical manufacturers for shipment in interstate commerce. Pursuant to the FDA Modernization Act of 1997 (FDAMA), Section 503A of the Food, Drug, and Cosmetic Act states that pharmacy compounding must comply with an applicable *USP* monograph, if one exists, and the *USP* chapter on pharmacy compounding[14] or be a component of an FDA-approved drug product; or, if neither of these apply to the ingredient being compounded, the substance must appear on a list of bulk drug substances developed by FDA and must be accompanied by a valid certificate of analysis and be manufactured in an FDA-registered establishment.[23] Inactive ingredients compounded by licensed pharmacies must comply with applicable *USP* monographs, if they exist, and the *USP* chapter on pharmacy compounding.[14] FDAMA prohibits pharmacists from compounding drug products that appear on a list of products that have been withdrawn or removed from the market because they have been found unsafe or ineffective. FDAMA also says that pharmacists may not compound, regularly or in inordinate amounts, drug products that are essentially copies of commercially available drug products; nor may they compound drug products identified by regulation as presenting demonstrable difficulties for compounding that reasonably demonstrate an adverse effect on safety or effectiveness.

The Centers for Disease Control and Prevention (CDC) has published guidelines for hand washing, prevention of intravascular infections, and hospital environmental control.[24,25]

The ASHP Guidelines on Quality Assurance for Pharmacy-Prepared Sterile Products are applicable to pharmaceutical services in various practice settings, including, but not limited to, hospitals, community pharmacies, nursing homes, ambulatory care infusion centers, and home care organizations. ASHP has also published practice standards on handling cytotoxic and hazardous drugs[26] and on pharmacy-prepared ophthalmic products.[27] These ASHP guidelines *do not* apply to the *manufacture* of sterile pharmaceuticals as defined in state and federal laws and regulations, *nor* do they apply to the preparation of medications by pharmacists, nurses, or physicians in emergency situations for *immediate* administration to patients (e.g., cardiopulmonary resuscitation). All guidelines may not be applicable to the preparation of radiopharmaceuticals.

These guidelines are referenced with supporting scientific data when such data exist. In the absence of published supporting data, guidelines are based on expert opinion or generally accepted pharmacy procedures. Pharmacists are urged to use professional judgment in interpreting these guidelines and applying them in practice. It is recognized that, in certain emergency situations, a pharmacist may be requested to compound products under conditions that do not meet these guidelines. In such situations, it is incumbent upon the pharmacist to employ professional judgment in weighing the potential patient risks and benefits associated with the compounding procedure in question.

Objectives. The objectives of these guidelines are to provide

1.   Information on quality assurance and quality control activities that should be applied to the preparation of sterile products in pharmacies and

2.   A method to match quality assurance and quality control activities

with the potential risks to patients posed by various types of products.

Multidisciplinary Input. Pharmacists are urged to participate in the quality or performance improvement, risk management, and infection control programs of their health care organizations, including developing optimal sterile product procedures.

Definitions. Definitions of selected terms, as used in this document, are provided in Appendix A. For brevity in this document, the term *quality assurance* will be used to refer to both quality assurance and quality control (as defined in Appendix A), as befits the circumstances.

Risk-Level Classification

In this document, sterile products are grouped into three levels of risk to the patient, increasing from least (level 1) to greatest (level 3) potential risk based on the danger of exposing multiple patients to inaccurate ingredients or pathogens and based on microbial growth factors influenced by product storage time, temperature and product ability to support microbial growth, surface and time exposure of critical sites, and microbial bioload in the environment. When circumstances make risk-level assignment unclear, guidelines for the higher risk level should prevail. Consideration should be given to factors that increase potential risk to the patient such as high-risk administration sites and immunocompromised status of the patient. A comparison of risk-level attributes appears in Appendix B.

Risk Level 1. Risk level 1 applies to compounded sterile products that exhibit characteristics 1, 2, *and* 3, stated below. All risk level 1 products should be prepared with sterile equipment (e.g., syringes and vials), sterile ingredients and solutions, and sterile contact surfaces for the final product. Risk level 1 includes the following:

1. Products
   a. Stored at room temperature (see Appendix A for temperature definitions) and completely administered within 28 hours after preparation or
   b. Stored under refrigeration for 7 days or less before complete administration to a patient over a period not to exceed 24 hours (Table 1) or
   c. Frozen for 30 days or less before complete administration to a patient over a period not to exceed 24 hours.
2. Unpreserved sterile products prepared for administration to one patient or batch-prepared products containing suitable preservatives prepared for administration to more than one patient.
3. Products prepared by closed-system aseptic transfer of sterile, nonpyrogenic, finished pharmaceuticals (e.g., from vials or ampuls)[b] obtained from licensed manufacturers into sterile final containers (e.g., syringes, minibags, elastomeric containers, portable infusion-device cassettes) obtained from licensed manufacturers.

Examples of risk level 1 processes include transferring a sterile drug product from a vial into a commercially produced i.v. bag; compounding total parenteral nutrient (TPN) solutions by combining dextrose injection and amino acids injection via gravity transfer into a sterile empty container, with or without the subsequent addition of sterile drug products to the final container with a sterile needle and syringe; and transferring a sterile, preserved drug product into sterile syringes with the aid of a mechanical pump and appropriate sterile transfer tubing device.

Risk Level 2. Risk level 2 sterile products exhibit characteristic 1, 2, *or* 3, stated below. All risk level 2 products should be prepared with sterile equipment, sterile ingredients and solutions, and sterile contact surfaces for the final product and with closed-system transfer methods. Risk level 2 includes the following:

1. Products stored beyond 7 days under refrigeration, stored beyond 30 days frozen, or administered beyond 28 hours after preparation and storage at room temperature (Table 1, see page 319).
2. Batch-prepared products *without preservatives* (e.g., epidural products) that are intended for use by more than one patient. (Note: Batch-prepared products without preservatives that will be administered to multiple patients carry a greater risk to the patients than products prepared for a single patient because of the potential effect of inaccurate ingredients or product contamination on the health and well-being of a larger patient group.)
3. Products compounded by complex or numerous manipulations of sterile ingredients obtained from licensed manufacturers in a sterile container or reservoir obtained from a licensed manufacturer by using closed-system aseptic transfer; for example, TPN solutions prepared with an automated compounder. (Note: So many risks have been associated with automated compounding of TPN solutions that its complexity requires risk level 2 procedures.[18])

Examples of risk level 2 processes include preparing portable-pump reservoirs for multiday (i.e., ambient temperature) administration; subdividing the contents of a bulk, sterile injectable (without preservatives) into single-dose syringes; and compounding TPN solutions with an automated compounding device involving repeated attachment of fluid containers to proximal openings of the compounder tubing set and of empty final containers to the distal opening, the process concluding with the transfer of additives into the filled final container from individual drug product containers or from a pooled additive solution.

Risk Level 3. Risk level 3 products exhibit either characteristic 1 *or* 2:

1. Products compounded from nonsterile ingredients or compounded with nonsterile components, containers, or equipment before terminal sterilization.
2. Products prepared by combining multiple ingredients—sterile or nonsterile—by using an open-system transfer or open reservoir before terminal sterilization.

Examples of risk level 3 products are calcium levulinate injection, estradiol in oil injection, and morphine sulfate 50-mg/mL injection.[32]

Quality Assurance for Risk Level 1

RL 1.1: Policies and Procedures.[33] Up-to-date policies and procedures for compounding sterile products should be written and available to all personnel involved in these activities. When policies and procedures are changed they should be updated, as necessary, to reflect current standards of practice and quality. Additions, revisions, and deletions should be communicated to all personnel involved in sterile compounding and related activities. These policies and procedures should address personnel education and training requirements, competency evaluation, product acquisition, storage and handling of products and supplies, storage and delivery of final products, use and maintenance of facilities and equipment,[34] appropriate garb and conduct for personnel working in the controlled area, process validation, preparation technique,[35] labeling, documentation, and quality control.[36] Further, written policies and procedures should address personnel access and movement of materials into and near the controlled area. Policies and procedures for monitoring environmental conditions in the controlled area should take into consideration the amount of exposure of the product to the environment during compounding and the environmental control devices used to create the critical area. Sources of information include vendor-supplied inservice programs and multimedia training programs, such as videotapes and Internet-site information. Before compounding sterile products, all personnel involved should read the policies and procedures. Written policies and procedures are required for all environmental control devices used to create the critical area for manipulation of sterile products. Examples of such devices are laminar-airflow workstations, biological safety cabinets, class 100 cleanrooms, and barrier isolator workstations (see Appendix A).[c]

RL 1.2: Personnel Education, Training, and Evaluation. Training is the most important factor in ensuring the quality of sterile products. Pharmacy personnel preparing or dispensing sterile products must receive suitable didactic and experiential training and competency evaluation through demonstration, testing (written or practical), or both. Some aspects that should be included in training programs include aseptic technique; critical-area contamination factors; environmental monitoring; facilities, equipment, and supplies; sterile product calculations and terminology; sterile product compounding documentation; quality assurance procedures; aseptic preparation procedures; proper gowning and gloving technique; and general conduct in the controlled area. In addition to knowledge of chemical, pharmaceutical, and clinical properties of drugs, pharmacists should be knowledgeable about the principles of pharmacy compounding.[14] Videotapes[37,38] and additional information on the essential components of a training, orientation, and evaluation program are described elsewhere.[39,40] All pharmacy and non-pharmacy personnel (e.g., environmental services staff) who work in the controlled area should receive documented training on cleaning, sanitizing, and maintaining equipment used in the controlled area. Training should be specific to the environmental control device and equipment present in the controlled area and should be based on current procedures.

The aseptic technique of each person preparing sterile products should be observed and evaluated as satisfactory during orientation and training and at least annually thereafter.[41] In addition to observation, methods of evaluating the knowledge of personnel include written or practical tests and process validation.[42,43]

RL 1.3: Storage and Handling within the Pharmacy.[44] Solutions, drugs, supplies, and equipment used to prepare or administer sterile products should be stored in accordance with manufacturer or *USP* requirements. Temperatures in refrigerators and freezers used to store ingredients and finished sterile preparations should be monitored and documented daily to ensure that compendial storage requirements are met. Warehouse and other pharmacy storage areas where ingredients are stored should be monitored to ensure that temperature, light, moisture, and ventilation remain within manufacturer and compendial requirements. To permit adequate floor cleaning, drugs, supplies, and compounding equipment should be stored on shelving, cabinets, and carts above the floor. Products that have exceeded their expiration dates should be removed from active storage areas. Before use, each drug, ingredient, and container should be visually inspected for damage, defects, and expiration date.[45]

Unnecessary personnel traffic in the controlled area should be minimized. Particle-generating activities, such as removal of intravenous solutions, drugs, and supplies from cardboard boxes, should not be performed in the controlled area. Products and supplies used in preparing sterile products should be removed from shipping containers outside the controlled area before aseptic processing is begun. Packaging materials and items generating unacceptable amounts of particles (e.g., cardboard boxes, paper towels [unless lint-free], reference books) should not be permitted in the controlled area or critical area. The removal of immediate packaging designed to retain the sterility or stability of a product (e.g., syringe packaging, light-resistant pouches) is an exception; obviously, this type of packaging should not be removed outside the controlled area. Disposal of packaging materials, used syringes, containers, and needles should be performed at least daily, and more often if needed, to enhance sanitation and avoid accumulation in the controlled area. Trash cans should be below the level of the laminar-airflow workbench and should be removed from the controlled area before being emptied. Sharps containers should be safely placed into the waste stream, according to policies developed by the institution to comply with regulations of the Occupational Safety and Health Administration (OSHA).

In the event of a product recall, there should be a mechanism for tracking and retrieving affected products from specific patients to whom the products were dispensed.

RL 1.4: Facilities[46] and Equipment.[47] The controlled area should be a limited-access area sufficiently separated from other pharmacy operations to minimize the potential for contamination that could result from the unnecessary flow of materials and personnel into and out of the area. The controlled area is a buffer from outside air that is needed because strong air currents from briefly opened doors, personnel walking past the laminar-airflow workbench, or the air stream from the heating, ventilating, and air conditioning system can easily exceed the velocity of air from the laminar-airflow workbench. Also, operators introducing supplies into the laminar-airflow workbench or reaching in with their arms can drag contaminants from the environment surrounding the workbench.[15] Cleanliness of the controlled area can be enhanced by (1) limiting access to those personnel assigned to work in the controlled area, (2) having those personnel wear the appropriate garb, (3) donning and removing garb outside the controlled area, (4) keeping doors to the controlled area closed, (5) limiting storage in the controlled area to items in constant use, (6) using low-particulate shelving, counters, and carts (e.g., stainless steel) in the controlled area, (7) not allowing cardboard and other particle-generating materials in the controlled area, (8) controlling the temperature and humidity inside the room, and (9) implementing a regular cleaning (e.g., nightly floor disinfection) and maintenance schedule.[48]

Barrier isolator workstations are closed systems and are not as sensitive to their external environment as laminar-airflow equipment. It is good practice to (1) place barrier isolator workstations in limited-access areas, (2) control the temperature and humidity of the surrounding area, and (3) clean and sanitize the surrounding area on a routine basis.[49]

Special precautions should be taken to clean equipment and compounding areas meticulously after preparing products that contain allergenic ingredients (e.g., sulfonamides and penicillins). Equipment should be of appropriate design and size for compounding and suitable for the intended uses. Equipment and accessories used in compounding should be inspected, maintained, and cleaned at appropriate intervals to ensure the accuracy and reliability of their performance.[14]

Computer entry, order processing, label generation, and record keeping should be performed outside the critical area. The controlled area should be well organized[50] and lighted[51] and of sufficient size to support sterile compounding activities. For hand washing, a sink with hot and cold running water should be in close proximity to but outside the controlled area. Refrigeration, freezing, ventilation, and room temperature control capabilities appropriate for storage of ingredients, supplies, and pharmacy-prepared sterile products in accordance with manufacturer, USP, and state or federal requirements should exist. The controlled area should be cleaned and disinfected at regular intervals with appropriate agents, according to written policies and procedures.[52] Disinfectants should be alternated periodically to prevent development of resistant microorganisms.[d] The floors of the controlled area should be nonporous and washable to enable regular disinfection. Active work surfaces in the controlled area (e.g., carts, compounding devices, counter surfaces) should be disinfected, in accordance with written procedures. Refrigerators, freezers, shelves, and other areas where pharmacy-prepared sterile products are stored should be kept clean.

Sterile products must be prepared in a class 100 environment (i.e., the critical area).[29] Such an environment exists inside a certified horizontal- or vertical-laminar-airflow workbench, a class 100 cleanroom, or a barrier isolator.[53] Cytotoxic and other hazardous products should be prepared in a vented class II biological safety cabinet or a barrier isolator of appropriate design to meet the personnel exposure limits described in product material safety data sheets (MSDS).[54] Barrier isolators are gaining favor as clean environments, especially for cytotoxic drug compounding.[55-57] Properly maintained barrier isolators provide suitable environments for the preparation of risk level 1, 2, and 3 sterile products.[58]

Laminar-airflow workbenches are designed to be operated continuously. If a laminar-airflow workbench is turned off between aseptic processes, it should be operated long enough to allow complete purging of room air from the critical area (e.g., at least 30 minutes), then disinfected before use. Barrier isolators, because of their closed nature, require less start-up time. If the barrier isolator has been turned off for less than 24 hours, a two-minute start-up time is sufficient. For periods greater than 24 hours, the chamber should be sanitized and the isolator should not be used for a minimum of 10 minutes after application of the sanitizing agent. The critical-area work surface and all accessible interior surfaces of the workbench should be disinfected with an appropriate agent before work begins and periodically thereafter, in accordance with written policies and procedures.[52] The exterior surfaces of the laminar-airflow workbench should be cleaned periodically with a mild detergent or suitable disinfectant; 70% isopropyl alcohol may damage the workbench's clear plastic surfaces. The laminar-airflow workbench should be certified by a qualified contractor[59] every six months[53] or when it is relocated to ensure operational efficiency and integrity. Prefilters in the laminar-airflow workbench should be changed (or cleaned, if they are washable) periodically (e.g., monthly), in accordance with written policies and procedures.

A method should be established for calibrating and verifying the accuracy of automated compounding devices used in aseptic processing (e.g., routine reconstitution of bulk or individual vials, transferring of doses from a bulk container to a minibag, syringe, or other single-dose container).

RL 1.5: Garb.[60] Procedures should require that personnel wear clean gowns or coveralls that generate few particles in the controlled area.[53] Scrub attire by itself is not acceptable (but can, like street clothes, be covered by a gown or coverall). Hand, finger, and wrist jewelry should be minimized or eliminated. Fingernails should be kept clean and trimmed. Head and facial hair should be covered. Masks are recommended because most personnel talk[61] or may cough or sneeze. Gloves are recommended. Personnel who have demonstrated sensitivity to latex should use either powder-free, low-latex protein gloves or, in the case of severe allergy, latex-free (synthetic) gloves.[62,63]

RL 1.6: Aseptic Technique[64,65] *and Product Preparation.*[66] Sterile products must be prepared with aseptic technique in a class 100 environment. Personnel should scrub their hands and forearms for an appropriate length of time with a suitable antimicrobial skin cleanser at the beginning of each aseptic compounding process and when reentering the controlled area, in accordance with written procedures. Personnel should wear appropriate attire (see RL 1.5: Garb). Eating, drinking, and smoking are prohibited in the controlled area. Talking should be minimized in the critical area during aseptic preparation (even when masks are worn).

Ingredients used to compound sterile products should be determined to be

stable, compatible, and appropriate for the product to be prepared, according to manufacturer or USP guidelines or appropriate scientific references. The ingredients of the preparation should be predetermined to result in a final product that meets physiological norms for solution osmolality and pH, as appropriate for the intended route of administration. Each ingredient and container should be inspected for defects, expiration date, and product integrity before use. Expired, inappropriately stored, or defective products must not be used in preparing sterile products. Defective products should be promptly reported to the FDA MedWatch Program.[67]

Only materials essential for preparing the sterile product should be placed in the laminar-airflow workbench or barrier isolator. The surfaces of ampuls, vials, and container closures (e.g., vial stoppers) should be disinfected by swabbing or spraying with an appropriate disinfectant solution (e.g., 70% isopropyl alcohol or 70% ethanol) before placement in the workbench. Materials used in aseptic preparation should be arranged in the critical area (within the laminar-airflow workbench or barrier isolator) in a manner that prevents interruption of the unidirectional airflow between the high-efficiency particulate air (HEPA) filter and critical sites of needles, vials, ampuls, containers, and transfer sets. All aseptic procedures should be performed at least 6 inches inside the front edge of the laminar-airflow workbench, in a clear path of unidirectional airflow between the HEPA filter and work materials (e.g., needles, closures). The number of personnel preparing sterile products in the workbench at one time should be minimized. Overcrowding of the critical work area may interfere with unidirectional airflow and increase the potential for compounding errors. Likewise, the number of units being prepared in the workbench at one time should allow unobstructed airflow over critical areas. Automated compounding devices and other equipment placed in or adjacent to the critical area should be cleaned, disinfected, and placed to avoid contamination or disruption of the unidirectional airflow between the HEPA filter and sterile surfaces. Closed systems like barrier isolators require less stringent placement of sterile units and equipment because the critical area encompasses the entire work surface. Hand and arm movements are not critical because the walls of the barrier isolator provide protection from the outside environment.[50]

Aseptic technique should be used to avoid touch contamination of sterile needles, syringe parts (e.g., plunger, syringe tip), and other critical sites. Solutions from ampuls should be properly filtered to remove particles. Solutions of reconstituted powders should be mixed carefully, ensuring complete dissolution of the drug with the appropriate diluent. Needle entry into vials should be performed in such a manner as to avoid coring of the vial closure. Some patients may require a latex-free admixture to avoid severe allergic reactions.[68] Latex-related policies and procedures should be developed by each institution, given the paucity of evidence that latex closures and syringe plungers are implicated in patient reactions to latex.[69,70] Before, during, and after the preparation of sterile products, the pharmacist should carefully check the identity and verify the amounts and sequence of the additives in sterile preparations against the original prescription, medication order, or other appropriate documentation (e.g., computerized patient profile, label generated from a pharmacist-verified order) before the product is released or dispensed.

RL 1.7: Process Validation.[71] Validation of aseptic processing procedures provides a mechanism for ensuring that processes consistently result in sterile products of acceptable quality.[10] In risk level 1, process validation (or process simulation) of compounding procedures is actually a method of assessing the adequacy of an operator's aseptic technique. Each individual involved in the preparation of sterile products should successfully complete a validation process on technique before being allowed to prepare sterile products. The validation process should follow written procedures.[42,43,45] Commercial kits are available for process validation; however, their ability to support microbial growth should be tested by challenging the intended kit with an indicator organism (e.g., *Bacillus stearothermophilus*) that can be purchased in known concentrations, is known not to be pathogenic, and grows only at relatively high temperatures.

Process simulation allows for the evaluation of opportunities for microbial contamination during all steps of sterile product preparation. The sterility of the final product is a cumulative function of all processes involved in its preparation and is ultimately determined by the processing step providing the lowest probability of sterility.[31] Process simulation testing is carried out in the same manner as normal production, except that an appropriate microbiological growth medium is used in place of the actual product used during sterile preparation. The same personnel, procedures, equipment, and materials are involved. Completed medium samples are incubated. If no microbial growth is detected, this provides evidence that adequate aseptic technique was used. If growth is detected, the entire sterile preparation process must be evaluated, corrective action taken, and the process simulation test performed again. No products intended for patient use should be prepared by an individual until the process simulation test indicates that the individual can competently perform aseptic procedures. It is recommended that personnel competency be revalidated at least annually, whenever the quality assurance program yields an unacceptable result, and whenever unacceptable techniques are observed; this revalidation should be documented.

RL 1.8: Expiration Dating.[72] All pharmacy-prepared sterile products should bear an appropriate expiration date. The expiration date assigned should be based on currently available drug stability information and sterility considerations. Sources of drug stability information include references (e.g., *AHFS Drug Information,*[73] *Extended Stability for Parenteral Drugs,*[74] *Handbook on Injectable Drugs,*[75] *King Guide to Parenteral Admixtures*[76]), manufacturer recommendations, and reliable, published research. When interpreting published drug stability information, the pharmacist should consider all aspects of the final sterile product being prepared (e.g., drug reservoir, drug concentration, storage conditions). Methods used for establishing expiration dates should be documented. Appropriate inhouse (or contract service) stability testing may be used to determine expiration dates when drug stability data are not readily available. Home care pharmacies are often required to assign extended beyond-use dates to sterile products, so ASHP has published guidelines for home care pharmacies that address beyond-use dating.[74,77]

RL 1.9: Labeling.[78] Sterile products should be labeled with at least the following information:

1. For patient-specific products: the patient's name and any other appropriate patient identification (e.g., location, identification number); for batch-prepared products: control or lot number,
2. All solution and ingredient names, amounts, strengths, and concentrations (when applicable),
3. Expiration date and time, when applicable,
4. Prescribed administration regimen, when appropriate (including rate and route of administration),
5. Appropriate auxiliary labeling (including precautions),
6. Storage requirements,
7. Identification (e.g., initials) of the responsible pharmacist (and technician),
8. Device-specific instructions (when appropriate), and
9. Any additional information, in accordance with state or federal requirements; for example, a prescription number for products

dispensed to ambulatory care, long-term-care, and home care patients.

The label should be legible and affixed to the final container in a manner enabling it to be read while the sterile product is being administered (when possible). Written policies and procedures should address proper placement of labels on containers.[79]

RL 1.10: End-Product Evaluation.[80] The final product should be inspected when preparation is completed and again when the product is dispensed. This inspection includes an evaluation for container leaks, container integrity, solution cloudiness or phase separation, particulates in the solution, appropriate solution color, and solution volume. The responsible pharmacist should verify that the product was compounded accurately with the correct ingredients, quantities of each ingredient, containers, and reservoirs; different methods may be used for end-product verification (e.g., observation, calculation checks, documented records). Refractive index measurement may also be used to verify the addition of dextrose, for example in parenteral nutrient solutions.[81]

RL 1.11: Handling of Sterile Products Outside the Pharmacy.[82] Pharmacists should participate in developing procedures for the safe use (e.g., stability, sterility) of sterile products once they are distributed outside the pharmacy. How the product is transported from the pharmacy, how it is stored outside the pharmacy, and methods for return, recycling, and disposal should be addressed in written policies and procedures.[15,83] Sterile products should be transported so as to be protected from extremes of temperature outside their range of stability and from light if they are photosensitive. Storage containers and packaging verified as suitable for protection during transport should be specified. Transit time and conditions should also be specified and controlled. Delivery personnel should be instructed on special handling procedures. Once delivered to the end user, sterile products should be appropriately stored before use. Pharmacists should ascertain that the user has appropriate locations and equipment for storage (e.g., a refrigerator with a suitable thermometer). Special instructions for storage should be a part of the label or a separate information sheet (e.g., instructions for cleanliness, proper storage, interpretation of the expiration date and how to look for signs of product deterioration). The pharmacist should be notified if storage conditions do not remain suitable so that the pharmacist can give advice as to the disposition of the sterile products and remedies for storage problems. Pharmacists should participate in training end users on the proper care and storage of sterile products, either directly or through written instructional materials.

RL 1.12: Documentation.[84] The following should be documented and maintained on file for an adequate period of time, according to organizational policies and state regulatory requirements: (1) the training and competency evaluation of employees in sterile product procedures, (2) refrigerator and freezer temperatures, (3) certification of laminar-airflow workbenches, and (4) other facility quality control logs specific to the pharmacy's policies and procedures (e.g., cleaning logs for facilities and equipment). Pharmacists should also maintain appropriate dispensing records for sterile products, in accordance with state regulatory requirements.

Quality Assurance for Risk Level 2

Because the risks of inaccurate products are associated with more complex procedures and because instability and contamination are more likely with long-term storage and administration, more stringent requirements are appropriate for risk level 2 preparations. These requirements may be viewed as more important in circumstances where the medical need is *routine.* In circumstances where the medical need for a product is immediate (and there is not a suitable alternative) or when the preparation of such a product is rare, professional judgment should be applied to the extent to which some guidelines (e.g., cleanroom design and final product testing before product dispensing) must be applied.

RL 2.1: Policies and Procedures. In addition to all guidelines for risk level 1, a written quality assurance program should define and identify necessary environmental monitoring devices and techniques to be used to ensure an adequate environment for risk level 2 sterile product preparation. Examples include the use of airborne particle counters, air velocity and temperature meters, viable particle samplers (e.g., slit samplers), agar plates, and swab sampling of surfaces and potential contamination sites. All aspects of risk level 2 sterile product preparation, storage, and distribution, including such details as the choice of cleaning materials and disinfectants and the monitoring of equipment accuracy, should be addressed in written policies and procedures. Limits of acceptability (threshold or action levels) for environmental monitoring and process validation and actions to be implemented when thresholds are exceeded should be defined in written policies. For sterile batch compounding, written policies and procedures should be established for the use of master formulas and work sheets and for appropriate documentation. Policies and procedures should also address personnel attire in the controlled area, lot number determination and documentation, and any other quality assurance procedures unique to compounding risk level 2 sterile products.

RL 2.2: Personnel Education, Training, and Evaluation. All guidelines for risk level 1 should be met. In addition to guidelines for risk level 1, assessment of the competency of personnel preparing risk level 2 sterile products should include appropriate process validation (as described in RL 1.7: Process validation). However, process simulation procedures for assessing the preparation of risk level 2 sterile products should be representative of all types of manipulations, products, and batch sizes personnel preparing risk level 2 products are likely to encounter.[15] Personnel should also be taught which products are to undergo end-product quantitative analysis (see RL 2.10).

RL 2.3: Storage and Handling. All storage and handling guidelines for risk level 1 should be met.

RL 2.4: Facilities and Equipment. In addition to all guidelines for risk level 1, the following guidelines should be followed for risk level 2 sterile product preparation:

1. The controlled area should meet the standards of a class 10,000 cleanroom,[e] as defined by Federal Standard 209E.[85,f] A positive air pressure relative to adjacent pharmacy areas is required, as are an appropriate number of air exchanges per hour and appropriate humidity and temperature levels.[86] For open-architecture cleanrooms, it is appropriate to measure the volume of air entering the cleanroom versus the volume of air entering adjacent rooms, so as to ensure a positive pressure gradient for the cleanroom. To allow proper cleaning and disinfection, walls, floors, and ceilings in the controlled area should be nonporous. To help reduce the number of particles in the controlled area, an adjacent support area (e.g., anteroom) should be provided. A properly maintained barrier isolator also provides an acceptable environment.[57] A barrier isolator provides a class 100 environment for product preparation; therefore, the isolator itself can be in a separate area of the pharmacy but need not actually be in a cleanroom.

2. Cleaning materials (e.g., mops, sponges, and germicidal disinfectants) for use in the cleanroom should be carefully selected. They should be made of materials that generate a low amount of particles. If reused, cleaning materials should be cleaned and disinfected between uses.

3. The critical-area work surfaces (e.g., interior of the laminar-airflow workbench) should be disinfected frequently and before and after each batch-preparation process with an appropriate agent, according to written policies and procedures. Floors should be disinfected at least daily. Carpet or porous floors, porous walls, and porous ceiling tiles are not suitable in the controlled area because these surfaces cannot be properly cleaned and disinfected. Exterior workbench surfaces and other hard surfaces in the controlled area, such as shelves, carts, tables, and stools, should be disinfected weekly and after any unanticipated event that could increase the risk of contamination. Walls should be cleaned at least monthly.

4. To ensure that an appropriate environment is maintained for risk level 2 sterile product preparation, an effective written environmental monitoring program is recommended.[87] Sampling of air and surfaces according to a written plan and schedule is recommended.[31] The plan and frequency should be adequate to document that the controlled area is suitable and that the laminar-airflow workbench or biological safety cabinet meets class 100 requirements. Limits of acceptability (thresholds or action levels) and appropriate actions to be taken in the event thresholds are exceeded should be specified. *USP* presents examples of environmental monitoring.[15] Settle plates or wipe samples can provide a simple but effective means of routinely monitoring airborne microbial contamination in controlled and critical areas.[45,88,89]

5. To help reduce the number of particles in the controlled area, an adjacent support area (e.g., anteroom) of high cleanliness, separated from the controlled area by a barrier (e.g., plastic curtain, partition, wall), is recommended. Appropriate activities for the support area include, but are not limited to, hand washing, gowning and gloving, removal of packaging and cardboard items, and cleaning and disinfecting hard-surface containers and supplies before placing these items into the controlled area.

6. Methods should be established for calibrating and verifying the accuracy and sterility of automated compounding methods used in aseptic processing.[90–96]

RL 2.5: Garb. All guidelines for risk level 1 should be met. Gloves, gowns, and masks are required for the preparation of all risk level 2 sterile products. Even when sterile gloves are used, they do not remain sterile during aseptic compounding; however, they do assist in containing bacteria, skin, and other particles that may be shed even from scrubbed hands. Clean gowns, coveralls, or closed jackets with sleeves having elastic binding at the cuff are recommended; these garments should be made of low-shedding materials. Shoe covers may be helpful in maintaining the cleanliness of the controlled area. Barrier isolators do not require the same level of gowning as laminar-airflow workstations as long as they operate as closed systems with HEPA filtration of air entering and leaving the barrier isolator and a separate area for entrance, such as an air lock for product transfers.

During sterile product preparation, gloves should be rinsed frequently with a suitable agent (e.g., 70% isopropyl alcohol) and changed when their integrity is compromised (i.e., when they are punctured or torn). Personnel should discard gloves upon leaving the cleanroom and don new gloves upon reentering the cleanroom.

RL 2.6: Aseptic Technique and Product Preparation.[97–99] All guidelines for risk level 1 sterile product preparation should be met. Relative to batch-prepared products, a master work sheet should be developed for a batch of each discrete identity and concentration of sterile product to be prepared. The master work sheet should consist of the formula, components, compounding directions or procedures, a sample label, and evaluation and testing requirements. Once the original master work sheet is approved by the designated pharmacist, a verified duplicate (e.g., a photocopy) of the master work sheet should be used as the preparation work sheet from which each batch is prepared and on which all documentation for each batch occurs. (For small-formula, frequently prepared batches, it may be more efficient to have multiple lines on the preparation work sheet for documenting more than one batch.) The preparation work sheet should be used to document the following:

1. Identity of all solutions and ingredients and their corresponding amounts, concentrations, or volumes,
2. Manufacturer lot number and expiration date for each component,
3. Component manufacturer or suitable manufacturer identification number,
4. Container specifications (e.g., syringe, pump cassette),
5. Lot or control number assigned to batch,
6. Expiration date of batch-prepared products,
7. Date of preparation,
8. Identity (e.g., initials, codes, signatures) of personnel involved in preparation,
9. End-product evaluation and testing specifications and results,
10. Storage requirements,
11. Specific equipment used during aseptic preparation (e.g., a specific automated compounding device), and
12. Comparison of actual yield with anticipated yield, when appropriate.

However documentation is done, a procedure should exist for easy retrieval of all records pertaining to a particular batch. Each batch of sterile products should bear a unique lot number. Identical lot numbers must never be assigned to different products or different batches of the same product. Lot numbers may be alphabetic, numeric, or alphanumeric.

The process of combining multiple sterile ingredients into a single sterile reservoir for subdivision into multiple units for dispensing may necessitate additional quality control procedures. A second pharmacist should verify calculations associated with this process, when possible; this verification should be documented. Because this process often involves making multiple entries into the intermediate sterile reservoir, the likelihood of contamination may be greater than that associated with the preparation of other risk level 2 sterile products.

For preparation involving automated compounding devices, a pharmacist should verify data entered into the compounding device before compounding begins. End-product checks should be performed to verify accuracy of ingredient delivery. These checks may include weighing and visually verifying the final product. For example, the expected weight (in grams) of the final product, based on the specific gravities of the ingredients and their respective volumes, can be documented on the compounding formula sheet, dated, and initialed by the responsible pharmacist. Once compounding is completed, each final product can be weighed and its weight compared with the expected weight. The product's actual weight should fall within a preestablished threshold for variance. Visual verification may be aided by marking the beginning level of each bulk container before starting the automated mixing process and checking each container after completing the mixing process to determine whether the final levels appear reasonable in comparison with expected volumes. The operator should also periodically observe the device during the mixing process to ensure that the device is operating properly (e.g., check to see that all stations are operating). If there are doubts whether a product or component has been properly prepared or stored, the product should not be used.

RL 2.7: Process Validation. Each individual involved in the preparation of risk level 2 sterile products should successfully complete a validation process, as recommended for risk level 1. Process simulation for compounding risk level 2 sterile products should be representative of all types of manipulations, products, and batch sizes that personnel preparing risk level 2 sterile products are likely to encounter.

RL 2.8: Expiration Dating. All guidelines for risk level 1 should be met.

RL 2.9: Labeling. All guidelines for risk level 1 should be met.

RL 2.10: End-Product Evaluation. All guidelines for risk level 1 should be met. For complex or toxic products, it is appropriate, when possible, to obtain quantitative testing of the accuracy of sterile additives; for example, the dextrose concentration in pediatric parenteral nutrient solutions or the potassium concentration in cardioplegia solutions.[g]

RL 2.11: Handling of Sterile Products Outside the Pharmacy. All guidelines for risk level 1 should be met.

RL 2.12: Documentation. All guidelines for risk level 1 should be met. Additionally, documentation of end-product sampling and batch-preparation records should be maintained for an adequate period, in accordance with organizational policies and procedures and state regulatory requirements.[100] Documentation for sterile batch-prepared products should include the

1. Master work sheet,
2. Preparation work sheet, and
3. End-product evaluation and testing results.

Quality Assurance for Risk Level 3

Risk level 3 addresses the preparation of products that pose the greatest potential risk to patients. The quality assurance activities described in this section are clearly more demanding—in terms of processes, facilities, and final product assessment—than for risk levels 1 and 2. Ideally, the activities described for risk level 3 would be used for all high-risk products. However, the activities may be viewed as most important in circumstances where the medical need for such high-risk products is *routine*. In circumstances where the medical need for such a product is immediate (and there is not a suitable alternative) or when the preparation of such a product is rare, professional judgment must be applied as to the extent to which some activities (e.g., strict facility design, quarantine, and final product testing before product dispensing) should be applied.

RL 3.1: Policies and Procedures. There should be written policies and procedures related to every aspect of preparation of risk level 3 sterile products. These policies and procedures should be detailed enough to ensure that all products have the identity, strength, quality, and purity purported for the product.[14,101] All policies and procedures should be reviewed and approved by the designated pharmacist. There should be a mechanism designed to ensure that policies and procedures are communicated, understood, and adhered to by personnel cleaning or working in the controlled area or support area. Written policies and procedures should define and identify the environmental monitoring activities necessary to ensure an adequate environment for risk level 3 sterile product preparation.

In addition to the policies and procedures required for risk levels 1 and 2, there should be written policies and procedures for the following:

1. Component selection, handling, and storage,
2. Any additional personnel qualifications commensurate with the preparation of risk level 3 sterile products,
3. Personnel responsibilities in the controlled area (e.g., sterilization, cleaning, maintenance, access to controlled area),
4. Equipment use, maintenance, calibration, and testing,

5. Sterilization and expiration dating,

6. Master formula and master work sheet development and use,

7. End-product evaluation and testing,

8. Appropriate documentation for preparation of risk level 3 sterile products,

9. Use, control, and monitoring of environmentally controlled areas and calibration of monitoring equipment,

10. Process simulation for each risk level 3 sterile product,

11. Quarantine of products and release from quarantine, if applicable,

12. A mechanism for recalling products from patients in the event that end-product testing procedures yield unacceptable results, and

13. Any other quality control procedures unique to the preparation of risk level 3 sterile products.

RL 3.2: Personnel Education, Training, and Evaluation. Persons preparing sterile products at risk level 3 must have specific education, training, and experience to perform all functions required for the preparation of risk level 3 sterile products. However, final responsibility should lie with the pharmacist, who should be knowledgeable in pharmacy compounding practice[14] and proficient in quality assurance requirements, equipment used in the preparation of risk level 3 sterile products, and other aspects of sterile product preparation. The pharmacist should have sufficient education, training, experience, and demonstrated competency to ensure that all sterile products prepared from sterile or nonsterile components have the identity, strength, quality, and purity purported for the products.[101] In addition to the body of knowledge required for risk levels 1 and 2, the pharmacist should possess sufficient knowledge in the following areas:

1. Aseptic processing,

2. Quality control and quality assurance as related to environmental, component, and end-product testing,

3. Sterilization techniques,[98] and

4. Container, equipment, and closure system selection.

All pharmacy personnel involved in the cleaning and maintenance of the controlled area should be specially trained and thoroughly knowledgeable in the special requirements of class 100 critical-area technology and design. There should be documented, ongoing training for all employees to enable retention of expertise.

RL 3.3: Storage and Handling. In addition to guidelines for risk levels 1 and 2, risk level 3 policies and procedures for storage and handling should include procurement, identification, storage, handling, testing, and recall of nonsterile components.[14,101]

Components and finished products ready to undergo end-product testing should be stored in a manner that prevents their use before release by a pharmacist, minimizes the risk of contamination, and enables identification. There should be identified storage areas that can be used to quarantine products, if necessary, before they are released.[15]

RL 3.4: Facilities and Equipment. Preparation of risk level 3 sterile products should occur in a class 100 horizontal- or vertical-laminar-airflow workbench that is properly situated in a class 10,000 cleanroom *or* in a properly maintained and monitored class 100 cleanroom (without the workbench).[102] The cleanroom area should have a positive pressure differential relative to adjacent, less clean areas of at least 0.05 inch of water. A properly designed and maintained barrier isolator provides an aseptic environment for risk level 3 products.

To allow proper cleaning and disinfection, walls, floors, and ceilings in the controlled area should be nonporous. To help reduce the number of particles in the controlled area, an adjacent support area (e.g., anteroom) should be provided.

During the preparation of risk level 3 sterile products, access to the controlled area or cleanroom should be limited to those individuals who are required to be in the area and are properly attired. The environment of the main access areas directly adjacent to the controlled area (e.g., anteroom) should meet at least Federal Standard 209E class 100,000 requirements. To help maintain a class 100 critical-area environment during compounding, the adjacent support area (e.g., anteroom) should be separated from the controlled area by a barrier (e.g., plastic curtain, partition, wall). Written policies and procedures for monitoring the environment of the controlled area and adjacent areas should be developed.

No sterile products should be prepared in the controlled area if it fails to meet established criteria specified in the policies and procedures. A calibrated particle counter capable of measuring air particles 0.5 mm and larger should be used to monitor airborne particulate matter.[103] Before product preparation begins, the positive-pressure air status should meet or exceed the requirements. Air samples should be taken at several places in the controlled area with the appropriate environmental monitoring devices (e.g., nutrient agar plates). Surfaces on which work actually occurs, including laminar-airflow workbench surfaces and tabletops, should be monitored by using surface contact plates, the swab-rinse technique, or other appropriate methods.[104]

Test results should be reviewed and criteria should be preestablished to determine the point at which the preparation of risk level 3 sterile products will be disallowed until corrective measures are taken. When the environment does not meet the criteria specified in the policies and procedures, sterile product processing should immediately cease and corrective action should be taken. In the event that this occurs, written policies and procedures should delineate alternative methods of sterile product preparation to enable timely fulfillment of prescription orders.

Equipment should be adequate to prevent microbiological contamination. Methods should be established for the cleaning, preparation, sterilization, calibration, and documented use of all equipment.

Critical-area work surfaces should be disinfected with an appropriate agent before the preparation of each product. Floors in the controlled area should be disinfected at least daily. Exterior workbench surfaces and other hard surfaces in the controlled area, such as shelves, tables, and stools, should be disinfected weekly and after any unanticipated event that could increase the risk of contamination. Walls and ceilings in the controlled area or cleanroom should be disinfected at least weekly.

Large pieces of equipment, such as tanks, carts, and tables, used in the controlled area or cleanroom should be made of a material that can be easily cleaned and disinfected; stainless steel is recommended. Stools and chairs should be cleanroom quality. Equipment that does not come in direct contact with the finished product should be properly cleaned, rinsed, and disinfected before being placed in the controlled area. All nonsterile equipment that will come in contact with the sterilized final product should be properly sterilized before introduction into the controlled area; this precaution includes such items as tubing, filters, containers, and other processing equipment. The sterilization process should be monitored and documented.[101]

RL 3.5: Garb. All guidelines for risk levels 1 and 2 should be met. Additionally, cleanroom garb should be worn inside the controlled area at all times during the preparation of risk level 3 sterile products. Attire should consist of a low-shedding coverall, head cover, face mask, and shoe covers. These garments may be either disposable or reusable. Head and facial hair should be covered. Before donning these garments over street clothes, personnel should thoroughly wash their hands and forearms with a suitable antimicrobial skin cleanser.[25] Sterile disposable gloves should be worn and rinsed frequently with an appropriate agent (e.g., 70% isopropyl alcohol) during processing. The gloves should be changed if their integrity is compromised. If persons leave the controlled area *or* support area during processing, they should regown with clean garments before reentering.

RL 3.6: Aseptic Technique and Product Preparation. All guidelines for risk levels 1 and 2 should be met. Methods should ensure that components and containers remain free from contamination and are easily identified as to the product, lot number, and expiration date. If components are not finished sterile pharmaceuticals obtained from licensed manufacturers, pharmacists should ensure that these components meet USP and FDA standards. Products prepared from nonsterile ingredients should be tested to ensure that they do not exceed specified endotoxin limits, unless the ingredient will denature all proteins (e.g., concentrated hydrochloric acid).[105] As each new lot of components and containers is received, the components should be quarantined until properly identified, tested, or verified by a pharmacist.[101]

The methods for preparing sterile products and using process controls should be designed to ensure that finished products have the identity, strength, quality, and purity they are intended to have. Any deviations from established methods should be documented and appropriately justified.

A master work sheet should be developed for the preparation of each risk level 3 sterile product. Once the pharmacist approves the master work sheet, a verified duplicate of the master work sheet should be used as the controlling document from which each sterile end product or batch of prepared products is compounded and on which all documentation for that product or batch occurs. The preparation work sheet should document all the requirements for risk level 2 plus the following:

1. Comparison of actual with anticipated yield,
2. Sterilization methods,[106,107]
3. Pyrogen testing,[108] and
4. Quarantine specifications.

The preparation work sheet should serve as the batch record for each time a risk level 3 sterile product is prepared. Each batch of pharmacy-prepared sterile products should bear a unique lot number, as described in risk level 2.

There should be documentation on the preparation work sheet of all additions of individual components plus the signatures or initials of those individuals involved in the measuring or weighing and addition of these components.

The selection of the final packaging system (including container and closure) for the sterile product is crucial to maintaining product integrity.[109] To the extent possible, presterilized containers obtained from licensed manufacturers should be used. If an aseptic filling operation is used, the container should be sterile at the time of the filling operation. If nonsterile containers are used, methods for sterilizing these containers should be established. Final containers selected should be capable of maintaining product integrity (i.e., identity, strength, quality, and purity) throughout the shelf life of the product.[110]

For products requiring sterilization, selection of an appropriate method of sterilization is of prime importance. Methods of product sterilization include sterile filtration, autoclaving, dry heat sterilization, chemical sterilization, and irradiation.[111,112] The pharmacist must ensure that the sterilization method used is appropriate for the product components and does not alter the pharmaceutical properties of the final product. A method of sterilization often used by pharmacists is sterile filtration.[113] In sterile filtration, the filter should be chosen to fit the chemical nature of the product, and the product should be filtered into presterilized containers under aseptic conditions. Sterilizing filters

of 0.22-μm or smaller porosity should be used in this process. Colloidal or viscous products may require a 0.45-μm filter; however, extreme caution should be exercised in these circumstances, and more stringent end-product sterility testing is essential.[114]

To ensure that a bacteria-retentive filter did not rupture during filtration of a product, an integrity test should be performed on all filters immediately after filtration. This test may be accomplished by performing a bubble point test, in which pressurized gas (e.g., air in a syringe attached to the used filter) is applied to the upstream side of the filter with the downstream outlet immersed in water and the pressure at which a steady stream of bubbles begins to appear is noted.[98] The observed pressure is then compared with the manufacturer's specification for the filter. To compare the used filter with the manufacturer's specifications, which would be based on the filtration of water through the filter, it is necessary to first rinse the filter with sterile water for injection. An observed value lower than the manufacturer's specification indicates that the filter was defective or ruptured during the sterilization process. Methods should be established for handling, testing, and resterilizing any product processed with a filter that fails the integrity test.

RL 3.7: Process Validation. In addition to risk level 1 and 2 guidelines, written policies and procedures should be established to validate all processes involved in the preparation of risk level 3 sterile products (including all procedures, equipment, and techniques) from sterile or nonsterile components. In addition to evaluating personnel technique, process validation provides a mechanism for determining whether a particular process will, when performed by qualified personnel, consistently produce the intended results.[115]

RL 3.8: Expiration Dating. In addition to risk level 2 guidelines, there should be reliable methods for establishing all expiration dates, including laboratory testing of products for sterility, nonpyrogenicity, and chemical content, when necessary. These tests should be conducted in a manner based on appropriate statistical criteria, and the results documented.

RL 3.9: Labeling. All guidelines for risk levels 1 and 2 should be met.

RL 3.10: End-Product Evaluation. For each preparation of a sterile product or a batch of sterile products, there should be appropriate laboratory determination of conformity (i.e., purity, accuracy, sterility, and nonpyrogenicity) to established written specifications and policies. Any reprocessed material should undergo complete final product testing. Additionally, process validation should be supplemented with a program of end-product sterility testing, according to a formal sampling plan.[116–127] Written policies and procedures should specify measurements and methods of testing. Policies and procedures should include a statistically valid sampling plan and acceptance criteria for the sampling and testing. The criteria should be statistically adequate to reasonably ensure that the entire batch meets all specifications. Products not meeting all specifications should be rejected and discarded. There should be a mechanism for recalling all products of a specific batch if end-product-testing procedures yield unacceptable results. On completion of final testing, products should be stored in a manner that ensures their identity, strength, quality, and purity.

It is advisable to quarantine sterile products compounded from nonsterile components, pending the results of end-product testing. If products prepared from nonsterile components must be dispensed before satisfactory completion of end-product testing, there must be a procedure to allow for immediate recall of the products from patients to whom they were dispensed.

RL 3.11: Handling of Sterile Products Outside the Pharmacy. All guidelines for risk levels 1 and 2 should be met.

RL 3.12: Documentation. In addition to the guidelines for risk levels 1 and 2, documentation for risk level 3 sterile products should include

1. Preparation work sheet,
2. Sterilization records of final products (if applicable),
3. Quarantine records (if applicable), and
4. End-product evaluation and testing results.

References

1. Hughes CF, Grant AF, Lick BD, et al. Cardioplegic solution: a contamination crisis. *J Thorac Cardiovasc Surg.* 1986; 91:296–302.

2. Pittsburgh woman loses eye to tainted drugs; 12 hurt. *Baltimore Sun.* 1990; Nov 9:3A.

3. ASHP gears up multistep action plan regarding sterile drug products. *Am J Hosp Pharm.* 1991; 48:386–90.

4. Dugleaux G, Coutour XL, Hecquard C, et al. Septicemia caused by contaminated parenteral nutrition pouches: the refrigerator as an unusual cause. *JPEN J Parenter Enteral Nutr.* 1991; 15:474–5.

5. Solomon SL, Khabbaz RF, Parker RH, et al. An outbreak of *Candida parapsilosis* bloodstream infections in patients receiving parenteral nutrition. *J Infect Dis.* 1984; 149:98–102.

6. Food and Drug Administration. Hazards of precipitation with parenteral nutrition. *Am J Hosp Pharm.* 1994; 51:427–8.

7. Pierce LR, Gaines A, Varricchio R, et al. Hemolysis and renal failure associated with use of sterile water for injection to dilute 25% human albumin solution. *Am J Health-Syst Pharm.* 1998; 55:1057,1062,1070.

8. Flynn EA, Pearson RE, Barker KN. Observational study of accuracy in compounding i.v. admixtures at five hospitals. *Am J Health-Syst Pharm.* 1997; 54:904–12.

9. Santell JP, Kamalich RF. National survey of quality assurance activities for pharmacy-prepared sterile products in hospitals and home infusion facilities—1995. *Am J Health-Syst Pharm.* 1996; 53:2591–605.

10. Kastango ES, Douglass K. Improving the management, operations and cost effectiveness of sterile-product compounding. *Int J Pharm Compd.* 1999; 3:253–8.

11. Guynn JB Jr, Poretz DM, Duma RJ. Growth of various bacteria in a variety of intravenous fluids. *Am J Hosp Pharm.* 1973; 30:321–5.

12. Hasegawa GR. Caring about stability and compatibility. *Am J Hosp Pharm.* 1994; 51:1533–4. Editorial.

13. Stability considerations in dispensing practice (general information chapter 1191). In: The United States pharmacopeia, 24th rev., and The national formulary, 19th ed. Rockville, MD: The United States Pharmacopeial Convention; 1999:2128–30.

14. Pharmacy compounding practices (general information chapter 1161). In: The United States pharmacopeia, 24th rev., and The national formulary, 19th ed. Rockville, MD: The United States Pharmacopeial Convention; 1999:2118–22.

15. Sterile drug products for home use (general information chapter 1206). In: The United States pharmacopeia, 24th rev., and The national formulary, 19th ed. Rockville, MD: The United States Pharmacopeial Convention; 1999:2130–43.

16. Good compounding practices applicable to state licensed pharmacies. *Natl Pharm Compliance News.* 1993; May:2–3, Oct:2–3.

17. Model rules for sterile pharmaceuticals. Chicago: National Association of Boards of Pharmacy; 1993:12.1–3.

18. National Advisory Group on Standards and Practice Guidelines for Parenteral Nutrition. Safe practices for parenteral nutrition formulations. *JPEN J Parenter Enteral Nutr.* 1998; 22:49–66.

19. Standard 3.3. Policies and procedures support safe medication prescription or ordering. In: 1999 Hospital accreditation standards. Chicago: Joint Commission on Accreditation of Healthcare Organizations; 1999:88.

20. Standard TX 5.1. Medications are prepared safely. In: 1999–2000 Comprehensive accreditation manual for home care. Chicago: Joint Commission on Accreditation of Healthcare Organizations; 1999:182.

21. Standard TX 2.3. The pharmacy organization maintains proper conditions of sanitation, temperature, light, moisture, ventilation, segregation, safety, and security for preparing medications. 1996–1998 Standards for long term care pharmacies. Chicago: Joint Commission on Accreditation of Healthcare Organizations; 1996:70–1.

22. Standard TX 3.3. Prescribing and ordering of medications follow established procedures. 1998–99 Comprehensive accreditation manual for ambulatory care. Chicago: Joint Commission on Accreditation of Healthcare Organizations; 1998:211.

23. Food and Drug Modernization Act of 1997, Pub. L. No. 105–115, 111 Stat. 2296.

24. Centers for Disease Control. Guideline for prevention of intravascular infections. *Am J Infect Control.* 1983; 11(5):183–93.

25. Centers for Disease Control. Guideline for handwashing and hospital environmental control. *Am J Infect Control.* 1986; 4(8):110–29.

26. American Society of Hospital Pharmacists. ASHP technical assistance bulletin on handling cytotoxic and hazardous drugs. *Am J Hosp Pharm.* 1990; 47:1033–49.

27. American Society of Hospital Pharmacists. ASHP technical assistance bulletin on pharmacy-prepared ophthalmic products. *Am J Hosp Pharm.* 1993; 50:1462–3.

28. Cleanrooms and associated controlled environments—part 1: classification of air cleanliness. International standard ISO 14644-1. 1st ed. New York: American National Standards Institute; 1999.

29. Federal standard no. 209E. Airborne particulate cleanliness classes in cleanrooms and clean zones. Washington, DC: General Services Administration; 1992.

30. Microbiological evaluation of clean rooms and other controlled environments (general information chapter 1116). In: The United States Pharmacopeia, 24th rev., and The national formulary, 19th ed. Rockville, MD: The United States Pharmacopeial Convention; 1999:2009–106.

31. Validation of aseptic filling for solution drug products. Technical monograph no. 22. Philadelphia: Parenteral Drug Association; 1996.

32. Formulations: *Int J Pharm Compd.* 1999; 2:297–307.

33. Buchanan EC. Policies and procedures for sterile product preparation. In: Principles of sterile product preparation. Bethesda, MD: American Society of Health-System Pharmacists; 1995:133–8.

34. Standard operating procedure of a horizontal laminar air flow hood. *Int J Pharm Compd.* 1997 (Sep/Oct); 1:344–5.

35. Standard operating procedure for general aseptic procedures carried out at a laminar air flow workbench. *Int J Pharm Compd.* 1998 (May/Jun); 2:242.

36. Standard operating procedure for particulate testing for sterile products. *Int J Pharm Compd.* 1997 (Jan/Feb); 2:78.

37. Quality assurance of pharmacy-prepared sterile products. Bethesda, MD: American Society of Hospital Pharmacists; 1994. Videotape and workbook.

38. Safe handling of cytotoxic and hazardous drugs. Bethesda, MD: American Society of Health-System Pharmacists; 1990. Videotape and study guide.

39. Schneider PJ, Buchanan EC. Personnel education, training and evaluation. In: Principles of sterile product preparation. Bethesda, MD: American Society of Health-System Pharmacists; 1995:9–15.

40. Hunt ML. Training manual for intravenous admixture personnel. 5th ed. Chicago: Precept; 1995.

41. Gallagher M. Home care pharmacist competency assessment program. *Am J Health-Syst Pharm.* 1999; 56:1549–53.

42. Dirks I, Smith FM, Furtado D, et al. Method for testing aseptic technique of intravenous admixture personnel. *Am J Hosp Pharm.* 1982; 39:457–9.

43. Brier KL. Evaluating aseptic technique of pharmacy personnel. *Am J Hosp Pharm.* 1983; 40:400–3.

44. McKinnon BT. Handling of sterile products within the pharmacy. In: Principles of sterile product preparation. Bethesda, MD: American Society of Health-System Pharmacists; 1995:111–6.

45. Morris BG, Avis KE. Quality-control plan for intravenous admixture programs. 1: Visual inspection of solutions and environmental testing. *Am J Hosp Pharm.* 1980; 37:189–95.

46. Buchanan EC. Sterile compounding facilities. In: Principles of sterile product preparation. Bethesda, MD: American Society of Health-System Pharmacists; 1995:25–35.

47. Schneider PJ. Equipment for sterile product preparation. In: Principles of sterile product preparation. Bethesda, MD: American Society of Health-System Pharmacists; 1995:37–43.

48. Lau D, Shane R, Yen J. Quality assurance for sterile products: simple changes can help. *Am J Hosp Pharm.* 1994; 51:1353. Letter.

49. Rahe H. Containment Technologies Group, Inc. Personal communication. 1999 Oct.

50. Hunt ML. Training manual for intravenous admixture personnel. 5th ed. Chicago: Precept; 1995:67–70.

51. Buchanan TL, Barker KN, Gibson JT, et al. Illumination and errors in dispensing. *Am J Hosp Pharm.* 1991; 48:2137–45.

52. Denny VF, Kopis EM, Marsik FJ. Elements for a successful disinfection program in the pharmaceutical environment. *PDA J Pharm Sci Technol.* 1999; 53:115–24.

53. Frieben WR. Control of the aseptic processing environment. *Am J Hosp Pharm.* 1983; 40:1928–35.

54. Scheckelhoff DJ. Handling, preparation and disposal of cytotoxic and hazardous agents. In: Principles of sterile product preparation. Bethesda, MD: American Society of Health-System Pharmacists; 1995:63–9.

55. Favier M, Hansel S, Bressole F. Preparing cytotoxic agents in an isolator. *Am J Hosp Pharm.* 1993; 50: 2335–9.

56. Mosko P, Rahe H. Barrier isolation technology: a labor-efficient alternative to cleanrooms. *Hosp Pharm.* 1999; 34:834–8.

57. Pilong A, Moore M. Conversion to isolators in a sterile preparation area. *Am J Health-Syst Pharm.* 1999; 56:1978–80.

58. Tillett L. Barrier isolators as an alternative to a cleanroom. *Am J Health-Syst Pharm.* 1999; 56:1433–6.

59. Bryan D, Marback RC. Laminar air flow equipment certification: what the pharmacist needs to know. *Am J Hosp Pharm.* 1984; 41:1343–9.

60. McKinnon BT. Personnel behavior and garb use. In: Principles of sterile product preparation. Bethesda, MD: American Society of Health-System Pharmacists; 1995:57–62.

61. Coriell LL, McGarrity GJ, Horneff J. Medical applications of dust-free rooms: I. Elimination of airborne bacteria in a research laboratory. *Am J Public Health.* 1967; 57:1824–36.

62. NIOSH recommends steps for reducing work-related exposure to latex. *Am J Health-Syst Pharm.* 1997; 54:1688,1691.

63. Dasher G, Dasher T. The growing problem of latex allergies. *Infusion.* 1996; 2(Jan):23–7.

64. Hunt ML. Techniques used in preparing intravenous admixtures. In: Training manual for intravenous admixture personnel. Chicago: Precept; 1995:87–103.

65. Scheckelhoff DJ. Use of aseptic technique. In: Principles of sterile product preparation. Bethesda, MD: American Society of Health-System Pharmacists; 1995:49–56.

66. Buchanan EC. Sterile product formulation and compounding. In: Principles of sterile product preparation. Bethesda, MD: American Society of Health-System Pharmacists; 1995:17–24.

67. Kessler DA. MedWatch: The new FDA medical products reporting program. *Am J Hosp Pharm.* 1993; 50:1921–36.

68. Rice SP, Gutfeld MB. Preparation of latex-safe products. *Am J Health-Syst Pharm.* 1998; 55:1462–7.

69. Holzman RS. Latex allergy: an emerging operating room problem. *Anesth Analg.* 1993; 76:635–41.

70. McDermott JS, Gura KM. Procedures for preparing injectable medications for latex-sensitive patients. *Am J Health-Syst Pharm.* 1997; 54:2516–7.

71. Schneider PJ. Process validation. In: Principles of sterile product preparation. Bethesda, MD: American Society of Health-System Pharmacists; 1995:121–4.

72. McKinnon BT. Factors influencing expiration dates. In: Principles of sterile product preparation. Bethesda, MD: American Society of Health-System Pharmacists; 1995:95–103.

73. McEvoy GK, ed. AHFS drug information 99. Bethesda, MD: American Society of Health-System Pharmacists; 1999.

74. Bing C, ed. Extended stability for parenteral drugs. Bethesda, MD: American Society of Health-System Pharmacists; in press.

75. Trissel LA. Handbook on injectable drugs. 10th ed. Bethesda, MD: American Society of Health-System Pharmacists; 1998.

76. Catania PN, ed. King guide to parenteral admixtures. St. Louis, MO: King Guide; 1999.

77. American Society of Health-System Pharmacists. ASHP guidelines: minimum standard for home care pharmacies. *Am J Health-Syst Pharm.* 1999; 56:629–38.

78. Scheckelhoff DJ. Labeling of sterile products. In: Principles of sterile product preparation. Bethesda, MD: American Society of Health-System Pharmacists; 1995:105–9.

79. Davis NM. Optimal checking of pharmacy-prepared sterile products. *Hosp Pharm.* 1996; 31:102. Editorial.

80. Schneider PJ. End-product evaluation. In: Principles of sterile product preparation. Bethesda, MD: American Society of Health-System Pharmacists; 1995:125–8.

81. Meyer GE, Novielli KA, Smith JE. Use of refractive index measurement for quality assurance of pediatric parenteral nutrition solutions. *Am J Hosp Pharm.* 1987; 44:1617–20.

82. Scheckelhoff DJ. Handling of sterile products outside the pharmacy. In: Principles of sterile product preparation. Bethesda, MD: American Society of Health-System Pharmacists; 1995:117–20.

83. Chamallas SN, Fishwick JJ, Riesenberg M. Special delivery, keeping the product stable during shipping. *Infusion.* 1997; 4(3):30–2.

84. McKinnon BT. Documentation of sterile product preparations. In: Principles of sterile product preparation. Bethesda, MD: American Society of Health-System Pharmacists; 1995:129–31.

85. Schumock GT, Kafka PS, Tormo VJ. Design, construction, implementation, and cost of a hospital pharmacy cleanroom. *Am J Health-Syst Pharm.* 1998; 55:458–63.

86. Gianino RR. Misconceptions about cleanrooms. *Am J Hosp Pharm.* 1994; 51:239–40. Letter.

87. Fundamentals of a microbiological environmental monitoring program. Technical report no. 13. Philadelphia: Parenteral Drug Association; 1990.

88. Whyte W. In support of settle plates. *PDA J Pharm Sci Technol.* 1996; 50:201–4.

89. Hyde HA. Origin of bacteria in the clean room and their growth requirements. *PDA J Pharm Sci Technol.* 1998; 52:154–8.

90. American Society of Health-System Pharmacists. ASHP guidelines on the safe use of automated compounding devices for the preparation of parenteral nutrition admixtures. *Am J Health-Syst Pharm.* 2000; 57:1343–8.

91. Davis NM. Unprecedented procedural safeguards needed with the use of automated iv compounders. *Hosp Pharm.* 1992; 27:488. Editorial.

92. Murphy C. Ensuring accuracy in the use of automatic compounders. *Am J Hosp Pharm.* 1993; 50:60. Letter.

93. Dickson LB, Somani SM, Herrmann G, et al. Automated compounder for adding ingredients to parenteral nutrient base solutions. *Am J Hosp Pharm.* 1993; 50:678–82.

94. Fishwick JJ, Murphy CC, Riesenberg MC, et al. Weight-based accuracy of parenteral nutrient solutions prepared with an automated compounder. *Am J Health-Syst Pharm.* 1997; 54:678–9.

95. Johnson R, Coles BJ, Tribble DA. Accuracy of three automated compounding systems determined by end-product laboratory testing and comparison with manual preparation. *Am J Health-Syst Pharm.* 1998; 55: 1503–7.

96. Combeau D, Rey JB, Rieutord A, et al. Accuracy of two filling systems for parenteral nutrient solutions. *Am J Health-Syst Pharm.* 1998; 55:1606–10.

97. Boylan JC. Essential elements of quality control. *Am J Hosp Pharm.* 1983; 40:1936–9.

98. McKinnon BT. Preparation and sterilization of batch compounds. In: Principles of sterile product preparation. Bethesda, MD: American Society of Health-System Pharmacists; 1995:71–7.

99. McKinnon BT. Batch preparation documentation. In: Principles of sterile product preparation. Bethesda, MD: American Society of Health-System Pharmacists; 1995:79–94.

100. Lima HA. Required documentation for home infusion pharmacies—compounding records. *Int J Pharm Compd.* 1998; 2:354–9.

101. Avis KE. Assuring the quality of pharmacy-prepared sterile products. *Pharmacopeial Forum.* 1997; 23:3567–76.

102. Fontan JE, Arnaud P, Brion F. Laminar-airflow ceiling in a hospital pharmacy cleanroom. *Am J Health-Syst Pharm.* 1998; 55:182–3. Letter.

103. Chandler SW, Trissel LA, Wamsley LM, et al. Evaluation of air quality in a sterile-drug preparation area with an electronic particle counter. *Am J Hosp Pharm.* 1993; 50:2330–4.

104. Schneider PJ. Environmental monitoring. In: Principles of sterile product preparation. Bethesda, MD: American Society of Health-System Pharmacists; 1995:45–8.

105. Bacterial endotoxins test (general tests and assays chapter 85). In: The United States pharmacopeia, 24th rev., and The national formulary, 19th ed. Rockville, MD: The United States Pharmacopeial Convention; 1999:1829–31.

106. Roberts JH, Wilson JD. Technical report no. 26: sterilizing filtration of liquids. *PDA J Pharm Sci Technol.* 1998; 52(suppl S1):1–31.

107. Akers MJ. Sterilization and depyrogenation: principles and methods. *Int J Pharm Compd.* 1999; 3:263–9.

108. Pyrogen test (general tests and assays chapter 151). In: The United States pharmacopeia, 24th rev., and The national formulary, 19th ed. Rockville, MD: The United States Pharmacopeial Convention; 1999:1850–1.

109. Aspects of container/closure integrity. Technical information bulletin no. 4. Philadelphia: Parenteral Drug Association; 1983.

110. Neidich RL. Selection of containers and closure systems for injectable products. *Am J Hosp Pharm.* 1983; 40:1924–7.

111. Validation of steam sterilization cycles. Technical information bulletin no. 1. Philadelphia: Parenteral Drug Association; 1978.

112. Turco S, ed. Sterile dosage forms: their preparation and clinical application. Philadelphia: Lea & Febiger; 1994:57–78.

113. McKinnon BT, Avis KE. Membrane filtration of pharmaceutical solutions. *Am J Hosp Pharm.* 1993; 50: 1921–36.

114. Eudailey WA. Membrane filters and membrane filtration processes for health care. *Am J Hosp Pharm.* 1983; 40:1921–3.

115. Wilson JD. Aseptic process monitoring—a better strategy. *PDA J Pharm Sci Technol.* 1999; 53:111–4.

116. Sterility tests (general tests and assays chapter 71). In: The United States pharmacopeia, 24th rev., and The national formulary, 19th ed. Rockville, MD: The United States Pharmacopeial Convention; 1999:1818–23.

117. Choy FN, Lamy PP, Burkhart VD, et al. Sterility-testing program for antibiotics and other intravenous admixtures. *Am J Hosp Pharm.* 1982; 39:452–6.

118. Doss HL, James JD, Killough DM, et al. Microbiologic quality assurance for intravenous admixtures in a small hospital. *Am J Hosp Pharm.* 1982; 39:832–5.

119. Posey LM, Nutt RE, Thompson PD. Comparison of two methods for detecting microbial contamination in intravenous fluids. *Am J Hosp Pharm.* 1981; 38:659–62.

120. Akers MJ. Progress toward a preferred method of monitoring the sterility of intravenous admixtures. *Am J Hosp Pharm.* 1982; 39:1297. Editorial.

121. Hoffman KH, Smith FM, Godwin HN, et al. Evaluation of three methods for detecting bacterial contamination in intravenous solutions. *Am J Hosp Pharm.* 1982; 39:1299–302.

122. Miller CM, Furtado D, Smith FM, et al. Evaluation of three methods for detecting low-level bacterial contamination in intravenous solutions. *Am J Hosp Pharm.* 1982; 39:1302–5.

123. DeChant RL, Furtado D, Smith FH, et al. Determining a time frame for sterility testing of intravenous admixtures. *Am J Hosp Pharm.* 1982; 39:1305–8.

124. Bronson MH, Stennett DJ, Egging PK. Sterility testing of home and inpatient parenteral nutrition solutions. *JPEN J Parenter Enteral Nutr.* 1988; 12:25–8.

125. Levchuk JW, Nolly RJ, Lander N. Method for testing the sterility of total nutrient admixtures. *Am J Hosp Pharm.* 1988; 45:1311–21.

126. Akers MJ, Wright GE, Carlson KA. Sterility testing of antimicrobial-containing injectable solutions prepared in the pharmacy. *Am J Hosp Pharm.* 1991; 48:2414–8.

127. Murray PR, Sandrock MJ. Sterility testing of a total nutrient admixture with a biphasic blood-culture system. *Am J Hosp Pharm.* 1991; 48:2419–21.

Footnotes

[a] Unless otherwise stated in this document, the term *sterile products* refers to sterile drugs or nutritional substances that are prepared (e.g., compounded or repackaged) by pharmacy personnel.

[b] Ampuls, swabbed and opened appropriately with contents filtered upon removal, should be considered part of a "closed" system.

[c]Isolator guidelines appear under risk level 1 sections because their greatest use is likely to be in the preparation of cytotoxic sterile products, most of which are risk level 1 processes.

[d]The need to alternate germicides is controversial. According to Akers and Moore (Microbiological monitoring of pharmaceutical cleanrooms: the need for pragmatism, *J Adv Appl Contam Control*. 1998; 1[1]:23–4,26,28,30), the data do not support alternating germicides. A literature search (Kopis EM. *Cleanrooms*. 1996; 10[10]:48–50) found little evidence for periodic alternation of disinfectants; the search did find that alternating use of acidic and alkaline phenolic disinfectants reduces resistance arising in pseudomonads adhering to hard surfaces. If ethanol 70% or isopropyl alcohol 70% is used as the primary disinfectant, it should be sterile filtered through a 0.22-µm filter before use.

[e]According to Trissel and Chandler (*Am J Hosp Pharm*. 1993; 50:1858–61), pharmacy air is nearly class 10,000 cleanroom quality already. However, true cleanrooms add HEPA air filtering and designate room air changes and room air pressure differentials to ensure cleanliness (*Am J Hosp Pharm*. 1994; 51:239–40. Letter).

[f]Note that the International Organization for Sanitation (ISO) is preparing documents that should replace Federal Standard 209E. The ISO documents (numbered 14644-1 through 14644-7 and 14698-1 through 14698-3) are being prepared by a technical committee consisting of members from six countries, including the United States. Document 14644-1 is published in final form and classifies the air cleanliness of cleanrooms and associated controlled environments. In 14644-1 ISO cleanroom class 5 is equivalent to Federal Standard 209E class 100, and ISO class 7 is equivalent to Federal Standard 209E class 10,000.

[g]As in general information chapter 1206 in *USP*, which does not require sterility testing until the third risk level, this assumes that sterile components remain sterile throughout preparation. Many sterile products are prepared in batches too small or used too quickly after preparation to make sterility testing meaningful. Also, one of the purposes of process validation is to determine that personnel and processes can produce a sterile product.

Supersedes the ASHP Technical Assistance Bulletin on Quality Assurance for Pharmacy-Prepared Sterile Products, dated September 24, 1993.

Approved by the ASHP Board of Directors, on April 27, 2000. Developed through the ASHP Council on Professional Affairs.

The bibliographic citation for this document is as follows: American Society of Health-System Pharmacists. ASHP Guidelines on Quality Assurance for Pharmacy-Prepared Sterile Products. *Am J Health-Syst Pharm*. 2000; 57:1150–69.

Appendix A—Glossary

Action Level: Established particulate or microbial counts or results that require corrective action when exceeded.

Aseptic Preparation or Aseptic Processing: The technique involving procedures designed to preclude contamination (of drugs, packaging, equipment, or supplies) by microorganisms during processing.

Batch Preparation: Compounding of multiple sterile product units, in a single discrete process, by the same individuals, carried out during one limited time period.

Cleanroom: A room (1) in which the concentration of airborne particles is controlled, (2) that is constructed and used in a manner to minimize the introduction, generation, and retention of particles inside the room, and (3) in which other relevant variables (e.g., temperature, humidity, and pressure) are controlled as necessary.[28] For example, the air particle count in a class 100 cleanroom cannot exceed a total of 100 particles 0.5 µm or larger per cubic foot of air.[29]

Clean Zone: Dedicated space (1) in which the concentration of airborne particles is controlled, (2) that is constructed and used in a manner that minimizes the introduction, generation, and retention of particles inside the zone, and (3) in which other relevant variables (e.g., temperature, humidity, and pressure) are controlled as necessary. This zone may be open or enclosed and may or may not be located within a cleanroom.[28] For example, an open-architecture controlled area should be a clean zone.

Closed-System Transfer: The movement of sterile products from one container to another in which the containers–closure system and transfer devices remain intact throughout the entire transfer process, compromised only by the penetration of a sterile, pyrogen-free needle or cannula through a designated closure or port to effect transfer, withdrawal, or delivery. Withdrawal of a sterile solution from an ampul through a particulate filter in a class 100 environment would generally be considered acceptable; however, the use of a flexible closure vial, when available, would be preferable.

Compounding: For purposes of these guidelines, compounding simply means the mixing of ingredients to prepare a medication for patient use. This activity would include dilution, admixture, repackaging, reconstitution, and other manipulations of sterile products.

Controlled Area: For purposes of these guidelines, a controlled area is the area designated for preparing sterile products. This is referred to as the buffer zone (i.e., the cleanroom in which the laminar-airflow workbench is located) by USP.[15]

Corrective Action: Action to be taken when the results of monitoring indicate a loss of control or when action levels are exceeded.

Critical Area: Any area in the controlled area where products or containers are exposed to the environment.

Critical Site: An opening providing a direct pathway between a sterile product and the environment or any surface coming into contact with the product or environment.

Critical Surface: Any surface that comes into contact with previously sterilized products or containers.

Designated Pharmacist: The pharmacist chosen by experience and training to be in charge of a sterile product preparation area or unit in a licensed pharmacy.

Expiration Date: The date (and time, when applicable) beyond which a product should not be used (i.e., the product should be discarded beyond this date and time). Expiration date and time should be assigned on the basis of both stability and risk level, whichever is the shorter period. **Note:** Circumstances may occur in which the expiration date and time arrive while an infusion is in progress. When this occurs, judgment should be applied in determining whether it is appropriate to discontinue that infusion and replace the product. Organizational policies on this should be clear.[15]

High-Efficiency Particulate Air (HEPA) Filter: A filter composed of pleats of filter medium separated by rigid sheets of corrugated paper or aluminum foil that direct the flow of air forced through the filter in a uniform parallel flow. HEPA filters remove 99.97% of all air particles 0.3 µm or larger. When HEPA filters are used as a component of a horizontal- or vertical-laminar-airflow workbench, an environment can be created consistent with standards for a class 100 cleanroom.

Isolator (or Barrier Isolator): A closed system made up of four solid walls, an air-handling system, and transfer and interaction devices. The walls are constructed so as to provide surfaces that are cleanable with coving between wall junctures.

The air-handling system provides HEPA filtration of both inlet and exhaust air. Transfer of materials is accomplished through air locks, glove rings, or ports. Transfers are designed to minimize the entry of contamination. Manipulations can take place through either glove ports or half-suits.

Media Fill: See process validation or simulation.

Preservatives: For purposes of these guidelines, preservatives refer to any additive intended to extend the content, stability, or sterility of active ingredients (e.g., antioxidants, emulsifiers, bacteriocides).

Process Validation or Simulation: Microbiological simulation of an aseptic process with growth medium processed in a manner similar to the processing of the product and with the same container or closure system.[30] Process simulation tests are synonymous with medium fills, simulated product fills, broth trials, and broth fills.

Quality Assurance: For purposes of these guidelines, quality assurance is the set of activities used to ensure that the processes used in the preparation of sterile drug products lead to products that meet predetermined standards of quality.

Quality Control: For purposes of these guidelines, quality control is the set of testing activities used to determine that the ingredients, components (e.g., containers), and final sterile products prepared meet predetermined requirements with respect to identity, purity, nonpyrogenicity, and sterility.

Repackaging: The subdivision or transfer of a compounded product from one container or device to a different container or device, such as a syringe or an ophthalmic container.

Sterilization: A validated process used to render a product free of viable organisms.

Sterilizing Filter: A filter that, when challenged with a solution containing the microorganism *Pseudomonas diminuta* at a minimum concentration of 10^{12} organisms per square centimeter of filter surface, will produce a sterile effluent.

Temperatures (USP): Frozen means temperatures between –20 and –10 °C (–4 and 14 °F). Refrigerated means temperatures between 2 and 8 °C (36 and 46 °F). Room temperature means temperatures between 15 and 30 °C (59 and 86 °F).

Validation: Documented evidence providing a high degree of assurance that a specific process will consistently produce a product meeting its predetermined specifications and quality attributes.

Worst Case: A set of conditions encompassing upper and lower processing limits and circumstances, including those within standard operating procedures, that pose the greatest chance of process or product failure when compared with ideal conditions. Such conditions do not necessarily induce product or process failure.[31]

Appendix B—Comparison of Risk-Level Attributes

This appendix does not show all details of the guidelines, nor does it tell whether an aspect of the sterile compounding process is "required" (must be) or "advisable" (should be). Regardless of the examples given, each compounding pharmacist must decide, according to the circumstances at the time, what conditions are appropriate for compounding a sterile product. In an emergency, it may be of more benefit to a patient to receive a sterile drug prepared under lower risk-level conditions. For the immunocompromised patient, even simple, single-patient admixtures may need to be compounded under higher risk-level conditions.

Table 1.

Assignment of Products to Risk Level 1 or 2 according to Time and Temperature before Completion of Administration

Risk Level	Room Temperature (15–30 °C)	No. Days Storage	
		Refrigerator (2–8 °C)	Freezer (−20 to −10 °C)
1	Completely administered within 28 hr	≤7	≤30
2	Storage and administration exceed 28 hr	>7	>30

Definition of Products by Risk Level

Risk Level 1	Risk Level 2	Risk Level 3
Products that are (1) stored at room temperature and completely administered within 28 hours from preparation, (2) unpreserved and sterile and prepared for administration to one patient, or batch prepared for administration to more than one patient and contain suitable preservatives, and (3) prepared by closed-system aseptic transfer of sterile, nonpyrogenic, finished pharmaceuticals obtained from licensed manufacturers into sterile final containers obtained from licensed manufacturers.	Products that are (1) administered beyond 28 hours after preparation and storage at room temperature, (2) batch prepared without preservatives and intended for use by more than one patient, or (3) compounded by complex or numerous manipulations of sterile ingredients obtained from licensed manufacturers in a sterile container obtained from a licensed manufacturer by using closed-system, aseptic transfer.	Products that are (1) compounded from nonsterile ingredients or with nonsterile components, containers, or equipment before terminal sterilization or (2) prepared by combining multiple ingredients (sterile or nonsterile) by using an open-system transfer or open reservoir before terminal sterilization.

Examples of Sterile Products by Risk Level

Risk Level 1	Risk Level 2	Risk Level 3
Single-patient admixture	Injections for use in portable pump or reservoir over multiple days	Alum bladder irrigation
Single-patient ophthalmic, preserved	Batch-reconstituted antibiotics without preservatives	Morphine injection made from powder or tablets
Single-patient syringes without preservatives used in 28 hours	Batch-prefilled syringes without preservatives	TPN solutions made from dry amino acids
Batch-prefilled syringes with preservatives	TPN solutions mixed with an automatic compounding device	TPN solutions sterilized by final filtration
Total parenteral nutrient (TPN) solution made by gravity transfer of carbohydrate and amino acids into an empty container with the addition of sterile additives with a syringe and needle		Autoclaved i.v. solutions

Policies and Procedures

Risk Level 1	Risk Level 2	Risk Level 3
Up-to-date policies and procedures for compounding sterile products should be available to all involved personnel. When policies are changed, they should be updated. Procedures should address personnel education and training, competency evaluation, product acquisition, storage and handling of products and supplies, storage and delivery of final products, use and maintenance of facilities and equipment, appropriate garb and conduct of personnel working in the controlled area, process validation, preparation technique, labeling, documentation, quality control, and material movement.	In addition to risk level 1 guidelines, procedures describe environmental monitoring devices and techniques, cleaning materials and disinfectants, equipment accuracy monitoring, limits of acceptability and corrective actions for environmental monitoring and process validation, master formula and work sheets, personnel garb, lot numbers, and other quality control methods.	Procedures cover every aspect of preparation of level 3 sterile products, so that all products have the identity, strength, quality, and purity purported for the product. Thirteen general policies and procedures, in addition to those in levels 1 and 2, are required.

Personnel Education, Training, and Evaluation

Risk Level 1	Risk Level 2	Risk Level 3
All pharmacy personnel preparing sterile products should receive suitable didactic and experiential training and competency evaluation through demonstration or testing (written or practical). In addition to the policies and procedures listed above, education includes chemical, pharmaceutical, and clinical properties of drugs and current good compounding practices.	In addition to guidelines in risk level 1, training includes assessment of competency in all types of risk level 2 procedures via process simulation. Personnel show competency in end-product testing as well.	Operators have specific education, training, and experience to prepare risk level 3 products. Pharmacist knows principles of good compounding practice for risk level 3 products, including aseptic processing; quality assurance of environmental, component, and end-product testing; sterilization; and selection and use of containers, equipment, and closures.

Storage and Handling in the Pharmacy

Risk Level 1	Risk Level 2	Risk Level 3
Solutions, drugs, supplies, and equipment must be stored according to manufacturer or USP requirements. Refrigerator and freezer temperatures should be documented daily. Other storage areas should be inspected regularly to ensure that temperature, light, moisture, and ventilation meet requirements. Drugs and supplies should be shelved above the floor. Expired products must be removed from active product storage areas. Personnel traffic in storage areas should be minimized. Removal of products from boxes should be done outside controlled areas. Disposal of used supplies should be done at least daily. Product-recall procedures must permit retrieving affected products from specific involved patients.	All guidelines for risk level 1 apply.	In addition to risk level 1 guidelines, procedures include procurement, identification, storage, handling, testing, and recall of components and finished products. Finished but untested products must be quarantined under minimal risk for contamination or loss of identity in an identified quarantine area.

Facilities and Equipment

Risk Level 1	Risk Level 2	Risk Level 3
The controlled area should be separated from other operations to minimize unnecessary flow of materials and personnel through the area. The controlled area must be clean, well lighted, and of sufficient size for sterile compounding. A sink with hot and cold water should be near, but not in, the controlled area. The controlled area and inside equipment must be cleaned and disinfected regularly. Sterile products must be prepared in a class 100 environment (the critical area), such as within a horizontal- or vertical-laminar-airflow workbench or barrier isolator. Computer entry, order processing, label generation, and record keeping should be performed outside the critical area. The critical area must be disinfected periodically. A workbench should be recertified every six months or when it is moved; prefilters should be changed periodically. Pumps should be recalibrated according to procedure.	In addition to risk level 1 guidelines, the following are recommended for risk level 2 products: controlled area must meet class 10,000 cleanroom standards; cleaning supplies should be selected to meet cleanroom standards; critical-area work surface must be cleaned between batches; floors should be disinfected daily, equipment surfaces weekly, and walls monthly; and there should be environmental monitoring of air and surfaces. An anteroom of high cleanliness is desirable. Automated compounding devices must be calibrated and verified as to accuracy, according to procedure.	Products must be prepared in a class 100 workbench in a class 10,000 cleanroom, in a class 100 cleanroom, or in a suitable barrier isolator. Access to the cleanroom must be limited to those preparing the products who are in appropriate garb. Methods are needed for cleaning, preparing, sterilizing, calibrating, and documenting the use of all equipment. Walls and ceilings should be disinfected weekly. All nonsterile equipment that is to come in contact with the sterilized final product should be sterilized before introduction into the cleanroom. An anteroom of high cleanliness (i.e., class 100,000) should be provided. Appropriate cleaning and disinfection of the environment and equipment are required.

Garb

Risk Level 1	Risk Level 2	Risk Level 3
In the controlled area, personnel wear low-particulate, clean clothing covers such as clean gowns or coverall with sleeves having elastic cuffs. Hand, finger, and wrist jewelry is minimized or eliminated. Nails are clean and trimmed. Gloves are recommended; those allergic to latex rubber must wear gloves made of a suitable alternative. Head and facial hair is covered. Masks are recommended during aseptic preparation. Personnel preparing sterile products scrub their hands and arms with an appropriate antimicrobial skin cleanser.	In addition to risk level 1 guidelines, gloves, gowns, and masks are required. During sterile preparation, gloves should be rinsed frequently with a suitable agent (e.g., 70% isopropyl alcohol) and changed when their integrity is compromised. Shoe covers are helpful in maintaining the cleanliness of the controlled area.	In addition to risk level 1 and 2 guidelines, cleanroom garb must be worn inside the controlled area at all times during the preparation of risk level 3 sterile products. Attire consists of a low-shedding coverall, head cover, face mask, and shoe covers. Before donning this garb, personnel must thoroughly wash their hands and arms. Upon return to the controlled area or support area during processing, personnel should regown with clean garb.

Aseptic Technique and Product Preparation

Risk Level 1	Risk Level 2	Risk Level 3
Sterile products must be prepared in a class 100 environment. Personnel scrub their hands and forearms for an appropriate period at the beginning of each aseptic compounding process. Eating, drinking, and smoking are prohibited in the controlled area. Talking is minimized to reduce airborne particles. Ingredients are determined to be stable, compatible, and appropriate for the product to be prepared, according to manufacturer, USP, or scientific references. Ingredients result in final products that meet physiological norms as to osmolality and pH for the intended route of administration. Ingredients and containers are inspected for defects, expiration, and integrity before use. Only materials essential for aseptic compounding are placed in the workbench. Surfaces of ampuls and vials are disinfected before placement in the workbench. Sterile components are arranged in the workbench to allow uninterrupted laminar airflow over critical surfaces of needles, vials, ampuls, etc. Usually only one person and one preparation are in the workbench at a time. Automated devices and equipment are cleaned, disinfected, and placed in the workbench to enable laminar airflow. Aseptic technique is used to avoid touch contamination of critical sites of containers and ingredients. Sterile powders are completely reconstituted. Particles are filtered from solutions. Needle cores are avoided. The pharmacist checks before, during, and after preparation to verify the identity and amount of ingredients before release.	In addition to risk level 1 guidelines, a master work sheet containing formula, components, procedures, sample label, final evaluation, and testing is made for each product batch. A separate work sheet and lot number are used for each batch. When combining multiple sterile ingredients, a second pharmacist should verify calculations. The pharmacist should verify data entered into an automatic compounder before processing and check the end product for accuracy.	In addition to risk level 1 and 2 guidelines, non-sterile components must meet USP standards for identity, purity, and endotoxin levels, as verified by a pharmacist. Batch master work sheets should also include comparisons of actual with anticipated yields, sterilization methods, and quarantine specifications. Presterilized containers should be used if feasible. Final containers must be sterile and capable of maintaining product integrity throughout shelf life. Sterilization method is based on properties of the product. Final filtration methods require attention to many elements of product, filter, and filter integrity.

Process Validation

Risk Level 1	Risk Level 2	Risk Level 3
All persons who prepare sterile products should pass a process validation of their aseptic technique before they prepare sterile products for patient use. Personnel competency should be reevaluated by process validation at least annually, whenever the quality assurance program yields an unacceptable result, and whenever unacceptable techniques are observed. If microbial growth is detected, the entire sterile process must be evaluated, corrective action taken, and the process simulation test performed again.	All risk level 1 guidelines apply, and process-simulation procedures should cover all types of manipulations, products, and batch sizes that are encountered in risk level 2.	In addition to risk level 1 and 2 guidelines, written policies should be made to validate all processes (including all procedures, components, equipment, and techniques) for each risk level 3 product.

Handling Sterile Products Outside the Pharmacy

Risk Level 1	Risk Level 2	Risk Level 3
Sterile products are transported so as to be protected from excesses of temperatures and light. Transit time and condition should be specified. Delivery personnel should be trained as appropriate. Pharmacists ascertain that the end user knows how to properly store products. End users notify pharmacists when storage conditions are exceeded or when products expire so that pharmacists can arrange safe disposal or return.	All guidelines for risk level 1 should be met.	All guidelines for risk level 1 should be met.

Documentation

Risk Level 1	Risk Level 2	Risk Level 3
The following must be documented according to policy, laws, and regulations: (1) training and competency evaluation of employees, (2) refrigerator and freezer temperature logs, (3) certification of workbenches, and (4) other facility quality control logs as appropriate. Pharmacists maintain appropriate records for the compounding and dispensing of sterile products.	In addition to the guidelines in risk level 1, documentation of end-product testing and batch-preparation records must be maintained according to policies, laws, and regulations.	In addition to the guidelines in risk levels 1 and 2, documentation for risk level 3 products must include (1) preparation work sheet, (2) sterilization records if applicable, (3) quarantine records if applicable, and (4) end-product evaluation and testing records.

Expiration Dating

Risk Level 1	Risk Level 2	Risk Level 3
All sterile products must bear an appropriate expiration date. Expiration dates are assigned based on current drug stability information and sterility considerations. The pharmacist considers all aspects of the final product, including drug reservoir, drug concentration, and storage conditions.	All guidelines for risk level 1 should be met.	In addition to risk level 1 and 2 guidelines, there must be a reliable method for establishing all expiration dates, including laboratory testing of product stability, pyrogenicity, and chemical content when necessary.

Labeling

Risk Level 1	Risk Level 2	Risk Level 3
Sterile products should be labeled with at least the following information: (1) for patient-specific products, the patient's name and other appropriate patient identification; for batch-prepared products, control or lot numbers, (2) all solution and ingredient names, amounts, strengths, and concentrations, (3) expiration date (and time when applicable), (4) prescribed administration regimen, (5) appropriate auxiliary labeling, (6) storage requirements, (7) identification of the responsible pharmacist, (8) any device-specific instructions, and (9) any additional information, in accordance with state and federal regulations. A reference number for the prescription or order may also be helpful. The label should be legible and affixed to the product so that it can be read while being administered.	All guidelines for risk level 1 must be met.	All guidelines for risk levels 1 and 2 must be met.

End-Product Evaluation

Risk Level 1	Risk Level 2	Risk Level 3
The final product must be inspected for container leaks, integrity, solution cloudiness or phase separation, particulates in solution, appropriate solution color, and solution volume. The pharmacist must verify that the product was compounded accurately as to ingredients, quantities, containers, and reservoirs.	In addition to risk level 1 guidelines, toxic products, like concentrated glucose and potassium chloride, should be tested for accuracy of concentration.	In addition to risk level 1 and 2 guidelines, the medium-fill procedure should be supplemented with a program of end-product sterility testing according to a formal sampling plan. Samples should be statistically adequate to reasonably ensure that batches are sterile. A method for recalling batch products should be established if end-product testing yields unacceptable results. Each sterile preparation or batch must be laboratory tested for conformity to written specifications (e.g., concentration, pyrogenicity). It is advisable to quarantine sterile products compounded from nonsterile components pending the results of end-product testing.

Medication Errors

JACQUELINE Z. KESSLER

Pharmacists are responsible for the safe and appropriate use of medications in all pharmacy practice settings. As part of the multidisciplinary health care team, the pharmacist's role is to cooperate to establish patient-specific drug therapy regimens designed to achieve predefined therapeutic outcomes without subjecting the patient to undue harm.

As pharmacists become more involved in patient-specific care, technicians are asked to perform tasks that have previously been restricted to pharmacists. As their responsibilities expand, technicians need to be aware of the significance and causes of medication errors and to recognize their role in preventing those errors.

Numerous terms are used to describe drug-related incidents. The term *drug misadventures* is used to describe both adverse drug reactions (unintended responses to drugs used at normal doses) and medication errors (errors related to the medication use process that may or may not result in adverse drug outcomes).[1] This chapter focuses on errors that occur during the medication use process, which includes the prescribing, dispensing, and administration phases of medication use; monitoring the patient for expected and unexpected outcomes; and patient compliance.

This chapter provides insight into the incidence and significance of medication errors. It reviews common causes of medication errors and suggests measures to minimize errors. In addition, it highlights the importance of medication error reporting and monitoring.

Types of Medication Errors

Medication errors can occur at any point during the medication use process. They do not occur only in the pharmacy. For example, medication errors can occur when a physician writes an order (during the prescribing process), when a nurse transcribes a medication order, when

After completing this chapter, the technician should be able to

1. Describe the different types of medication errors.

2. Identify causes or factors that contribute to medication errors.

3. List five "high alert" medications.

4. Describe things that can be done to prevent medication errors from occurring.

5. List examples of common errors.

6. Recognize possible consequences of actual medication errors.

7. Describe steps to be taken when an error has been identified.

8. Understand the role of quality assurance monitoring of medication errors.

office personnel phone in a prescription to the pharmacy, or when patients do not take their medication as directed (patient compliance).

Pharmacy technicians should be aware of and concerned with all types of errors, not just those specifically occurring in the pharmacy. Sometimes a pharmacist may miss an error and a technician may notice it. According to the *ASHP Guidelines on Preventing Medication Errors in Hospitals*,[2] medication errors can be categorized into 11 types. The specific category to which an error belongs is not always obvious, because of the complex nature of the medication use process. Errors may occur because of multiple factors, and therefore may fit several categories.

Prescribing Errors

A prescribing error occurs at the time a prescriber orders a drug for a specific patient. Errors may include the selection of an incorrect drug, dose, dosage form, route of administration, length of therapy, or number of doses. Other prescribing errors are an inappropriate rate of administration, a wrong drug concentration, or inadequate or wrong instructions for use. When evaluating whether a medication was prescribed in error, it is important to consider patient characteristics, such as allergies, weight, age, medical indication (condition being treated), and concurrent drug therapy, among other factors. For example, a prescription for amoxicillin 250 mg PO TID may be appropriate to treat a middle ear infection in a 5-year-old child but would be too high a dose for a 12-month-old infant and thus would be considered a prescribing error. Prescriptions that are filled incorrectly because of illegible handwriting are also considered prescribing errors.

Omission Errors

Failure to administer an ordered dose to a patient in a hospital, nursing home, or other facility before the next scheduled dose is considered an omission error. An omission error occurs when a dose is completely omitted as opposed to administered late. If a dose is ordered to be held for medical reasons, it is not considered an error. Examples of times when an omitted dose is not an error are when the patient cannot take anything by mouth (NPO) prior to a procedure or when health care providers are waiting for drug level results to be reported. In addition, not administering medications because a patient refuses to take them is not considered an error.

Wrong Time Errors

Timing of administration is critical to the effectiveness of some medications. Maintaining an adequate blood level of some drugs, such as antibiotics, frequently depends on evenly spaced, around-the-clock dosing. Administering doses too early or too late may affect the drug serum level and consequently the efficacy of the drug. Nursing homes and hospitals frequently have predefined administration times to establish consistency. It could be harmful to a patient if a daily dose is administered inconsistently. It would not be realistic to expect all morning doses to be administered at exactly 0800. Therefore, an acceptable interval surrounding the scheduled time is usually established. An institution may determine that administering medications within 30 minutes of the scheduled time (30 minutes before or after) is acceptable. Medications administered outside this window would be considered wrong time errors. Wrong time errors are occasionally unavoidable because the patient is away from the patient care area for a test or the medication is not available at the time it is due.

Unauthorized Drug Errors

Administration of a medication to a patient without proper authorization by the prescriber is categorized as an unauthorized drug error. An unauthorized drug error might occur if a medication for one patient was given mistakenly to another patient or if a nurse gave a medication without a physician order. Another cause is patients at home who sometimes "share" prescriptions. Refilling a prescription that has no refills remaining without authorization from the physician is another example of an unauthorized drug error.

Some health care facilities have guidelines or protocols that allow flexibility in administering medications on the basis of specific patient parameters. For example, a post-surgical protocol may allow a nurse to administer a potassium chloride injection when a patient's serum potassium level falls below a specified level. The dose of potassium chloride may vary depending on how low the serum level is. Administration of medications outside the established guidelines is another example of an unauthorized drug error.

Improper Dose Errors

Improper dose errors occur when a patient is given a dose that is greater or less than the prescribed dose. This type of error may occur if there is a delay in documenting a dose—or absence of documentation—that results in an additional dose being administered. Inaccurate measurement of an oral liquid is also an improper dose error. Excluded from this category are doses that cannot be accurately measured or are not specified, as in topical applications. Variances that occur from apothecary to metric conversions are excluded as well.

Wrong Dosage Form Errors

Doses administered or dispensed in a different form from that ordered by the prescriber are classified as wrong dosage form errors. Depending on state laws and health care facility guidelines, dosage form changes may be acceptable to accommodate particular patient needs. For example, dispensing a liquid formulation without a specific prescription to a patient who has difficulty swallowing tablets might be an acceptable dosage form change.

Wrong Drug Preparation Errors

Drugs requiring reconstitution (adding liquid to dissolve a powdered drug), dilution, or special preparation prior to dispensing or administration are subject to drug preparation errors. Examples include reconstituting a cephalexin oral suspension with an incorrect volume of water, using bacteriostatic saline for injection instead of sterile water for injection to reconstitute a lyophilized powder for injection, or not breaking the seal of a ready-to-mix heparin bag. Using a wrong base product when compounding an ointment is another example of a wrong drug preparation error.

Wrong Administration Technique Errors

Doses that are administered using an inappropriate procedure or incorrect technique are categorized as wrong administration technique errors. A subcutaneous injection that is given too deep and an intravenous (IV) drug that is allowed to infuse via gravity instead of using an IV pump are classified in this category. Instilling eye drops in the wrong eye is another example of an error in this category.

Deteriorated Drug Errors

Although sometimes cumbersome, monitoring expiration dates of products is very important. Drugs used past their expiration date may have lost potency and may be less effective or ineffective. Refrigerated drugs stored at room temperature may decompose to the point that their efficacy is less than optimal. Medications that are dispensed or administered beyond their expiration date or medications that have deteriorated because of improper storage are listed as deteriorated drug errors.

Monitoring Errors

Monitoring errors result from inadequate drug therapy review. Ordering serum drug levels for a patient on phenytoin (seizure medication) but not reviewing them or not responding to a level outside of the therapeutic range is a monitoring error. Not ordering drug levels when required or prescribing an antihypertensive agent, which lowers blood pressure, and failing to check blood pressure are monitoring errors as well.

Compliance Errors

Medication errors are committed by patients, too, when they fail to adhere to a prescribed drug regimen. These errors may be detected when a patient requests refills for prescriptions at unreasonable intervals (too long after or too soon before a refill is due) without a reasonable explanation.

Other Errors

Errors that cannot be placed into one of the 11 categories are grouped together in a miscellaneous category. Some of the errors as defined in the ASHP guidelines seem to apply primarily to patients in a health care facility. These same definitions actually can be applied to home health care, clinic, or physician office settings, as well as the outpatient pharmacy practice setting.

Incidence

Although medication errors are not uncommon, determining their actual numbers is difficult. Few studies provide a complete and thorough evaluation of errors within the entire medication use process. It is hard to project data from studies on medication errors because of the different methods used to detect errors and the various definitions of errors. In addition, the focus of some studies is on just physician, nursing, or pharmacy errors or just one component of the medication use process.

Medication errors can occur at any point in the medication use process. Millions of doses are administered daily in health care facilities and patient homes, and the volume of prescriptions filled annually in community-based pharmacies, including mail order, is more than 3.1 billion.[3] On the basis of these estimates alone, it is apparent that even with a high rate of accuracy, a small percentage of errors can result in a large number of medication errors.

The number of new drugs and dosage forms available continues to grow, making it difficult to keep up with new developments in pharmacy. Staying abreast of technological advances and complex medication regimens requires professional commitment. Medication error awareness and prevention must be a high priority in all health care facilities and pharmacies.

Medication Error Rates

This section describes medication error rates reported in some studies. It provides an overview of the complexity of studying medication errors owing to the different monitoring, measuring, and reporting techniques used. It also reviews differences in the studies that contribute to varying medication error rates reported in the literature.

The Harvard Medical Study[4] that looked at the incidence of adverse events in hospitalized patients found that 19 percent of the adverse events that occurred in hospitalized patients were related to drug complications. This study demonstrates that complications from drugs, including those caused by errors, are a significant cause of medical management injuries in hospitalized patients.

Physician prescribing error rates in hospital and community settings have been reported to be 0.3 to 1.9 percent.[5–7] One study determined that almost one-third (28.3 percent) of the prescribing errors were potentially harmful if not followed up by a pharmacist.[6] An evaluation of causes of prescribing errors in hospitals found that the majority of potentially serious prescribing errors were made because of performance lapses (knowing the right thing to do, but accidentally doing something else) by the physician or because of failure to adhere to established procedures.[8] Further, it has been observed that errors occurring earlier in the medication use process (in the prescribing phase) are more likely to be detected and corrected than those occurring later in the process (in administration).[9]

Physician prescribing is only the first step in the medication use process. Other studies have evaluated medication errors occurring at various other stages. Error rates of pharmacist dispensing in the outpatient setting have been reported to be approximately 12 percent.[10,11] There are conflicting data evaluating the relationship between the number of serious errors and the number of prescriptions filled.[10–12] The medication error rate in health care institutions not using a unit dose system has been estimated to be one error per patient per day.[13] One study evaluated the number of errors occurring in the drug administration phase in 36 hospitals and skilled nursing facilities and found that 19

percent of all doses were not administered correctly. The majority (43 percent) of errors were due to wrong time of administration.[14]

Medication error studies report different error rates. The pharmacy technician should recognize that the differences in error rates may be due to differences in how studies were performed, the various techniques and definitions used, and the scope of a study. Many errors are identified and corrected before medications reach the patient. Studies also show that a small percentage of errors lead to adverse events in patients.[15]

Medication Error Reporting

The rate of medication errors is often based on incident reports. Ideally, health care providers complete incident reports when a medication error is discovered. That does not always happen, however, because many health care personnel lack the knowledge to identify errors, lack the time to document them, or are afraid of negative consequences.

Many times errors are discovered when a pharmacist checks a prescription or medication order prior to dispensing, and the error is corrected promptly before the medication reaches the patient. Often, the error is not documented because it is not recognized as an error or the reporting process is cumbersome. For these reasons, the number of medication errors is probably higher than reported.

Reporting medication errors can sometimes be a frightening experience. Health care personnel may be afraid of disciplinary or punitive actions or of the backlash of reporting an error made by a coworker. They may also be concerned about liability issues should a negative outcome occur because of an error.

It is apparent that medication errors occur every day in all practice settings. Fortunately, most of these errors are detected and corrected before the medication ever reaches the patient. Some medication errors do, however, reach the patient, and some errors result in negative outcomes.

Impact of Medication Errors

The outcomes of medication errors range from no effect to minor discomfort to devastating long-term disability or death.[16,17] Often, predicting the outcome and significance of a medication error is difficult because so many factors are involved. Such factors include the type of medication error, the health status of the patient, the pharmacologic classification of the drug involved, the route of drug administration, the timing of drug administration, the cost to the health care system, and the damage to the patient's trust in care providers.

Impact on the Patient

In a report of five pediatric patients who received overdoses of vincristine (a chemotherapy drug), three patients died and two recovered.[18] Of the three patients who died, two received a 10-fold overdose and the third was very ill with an advanced stage leukemia. The two children who recovered were in remission (their leukemia was under control) at the time and received smaller overdoses. In this situation, the health status of the patients and magnitude of the overdose helped determine the significance of the error.

Sometimes, not receiving a drug or receiving it late may harm patients as well. Administration of a phenytoin (seizure medication) dose was delayed 28 hours in an elderly patient and resulted in a seizure.[19] The patient subsequently underwent extensive surgery to repair a jaw fracture that resulted from a fall during the seizure. All these events can be attributed to one medication error—late administration of the phenytoin. Many case reports describe adverse drug events caused by medication errors.

Financial Impact of Medication Errors

Not only can medication errors lead to negative patient outcomes, they can prolong hospital stays and increase health care expenses.[20] Treating adverse events is estimated to cost billions of dollars annually.[16,21,22] It was estimated that $1.5 million was spent in a single year to treat adverse drug events at one hospital.[21] Another study evaluated the cost of drug-related morbidity and mortality in the ambulatory setting. That study estimated that the United States spends $76.6 billion annually to manage those drug-related occurrences, some of which were due to medication errors.[22] Not only the cost of additional medical management but also the legal fees or out-of-court settlements resulting from malpractice claims must be considered.

In one case, almost $14,000 in medical costs were incurred to treat a patient who experienced recurrent hypoglycemia (low blood sugar) because of a prescription error.[23] The pharmacist inadvertently dispensed glyburide (Diabeta®, a drug for high blood sugar) instead of diazepam (Valium®, an anti-anxiety medication).

Loss of Trust

Patients may lose faith in the medical community as a result of experiencing or reading about an adverse drug event. They may choose to switch pharmacies or physicians or even hesitate to seek medical help for fear of not receiving quality care. Patients may also seek nonconventional treatments from outside the medical community. Personnel responsible for medication errors that result in significant patient injury may lose confidence in themselves as practitioners as well.

Fortunately, most medication errors are detected and corrected before the medication is dispensed to the patient or the patient care area. However, medication errors do occur and may result in reversible or permanent negative patient outcomes. They can also be associated with a financial impact to an individual, an institution, and the overall health care system.

Causes of Medication Errors and Ways to Prevent Them

Medication errors can be attributed to a number of different causes. It would be unfair to place blame solely on an individual without considering factors that might contribute to an error. Administrators of health systems constantly strive to decrease the presence of factors in the medication use system that contribute to medication errors. In turn, each health care provider must also strive to minimize the occurrence of medication errors. One of the best ways to do this is to become familiar with the most common causes of medication errors. Medication errors are most often attributed to one or more of the following: calculation errors, careless use of zeros and decimal points, inappropriate use of abbreviations, careless prescribing, illegible handwriting, missing information, drug product characteristics, compounding/drug preparation errors, prescription labeling, and work environment or staffing issues.

Calculation Errors

Reports show that numerous medication errors are caused by errors in mathematical calculations. In some cases, patients have died as a result of miscalculated doses.[17,24] Calculation errors are made by prescribers, pharmacists checking doses for appropriateness or calculating doses, technicians compounding products, and nurses preparing or administering doses. Even with the use of calculators, health care personnel frequently make calculation errors.[25]

The pediatric population is particularly at risk. It is not uncommon for pediatric doses to be determined by the patient's weight, requiring an interim step to calculate the final dose. Many drugs are not available in pediatric formulations, so adult formulations must be diluted or manipulated multiple times to get the appropriate dose. One study evaluated errors in drug computations for health care personnel in a neonatal intensive care unit. Test scores were 75.6 percent (range of 45–95 percent) correct answers for nurses, 89.1 percent for physicians, and 96 percent for pharmacists.[26] Many of the errors found in this study would have resulted in doses 10 times higher or lower than the dose ordered.

Personnel with multiple years of experience are just as likely to make mathematical errors as inexperienced personnel.[26-28] Calculation errors are often made by using the wrong concentration of stock solutions, misplacing a decimal point, or using wrong conversions. Personnel also neglect to double-check their work, rely on their memory instead of looking up a conversion, or do not ask themselves, "Does the answer seem reasonable?"

Another way to decrease the risk of a calculation error is to ask a pharmacist or another technician to double check the calculation prior to preparing the product. The calculation should be performed independently and compared with the original answer. This system is an effective way to prevent calculation errors.

Decimal Points and Zeros

Misplacing a decimal point by one place results in errors 10-fold greater than or less than intended. For drugs with a narrow therapeutic range (e.g., digoxin, phenytoin, lidocaine, aminoglycoside antibiotics), the consequences can be significant.

Decimal point errors can occur as a result of a miscalculation, as described above, and also when writing orders or instructions. Failure to write a leading zero in front of a number less than one (e.g., .1 mg instead of 0.1 mg) might cause the number to be read as a whole number (1 mg). Writing unnecessary trailing zeros can also be confusing (e.g., 10.0 mg instead of 10 mg may be interpreted as 100 mg). Medication order sheets with lines can sometimes cause a decimal point to be overlooked on the duplicate copy that is usually sent to a pharmacy. Therefore, when writing numbers, a leading zero should always be used with a decimal point for numbers less than one (0.1 mg, not .1 mg) and a decimal point and trailing zero should never be used for whole numbers (10 mg, not 10.0 mg).

Technicians must be aware of the potential for decimal point errors due to misplaced or missing decimal points when interpreting orders. Questionable orders should be brought to the attention of the pharmacist.

Abbreviations

The abbreviation of medical terms and drug names can lead to medication errors. Use of the abbreviation "AZT" for zidovudine (Retrovir®—an antiretroviral agent) for a patient with AIDS could be detrimental if the patient received azathioprine (Imuran®—an immunosuppressant sometimes abbreviated AZT) instead of zidovudine.

Another example of an abbreviation error is the use of "U" as an abbreviation for units. This abbreviation might result in a 10-fold error were the "U" to be read as a "zero" (e.g., 10 U insulin may be read as 100 insulin). A daily order written as "QD" instead of "daily" may be troublesome because it could be read as "QID" (four times a day) or "OD" (every other day).

The Institute for Safe Medication Practices (ISMP) has developed a table (**Table 15-1**) listing dangerous abbreviations and dose designations.

There are many accepted abbreviations in health care, and use of abbreviations can be efficient if everyone understands and agrees on the definitions. The Joint Commission on Accreditation of Healthcare Organizations (JCAHO) recommends that institutions maintain an approved list of acceptable abbreviations and terms.[29] Their 2003 National Patient Safety Goals include a recommendation that organizations create a list of abbreviations, acronyms, and symbols that should *not* be used as well.[30] Being unaware of the accepted interpretation of abbreviations can lead to errors. Creating new abbreviations that others may not understand should be avoided.[31] ASHP recommends that an approved list be developed by the Pharmacy and Therapeutics Committee (or its equivalent).[2] Abbreviations not on the approved list should be reviewed carefully before processing an order. Another recommendation from ASHP is to write out directions for medication use rather than using nonstandard or ambiguous abbreviations. The complete drug name, preferably the generic, should be used.

Technicians should become familiar with the list of abbreviations approved for their pharmacy. Such a

TABLE 15-1. DANGEROUS ABBREVIATIONS AND DOSE DESIGNATIONS

Abbreviation/Dose Expression	Intended Meaning	Misinterpretation	Correction
Apothecary symbols	dram, minim	Misunderstood or misread (symbol for dram misread for "3" and minim misread as "mL").	Use the metric system.
AU	aurio uterque (each ear)	Mistaken for OU (oculo uterque—each eye).	Do not use this abbreviation.
D/C	discharge discontinue	Premature discontinuation of medications when D/C (intended to mean "discharge") has been misinterpreted as "discontinued" when followed by a list of drugs.	Use "discharge" and "discontinue."

Drug names	Use the complete spelling for drug names		
ARA°A		vidarabine	cytarabineARA°C
AZT		zidovudine (RETROVIR)	azathioprine
CPZ		COMPAZINE (prochlorperazine)	chlorpromazine
DPT		DEMEROL-PHENERGAN-THORAZINE	diphtheria-pertussis-tetanus (vaccine)
HCl		hydrochloric acid	potassium chloride (The "H" is misinterpreted as "K.")
HCT		hydrocortisone	hydrochlorothiazide
HCTZ		hydrochlorothiazide	hydrocortisone (seen as HCT250 mg)
MgSO4		magnesium sulfate	morphine sulfate
MSO4		morphine sulfate	magnesium sulfate
MTX		methotrexate	mitoxantrone
TAC		triamcinolone	tetracaine, ADRENALIN, cocaine
ZnSO4		zinc sulfate	morphine sulfate

Stemmed names			
"Nitro" drip	nitroglycerin infusion	sodium nitroprusside infusion	
"Norflox"	norfloxacin	NORFLEX	

Abbreviation/Dose Expression	Intended Meaning	Misinterpretation	Correction
mg	microgram	Mistaken for "mg" when handwritten.	Use "mcg."
o.d. or OD	once daily	Misinterpreted as "right eye" (OD—oculus dexter) and administration of oral medications in the eye.	Use "daily."
TIW or tiw	three times a week.	Mistaken as "three times a day."	Do not use this abbreviation.
Per os	orally	The "os" can be mistaken for "left eye."	Use "PO," "by mouth," or "orally."
q.d. or QD	every day	Mistaken as q.i.d., especially if the period after the "q" or the tail of the "q" is misunderstood as an "i."	Use "daily" or "every day."
Qn	nightly or at bedtime	Misinterpreted as "qh" (every hour).	Use "nightly."

cont'd

Abbreviation/Dose Expression	Intended Meaning	Misinterpretation	Correction
Qhs	nightly at bedtime	Misread as every hour.	Use "nightly."
q6PM, etc.	every evening at 6 PM	Misread as every six hours.	Use 6 PM "nightly."
q.o.d. or QOD	every other day	Misinterpreted as "q.d." (daily) or "q.i.d. (four times daily) if the "o" is poorly written.	Use "every other day."
sub q	subcutaneous	The "q" has been mistaken for "every" (e.g., one heparin dose ordered "sub q 2 hours before surgery" misunderstood as every 2 hours before surgery).	Use "subcut." or write "subcutaneous."
SC	subcutaneous	Mistaken for SL (sublingual).	Use "subcut." or write "subcutaneous."
U or u	unit	Read as a zero (0) or a four (4), causing a 10-fold overdose or greater (4U seen as "40" or 4u seen as 44").	"Unit" has no acceptable abbreviation. Use "unit."
IU	international unit	Misread as IV (intravenous).	Use "units."
cc	cubic centimeters	Misread as "U" (units).	Use "mL."
x3d	for three days	Mistaken for "three doses."	Use "for three days."
BT	bedtime	Mistaken as "BID" (twice daily).	Use "hs."
ss	sliding scale (insulin) or ½ (apothecary)	Mistaken for "55."	Spell out "sliding scale." Use "one-half" or use "½."
> and <	greater than and less than	Mistakenly used opposite of intended.	Use "greater than" or "less than."
/ (slash mark)	separates two doses or indicates "per"	Misunderstood as the number 1 ("25 unit/10 units" read as "110" units).	Do not use a slash mark to separate doses. Use "per."
Name letters and dose numbers run together (e.g., Inderal40 mg)	Inderal 40 mg	Misread as Inderal 140 mg.	Always use space between drug name, dose, and unit of measure.
Zero after decimal point (1.0)	1 mg	Misread as 10 mg if the decimal point is not seen.	Do not use terminal zeros for doses expressed in whole numbers.
No zero before decimal dose (.5 mg)	0.5 mg	Misread as 5 mg.	Always use zero before a decimal when the dose is less than a whole unit.

Reprinted with permission from www.ismp.org

list can be obtained from a pharmacy supervisor. Community pharmacies generally do not have a formal, approved list of abbreviations. However, posting a list of commonly accepted medical abbreviations in the pharmacy may be beneficial. Technicians should also be familiar with the abbreviations and dose designations that are considered dangerous and pay particular attention to them when filling orders.

High Alert Medications

Several medications or drug classes have been categorized as high alert medications because of their high risk of causing serious harm to patients when given in error. According to the ISMP, the following are considered high alert medications:[32]

1. insulin

2. narcotics and opiates

3. potassium chloride injection

4. heparin

5. concentrated sodium chloride (> 0.9%)

A complete list of high alert medications can be found on the ISMP website.[32] Technicians should pay special attention when processing orders involving these medications because of their potential for serious harm if given in error.

Prescribing Issues

Medication errors may result from the way a drug is prescribed. Issues associated with the prescribing component of the medication use process that may contribute to an error include verbal orders, confusion with the concentration of a product, illegible handwriting, missing information, use of the apothecary system, and writing doses based on the course of therapy as opposed to a daily dose. This section describes how these prescribing issues may lead to errors and ways to minimize such errors.

Verbal Orders

Verbal orders can lead to medication errors when the orders are not transmitted clearly, and the use of car phones and static connections can make verbal orders even more difficult to understand. With the number of similar-sounding products available, it is easy to misunderstand a verbal order. In one case report, a verbal order was received by a nurse from a physician and then transmitted to a community pharmacy. The nurse inadvertently confused *Ismelin*® (guanethidine—potent antihypertensive agent) for *Hismanal*® (astemizole—antihistamine), and the patient received the potent antihypertensive agent for his allergy symptoms.[33]

Verbal orders should be reserved for situations when it is impossible or impractical for the prescriber to write the order or enter it via computer. The recipient should immediately write down the order and read it back to the prescriber to ensure clarity of the order. A written copy of the order should be placed in the pharmacy's prescription file or the patient's medical record. Institutional pharmacies routinely require the prescriber to confirm verbal orders by signature. The use of verbal orders should be avoided in chemotherapy prescribing because of the complexity of these orders and the potentially lethal impact of mistakes with these drugs.

Although car phones, foreign terminology, accents, and poor connections can make taking a verbal order difficult, it is the responsibility of the technician to ask the other party to clarify parts of the order that are not clear. Simply asking the other party to spell the names of the drugs or other words that are unclear and repeating the order back to the other party can help ensure that the right order is received. Many states limit the acceptance of verbal medication orders to registered pharmacists. State law and pharmacy policy should be consulted to determine what role, if any, technicians may play in accepting verbal orders.

Drug Concentration

Failure to include the concentration of a liquid formulation in a prescription could result in a wrong dose being dispensed. For example, an order for amoxicillin suspension ½ tsp (2.5 ml) TID does not specify the concentration of the suspension, causing confusion as to the actual dose ordered. It is unclear whether the physician ordered 62.5 mg (½ tsp of 125 mg/5 ml) or 125 mg (½ tsp of 250 mg/5 ml).

Writing "1 amp," "1 vial," or "1 cap" can lead to errors when products come in multiple strengths, doses, or vial sizes. An amp of magnesium sulfate might be filled with a 2 ml amp (8 mEq), a 20 ml amp (16 mEq), or 10 ml amp of 50% concentration (40 mEq). The pharmacist should clarify ambiguous doses before the technician processes the order.

Illegible Handwriting

The poor handwriting of physicians frequently is joked about. However, illegible handwriting of any health care provider is no laughing matter when it contributes to medication errors. With the many sound-alike and look-alike drug names on the market, it is easy to understand how illegible handwriting can lead to errors. One report describes a poorly written order for Aredia® (pamidronate—a blood calcium lowering agent) 60 mg IV that was filled and administered as Adria, a commonly spoken name for Adriamycin® (doxorubicin—a chemotherapy agent). The patient received approximately 20 percent of the dose before the error was noticed. The patient experienced bone marrow toxicity (decrease in blood cell counts) as a consequence.[34] Both agents are reasonable drugs for a cancer patient and are prescribed in doses of 60 mg, but the poorly written drug name led to the mix-up. Facsimile transmission of handwritten orders may further complicate interpretation of illegible handwriting.

The entire order should be carefully evaluated when trying to decipher illegible handwriting. Sometimes the dose or route of administration may be helpful in determining what drug was ordered. Assistance should be obtained from a pharmacist when orders are difficult to interpret because of illegible handwriting. The pharmacist should contact the prescriber to clarify orders that are difficult to interpret. In some practice settings, technicians may have a role in obtaining order clarifications.

Using standardized preprinted order forms for complex drug regimens is one way to minimize illegible handwriting.[2] Computerization and typewritten labeling can reduce medication errors by making the medication labels easier to read for both health care personnel and patients. The use of upper- and lowercase lettering also improves readability.

Missing Information

Lack of medical information about the patient, such as age, weight, height, and diagnosis, can contribute to medication errors. Medical information is important because dose usually depends on indication and severity of the condition. Unfortunately, physicians do not routinely write the indication on prescriptions, and patients do not always fully understand their conditions. In some hospital pharmacies, medical information is available only in the chart because the pharmacy computer system does not interface with the main hospital computer.

Thorough and complete medication profiles should be maintained for all patients. These profiles should include current prescription and nonprescription medications, allergies, age, height, and weight of the patient. Previous medication use is also helpful. Profiles should be kept current and referred to routinely. It may be necessary to question the patient or contact the prescriber to obtain this information, because pharmacists often need it to check an order for appropriateness.

Apothecary System

The apothecary system is a system of measurement that some physicians continue to use out of habit. This system can lead to errors because it is unfamiliar to many health care personnel or because it must be converted to the metric system. The fact that "1 gr" (grain) may be interpreted as 60 mg or 65 mg is confusing enough, but if it is written sloppily, it could be misread as "1 gm" (1 gram = 1000 mg). Prescribers should be discouraged from using the apothecary system.

Apothecary conversion charts should be readily available in the pharmacy. Technicians should become familiar with commonly used apothecary symbols and their metric equivalents, which are available in Chapter 5.

Course Dose vs. Daily Dose

Chemotherapy drug regimens are commonly prescribed on a per course, or cycle of treatment, basis, as opposed to a per dose basis. This practice increases the chances for medication errors because the orders are often difficult to interpret.[35] Many chemotherapy treatments require a patient to receive medication over several days and then rest (receive no drug treatment) for several days or weeks. This allows time for the patient to recover from the side effects and for the drugs to work in the optimal phase of the tumor cell cycle. One course of treatment may consist of several drugs given on one or more days during a specified time period.

An example of a course dose is flourouracil 4 g/m^2 IV on days 1, 2, 3, and 4. This order might be interpreted as 4 g/m^2 of flourouracil (a cytotoxic agent) daily for four days—a total of 16 g/m^2. One could also interpret it as 4 g/m^2 to be divided into four daily doses (1 g/m^2 daily on days 1, 2, 3, and 4). It is easy to see how course doses can be misinterpreted. Errors such as this can result in massive overdoses, leading to significant morbidity or death.

Manufacturer- and Drug Product–Related Causes

A review of medication errors reported to the United States Pharmacopeial Convention (USP) between August 1991 and April 1993 revealed that the most common error reported was related to a problem with drug product characteristics (e.g., drug name, packaging).[36] The USP has a medication error reporting program in conjunction with the ISMP. This program focuses on product design and characteristics. In addition to the USP program, the Food and Drug Administration (FDA) accepts reports of medication errors or potential errors via a toll-free telephone line. The FDA receives and reviews all medication error reports, whether made initially to the USP or the FDA. Potential errors can also be reported to the FDA. Among other things, the FDA uses this information to alert health care providers before an actual error occurs.

Characteristics of drug products that may contribute to medication errors include look-alike and sound-alike drug names, the use of numbers or letters as part of the drug name, product labeling, and color coding.[37] Drug product problems identified by the USP are forwarded to pharmaceutical manufacturers, which can then address the problems by making appropriate modifications to the drug products.

Look-Alike and Sound-Alike Drug Names

Many case reports deal with medication errors caused by confusion surrounding drug names.[38-44] Approximately 15 percent of all medication errors reported to the USP have been associated with confusion regarding similar drug names.[45] Hundreds of drug names either sound or look like another trade or generic drug name. A list of more than 750 potentially confusing drug names that have been reported to the USP is available on the USP website. It includes pairs of similar-looking or -sounding drug names that have resulted in an error or could potentially lead to one.[46]

Sometimes errors occur because drug names look and sound similar and may even be used to treat a common condition. For example, amrinone (Inocor®—a cardiac agent) was inadvertently administered to a patient instead of amiodarone (Cordarone®—an antiarrythmic agent).[39] Both drugs may be used in treating cardiovascular conditions, and their generic names sound somewhat alike. Viracept® (nelfinavir) and Viramune® (nevirapine) are two antiretroviral agents used in the treatment of AIDS. Both the brand and the generic names are similar, increasing the risk for confusion.[47] Sloppy handwriting or misspelling can contribute to drug name confusion. An order carelessly written for interferon 1 ml (an immunologic agent) was interpreted and prepared as Imferon® 1 ml (iron dextran).[38] In this case, the patient's mother questioned the dark brown coloring of the drug before it was administered, and the mix-up was corrected before the patient received the wrong drug.

The likelihood of confusing two drugs with similar names is increased when the dosages of both drugs are the same. Lanoxin® (digoxin) and Levoxine® (a brand name for levothyroxine) have similar looking and sounding names and are both commonly prescribed at a dose of 0.125 mg daily.[41] Because of these similarities, the pharmaceutical manufacturer of Levoxine® changed the trade name to Levoxyl® in an effort to avoid confusion with Lanoxin®.

One report describes an error resulting from two ophthalmic ointment products having brand names that are spelled and pronounced identically.[44] One brand name, Ocu-Mycin® (gentamicin 3%), contains a hyphen, and the other, Ocumycin® (bacitracin/polymixin B) does not. Given as a verbal order with vague directions, such as "take as directed," there would be no way of knowing which drug was intended. Use of both the brand and generic name would help avoid confusion in this situation.

A frequently reported mix-up occurs between quinine (an antimalarial) and quinidine (an antiarrhythmic). The names are similar, routine doses are the same, and they are frequently stocked next to each other. It is easy to see how one drug could be picked instead of the other.

Confusion with sound-alike or look-alike names is a growing issue with the increasing number of drug products available. Pharmaceutical manufacturers are responsible for carefully selecting drug product names, keeping patient safety in mind. Approximately 30 percent of all new drug names reviewed by the FDA are rejected because they may lead to confusion.[45] **Table 15-2** lists examples of drug product names that were changed to reduce the risk of prescribing errors. Health care providers can help identify potentially confusing drug names by notifying the USP or FDA with their concerns.

TABLE 15-2		
Examples of Drug Product Names Changed to Reduce the Risk of Prescribing Errors		
Former Trade Name	Confused With	New Trade Name
Losec	Lasix	Prilosec
Larocin	Lanoxin	Larotid
Microx	Micro-K	MyKrox
Clonopin	Clonidine	Klonopin

Numbers or Letters as Part of the Drug Name

Manufacturers sometimes include numbers or letters as a prefix or suffix to the brand name (e.g., Tylenol #3®, Percocet-5®, Procardia-XL®). The intent may be to indicate a strength or that a product is an extended release formulation, but it can lead to errors. A case of such an error reported in the literature describes an ice pack applied to the chest of a patient hospitalized with pneumonia instead of administration of the antibiotic azithromycin. The physician wrote for a "Z-Pak," commonly prescribed this way on outpatient prescriptions. The specific dosage regimen was not written out because the product is available as a blister pack containing the entire course of therapy and is labeled with dosing instructions. The patient's pneumonia worsened until the error was discovered 2 days later and appropriate treatment was initiated.[48]

Numbers in the drug name may be misinterpreted as the dose. The prescription in **Figure 15-1** might be interpreted to take five tablets of Percocet every 4 hours as needed instead of one tablet of Percocet-5® every 4 hours as needed. A patient might become extremely drowsy or confused after taking five tablets of Percocet-5®.

Letters or numbers that are omitted from brand names when writing an order can contribute to errors. The immediate release form of Procardia® may be dispensed instead of the extended release formulation in **Figure 15-2** because the "XL" part of the name is left off. The extended release formulation is designed to release the drug slowly over the entire day, whereas the immediate release form releases the entire dose at once. A patient taking the wrong formulation of Procardia® might not have adequate control of his blood pressure throughout the entire day.

Product Labeling

As a marketing strategy, product labels often emphasize a manufacturer's name or logo, making it difficult to readily identify the drug name and dose. Manufacturers often use the same labeling scheme, including letter size, print, and background color, to associate the product with the manufacturer. Sometimes this strategy, which makes all labels look alike, can be detrimental.

Example 1: The dosage strength and total contents of liquid formulations are not always labeled clearly. Different vial sizes of injections may be similarly labeled with the concentration (mg/ml), but too little emphasis may be placed on the total contents of the

vial. When midazolam (Versed®) first appeared on the market, it was available in a 5 mg/ml concentration in 1 ml and 2 ml size vials. The vial size was not prominent on either label, which made it difficult to differentiate between the 10 mg (2 ml) and 5 mg (1 ml) vials.

Example 2: There have been numerous cases of a health care provider using potassium chloride (KCl) injection to flush an IV line instead of normal saline because the vial sizes and labeling of the two products were similar. Manufacturers of potassium chloride injection are now required to use black vial caps and overseals and prominently display a warning on the vial label that states "*must be diluted.*"[49]

Color Coding

Relying on the color of product packaging is not a safe practice. Manufacturers may change their packaging color scheme at any time, and color-coding schemes for similar products may differ among manufacturers. Drug products with similar colors may be misplaced in

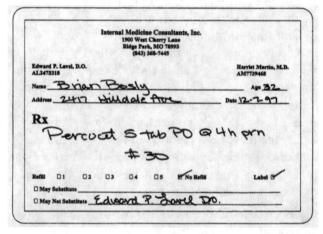

Figure 15-1. Example of a drug name that contains a number as a suffix.

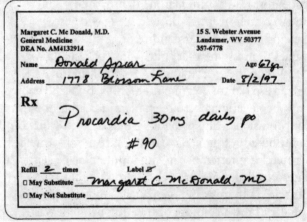

Figure 15-2. Example of a drug name that should contain letters as a suffix.

the stock areas and could easily be dispensed in error. For example, both daunorubicin (Cerubidine®) 20 mg and doxorubicin 10 mg are packaged in vials that are shaped similarly and have dark blue vial caps. They are both lyophilized powders that turn into red solutions upon reconstitution. Relying on the color of the vial cap or of the diluted solution could lead to very serious errors.

Advertising

Many practices that contribute to medication errors are perpetuated through pharmaceutical product advertising. Journal advertisements may include abbreviations, lack of adequate dosage strength identification, inappropriate use of decimal points, and so forth. The more frequently these things are seen, the more readily they are accepted by health care personnel and the more likely they may lead to errors. These issues must be kept in mind when reviewing drug literature.

Compounding/Drug Preparation Errors

Errors can occur during the compounding and drug preparation phase. These errors can be difficult for others to catch. Therefore, it is essential that technicians take steps to decrease the risk of making an error when compounding and preparing drug products. Such an approach includes reading the product labels carefully, not processing more than one prescription at a time, labeling prescriptions properly, storing drugs properly, maintaining a safe work environment, and keeping up with changes in the medical profession.

Reading the Label

Reading drug product labels carefully when filling an order is a step that is often neglected. This step is extremely important because of the number of product names that sound or look alike, similar product packaging, illegible handwriting, and color-coding. The ISMP recommends that pharmacy personnel read drug product labels a minimum of three times before processing an order to help minimize errors caused by mistaking one product for another. The label should be read as the product is removed from the shelf, as the order is being prepared, and again as the finished product is set aside for the pharmacist to check.

Processing Multiple Products

Processing more than one prescription or order at the same time can result in errors. It is easy to add a drug to the wrong IVPB diluent if several orders are being compounded simultaneously in the laminar flow hood.

In this situation, filling a prescription for the wrong patient or confusing the quantities to be dispensed is just as easy.

Technicians should process only one prescription or common batch (e.g., all 0800 ampicillin 1 g IVPB orders) at a time. Supplies for multiple prescriptions should not be mixed together. Each prescription should be completed before starting the next one. Completed prescriptions waiting for a pharmacist check should be clearly separated from each other and from those that have not yet been completed.

Labeling

Technicians should be familiar with the labeling requirements for prescriptions in their pharmacy as dictated by state law and pharmacy policy. If a label is handwritten, it should be neat and legible. Ink cartridges and printer ribbons should be changed before the print is too faded to read, the label should be free of smudges, and the print should be aligned on the label appropriately. Labels that are difficult to read may result in miscommunication and ultimately a medication error.

Auxiliary labels give the patient or nursing personnel useful information. This information may be important in helping to prevent medication errors. Many pharmacy computer systems are designed to identify the appropriate auxiliary labels for prescriptions. Other pharmacies use reference charts as aids. Auxiliary labels should be placed carefully on the drug container so they do not cover up other pertinent information.

Deteriorated Medications

Because expired medications or improperly stored medications may have lost their potency and thus effectiveness, technicians should take steps to keep these medications out of the dispensing stock. In many cases, it is the technician's responsibility to rotate stock. Technicians should be familiar with the pharmacy's regular system for checking for expired medications. Although checking expiration dates is sometimes viewed as a tedious job, it is important because it reduces the risk of making deteriorated drug errors.

When replenishing stock, always remove expired medications and place the stock with the earliest expiration date near the front to be used first. Some drugs have a short expiration date once the container has been opened. Pharmacies usually have procedures that require the date of opening or the expiration date to be written on the label to help prevent use of an expired drug. Examples of drugs that usually require dating include reconstituted oral suspensions and injectable drugs. Technicians should be familiar with the drugs that have short expiration dates and the procedures for indicating date of first use or expiration. Marking opened containers with an "X" to readily identify the container that should be used first is also recommended.

Medications that require special storage conditions, such as refrigeration or freezing, should be kept in those conditions as long as possible. Drugs stored under refrigeration may be stable for only a short time out of the refrigerator. When filling an order for a pharmacist to check, the technician must comply with the institution's policy. Some pharmacies/pharmacists require that refrigerated medications be left in the refrigerator and not on the counter, whereas others allow them to stay on the counter briefly.

Work Environment

Factors within the workplace may contribute to medication errors. Inadequate lighting,[11] poorly designed work spaces, or inefficient workflow can make it difficult to perform assigned duties accurately. Cluttered work spaces or stock areas might increase the chances of picking up the wrong drug. The many distractions and interruptions, including phone calls, in a busy pharmacy can cause loss of concentration.

Many modern pharmacies rely on specialized equipment and computers to assist in filling prescriptions. Improper maintenance of this equipment may result in unacceptable performance or may necessitate the use of older, unfamiliar, or cumbersome manual systems when the equipment breaks down. Failure to properly maintain a balance might result in an inaccurate measure of drug components for a compounded prescription and ultimately a wrong dose error. Routine maintenance schedules should be followed to prevent equipment malfunction. Technicians should be trained on the use and maintenance of such equipment. Operating manuals should be available in the pharmacy for troubleshooting when a problem occurs.

Scheduling of staff members and the frequency of rotating shifts have been shown to correlate with error rates.[50] Other factors, such as staffing levels and amount of supervision, may also be work environment issues to consider.

The frequency with which drug products are changed because of changes in purchasing contracts may lead to unfamiliarity with products among the staff. Significant changes should be communicated to the staff, and product labels should be read carefully.

Personnel-Related Factors

Untrained, inadequately trained, or inexperienced personnel may be unfamiliar with drug names, doses, or uses of agents, which limits their ability to recognize inappropriate orders and circumstances. New technological advances make keeping up with drug use difficult even for experienced health care practitioners. The important thing is for technicians to recognize their limits and work within them, just as nurses, pharmacists, and physicians are trained to do. Relying on memory instead of checking references (e.g., dilution charts, maximum dosage ranges) or performing complicated calculations without a double-check may result in errors. It is a technician's responsibility to help prevent medication errors by questioning unusual or unfamiliar orders. When abnormal or unfamiliar situations arise, it is always best to consult references and others before making a decision or taking action. Being aware of a potential error and not knowing what to do about it, thinking that someone else will catch it, or feeling intimidated by a pharmacist or supervisor certainly increases the chances that an actual error will take place.

The lack of knowledge of medication errors and how to avoid them also contributes to medication errors. Not being familiar with common errors or medications most frequently involved in errors might cause one to think that medication errors are infrequent. The medication errors most frequently reported to the USP from August 1991 to April 1993 involved heparin, lidocaine, potassium chloride injection, and epinephrine.[36]

Deficiencies in Medication Use Systems

Medication errors cannot be attributed to human error alone. Errors are frequently due in part to defective or inadequate systems.[51] For example, stocking dangerous drugs in patient care areas (i.e., floor stock) increases the chances of an error because the drugs are available to nurses without a pharmacy check. Floor stock mix-ups between potassium chloride injection and normal saline injection for flushing IV tubing, potassium chloride and furosemide injections, premixed lidocaine in D5W 500 ml and plain D5W 500 ml bags, and so on, can lead to serious consequences.

Pharmacy unit dose and IV admixture systems have been shown to reduce medication errors, yet many hospitals in the United States still do not have these systems in place. The unavailability of or difficulty in obtaining patient data, such as current body weight, allergy information, or laboratory results, also contributes to medication errors.

Inefficient processes with too many or too few checks along the way or checks at inappropriate times can cause errors. Lack of standardized procedures or outdated procedures might also lead to errors.

Being familiar with factors that may lead to medication errors and things that can be done to prevent them is the first step in reducing medication errors.

Failure Mode and Effects Analysis

It is impossible to eliminate all potential for error. People are not perfect, and even the most conscientious and knowledgeable staff makes mistakes. Sometimes the systems that people work within present numerous opportunities for errors. Failure mode and effects analysis (FMEA), also called failure mode effect and criticality analysis (FMECA), is a systematic evaluation of a process or system used to predict the opportunity for and severity of errors at various steps in the process.[52,53] FMEA focuses on finding flaws within a system that create opportunities for individuals to make errors. It evaluates the "how" and "why" of an error instead of the "who."

The first step in evaluating a system or process using FMEA is to describe in detail the individual steps involved in the overall process from start to finish. Use of a flow diagram is helpful to create a visual representation of the process. The next step is to list the potential opportunities for failure at each stage. Then, the effects of these failures on the process and their root causes are described. The severity, likelihood of occurrence, and probability of actually identifying the failure are then estimated. The criticality index is determined by multiplying these three estimates. Steps that have the highest criticality index should be addressed first, because improvements in these areas have the greatest potential of reducing the risk for error. After making changes to the process, FMEA should be performed again to determine the effectiveness of these changes.

An Australian hospital used the FMEA system to modify its medication use system and developed a new system that resulted in a decreased medication error rate. The hospital went from a ward stock system to a 5-day, patient-specific drug distribution system with pharmacist review of orders prior to dispensing.[54]

Systems Designed to Prevent Medication Errors

There are many ways to reduce the chance of a medication error. Institutions help minimize medication errors by fostering a well-trained and knowledgeable staff, maintaining a favorable work environment, and instituting effective policies and procedures, among other things. Technicians must be familiar with the systems designed to provide additional checks in the medication use process. It is also essential that technicians ask questions when they are not familiar with the proper procedures.[5]

Well-designed systems help prevent medication errors. Such systems adhere to legal requirements and include licensed personnel, policies and procedures, multiple check systems, standardized order forms and checklists, and quality assurance activities and monitoring systems, which will be addressed later in this chapter.

Another system designed to help prevent medication errors in the outpatient setting is patient counseling. When a patient or designee drops off a prescription to be filled at the pharmacy, the pharmacist or pharmacy technician asks if the patient is allergic to any medications and asks for the proper spelling of the patient's name and address, among other things. When the prescription is picked up, the pharmacist and the patient discuss how to take the medication, any possible side effects, and why it is important for the patient to take the medication exactly as the physician has prescribed it. The patient has the opportunity to ask questions or discuss any concerns about the medication with the pharmacist. Patient counseling plays a very important role in reducing medication errors because it increases the likelihood that patients will take their medication as prescribed.

Legal Requirements

Pharmacy laws are designed to protect the public by ensuring that a knowledgeable individual double-checks the results of the prescribing process and oversees the use of medications. The laws help prevent medication errors. The law requires a licensed pharmacist to be on duty during pharmacy business hours. Licensed pharmacists must graduate from an accredited school of pharmacy, pass a licensure examination, and pass the state pharmacy examination to practice pharmacy in that state.

Policies and Procedures

Another system designed to prevent medication errors is establishing policies and procedures. Policies and procedures manuals formally establish a system to prevent medication errors. Therefore, technicians should be familiar with the workplace's policies and procedures manual. A study of dispensing errors in an outpatient pharmacy concluded that approximately 33 percent of the errors discovered were due to noncompliance with company or department policies and procedures.[11]

Multiple Check Systems

Another system designed to prevent medication errors is a multiple check system. This can include the pharmacist reviewing a physician order, a pharmacy technician preparing a medication for the pharmacist to check, a nurse inspecting the dose from the pharmacy, and a patient asking questions and examining the medication before taking it. A popular check system encourages each person to read the label three times, which reminds health care professionals to spend more time reviewing medication labels carefully to prevent medication errors. A multiple check system is especially important when dealing with potentially lethal drugs, such as cancer chemotherapeutic agents.[35]

Standardized Order Forms

Standardized preprinted order forms have been developed to prevent medication errors by making medication orders easier for the prescriber to read and easier for the pharmacist and nurse to interpret. **Figure 15-3** is an example of a standardized, preprinted order form. Note that the chemotherapy agents are listed in alphabetical order with the exception of those beginning with the letter "v." Vinblastine, vinorelbine, and vincristine are separated on the form because of the similarity in their names. Also note that the nonchemotherapy agents mesna and leucovorin are listed adjacent to their companion chemotherapy drugs to prompt the physician to remember to order them when appropriate. Chemotherapeutic agents have been designated as high alert medications by ISMP, making them ideal drugs to be included on a standardized order form.[32] The use of preprinted order forms for other complicated drug therapies or high-risk drugs can also be beneficial. Preprinted forms are neatly typewritten and more legible. They generally make it easier for other health care personnel to double-check the prescriber's order and calculations. The forms help reduce errors primarily associated with illegible handwriting and also informally educate the prescriber about which medications are on the hospital formulary.

Checklists

Checklists can be included on a standard preprinted order form. This system ensures that personnel use a systematic, thorough procedure to check medications before they are prescribed, dispensed, or administered to a patient.[35]

Education and Training

Education and training are important in reducing medication errors. Technicians receive formalized training at a community college, in organized departmental programs, or through on-the-job training. Training can include pharmacy calculations, compounding techniques, pharmacy abbreviations, preparation of IV medications, and computer operation skills. Health care personnel should be familiar with the classes of medications, their generic and trade names, and their forms and doses. Some pharmacy technician applicants complete certificate or associate degree programs in pharmacy technology at a community college before applying for a pharmacy technician position. In this situation, it is still important for the technician to complete pharmacy department training programs, because they are specific for the institution and the new technician's position.

Technicians also receive training on the job. JCAHO requires organizations to prove that their personnel are competent. Ideally, on-the-job training will include instruction and demonstrations. After technicians have been instructed and have witnessed a demonstration of a task, they are usually asked to perform the task while the educator observes. This procedure allows the health system to document the technicians' competency.

To complement formal and on-the-job training, technicians should read pharmacy literature, participate in local pharmacy organizations, and attend continuing education lectures to improve their knowledge base. At a minimum, these programs and activities help technicians keep up with changes in formulations and recognize the differences among various medication products.[2]

Computerization and Automation

Proper use of computerization and automation are good ways to prevent medication errors. Many health care facilities use bar coding, automatic dispensing machines, and robots to reduce medication errors.

Cancer Chemotherapy Order Form/ADULT

Part 1 - Chemotherapy

Orders must be received in pharmacy by 2100 for administration between 2300 and 0900

☐ Protocol # _____ 1 2 3 4 5 6 7 8 Course (Circle One)	Diagnosis	BSA m² ☐ Dose reduction_____ %	Height	Weight

CHEMOTHERAPY

Provide dose, select a route, and designate the frequency and duration for each chemotherapy ordered.
Designate day number, sequence and time in column A.   Cont. Inf. = Continuous Infusion over 24 hours

A	DRUG	DOSE	ROUTE	FREQUENCY/DURATION				Total Dose per Course
	Asparaginase	units/m² = ____ U	☐ IVPB over 30 min	☐ SC ☐ IM	q	X	doses	unit
	Bleomycin	units/m² = ____ U	☐ IVP over 10 min ☐ IVPB over ____ h	☐ Cont Inf	q	X	doses	unit
	Carboplatin	AUC of _____ = mg/m² = ____ mg	☐ IVPB over 30 min Creat= ____ mg/dl		q	X	doses	mg/m²
	Carmustine	mg/m² = ____ mg	☐ IVPB over 60 min in GLASS container	☐ Cont Inf	q	X	doses	mg/m²
	Cisplatin	mg/m² = ____ mg	☐ IVPB over 60 min ☐ IVPB over ____ h with ____ g mannitol	☐ Cont Inf	q	X	doses	mg/m²
	Cyclophosphamide	mg/m² = ____ mg	☐ IVP over 5 - 10 min ☐ IVPB over 30 - 60 min	☐ Cont Inf	q	X	doses	mg/m²
	Cytarabine	mg/m² = ____ mg	☐ Intrathecal ☐ IVPB over ____ h	☐ Cont Inf	q	X	doses	mg/m²
	Dacarbazine	mg/m² = ____ mg	☐ IVP over 2-3 min ☐ IVPB over 15 - 30 min	☐ Cont Inf	q	X	doses	mg/m²
	Daunorubicin	mg/m² = ____ mg	☐ IVP over 2 - 3 min ☐ IVPB over 15 min		q	X	doses	mg/m²
	Docetaxel	mg/m² = ____ mg	☐ IVPB over 60 min in glass container		q	X	doses	mg/m²
	Doxorubicin	mg/m² = ____ mg	☐ IVP over 10 - 15 min ☐ IVPB over 30 min	☐ Cont Inf	q	X	doses	mg/m²
	Etoposide	mg/m² = ____ mg	☐ IVPB over 1 -2 h	☐ Cont Inf	q	X	doses	mg/m²
	Fluorouracil	mg/m² = ____ mg	☐ IVP over 2 - 3 min ☐ IVPB over 30 - 60 min		q	X	doses	mg/m²
	Gemcitabine	mg/m² = ____ mg	☐ IVPB over ____ h ☐ IVPB over 30 min	☐ Cont Inf	q	X	doses	mg/m²
	Idarubicin	mg/m² = ____ mg	☐ IVPB over 15 min		q	X	doses	mg/m²
	Ifosfamide	mg/m² = ____ mg	☐ IVPB over 30 - 60 min	☐ Cont Inf	q	X	doses	mg/m²
	Mesna	mg/m² = ____ mg	☐ IVPB over 15 -20 min, 30 min prior to, 4h & 8h after start of ifosfamide	☐ Mix with ifosfamide	q	X	doses	mg/m²
	Mesna	mg/m² = ____ mg	☐ IVPB over 15 - 20 min, 4h and 8h after last ifosfamide					
	Methotrexate	mg/m² = ____ mg	☐ Intrathecal ☐ IVPB over ____ h	☐ Cont Inf	q	X	doses	mg/m²
	Leucovorin	mg/m² = ____ mg	☐ IVP over 3 min ☐ 24 h after methotrexate ☐ Prior to fluorouracil	☐ PO	q	X	doses	mg/m²
	Vinblastine	mg/m² = ____ mg	☐ IVP over 2 - 3 min	☐ Cont Inf	q	X	doses	mg/m²
	Mitoxantrone	mg/m² = ____ mg	☐ IVPB over 15 min		q	X	doses	mg/m²
	Paclitaxel	mg/m² = ____ mg	☐ IVPB over ____ h in GLASS container	☐ Cont Inf	q	X	doses	mg/m²
	Vincristine	mg/m² = ____ mg	☐ IVP over 2 - 3 min	☐ Cont Inf	q	X	doses	mg/m²
	Topotecan	mg/m² = ____ mg	☐ IVPB over 30 min	☐ Cont Inf	q	X	doses	mg/m²
	Vinorelbine	mg/m² = ____ mg	☐ IVP over 6 - 10 min		q	X	doses	mg/m²

Other:

Date:	Time:	Prescriber's signature		Pager #:

91-4123-1 05/02
Page 1 of 3

Gold - Chart   White - Pharmacy   White - Pharmacy   © 2002 Advocate Health Care

Figure 15-3. Example of a preprinted chemotherapy order form.

Source: *Advocate* Lutheran General Hospital, Park Ridge, Illinois.

cont'd

CHEMOTHERAPY FLUID/VOLUME CHART

The following table provides information for the dilution and administration of chemotherapy. This table may be utilized as a guideline when fluids, volumes and/or rates are not specified on the physicians orders.

DRUG	ROUTE	DOSE	FLUID	VOLUME	RATE
Asparaginase (Elspar)	IVPB	All[1]	D5 (or NS)	50 ml	30 min
	SubQ		-	-	-
Bleomycin (Blenoxane)	IVPB	All[2]	NS	50 ml	1 UNIT / min
	SubQ		-	-	-
Carboplatin (Paraplatin)	IVPB	All	D5	250 ml	30 min
Carmustine (BCNU)					
	IVPB		D5	250 ml (GLASS)	60 min
Cisplatin (Platinol) (CDDP)	IVPB over 1h	All	NS	250 ml	1 h
	IVPB over 6h		D5.45NS	1000 ml	6 h
Cyclophosphamide	IVPB	≤ 1 gm	D5	100 ml	30 - 60 min
		> 1 gm	D5	250 ml	30 - 60 min
	IVPush	All	-	-	5 - 10 min
Cytarabine (Cytosar) (Ara-C)	Cont. Inf.	<500 mg	D5 (or NS)	250 ml	24 h
	IVPB	≤1 gm	D5 (or NS)	50 ml	30 - 60 min
		> 1 gm	D5 (or NS)	250 ml	30 - 60 min
	Intrathecal	-	NS*	3 - 6 ml	
Cladribine (Leustatin) (2-CdA)	Cont. Inf.	All	NS	500 ml	24 h
Dacarbazine (DTIC)	IVPB	All	D5 (or NS)	250 ml	15 min
Dactinomycin (Cosmogen)	IVPB	All	D5 (or NS)	50 ml	10 - 15 min
	IV Push			-	10 - 15 min
Daunorubicin (Cerubidine)	IVPB	All	NS	50 ml	15 min
	IV Push		D5 (or NS)	-	2 - 3 min
Docetaxel (Taxotere)	IVPB.	All	D5 (or NS)	250 ml (Glass)	60 min
Doxorubicin (Adriamycin)	IVPB	All	D5 (or NS)	100 ml	30 min
	IV Push		-	-	10 - 15 min
Doxorubicin/Vincristine	Cont. Inf.	All	D5	500 ml	24 h
Etoposide (Vepesid) (VP-16)	IVPB	All	D5 (or NS)	<0.6, 0.4, 0.2 mg/ml	1 - 2 h
Floxuridine (FUDR)	Cont. Inf.	All	D5 (or NS)	1000 ml	24 h
Fludarabine (Fludara)	IVPB	All	D5 (or NS)	50 ml	30 min
Fluorouracil (5-FU)	Cont. Inf.	All	D5 (or NS)	500 or 1000 ml	12 or 24 h
	IVPB		D5 (or NS)	50 ml	30 - 60 min
	IV Push		-	-	2 - 3 min
Gemcitabine (Gemzar)	IVPB	≥ 1 gm/m²	NS	100 ml	30 min
		<1 gm/m²		250 ml	over 6 - 24 h
Idarubicin (Idamycin)	IVPB	All	D5 (or NS)	50 ml	15 min
Ifosfamide (Ifex)	IVPB	All	D5 (or NS)	250 ml	30 - 60 min
Ifosfamide/Mesna	Cont. Inf.	All	D5 (or NS)	1000 ml	24 h
Leucovorin	IV Push	All	D5 (or NS)	-	2 - 3 min
Mechlorethamine (Mustargen)	IVPB	All	D5 (or NS)	100 ml	15 min
Melphalan (Alkeran)	IVPB	All	NS	≤0.45mg/ml	15 -30 min
Mesna (Mesnex)	IVPB	All	D5 (or NS)	100 ml	20 min
Methotrexate (MTX)	IVPB	All	D5 (or NS)	250 ml	15 - 30 min
	Intrathecal		NS*	3 -6 ml	
Mitomycin (Mutamycin)	IVPB	All	NS	50 ml	15 min
Mitoxantrone (Novantrone)	IVPB	All	D5 (or NS)	50 ml	15 min
Paclitaxel (Taxol)	Cont Inf.	All	D5 (or NS)	500 ml (GLASS)	1, 3, 24 or 96 h
Teniposide (Vumon)	IVPB	All	NS	100 ml	45 - 60 min
Thiophosphoramide (Thiotepa)	IVPB	All	D5 (or NS)	50 ml	15 min
Topotecan (Hycamptin)	IVPB	All	D5 (or NS)	50 ml	30 min
	Cont Inf.			250 ml	24h
Vinblastine (Velban)	IV Push	All	-	-	2 - 3 min
Vincristine (Oncovin)	IV Push	All	-	-	2 - 3 min
Vinorelbine (Navelbine)	IV Push	All	-	-	6 - 10 min

[1] Asparaginase test dose: 2 IU (0.1ml) INTRADERMAL at least 1 hour prior to dose
[2] Bleomycin test dose: 2 units in 50 ml D5W IVPB OVER 15 - 20 min at least 1 hour prior to dose
*Preservative Free

Figure 15-3. Example of a preprinted chemotherapy order form.

Source: *Advocate* Lutheran General Hospital, Park Ridge, Illinois.

They reduce the number of health care personnel who handle the medications, which may in turn reduce the chance for human error.[55] Pharmacy-generated medication administration records or labels are recommended to assist nurses in interpreting and documenting medication activities.[2] Packaging is getting more sophisticated; one company recently introduced barcoded unit-dose packaging for use with an automated dispensing machine. Bar coding may help health care personnel avoid mistaking one patient for another. An automated final check and sortation device using barcode technology helped to reduce medication dispensing errors in a correctional health care system.[56] It is recommended that computerized pharmacy systems be in place to enable automated checking of doses, duplicate therapies, allergies, drug interactions, and other aspects of use.

Computerized Physician Order Entry (CPOE) has been shown to reduce the rate of serious errors in an inpatient setting by 55 percent.[57] CPOE is also being investigated at some institutions to decrease the number of personnel involved in the ordering process and the medication errors in the transcription process (where medication orders are written down by a nurse or unit clerk and sent to the pharmacy). Computer systems designed to alert physicians about possible allergy problems or overdoses have been shown to prevent potential adverse events before the order reaches the pharmacist.[58]

The Quality Assurance Process

What to Do When an Error Occurs

When a potential medication error occurs—for example, a pharmacy technician incorrectly fills a unit dose order—and the pharmacist catches the error in the pharmacy, usually the pharmacist will tell the technician of the error and ask the technician to correct it. It is important for the technician to realize that the pharmacist's intent is to make the mistake a learning experience for the technician as well as give the technician an opportunity to ask questions. Although making a mistake is frustrating, focusing on improving work habits so the same error will not be made again is important.

Whatever the circumstances surrounding an actual medication error, the pharmacy technician has a responsibility to inform the pharmacist about any known details. Pharmacists usually investigate the error and the severity of the consequences and gather the details before contacting the nurse and the physician.

If the error is caught before the patient receives the medication, it can be corrected within the pharmacy. If the patient has received the medication, the course of action depends on the details of the error. The pharmacist may refill the medication for free and have it delivered to the patient or send a formal letter of apology to the patient. If the error has caused patient harm, the pharmacist may seek legal advice.

Documentation

When a medication error occurs, the organization's medication error reporting form should be completed according to the organization's established reporting procedures. **Figure 15-4** is an example of a medication error reporting form.

The medication error reporting form should be filled out and reviewed by those involved in the error to ensure that the content is accurate and correct. Once the form is complete, it is usually sent to the pharmacy supervisor and, if necessary, to the risk management department for review. These forms are reviewed periodically by the organization's designated committee (quality assurance, for example), which may consist of pharmacy, medicine, nursing, risk management, quality assurance, staff education, and legal counsel staff members.[2]

Identifying Trends

One of the purposes of medication error review is to look for medication errors that occur frequently or involve high-risk medications. The reviewers look for trends in the medication error process and evaluate the systems involved in the errors. Many quality assurance committees focus on the institution's systems (e.g., staff orientation and education) instead of on individual staff members, because most medication errors are due more to poor drug distribution systems, miscommunications, faulty pharmaceutical packaging, labeling, nomenclature, and lack of information than to any one person. When there is a chance of serious errors, action is taken to improve the system and minimize the possibility of errors.[59]

Making Necessary Changes

Once a trend has been identified, action must be taken to reduce the possibility of future errors. Changes may involve educating staff, purchasing a more appropriately labeled medication from another company, revising department policies and procedures, or purchasing a piece of equipment.

Advocate Health Care

Confidential Patient Safety Event Form
Do Not Copy (NOT PART OF THE MEDICAL RECORD)

☐ Advocate North Side
☐ Bethany
☐ Christ
☐ Good Samaritan

☐ Good Shepherd
☐ Lutheran General
☐ South Suburban
☐ Trinity

Include name & Medical Record No.

Date of Occurrence	Mental Status	Identification:
	☐ Normal/Alert ☐ Unconscious ☐ Sedated ☐ Asleep ☐ Disoriented	☐ Inpatient ☐ ER Patient ☐ Visitor ☐ Out-patient ☐ Other

Time of Occurrence _____
☐ Day
☐ PM
☐ Nite

Medicated Past 2 Hrs?
☐ Yes   ☐ No

Primary Diagnosis

_____

Attending Physician

_____

Unit/Room No.

_____

Area Incident Occurred
☐ Operating Room
☐ Emergency Room
☐ Intensive Care Unit
☐ Recovery Room
☐ Labor & Delivery
☐ X-Ray
(specify)
☐ Pharmacy
☐ Physician Office
☐ Bathroom
☐ Hallway
☐ Facility Grounds
☐ Patient Room

| Types of Medication | Age | ☐ Male | |
| | | ☐ Female | |

Event/Occurrence   Please check as many items as needed to fully explain event

Safety/Fall Related
☐ Found on floor
☐ Fall from bed/chair/table
☐ Fall while ambulating
☐ Removed restraints
☐ Climbed over side rails
☐ Reported fall/not observed
☐ Assisted Fall
☐ Other _____

_____

Bedrails ☐ Up   ☐ Down

Restraints On   ☐ Yes   ☐ No

Equipment Related (include Medical Device Reporting Form)
☐ Patient burned
☐ Function
☐ Availability
☐ Other _____
Type: _____

_____

Communication Related
☐ MD notification/MD response
☐ Orders/instructions
☐ Chart documentation
☐ Informed consent
☐ Other _____

Diagnosis/Testing/Treatment Related
☐ Blood administration
☐ Catheter/tube/drain
☐ Complications of procedure
☐ Consult
☐ Extubation
☐ ID band
☐ Return to surgery
☐ Specimen collection
☐ Specimen label
☐ Test or procedure timing
☐ X-Rays
☐ Other _____

Arrest ☐ Intubation required
☐ Resuscitated
☐ Expired

Non-Medical
☐ Altercation
☐ Suicide attempt/self inflicted injury
☐ Left AMA
☐ Left without being seen

☐ Elopement
☐ Pt./family dissatisfaction
☐ Refused treatment
☐ Lost Property

☐ Pt. non-compliance
☐ Other _____

Initiator's Report/Comments

_____

_____

_____

_____

_____

Name (print) Dept/Unit Ext.	Signature	Date

PS 239 12/01

© 2002 Advocate Health Care

Figure 15-4. Sample of a medication error reporting form.

Source: Advocate Health Care, Oakbrook, Illinois.

cont'd

Medication Error Information Report

Risk Management # _____   MedMarx # _____

*Severity Level/Outcome

Errors did not reach the patient
- ☐ Category A: capacity to cause error
- ☐ Category B: did not reach the patient

Errors that reach the patient
- ☐ Category C: did not cause patient harm
- ☐ Category D: increased patient monitoring, no patient harm
- ☐ Category E: need for treatment or intervention and caused temporary patient harm (dextrose, narcan, etc)
- ☐ Category F: resulted in initial or prolonged hospitalization and caused temporary patient harm (transferred to ICU)

Errors causing permanent harm
- ☐ Category G: permanent patient harm
- ☐ Category H: resulted in a near-death event (e.g., anaphylaxis, cardiac arrest)
- ☐ Category I: patient death

*Background

Medication(s) & dosage form involved:
_____
_____

*Where did the **initial** error occur? ☐
- Prescribing ☐   Administering ☐
- Documenting ☐   Monitoring ☐
- Dispensing ☐

Level of staff that made the initial error:
- ☐ Pharmacy Technician   ☐ Physician
- ☐ Nurse Practitioner   ☐ Physician Assistant
- ☐ Nurse, LPN   ☐ Unit Secretary/Clerk
- ☐ Nurse, RN   ☐ Pharmacist
- ☐ **Other: _____

*Type of Error
- ☐ Prescribing   ☐ Extra dose
- ☐ Omission   ☐ Wrong administration technique
- ☐ Wrong patient   ☐ Wrong dosage form
- ☐ Wrong route   ☐ Wrong dosage form
- ☐ Improper dose/quantity
  - enter dose ordered: _____
  - enter dose given: _____
- ☐ Unauthorized (wrong) drug
  - name of medication ordered: _____
  - name of medication given: _____
- ☐ Other _____

- ☐ Abbreviations (e.g. AZT)
- ☐ Calculation error
- ☐ Communication confusing/ intimidating/lacking
- ☐ Computer entry error

Decimal point
- ☐ leading zero missing (e.g. .20mg)
- ☐ trailing zero (e.g.20.0mg)

- ☐ Diluent wrong (e.g. NS vs D5W)
- ☐ Dispensing device involved (e.g. pump)
- ☐ Documentation inaccurate/lacking
- ☐ Dosage form confusion
- ☐ Drug distribution system (e.g. not unit dose)

Possible cause(s) or error (check all that apply):
- ☐ Equipment design confusing
- ☐ Failure to activate medication (e.g. advantage vials)
- ☐ handwriting illegible/unclear
- ☐ Knowledge deficit

Label
- ☐ facilities
- ☐ manufacturers
- ☐ Measuring device inaccurate/inappropriate
- ☐ Monitoring inadequate/lacking

Names
- ☐ look alike
- ☐ sound alike
- ☐ Non-metric units (grains vs. mg)
- ☐ Other: _____

Orders – inaccurate/confusing/incomplete
- ☐ verbal order
- ☐ written order
- ☐ facsimile order
- ☐ preprinted order form
- ☐ Packaging design
- ☐ Performance deficit (i.e., person trained/ expectation not met)
- ☐ Procedure / protocol not followed
- ☐ Pump, mis-program, improper use
- ☐ Reference manual confusing/inaccurate/ unclear/outdated
- ☐ System safeguard(s) inadequate/lacking
- ☐ Transcription inaccurate/omitted

NATURE OF INJURY: PLEASE CHECK AS MANY ITEMS AS NEEDED TO FULLY EXPLAIN NATURE OF INJURY

☐ **No Apparent Injury**

Musculoskeletal
- ☐ Broken teeth/dental work
- ☐ Fracture/dislocation
- ☐ Strain/sprain
- ☐ Other _____

Central Nervous System
- ☐ Cerebral vascular accident
- ☐ Neuro damage/deficit/loss/change
- ☐ Seizure
- ☐ Other _____

Cardiopulmonary
- ☐ Death
- ☐ Hemorrhage
- ☐ Other _____

Skin/Tissue/Systemic
- ☐ Abscess/decubitus ulcer
- ☐ Allergic/adverse reaction (non medication)
- ☐ Bleeding, additional
- ☐ Burn
- ☐ Contusion/abrasion
- ☐ Edema/swelling
- ☐ Hematoma
- ☐ Laceration/perforation
- ☐ Rash
- ☐ Sloughing/scarring/necrosis
- ☐ Wound infection
- ☐ Other _____

Comments:
_____
_____
_____

Severity
- Level 0: Potential for error, no error occurred.
- Level 1: An error occurred, no patient harm.
- Level 2: Error resulted in increased monitoring but no change in VS/labs and no harm to the patient noted.
- Level 3: Error resulted in increased monitoring with change in VS, but no harm to the patient noted.
- Level 4: Error resulted in the need for treatment with another drug or an increased length of stay.
- Level 5: Error resulted in potentially permanent patient harm.
- Level 6: Error resulted in patient death.

Does this occurrence pertain to another department/unit?   ☐ Yes   ☐ No
If so, have you discussed this occurrence with the appropriate manager?   ☐ Yes   ☐ No

Reviewed by Unit/Dept. Supervisor	Signature	Date
Dept/Unit _____ Ext. _____		

SEND THIS REPORT TO THE RISK MANAGEMENT DEPARTMENT

This report has been prepared at the direction of the Risk Management Department for review, analysis and process improvement by the internal Quality Assurance/Improvement Departments. This report is confidential and is subject to the Medical Studies Act.

PS 239 12/01   © 2002 Advocate Health Care

Figure 15-4. Sample of a medication error reporting form.

Source: Advocate Health Care, Oakbrook, Illinois.

Three ways the pharmacy department can educate its staff on a continual basis about actual medication errors are (1) by publishing in staff newsletters summaries of errors that have occurred, (2) by conducting educational programs, and (3) by discussing medication errors as a regular agenda item at staff meetings.[2] It is important for technicians to pay close attention to newsletters, educational programs, and discussions of errors to help reduce them.

If product labeling contributed to a medication error, the pharmacist usually contacts the drug company and communicates how the labeling contributed to the error. The problem should also be reported to either the USP Medication Errors Reporting Program or the FDA MedWatch Program, both of which are national programs to monitor medication errors. Both programs collect data on drug product problems and report them to the manufacturers and may even distribute an alert to the medical community when necessary. Problems with product labeling or packaging can be reported to either program using the Internet, by telephone, or by mailing or faxing in a completed report form. Report forms can be downloaded from the Internet and can be found in many pharmacy journals.

Once a system has been identified as a contributor to medication errors, the policies and procedures are revised to eliminate or reduce the chance of future errors. The staff is given in-service training or informed about the changes in procedures and the reasons for the changes.

Monitoring the Impact of Change

After a system has been modified, the committee will continue to monitor it for medication errors to determine the impact of the changes.[59]

Technician/Pharmacist Liability Issues

Technicians and pharmacists need to be informed about how to prevent medication errors. In addition to the institution or company liability, they may be held accountable for a medication error involving injury to a patient.[60]

Summary

The ultimate goal of pharmacy services must be the safe use of medications by the public.[61] Medication errors can occur in many ways and also can be prevented in many ways. Pharmacy technicians play an important role in ensuring the safe use of medications.

Recommended Reading

American Society of Hospital Pharmacists. ASHP guideline on preventing medication errors in hospitals. *Am J Hosp Pharm.* 1993; 50: 305–14.

Brennan TA, Leape LL, Laird NM et al. Incidence of adverse events and negligence in hospitalized patients–results of the Harvard medical practice study I. *N Engl J Med.* 1991; 324: 370–6.

Cohen JR, Anderson RW, Attilio RM et al. Preventing medication errors in cancer chemotherapy. *Am J Health-Syst Pharm* 1996; 53: 737–46.

Cohen MR, Senders J, Davis NM. Failure mode and effects analysis: a novel approach to avoiding dangerous medication errors and accidents. *Hosp Pharm.* 1994; 29: 319–24, 326–28, 330.

Cohen MR, ed. Medication errors. Washington, DC: American Pharmaceutical Association; 1999.

Johnson JA, Bootman JL. Drug-related morbidity and mortality and the economic impact of pharmaceutical care. *Am J Health-Syst Pharm.* 1997; 54: 554–8.

Kistner UA, Keith MR, Sergeant KA et al. Accuracy of dispensing in a high-volume, hospital-based outpatient pharmacy. *Am J Hosp Pharm.* 1994; 51: 2793–7.

Allan EL, Barker KN. Fundamentals of medication error research. *Am J Hosp Pharm.* 1990; 47: 555–71.

Kenagy JW, Stein GC. Naming, labeling, and packaging of pharmaceuticals. *Am J Health-Syst Pharm.* 2001; 58: 2033–41.

Recommended Websites

www.ashp.org

www.fda.gov/cder/drug/MedErrors/nameDiff.htm

www.fda.gov/medwatch

www.ismp.org

www.jcaho.org

www.usp.org

References

1. Manasse HR Jr. Medication use in an imperfect world: drug misadventuring as an issue of public policy, part I. *Am J Hosp Pharm.* 1989; 46: 929–44.

2. American Society of Hospital Pharmacists. ASHP guideline on preventing medication errors in hospitals. *Am J Hosp Pharm.* 1993; 50: 305–14.

3. National Association of Chain Drug Stores. 2002

community pharmacy results. http://www.nacds.org/user-assets/PDF_files/2002_results.PDF (accessed 2003 May 30).

4. Brennan TA, Leape LL, Laird NM et al. Incidence of adverse events and negligence in hospitalized patients—results of the Harvard medical practice study I. *N Engl J Med.* 1991; 324: 370–6.

5. Lesar TS, Briceland LL, Delcoure K et al. Medication prescribing errors in a teaching hospital. *JAMA.* 1990; 263: 2329–34.

6. Rupp MT, DeYoung M, Schondelmeyer SW. Prescribing problems and pharmacist interventions in community practice. *Medical Care.* 1992; 30: 926–40.

7. Blum KV, Abel SR, Urbanski CJ et al. Medication error prevention by pharmacists. *Am J Hosp Pharm.* 1988; 45: 1902–3.

8. Dean B, Schachter M, Vincet C et al. Causes of prescribing errors in hospital inpatients: a prospective study. *Lancet.* 2002; 359: 1373–8.

9. Bates DW, Cullen DJ, Laird N et al. Incidence of adverse drug events and potential adverse drug events. *JAMA.* 1995; 274: 29–34.

10. Guernsey BG, Ingrim NB, Kokanson JA et al. Pharmacists' dispensing accuracy in a high-volume outpatient pharmacy service: focus on risk management. *Drug Intell Clin Pharm.* 1993; 17: 742–6.

11. Kistner UA, Keith MR, Sergeant KA et al. Accuracy of dispensing in a high-volume, hospital-based outpatient pharmacy. *Am J Hosp Pharm.* 1994; 51: 2793–7.

12. Buchanan TL, Barker KN, Gibson JT et al. Illumination and errors in dispensing. *Am J Hosp Pharm.* 1991; 48: 2137–45.

13. Allan EL, Barker KN. Fundamentals of mediation error research. *Am J Hosp Pharm.* 1990; 47: 555–71.

14. Barker KN, Flynn EA, Pepper GA et al. Medication errors observed in 36 health care facilities. *Arch Intern Med.* 2002; 162: 1897–1903.

15. Bates DW, Boyle DL, Vander Vliet MB et al. Relationship between medication errors and adverse drug events. *J Gen Intern Med.* 1995; 10: 199–205.

16. Leape LL. Error in medicine. *JAMA.* 1994; 272: 1851–7.

17. Phillips J, Beam S, Brinker A et al. Retrospective analysis of mortalities associated with medication errors. *Am J Health-Syst Pharm.* 2001; 58: 1835–41.

18. Kaufman A, Kung FH, Koenig HM et al. Overdosage with vincristine. *J Pediatr.* 1976; 89: 671–4.

19. Davis NM. Preventing omission errors. *Am J Nursing.* 1195; 95: 17.

20. Classen DC, Pestotnik SL, Evans RS, et al. Adverse drug events in hospitalized patients. *JAMA.* 1997; 277: 301–6.

21. Schneider PJ, Gift MG, Lee Y, et al. Cost of medication-related problems at a university hospital. *Am J Health-Syst Pharm.* 1995; 52: 2415–8.

22. Johnson JA, Bootman JL. Drug-related morbidity and mortality. A cost of illness model. *Arch Intern Med.* 1995; 155: 1949–56.

23. Wou K. Costs associated with recurrent hypoglycemia caused by dispensing error. *Ann Pharmacother.* 1994; 28: 965–6. Letter.

24. Koren G, Barzilay Z, Greenwald M. Tenfold errors in administration of drug doses: a neglected iatrogenic disease in pediatrics. *Pediatrics.* 1986; 77: 848–9.

25. Koren G, Barzilay Z, Modan M. Errors in computing drug doses. *Can Med Assoc J.* 1983; 129: 721–3.

26. Perlstein PH, Callison C, White M et al. Errors in drug computations during newborn intensive care. *Am J Dis Child.* 1979; 133: 376–9.

27. Bindler R, Bayne T. Medication calculation ability of registered nurses. *IMAGE: J Nursing Scholarship.* 1991; 23: 221–4.

28. Bayne T, Bindler R. Medication calculation skills of registered nurses. *J of Continuing Education in Nursing.* 1988; 19: 258–62.

29. Joint Commission on Accreditation of Healthcare Organizations. 2002 comprehensive accreditation manual for hospitals: the official handbook (CAMH). IM.3. Oakbrook Terrace, IL: Joint Commission on Accreditation of Healthcare Organizations, 2002.

30. Joint Commission on Accreditation of Healthcare Organizations. 2003 national patient safety goals. http://www.jcaho.org/accreditedorganizations/patient+safety/npsg/npsg_03.htm (accessed 2003 May 30).

31. Robertson WO. Alphabet soup: more or less? *JAMA.* 1980; 244: 1902. Letter.

32. Institute for Safe Medication Practices. High alert medications. http://www.ismp.org/MSArticles/HighAlertMedications.htm (accessed 2003 June 12).

33. Cohen MR, Davis NM. Errors caused by medical office personnel. *Am Pharm.* 1993; NS33:18.

34. Davis NM. Confusion over illegible orders. *Am J Nursing.* 1994; 94(1): 9.

35. Cohen JR, Anderson RW, Attilio RM et al. Pre-

venting medication errors in cancer chemotherapy. *Am J Health-Syst Pharm.* 1996; 53: 737–46.

36. Edgar RA, Lee DS, Cousins DD. Experience with a national medication error reporting program. *Am J Hosp Pharm.* 1994; 51: 1335–8.

37. Kenagy JW, Stein GC. Naming, labeling, and packaging of pharmaceuticals. *Am J Health-Syst Pharm.* 2001; 58: 2033–41.

38. Davis NM. A well-informed patient is a valuable asset. *Am J Nursing.* 1994; 94: 16.

39. Cohen MR. Amrinone-amiodarone mix-up reported. *Hosp Pharm.* 1996; 31: 64.

40. Rodriquez G, Poretsky L. Toradol instead of tapazole. *Am J Health-Syst Pharm.* 1995; 52: 1098. Letter.

41. Pourmotabbed G. The naming of drugs is a difficult matter. *N Engl J Med.* 1994; 331: 1163.

42. Chu G, Mantin R, Shen Y et al. Massive cisplatin overdose by accidental substitution for carboplatin. *Cancer.* 1993; 72: 3707–14.

43. Malcolm KE, Hogan TT, Wyatt TL. Is the prescription really for selegiline? *Am J Hosp Pharm.* 1994; 51: 930. Letter.

44. Cohen MR, Davis NM. Trademark similarities can cause problems. *Am Pharm.* 1993; NS33: 16–7.

45. Look-alike, sound-alike drug names. *Jt Comm Persp.* 2001; 19: 10–11.

46. Use caution—avoid confusion. *USP Quality Rev.* 2001; 76.

47. Raffalli J, Nowakowski J, Wormser GP. "Vira something": a taste of the wrong medicine. *Lancet.* 1997; 350: 887. Letter.

48. Lawyer C, Despot J. 'Z-Pak' vs ice pack: need for clarity and continuous quality assurance. *JAMA.* 1997; 278: 1405. Letter.

49. Rheinstein PH, McGinnis TJ. Medication errors. *Am Fam Physician.* 1992; 45:2720–22.

50. Gold DR, Rogacz S, Bock N et al. Rotating shift work, sleep and accidents related to sleepiness in hospital nurses. *Am J Public Health.* 1992; 82: 1011–4.

51. Leape LL, Bates DW, Cullen DJ et al. Systems analysis of adverse drug events. *JAMA.* 1995; 274: 35–43.

52. Cohen MR, Senders J, Davis NM. Failure mode and effects analysis: a novel approach to avoiding dangerous medication errors and accidents. *Hosp Pharm.* 1994; 29: 319–24, 326–28, 330.

53. Williams E, Talley R. The use of failure mode effect and criticality analysis in a medication error subcommittee. *Hosp Pharm.* 1994; 29: 331–2, 334–7.

54. McNally KM, Page MA, Sunderland VB. Failure-mode and effects analysis in improving a drug distribution system. *Am J Health-Syst Pharm.* 1997; 54: 171–7.

55. Borel JM, Rascati KL. Effect of an automated, nursing unit-based drug dispensing device on medication errors. *Am J Health-Syst Pharm.* 1995; 52: 1875–9.

56. Carmenates J, Keith MR. Impact of automation on pharmacist interventions and medication errors in a correctional health care system. *Am J Health-Syst Pharm.* 2001; 58: 770–83.

57. Bates DW, Leape LL, Cullen DJ et al. Effect of computerized physician order entry and a team intervention on prevention of serious medication errors. *JAMA.* 1998; 280: 1311–16.

58. Raschke RA, Gollihare B, Wunderlich RA et al. A computer alert system to prevent injury from adverse drug events: development and evaluation in a community teaching hospital. *JAMA.* 1998; 280: 1317–20.

59. Cohen MR. Risk management of medication errors must include a careful look at the specific systems involved. *Hosp Pharm.* 1996; 31: 454, 458, 461–2.

60. Brushwood DB. Patient injury and attempted link with pharmacist's negligence. *Am J Hosp Pharm.* 1993; 50: 2382–5.

61. Brodie DC. The challenge to pharmacy in times of change—a report of the Commission on Pharmaceutical Services to Ambulant Patients by Hospitals and Related Facilities. Washington, DC: American Pharmaceutical Association and American Society of Hospital Pharmacists; 1966.

Self-Assessment Questions

1. A medication error is defined as "an error made by a pharmacist or pharmacy technician at any time during the dispensing process." True or False

2. Which of the following might increase the likelihood of a medication error?
   a. reading the drug label carefully when obtaining the drug from the shelf
   b. reviewing recent medication errors at a pharmacy staff meeting
   c. asking another pharmacy technician to double-check a calculation
   d. having a nurse phone in a prescription order that was communicated verbally by the doctor

3. Manufacturers are required to print the warning, "MUST BE DILUTED," on the container cap and label for which of the following products?
   a. potassium chloride injection
   b. vincristine injection
   c. digoxin liquid
   d. amoxicillin suspension

4. Manufacturers have made modifications to products in response to medication error occurrences. Which of the following changes could a manufacturer make to help prevent medication errors?
   a. Place a "hood" (stopper) on a syringe that is designed to prevent direct injection into a vein.
   b. Change the trade name of a product.
   c. Decrease the size of the manufacturer's logo on the label to make it less prominent than the drug name.
   d. all of the above

5. A prescription for diazepam (Valium®—an antianxiety agent) was erroneously filled with Diabeta® (glyburide—a drug that lowers blood sugar). Possible consequences resulting from this dispensing error include which of the following?
   a. Patient experiences hypoglycemia (too low blood sugar) and faints.
   b. Unnecessary health care expenses are incurred.
   c. Patient experiences no ill effects.
   d. all of the above

6. Jane Smith received the following prescription for an antibiotic to treat a respiratory tract infection on January 1:

   Amoxicillin 500 mg TID X 10 days

   After taking the drug for 3 days, Ms. Smith felt much better and stopped taking her medication.

   On January 12, Ms. Smith presents to the pharmacy with the following prescription for another antibiotic:

   Clarithromycin 500 mg PO BID X 10 days

   The medication error that has occurred would be categorized as which of the following medication errors?
   a. patient noncompliance
   b. prescribing error
   c. wrong drug dispensed
   d. deteriorated drug error

7. The pharmacist asks you to prepare the following medications:
   Gentamicin 1 g IVPB Q 8 hr
   Cefazolin 60 mg IVPB Q 12 hr

   After obtaining the necessary supplies from the shelf, you are puzzled by the number of vials needed for the gentamicin dose (13 vials). You should:
   a. Prepare the doses as requested.
   b. Prepare the doses as requested, but ask another technician to check your calculations.
   c. Question the pharmacist about the order because you have never had to use so many vials to prepare a gentamicin dose before.
   d. Prepare the doses as requested because the order has already been reviewed by a pharmacist.
   e. Contact the doctor to clarify the order.

8. Katie Loden presents to your pharmacy with the prescription in **Figure 15-5**, and Lanoxin® (digoxin—heart medication) is dispensed. She calls the pharmacy several hours later and asks why her thyroid medication is a yellow instead of a light brown round tablet.

   How would this medication error most likely be categorized?
   a. patient compliance error
   b. prescribing error
   c. wrong drug preparation error
   d. physician error

Self-Assessment Questions

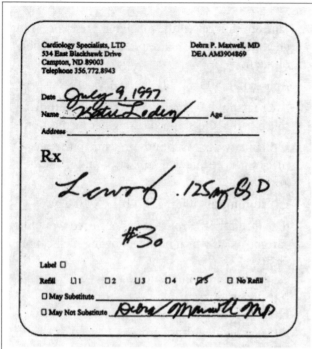

Figure 15-5. Pharmacy prescription from which Lanoxin is prescribed.

9. Susan Baker was in the radiology department when the nurse came to her room to administer the 0900 dose of captopril 25 mg PO 3 times daily (scheduled for 0900, 1600, and 2200). Because of the complexity of the procedure and a number of delays in radiology, Ms. Baker did not return to her room until 1630, at which time her captopril was administered.

   Which of the following is a TRUE statement regarding Ms. Baker's captopril?
   a. A nursing error has been committed.
   b. The medication delay resulted in a wrong time error for the 0900 dose.
   c. An omission error occurred.
   d. No medication error has occurred.

10. When compounding the following order, the technician inadvertently used 1 ml of the 40 mg/ml concentration solution instead of the pediatric concentration (10 mg/ml).

   Gentamicin 10 mg IVPB Q 8 hr

   Identify the category or categories in which this error could be classified.
   a. wrong dosage form error
   b. calculation error
   c. improper dose error
   d. wrong administration technique error
   e. b and c

11. As a technician undergoing on-the-job training, you are falling behind in putting away the drug shipment that arrived earlier this morning. In an effort to save time, you fail to rotate the stock and put all the new stock in front of the containers already in the stock area.

   Failure to rotate stock could lead to which of the following medication errors?
   a. deteriorated drug error
   b. improper dose error
   c. inventory error
   d. monitoring error

12. Which of the following would be considered a wrong drug preparation error?
   a. using the wrong base product to compound a skin ointment
   b. adding an incorrect volume of water to reconstitute a 80 ml bottle of amoxicillin oral suspension 125 mg/5 ml.
   c. using the wrong diluent to reconstitute a lyophilized powder for injection
   d. all of the above

13. Experienced pharmacy technicians are less likely than technicians-in-training to make calculation errors.
   True or False

14. Which of the following may lead to a calculation error?
   a. not verifying that the final answer is reasonable
   b. using an inaccurate conversion
   c. misplacing the decimal point
   d. all of the above

15. Which of the following is least likely to lead to a wrong dose error?
   a. 4 mg
   b. .4 g
   c. 4U
   d. 4.0 units

16. Using abbreviations that have been published in reputable medical journals is acceptable because only widely accepted abbreviations are used in publications.
   True or False

17. The best way to write "five thousand units of heparin" is _____.

18. Identify four things from the following order

Self-Assessment Questions

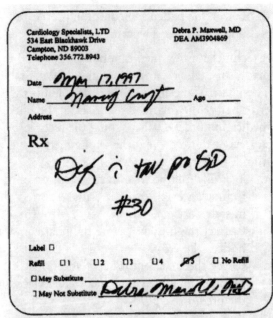

Figure 15-6. Identify four things in the order that might contribute to a medication error.

(**Figure 15-6**) that might contribute to a medication error.

19. One morning you are busy preparing IVPB antibiotic orders for the 1000 delivery. The orders are:
    Pat Carlson Cefazolin 1 g IVPB Q 8 hr
    Paul Cariton Ceftazidime 1 g IVPB Q 8 hr

    You decide to prepare both orders simultaneously to save time and avoid missing the delivery.

    List four reasons that the chances of making an error this morning are increased.

20. Name at least five things the pharmaceutical manufacturer could do to improve labeling for this new drug product (**Figure 15-7**).

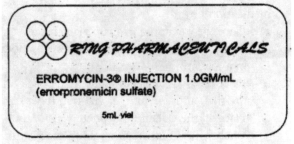

Figure 15-7. Drug product label.

21. Which of the following statements are TRUE regarding the practice of color coding drug product packaging and its relationship to medication errors?
    a. Color-coding the vial caps red for all injectable solutions that turn red upon reconstitution would decrease the likelihood of medication errors.
    b. Developing a color-coding scheme unique to a specific manufacturer would decrease the likelihood of a medication error.
    c. Color-coding saves time because you do not have to read the product label.
    d. In general, color-coding is an unsafe practice.

22. Which could be considered a contributing factor (or factors) to medication errors?
    a. performing routine maintenance procedures on the tablet counting machine
    b. failing to read current pharmacy literature about new drug products
    c. scheduling additional staff to work during periods of heavy workload
    d. all of the above

23. Why are medication error rates reported in studies probably underestimated?
    a. Only errors that result in patient injury are reported.
    b. Some errors go undetected.
    c. Few errors are identified and corrected during the prescribing phase.
    d. Efficient anonymous reporting systems are common.

24. Which of the following statements is **TRUE** regarding the impact of medication errors on health care expenses?
    a. Medication errors are usually insignificant, easily corrected, and inexpensive.
    b. Medical care costs for treating negative outcomes due to medication errors are usually paid for by the health care worker responsible for the error.
    c. Health care expenses associated with medication errors cost billions of dollars each year.
    d. Malpractice claims for medication errors are usually thrown out in court.

25. Omission errors are less likely to result in negative outcomes than improper dose errors because the patient is not receiving a harmful dose.
    True or False

26. Judy Jones, a technician working in the unit dose

cartfill area, notices the 25 mg and 50 mg strengths of Benadryl® are mixed together in the same storage bin. What can Judy do to correct this problem?

a. Make no changes, because technicians are responsible for reading labels carefully.

b. Modify the stock shelf so each strength has its own section or bin.

c. Change the label to indicate that both strengths are in the bin.

d. Store the 25 mg strength under Benadryl® and the 50 mg strength under Diphenhy-dramine.

27. The technician filling a prescription for Mr. Hill notices that the print on the label is faded and hard to read. What is the best way for the technician to correct this problem?

a. Hand write the patient name and directions on the label.

b. Ask the pharmacist to change the printer ribbon before the next label is printed.

c. Change the printer ribbon, and reprint the label for Mr. Hill's prescription.

d. all of the above

28. Anonymous self-reporting of medication errors may be used in some institutions or companies as a means of determining the numbers/severity of medication errors.
True or False

29. A technician compounds a continuous infusion of Heparin 25,000 units in 500 ml of 5% Dextrose in Water (D5W) and places the bag on the counter for the pharmacist to check. The technician then begins to fill other medication orders. One of the orders the technician fills calls for two Heparin 5,000 unit syringes for subcutaneous injection. The technician notices the same patient name on the continuous infusion label and the subcutaneous injection label. What should the technician do?

a. Fill the other medication orders and assume the pharmacist will evaluate the doses.

b. Inform the pharmacist that both Heparin prescriptions have the same patient name and ask if both orders are correct.

c. Ask another technician what the standard dose of Heparin is and fill both orders.

d. Check the patient's medication profile and fill both orders for Heparin.

30. A technician fills a medication order for a 20 mg prednisone tablet with a propranolol 20 mg tablet. The pharmacy technician supervisor notices the error before the pharmacist checks all the filled medication orders. What should the technician supervisor do to prevent the wrong medication from leaving the pharmacy?

a. Tactfully call the error to the attention of the technician who made the error to correct the mistake.

b. Correct the mistake before the pharmacist also notices the error.

c. Check the stock bin to see if additional propranolol tablets were incorrectly placed in the prednisone bin.

d. Both a and c

31. A newly employed technician begins training in the pharmacy. A senior technician is training the new technician about the duties of the position. Which of the following ideas can the senior technician discuss or demonstrate that can prevent medication errors?

a. Discuss experiences the senior technician has had with making and preventing medication errors.

b. Demonstrate the use of the credit card verification machine.

c. Demonstrate how to fill medication orders and talk on the telephone at the same time.

d. Both a and c

32. A technician compounding an IV preparation of calcium gluconate and 5% Dextrose in Water (D5W) notices the calcium gluconate injection looks slightly cloudy before preparing the bag. What should the technician do to prevent a medication error?

a. Place the calcium gluconate vials in the refrigerator to see if the cloudiness disappears in a few minutes.

b. Place that vial of calcium gluconate back on the shelf and use another vial that looks clear.

c. Place all the calcium gluconate vials in the "shaker," the machine that helps reconstituted medications dissolve more quickly before preparation.

d. Inform the pharmacist that the calcium

Self-Assessment Questions

gluconate vials look cloudy and inspect all the calcium gluconate vials in stock.

e. Discard the vials of calcium gluconate that look cloudy.

33. The background music in the pharmacy is too loud where two technicians and a pharmacist are working. The first technician likes to work to loud music because he says it makes his job more fun. The second technician is having trouble hearing the phone ring. The second technician is also having trouble concentrating on his work and is worried about making a medication error because he cannot concentrate. What should the second technician do?

a. Try harder to concentrate with the music on and tell the callers on the phone to speak louder so he can hear them.

b. Tactfully ask the first technician and the pharmacist if he can turn the radio volume lower.

c. Remind himself to bring ear plugs to the pharmacy next time he is scheduled to work.

d. Wear a headset radio in the pharmacy and tell the first technician he has to answer the phone because he's the only one who can hear it ring.

34. Nancy Andrews, a pharmacy technician, notices that the nifedipine capsules in the automated tablet and capsule machine (ATC Machine®) are almost gone. She also notices that there are no more nifedipine capsules in the pharmacy to restock the machine. What is the next action she can take to reduce the chance of a medication error?

a. Inform the technician on the next shift that the nifedipine capsules are almost gone.

b. Remind herself to order nifedipine capsules the next time she is scheduled to work.

c. Inform the pharmacist that the pharmacy is almost out of nifedipine capsules.

d. Determine the immediate needs of the patients and inform the purchasing personnel of the situation.

35. Roger Young, a pharmacy technician at Hometown Pharmacy, has the flu and has been taking antihistamines to dry his runny nose. He chose to work his scheduled shift because he knows

how busy the pharmacy has been this week. However, he feels terrible and the antihistamine is making him sleepy. Roger is trying to fill prescriptions accurately, but his eyes are watery and he is having trouble reading. What should Roger do to prevent medication errors from occurring?

a. Drink a few cups of coffee to wake up.

b. Ask the pharmacist if he can go home because he is ill.

c. Drink lots of water and have chicken soup for lunch.

d. Ask the patients to read their prescriptions to him.

36. Match the medications in the first column that are commonly mistaken with the ones in the second column:

Amoxicillin 250 mg capsule	Percodan® tablet
Hydroxyzine 25 mg tablet	Digitoxin 0.1 mg capsule
Potassium Chloride 20 mEq injection	Quinidine 200 mg tablet
Desipramine 25 mg tablet Ampicillin	Lidocaine 1 gm prefilled syringe
Digoxin 0.125 mg tablet	Ampicillin 250 mg capsule
Quinine 200 mg capsule	Dimenhydrinate 50 mg capsule
Epinephrine 1:1,000 injection	Hydralazine 25 mg tablet
Percocet® tablet	Furosemide 20 mg injection
Diphenhydramine 50 mg capsule	Imipramine 25 mg tablet
Lidocaine 100 mg prefilled syringe	Epinephrine 1:10,000 injection

37. The pharmacy receives a prescription for hydrocortisone 2.5% cream. The technician notices the pharmacy is out of stock in that item. The pharmacy can substitute hydrocortisone 2.5% ointment without calling the doctor.
True or False

38. A nurse discovers the continuous infusion being administered to Mr. Williams contains potassium chloride 40 mEq. Because of Mr. Williams' kidney problems, the continuous infusion prescribed for him was supposed to be without potassium chloride. After the nurse discontinues the incorrect

continuous infusion and hangs the ordered continuous infusion, the nurse is required to call the physician.
True or False

39. A pharmacy technician notices that two different-looking tablets are mixed together in the ciprofloxacin 500 mg tablet bin in the automatic tablet and capsule machine (ATC-212,® an automated dispensing device). The filling log indicates that the machine was refilled the day before, and the lot number is significantly different than the previous refill log entries. What should the technician do?
   a. Remove the different-looking tablets and discard them.
   b. Nothing; assume the manufacturer has changed the look of the tablets.
   c. Inform the pharmacist of the situation immediately.
   d. Nothing; the personnel who refilled the machine rarely make mistakes.

40. A pharmacy technician supervisor notices several technicians making the same calculation error. In the next technician staff meeting, the supervisor discusses the errors with the group without mentioning who made the mistakes. The supervisor also demonstrates how to perform the calculation correctly. This practice can help prevent medication errors.
True or False

41. The purpose of a national medication error reporting program is to share experiences among health care personnel so patient safety can be improved. It also can contribute to educational efforts to prevent future medication errors.
True or False

42. Name at least five departments or members of a quality assurance committee that are responsible for reviewing reports of medication errors.

43. Name three ways a pharmacy can educate the staff about actual medication errors on a continuous basis.

44. Technicians and pharmacists may be held legally responsible for a medication error that causes harm to a patient.
True or False

Self-Assessment Answers

1. False. A medication error may occur any time during the medication use process—prescribing, transcription, dispensing, administration (patient compliance)—and may be made by personnel other than pharmacists or pharmacy technicians.

2. d. Orally transmitted orders can easily be misunderstood, especially with the number of sound-alike drugs names on the market. In this case, the order was orally communicated twice—from the physician to the nurse and then again to the pharmacist.

3. a. Undiluted potassium chloride injection should never be injected directly into a patient's vein because of the potential for an irregular heartbeat and possibly death. The USP implemented this labeling requirement in response to the many potassium chloride injection errors reported.

4. d. All the changes may decrease the potential for a medication error. The hood would prevent direct IV injection of a dangerous concentration or dose and remind health care personnel that the drug must be diluted prior to injection. Changing a drug name to one that is distinctly different from others would decrease the chance of a sound-alike or look-alike error. Ancillary information on a drug label, such as a manufacturer logo, should be small enough that it does not distract from critical information (drug name, strength, concentration, route, etc.).

5. d. Outcomes of errors depend on many factors. Some patients may be more prone to ill effects because of their overall health, age, weight, or underlying diseases. Consequences may result from taking the wrong drug (low blood sugar) and from not taking the correct medication (increased anxiety due to not taking diazepam). Some patients may not experience any adverse effect from the incorrect medication.

6. a. Patients have a responsibility in the medication use process to take their medication as instructed. Not taking the entire prescription could have led to inadequate treatment, with symptoms reappearing a short time later. The newer, more costly agent may have been prescribed because the physician was not aware that Ms. Smith stopped taking her amoxicillin after 3 days. This may have led the physician to believe that amoxicillin was ineffective and an alternate agent was required. It is assumed that the pharmacist counseled Ms. Smith adequately when the amoxicillin was dispensed.

7. c. Technicians should not feel intimidated about questioning a pharmacist about orders. Pharmacists make errors just like everyone else. Remember to be tactful when posing the question.

8. b. The error was made because Levoxyl® (levothyroxine) was sloppily written by the prescriber and misread as Lanoxin® (digoxin).

9. c. An omission error occurred because the 0900 dose was not administered until the next scheduled dose was due. The patient would likely receive only two doses that day instead of three.

10. e. Improper dose error is the best classification for this error. The patient would have received 40 mg instead of the 10 mg prescribed. The 40 mg/ml gentamicin could have been used to prepare the IVPB accurately; however, by using 0.25 ml instead of 1 ml this could be classified as a calculation error.

11. a. Failure to rotate stock may result in drugs with longer expiration dates being used first. Older drugs on the back of the shelf may expire before being used.

12. d. All of the answers describe a problem in the preparation of a drug prior to administration.

13. False. Number of years of pharmacy experience does not correlate with frequency of calculation errors.

14. d. All examples may lead to calculation errors.

15. a. ".4 g" could be interpreted as 4 g and would best be written as 0.4 g or 400 mg. Both c and d would be best written as "4 units." Abbreviations should be avoided whenever possible because the "U" in "4U" could be read as "40." Trailing zeros after the decimal point should be avoided for the same reason.

16. False. Many times authors make up abbreviations for disease states or drug names/combinations to avoid having to write out lengthy terms numerous times. This practice is acceptable when writing an article for publica-

tion provided the full term is spelled out the first time the abbreviation is used. It is not an acceptable practice for writing medication orders or prescription labels.

17. "Heparin 5000 units" or "5000 units Heparin" would both be acceptable—remember to write legibly!

18. 1. use of "dig" as an abbreviation for digoxin
2. "QD" could be interpreted as QID, OD, or QOD and should, therefore, be written out as "daily."
3. "1 tab" is not appropriate because digoxin is available in two strengths.
4. sloppy handwriting

19. 1. The drug names are similar.
2. More than one order is being prepared at the same time.
3. The patients' names are similar.
4. It is a rushed work environment.

20. 1. Make the manufacturer name/logo less prominent (smaller).
2. Omit the trailing zero in the concentration strength.
3. Enlarge the total contents of the vial.
4. Enlarge the drug name.
5. Change the trade name to something that does not sound like erythromycin or E-Mycin.
6. Change the trade name to omit the suffix "3."
7. Use upper- and lowercase lettering for the drug name.

21. d. Matching vial cap colors with solution colors would not aid drug identification. Color-coding unique to a manufacturer would be confusing, as manufacturers may change with each new drug purchasing contract. Technicians should always read the drug product label three times.

22. b. Technicians have a responsibility to learn continuously about new drugs and therapies.

23. b. There is no way to account for errors that are not detected. Other reasons might be that errors that are corrected before the drug is administered to the patient are frequently not reported, and health care personnel are afraid to report errors.

24. c. Costs of treating adverse events caused by medication errors, out-of-court settle-

ments, and legal fees add up to billions of dollars annually.

25. False. Omission errors can be just as dangerous as those that result in too high a dose being given or taken, because the medical treatment for which the drug is prescribed has been withheld.

26. b. Medications with the same generic name but different strengths should be stored in separate bins next to each other on the shelf. There is an increased chance of error when different strengths are stored together in the same bin.

27. c. Hard-to-read medication labels may contribute to a medication error. The technician should try to change the printer ribbon and reprint the label first. Printer ribbons should be routinely changed as established by company/department policies and procedures. If this is not possible, the technician (with the pharmacist's approval) should type or legibly write the label in a manner that the patient can clearly understand.

28. True. Anonymous self-reporting may be used in some institutions.

29. b. The technician should question the pharmacist about the duplicate orders. One order may have been for another patient, or an order to discontinue the continuous infusion may have been overlooked.

30. d. The second technician should tactfully point out the error to the first technician and allow the first technician to correct it. This gives the first technician a chance to learn from the mistake and may prevent similar mistakes in the future. Checking the stock bin can also prevent future mistakes.

31. a. Generally, discussing previous medication errors and error correction from a senior technician's experience can help teach the new technician about medication errors. Answer c is wrong because it is important to concentrate on correctly filling medication orders without doing two things at once. Performing one task at a time can reduce the chance of medication errors.

32. d. The technician has a responsibility to be observant and inform the pharmacist about any potential medication errors. The technician should compound this IV admixture only

Self-Assessment Answers

if the calcium gluconate looks clear. The technician also has the responsibility to alert appropriate personnel so that all calcium gluconate vials in the pharmacy can be inspected for the cloudy appearance.

33. b. The work environment needs to be conducive to concentrating on the duties of the position. If the music in the pharmacy is preventing the second technician from performing his duties, he should speak up tactfully and take action to correct the situation. This can prevent medication errors by improving his ability to concentrate, hear the telephone ring, and hear the callers on the phone.

34. d. The technician has the responsibility to make sure the pharmacy has enough nifedipine capsules to prevent patients from missing their scheduled doses. If the pharmacy runs out of a medication, an error of omission may occur.

35. b. Roger should ask the pharmacist if he can go home because he is not feeling well. If Roger cannot concentrate on his work and is having difficulty reading, he is more likely to make a medication error.

36. Amoxicillin—Ampicillin
Hydroxyzine—Hydralazine
Potassium Chloride—Furosemide
Desipramine—Imipramine
Digoxin—Digitoxin
Quinine—Quinidine
Epinephrine—Epinephrine
Percocet—Percodan
Diphenhydramine—Dimenhydrinate
Lidocaine—Lidocaine

37. False. The physician must be contacted, and the prescription would need to be changed with physician approval before the ointment can be dispensed. Dispensing a cream instead of an ointment, or vice versa, is a common mistake. In many cases, the packaging only differs by only one word (ointment or cream). Most pharmacies store the ointment separately from the cream in an effort to prevent mistakes.

38. True. The nurse must immediately contact the physician and inform the physician about the medication error. The physician will determine if further action is needed.

39. c. Inform the pharmacist of the situation immediately. The pharmacist can help investigate and provide direction according to established policies and procedures.

40. True. This practice can educate the staff about the correct way to make the calculation and prevent future medication errors.

41. True. The United States Pharmacopeial Convention, Inc. (USP) Medication Errors Reporting Program is an example of a national program.

42. The committee should have representatives from pharmacy, medicine, nursing, risk management, quality assurance, staff education, and legal counsel.

43. The pharmacy can educate staff about actual medication errors with periodic newsletters, with educational programs, and by reviewing medication errors reports at staff meetings.

44. True. Technicians and pharmacists both contribute to the safe use of medications by the public. If their actions result in patient harm, they may be held legally liable for their actions, along with the institution and others involved.

Purchasing and Inventory Control

JERROD MILTON

An effective purchasing and inventory control system requires the understanding and active participation of all pharmacy staff; however, generally, certain staff are responsible for managing the pharmacy inventory and purchasing activities. As the primary handler of medication in the pharmacy medication preparation system, the pharmacy technician's performance is critical to the success of the purchasing and inventory control measures.

This chapter describes the basic principles of pharmaceutical purchasing and inventory control. It applies to all types of pharmacy settings, including decentralized, centralized, home infusion, and ambulatory care pharmacy operations.

For technicians interested in considering a specialized position within purchasing and inventory control, or for readers desiring more in-depth study, a reading list is included in the Recommended Reading section of this chapter.

The Formulary System

Most hospitals and health care systems develop a list of medications that may be prescribed for patients in the institution or health care system. This list is usually called a *formulary* and serves as the cornerstone of the purchasing and inventory control system. The formulary is developed and maintained by a committee of medical and allied health staff called the Pharmacy and Therapeutics (P&T) committee. This group generally comprises physicians, pharmacists, nurses, and administrators, although other disciplines may be present, including dieticians, risk managers, and case managers. They collaborate to ensure that the safest, most efficacious, and least costly medications are included on the formulary. The products on the hospital formulary dictate what the hospital pharmacy should keep in inventory. Third-party prescription drug benefit providers also will establish plan-specific formularies for their ambulatory patients. Ambulatory (retail) pharmacy staff frequently encounter insurance plan–specific drug formularies in serving their patients and adjust their inven-

Learning Objectives

After completing this chapter, the technician should be able to

1. Demonstrate an understanding of the formulary system and its application in a purchasing and inventory system.

2. Apply the proper principles and processes when receiving and storing pharmaceuticals.

3. Identify key techniques for reviewing packaging, labeling, and storage considerations when handling pharmaceutical products.

4. Demonstrate both an understanding and the application of appropriate processes for maintaining and managing a pharmaceutical inventory.

5. Complete the appropriate processes in the handling of pharmaceutical recalls and the disposal of pharmaceutical products.

6. Execute lending and borrowing pharmaceutical transactions between pharmacies.

7. Demonstrate an understanding of pharmaceutical products that require special handling within the purchasing and inventory system.

tory accordingly. Most retail pharmacies do not rigidly restrict items in their inventory, because in this setting, inventories are largely dependent on the dynamic needs of their patient population and, to some degree, their patients' respective insurance plans. Therefore, the concept of formulary management differs greatly depending on the perspective taken (e.g., that of the hospital compared with that of the retail pharmacy).

The hospital formulary usually is available in print form and may also be maintained in an on-line format. The formulary is produced exclusively for all health practitioners involved in prescribing, dispensing, and monitoring medications, and this tool is formatted generally to inform users of product availability, the appropriate therapeutic uses, and recommended dosing of medications. Most formularies are organized alphabetically by the generic drug's name, which is typically cross-referenced with the trade name products. In most cases, the drug storage areas in the pharmacy are arranged alphabetically by either the generic or trade name of the drug. Therefore, the formulary can help the pharmacy technician determine if a product is stocked in the pharmacy and where it would be.

Pharmacy technicians must learn how the formulary is updated and how and when changes in the formulary are communicated to the staff. Drugs are added and deleted from the formulary on a regular basis, but the frequency with which drugs are added or deleted varies among organizations. Formularies typically are updated every 12 to 18 months. Loose-leaf formularies and those maintained on-line can be updated continuously in a more timely manner, whereas bound formulary handbooks rely on supplementary updates or publication of serial editions.

Other important information that may be available in the formulary, specified under each listing, is the dosage form, strength, and concentration; package size(s); common side effects; and administration instructions. Some institutions also indicate the actual or relative cost of a given item. When selecting a drug product from inventory, the technician must consider all product characteristics, such as name, dosage form, strength, concentration, and package size (see **Figure 16-1**). Detailed review and consideration of each listing helps minimize errors in product selection.

Ordering Pharmaceuticals

Some pharmacies employ a dedicated purchasing agent to manage the procurement and inventory of pharmaceuticals; others employ a more general approach,

whereby a variety of staff are involved in ordering pharmaceuticals. The state-of-the-art practice involves the use of computer and Internet technology to manage the process of purchasing and receiving pharmaceuticals from a drug wholesaler. This technology includes using bar codes and hand-held computer devices for on-line procurement and purchase order generation and for electronic receiving processes. Using computer technology for these purposes has many benefits, including up-to-the-minute product availability information, comprehensive reporting capabilities, accuracy, and efficiency. It also encourages compliance with various pharmaceutical purchasing contracts.

Receiving and Storing Pharmaceuticals

One of the most useful experiences for a new pharmacy technician is to see the pharmacy department receive pharmaceuticals. This experience is useful for a number of reasons: (1) It helps the pharmacy technician become familiar with the various processes involved with the ordering and receiving of pharmaceuticals, (2) it may help the technician become familiar with formulary items, (3) it may demonstrate the system used to ensure that only formulary items are put into inventory, and (4) it helps familiarize the technician with the various locations in which drugs are stored.

Receiving is one of the most important parts of the pharmacy operation. A poorly organized and executed receiving system can put patients at risk and elevate health care costs. For example, if the wrong concentra-

---

CEFTAZIDIME[1]   8:12.06[2]
(Antibiotic)[3] (Fortaz®)[4]

Note: **This product is restricted to Pulmonary Medicine, Hematology/Oncology or Infectious Disease Service Approval.[5]**

DOSAGE[6]

Neonates:
   Postnatal age less than 7 days: 100 mg/kg divided q 12h
   Postnatal age greater than 7 days:
      Less than 1200 g: 100 mg/kg per day divided q 12h
      Greater than 1200 g: 150 mg/kg per day divided q 8h

Infants & children 1 month to 12 yr.: 100–150 mg/kg per day divided every 8 hours; Maximum = 6 g/day

Adjust dosage with creatinine clearance

INJECTION, 500 mg, 1 g & 2 g vials[7]

Formulary book listings usually include: [1] generic name, [2] numeric cross reference to the American Hospital Formulary Service, [3] class of drug, [4] proprietary/trade name, [5] restricted uses within the institution, [6] dosing information, and [7] dosage form and package sizes

Figure 16-1. Formulary listing.

tion of a product were received in error, it could lead to a dosing error or a delay in therapy. Misplaced products or out-of-stock products also jeopardize patient care as well as the efficiency of the department—both are undesirable and costly outcomes. To avoid these unfavorable outcomes, pharmacy technicians should become familiar with the process for receiving and storing pharmaceuticals.

The Receiving Process

Some pharmacies create processes whereby, as much as possible, the person receiving pharmaceuticals is different from the person ordering them. This process is especially important for controlled substances because it effectively establishes a check in the system to minimize potential drug-diversion opportunities.

In a reliable and efficient receiving system, the receiving personnel verify that the shipment is complete and intact (i.e., they check for missing or damaged items) before putting items into circulation or inventory. The receiving process begins with the verification of the boxes containing pharmaceuticals delivered by the shipper. The person receiving the shipment begins the process by verifying that the name and address on the boxes is correct and that the number of boxes matches the shipping manifest. Many drug wholesalers use rigid plastic crates because they protect the contents of each shipment better than foam or cardboard boxes. These crates are also environmentally friendly because they are returned to the wholesaler for cleaning and reuse. Regardless, each box should be inspected for gross damage.

Products with a cold storage requirement (i.e., refrigeration or freezing) should be processed first. The shipper is responsible for taking measures to ensure the cold storage environment is maintained during the shipment process and will generally package these items in a shippable foam cooler that includes frozen cold packs to keep products at the correct storage temperature during shipment.

Receiving personnel play a critical role in protecting the pharmacy from financial responsibility for products damaged in shipment, products not ordered, and products not received. Any obvious damage or other discrepancies with the shipment, such as a breach in the cold storage environment or an incorrect product, should be noted on the shipping manifest, and, if warranted, that part of the shipment should be refused. Ideally, identifying gross shipment damage or incorrect box-counts should be performed in the presence of the delivery person and should be well documented when signing for the order. Other problems identified after delivery personnel have left, such as mispicks, product dating, or internally damaged goods, must be resolved according to the vendor's policies. Most vendors have specific procedures to follow in reporting and resolving these sorts of discrepancies.

The next step of the receiving process entails checking the newly delivered products against the receiving copy of the purchase order. This generally occurs after the delivery person has left. A purchase order, created when the order is placed, is a complete list of the items that were ordered. Traditionally, a purchase order will be executed in multiple copies, including an original file copy, a copy used in the receiving process, and a copy for the supplier (see **Figure 16-2**).

The person responsible for checking products into inventory uses the receiving copy. This ensures that the products ordered have been received. The name, brand, dosage form, size of the package, concentration strength, and quantity of product must match the purchase order. Once the accuracy of the shipment is confirmed, the purchase order copy is generally signed and dated by the person receiving the shipment (Figure 16-2). At this point, the product's expiration date should be checked to ensure that it meets the department's minimum expiration date requirement. Frequently, departments will require that products received have a minimum shelf life of 6 months remaining before they expire. It is noteworthy to mention that on occasion, the manufacturer/wholesaler inadvertently may ship an excess quantity of an ordered product to the pharmacy. The ethical response is to notify the manufacturer or wholesaler of this situation immediately and subsequently arrange for the return of any excess quantity.

Controlled substances require additional processing on receipt. Regulations specific to Schedule II controlled substances require Drug Enforcement Administration (DEA) form 222 to be completed on receipt of these products and filed separately with a copy of the invoice and packing slip accompanying each shipment. If a pharmacist or pharmacy technician other than the receiving technician removes a product from a shipment before it has been properly received and cannot locate the receiving copy of the purchase order, then a written record of receipt should be created. This is done by listing the product, dosage form, concentration/strength, package size, and quantity on a blank

Department of Pharmacy Services
Community Hospital
1 Valley Road
Suburbia, MD 20777
(333) 555-1010

Purchase Order
No. 0849
THIS NUMBER MUST
APPEAR ON ALL INVOICES,
PACKING SLIPS, BILLS,
PACKAGES AND CARTONS

Vendor: Pharmaceutical Labs
185 Commerce Ave.
Ft. Washington, PA
1-800-555-3753
Acc# 123-12345

BY_____DIRECTOR
PHARMACY SERVICES/DESIGNEE

ORDER DATE	FOB			DATE REQUIRED IN HOSPITAL	TERMS	DEPARTMENT	SHIP VIA
4/1/97	☐ HOSPITAL		☐ SHIPPING POINT	ASAP	N/A	Pharmacy	Standard

QUANTITY RECEIVED	ORDERED	DESCRIPTION	UNIT PRICE	AMOUNT
4	5	Orimune 50 × 1	$450.00	$2,250.00
50	50	Haemophilus B Vaccine Via 4s	$ 52.92	
13	12	Piperacillin 40 g Vial each	$110.00	$2,646.00
30	30	DPT Vaccine Vial 7.5 ml each	$ 56.50	
				$1,320.00
				$1,695.00

Quantity received as indicated / one vial
of piperacillin broken in shipment.

Joe Johnson, Pharmacy Technician   4/15/97

1. Goods not in accordance with specifications will be rejected and held at vendor's risk awaiting disposal. Vendor must pay transportation both ways on all rejected material.
2. The right is reserved to cancel all or part of this order if not delivered within the time specified.
3. No price change allowed unless authorized by this office.
4. Packing slips must accompany all shipments.
5. All shipments must be prepaid.
6. Equipment supplied under this purchase order must meet all applicable O.S.H.A.. Standards.

The quantity received is recorded in the "received" column by the person receiving the order. Damaged merchandise is noted on the purchase order, and the receiver signs and dates the receipt. This information enables the purchasing agent to confirm back orders, address mechanisms for retaining or returning overages, and determine financial accountability for damaged merchandise.

Figure 16-2. Documenting receipt on a purchase order.

piece of paper (see **Figure 16-3**) or the supplier's packing slip/invoice and checking off the line item received (see **Figure 16-4**). In both cases, the name of the person receiving the product should be included, and the document should be given to the receiving technician to avoid confusion and an unnecessary call to the wholesaler or manufacturer.

The Storing Process

Once the product has been received properly, it must be stored properly. Depending on the size and type of the pharmacy operation, the product may be placed in a bulk, central storage area or into the active dispensing areas of the pharmacy. In any case, the expiration date of the product should be compared with the products currently in stock. Products already in stock that have expired should be removed. Products that will expire in the near future should be highlighted and placed in the front of the shelf or bin. This is a common practice known as *stock rotation*. The newly acquired products will generally have longer shelf lives and should be placed behind packages that will expire before them. Stock rotation is an important inventory management principle that encourages the use of products before they expire and helps prevent the use of expired products and waste. **Table 16-1** identifies the optimum storage temperatures and humidity.

Product Handling Considerations

Pharmacy technicians usually spend more time handling and preparing medications than do pharmacists. This presents pharmacy technicians with the critical responsibility of assessing and evaluating each product from both a content and a labeling standpoint. It also provides the technician with an opportunity to confirm that the receiving process was performed properly.

Just as checking the product label carefully at the time a prescription or medication order is filled is important, taking the same care when receiving pharmaceuticals and accurately placing them in their storage location is essential. The pharmacy technician should read product packaging carefully, rather than rely on the general appearance of the product (e.g., packaging type, size or shape, color, logo), because a product's appearance may change frequently and may be similar to other products. Technicians play a vital role in minimizing dispensing errors that may occur because of human fallibility. They are generally the first in a series of checks involved in an accurate dispensing process.

TABLE 16-1. DEFINED STORAGE TEMPERATURES AND HUMIDITY[†]		
Freezer	−25º to -10º C	−13º to 14º F
Cold (Refrigerated)	2º to 8º C	36º to 46º F
Cool	8º to 15º C	46º to 59º F
Room Temperature	The temperature prevailing in a working area.	
Controlled Room Temperature	20º to 25 C	68º to 77º F
Warm	30º to 40º C	86º to 104º F
Excessive Heat	Any temperature above 40º C (104º F)	
Dry Place	A place that does not exceed 40 percent average relative humidity at controlled room temperature or the equivalent water vapor pressure at other temperatures. Storage in a container validated to protect the article from moisture vapor, including storage in bulk, is considered a dry place.	

† United States Pharmacopeia 26/The National Formulary 21, pp. 9–10; 2003. United States Pharmacopeial Convention, Inc., Rockville, MD.

Invoice

Shipper	Buyer
Pharmaceutical Labs	Community Hospital
185 Commerce Avenue	1 Valley Road
Ft. Washington, PA	Suburbia, MD 20777

Invoice # 12346
Invoice Date 4/01/97

Quantity	Product #	Product Description	Unit Price	Amount
5 4 rec.	6190	Orimune 50 × 1	$450.00	$2,250.00
4 ✓	7183	Haemophilus B Vaccine	$ 52.92	$2,646.00
13 12 rec.	4391	Piperacillin 40 g Vial	$110.00	$1,320.00
30 ✓	2727	DPT Vaccine 7.5ml Vial	$ 56.50	$1,695.00

Quantity received as indicated
one vial Piperacillin broken in shipment.

Received 4 × 50's   Orimune
50   Haemophilus B Vaccine
13   Piperacillin 40 gm vial
30   DTP Vaccine 7.5 ml
4/15/97
Joe Johnson
Pharmacy Technician

Received to stock
4 × 50's Oral Polio Vaccine, 0.5 ml
50 × 4's Haemophilus B vaccine vials
13 each Piperacillin 40 gm vials
30 DTP vials, 7.5 ml
4/15/97
One vial Piperacillin broken in shipment.
Joe Johnson
Pharmacy Technician

Figure 16-3. Receipt of pharmaceutical on blank piece of paper.

Figure 16-4. Receipt of pharmaceutical on packing slip/invoice.

When performing purchasing or inventory management roles, the technician must pay close attention to the product's expiration date. For liquids or injectable products, the color and clarity of the items should also be checked for consistency with the product standard. Products with visible particles, an unusual appearance, or a broken seal should be reported to the pharmacist.

Because pharmacy technicians handle so many products each day, they are in a perfect position to identify packaging and storage issues that could lead to errors. The technician should pay close attention to these three main issues:

1. *Look-Alike/Sound-Alike Products.* Stocking products of similar color, shape, and size could result in error if someone fails to read the label carefully. All staff members should be alerted to look-alike or sound-alike products (see **Figure 16-5**).

2. *Misleading Labels.* Sometimes the company name or logo is emphasized on the label instead of the drug name, concentration, or strength (see **Figure 16-6**).

3. *Product Storage.* Storing products that are similar in appearance adjacent to one another can result in error if someone fails to read the label (see **Figure 16-7**).

Alerting other staff members to products that fall into one of these categories is essential. Some pharmacies routinely discuss product-handling considerations at staff meetings or in departmental newsletters—dispensing errors may be averted by simply relocating a look-alike/sound-alike product or by placing warning notes (i.e., auxiliary labeling or highlights) on the shelf or directly on the product itself. Pharmacy technicians should also discuss their concerns with coworkers and advocate changes to products with poor labeling.

Maintaining and Managing Inventory

An inventory management system is an organized approach designed to maintain just the right amount of pharmaceutical products in the pharmacy at all times. A variety of inventory management systems are used, ranging from simple to complex. They include the order book, the minimum/maximum (par) level, the Pareto (ABC) Analysis, the economic order quantity (EOQ), and, finally, the fully automated, computerized system.

Economic Models

The Pareto ABC analysis is also known as the 80/20 rule, and it essentially groups inventory products by aggregate value and volume of use into three groupings (A, B, and C). This analysis is useful in determining where inventory control efforts are best directed. For example, group A may include 10 percent of all items that make up 70 percent of the inventory cost. Tight control over these items would be sensible. Group B may include 20 percent of items and 15 percent of the

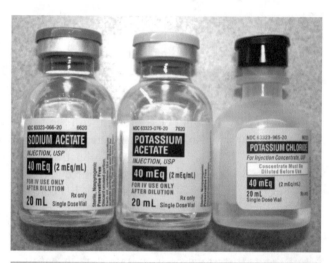

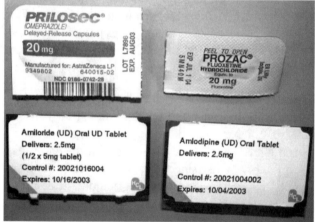

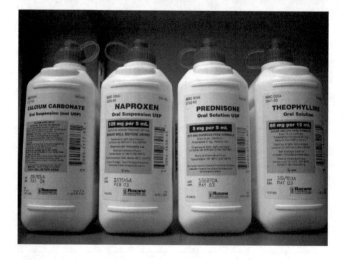

Figure 16-5. Look-alike/sound-alike products.

inventory cost. An automatic order cycle might be useful here based on well-established par levels. Group C may include 70 percent of items and 10 percent of the inventory cost. Less aggressive monitoring of these items may be justifiable.

The EOQ is a model for calculating inventory order quantities and is also known as the Minimum Cost Quantity approach. In essence, this approach is an accounting formula used to determine the point at which the combination of order costs and inventory holding costs are minimized. One variation of the EOQ formula is as follows:

$$EOQ = \sqrt{\frac{2(\text{Annual usage in units})(\text{Order cost})}{(\text{Annual carrying cost per unit})}}$$

EOQ relies heavily on the accuracy of various data inputs, such as annual product usage, fixed costs associated with each order (including processing the purchase order, receiving, inspection, processing the invoice, vendor payment, and inbound freight costs), and the annual cost per average on-hand inventory unit. If calculated accurately, it results in the most cost-efficient order quantity. Economists would argue that anytime one has repetitive purchasing tasks, EOQ should be considered. Some organizations may find EOQ useful in aspects of their operation; applying it universally is relatively difficult in pharmacy practice because of the wide variability of the individual patient's pharmaceutical needs. Therefore, some pharmacies may find it useful to use a combination of the systems mentioned here.

Automation

The ideal system for inventory management is an automated or computerized system that supports a *just-in-time* product inventory. *Just-in-time* inventory management is a philosophy that simply means products are ordered and delivered at just the right time—when they are needed for patient care—with a goal of minimizing wasted steps, labor, and cost. Pharmaceuticals are neither overstocked nor understocked. In pharmacy, this business philosophy couples responsible financial management of pharmaceutical purchasing with the clinical aspects of patient care. A related business philosophy is known as *maximizing inventory turns,* which means that, because a product should not sit on the shelf, unused for long periods of time, specific drug inventory ideally is purchased and used many times throughout the course of a year. A simple means of calculating inventory turns in a given period is to divide the total purchases in that period by the value of physical inventory taken at one point in time. For example, if total pharmaceutical purchases for fiscal year (FY) 2004 were $10,243,590, and the physical inventory value on 12/31/2003 was $521,550, then the calculated inventory turns for FY2004 would be 19.6 times ($10,243,590/$521,550 = 19.6). This method assumes a relatively constant volume of pharmaceutical purchases and constant residual inventory over time. The economic principle is simple: One does not want to buy pharmaceuticals that won't be used in a timely manner. Minimizing inventory carrying costs (or holding costs) is an important aspect of sound business administration. Carrying cost can be defined as all costs associated with inventory investment and storage costs, which might include interest, insurance, taxes, and storage expenses.

Although automated inventory management modalities are available, they are not the mainstay in practice today. Generally, today, a manual inventory management system is employed. Manual systems require the active oversight of pharmacy technicians and are usually based on a minimum/maximum, or par-level, system. Staff may create a pharmaceutical

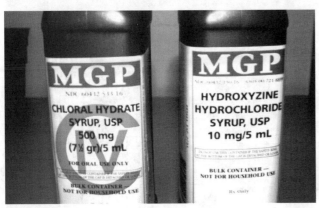

Figure 16-6. Product labeling—emphasis on manufacturer name.

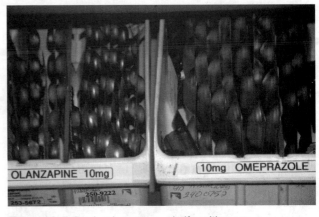

Figure 16-7. Product inventory—shelf position.

order using a hand-held bar-code scanning device or may enter product stock numbers directly into a personal computer. Manual systems typically involve a minimum/maximum, or par-level, shelf-sticker that corresponds to each product. The minimum and maximum inventory level is written on this label, and the information is used as a relative guide for pharmacy staff involved in purchasing. To that end, staff strive to maintain pharmaceutical inventories within the minimum to maximum range to avoid running short on a product or overstocking. Running short on a product may affect patient care, and overstocking adds unnecessary expense to the organization. This system requires pharmacy staff to routinely scan inventory levels and place orders accordingly. With either the electronic or manual system, pharmacy staff should realize that the diversity of their patients' specific needs may require modification in a particular product's par-level. In the fully computerized inventory system, each dispensing transaction is subtracted from the perpetual inventory log that is maintained electronically in the computer; conversely, all products received are added to the inventory log. When the quantity of a pharmaceutical product in stock reaches a predetermined point (often called *par* or *par-level*), a purchase order is automatically generated to order more of the product. The system does not depend on any one employee to monitor the inventory or to reorder pharmaceuticals. The technology is available to have a computerized inventory in most pharmacies, but interfacing a computerized inventory system with existing pharmacy computer systems designed for dispensing and patient management systems is often difficult. In addition, other variables, such as product availability, contract changes, and changing use patterns (either up or down), make relying on the fully computerized model challenging. Consequently, even the most sophisticated electronic or automated systems will require human oversight.

The use of automated dispensing devices in inpatient hospital nursing units, clinics, operating rooms, and emergency rooms has facilitated the use of computers for inventory management. Similar devices are evolving in retail pharmacy and hold promise for not only making the dispensing process safer and more efficient but also serving, possibly, to assist in inventory management. These devices are essentially repositories, or *pharmaceutical vending machines,* for medications that will be dispensed directly from a patient care area. A variety of manufacturers of automated dispensing devices are in the market today. The Pyxis Medstation, Meditrol, Omnicell, and SureMed are examples of products available to institutions today. These machines generally are networked via a dedicated computer file server within the facility, and they allow both unit-dose and bulk pharmaceuticals to be stocked securely on a given patient care unit location. Each unit's inventory is configurable and allows for variation and flexibility from device to device, depending on the unit's location. The machines are capable of tracking perpetual inventory at the product level. They also limit access to only authorized personnel, record the identities of those who access inventory, and record how much of a specific drug was removed for a given patient. A useful feature in many of these systems allows pharmacy personnel to automatically generate a fill-list of what needs to be replenished on the basis of a par-level system. In essence, the nursing and medical personnel who use these automated dispensing devices have a computerized inventory and billing system that the pharmacy staff manages. Medications used to restock these devices may be taken from the pharmacy's main inventory, or a separate purchase order may be executed for each device on a periodic basis.

The minimum/maximum, or par-level, inventory system relies on a predetermined order quantity and an order point. Shelf labels are placed on the storage bin or shelf to alert all staff to the minimum stock quantity (see **Figure 16-8**). The pharmacy technician should always determine if the minimum stock quantity has been reached when removing a product and inform the appropriate purchasing personnel or list the item on a designated order book as described below. An assigned staff member performs a periodic inventory of the stock to identify products that have a stock level at or below the reorder point. When the inventory is reduced to, or below, the order point, designated pharmacy personnel initiate a purchase order, or electronically transmit a purchase order, to a drug wholesaler.

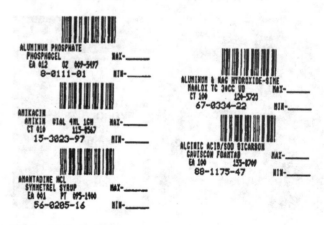

Figure 16-8. Shelf labels.

Many pharmacies will use an order book system, also called a *want list* or *want book*. When pharmacists or pharmacy technicians determine that a product should be reordered, they write the item in the order book. Although this approach is simple, it provides the least amount of organized control over inventory. Its success is highly dependent on the participation of staff. Therefore, the order book system is usually not the sole method of inventory management and is often used in conjunction with one of the other systems mentioned previously.

Regardless of the inventory system used, pharmacy technicians are vital contributors. The pharmacy technician may frequently identify changes in use or prescription patterns of pharmaceuticals. Examples might include high use of asthmatic medications (e.g., epinephrine, albuterol, or inhaled steroids) by the emergency department or various clinics, high doses of a particular antibiotic (e.g., chloramphenicol or liposomal amphotericin b) by a seriously ill patient who is likely to be hospitalized for an extended period, or high dose opioid use by one or more oncology patients. Alerting purchasing staff to orders for unusual amounts of medications helps avoid out-of-stock situations and facilitates optimal inventory management. Other, more sophisticated approaches toward inventory management include the ABC analysis and the economic order quantity, discussed above. For more detailed information on these inventory methods and to learn about inventory turnover rate calculation, see the third reference in the Recommended Reading section.

Drug Recalls

A manufacturer, on its own or at the direction of the Food and Drug Administration (FDA), will occasionally recall pharmaceuticals for such reasons as mislabeling, contamination, lack of potency, lack of adherence to the acceptable Good Manufacturing Practices, or other situations that may present a significant risk to public health. A pharmacy must have a system for rapid removal of any recalled products.

Role of the Food and Drug Administration[‡]

The FDA plays an active role in initiating the drug-recall process. It coordinates drug recall information, helps manufacturers and distributors develop specific recall plans, and performs health hazard evaluations to assess the risk facing the public by products being recalled. It also classifies recall actions in accordance with the level of risk and formulates recall strategies on the basis of the health hazard presented by the product in addition to other factors, including the extent of distribution of the

product to be recalled. It decides on the need for public warnings and assists the recalling agency with public notification about the recall as needed. The following are the top 10 reasons for drug recalls in 2002:

- Penicillin cross-contamination
- Lack of sterility assurance
- Incorrect expiration date on label
- Dissolution failure
- Expiration date out of accordance with stability data
- Mispacking (incorrect product in carton)
- Good Manufacturing Practice deviations (failure to perform or document performance of requirement)
- Foreign substance

[‡]Report to the nation—improving public health through human drugs. Center for Drug Evaluation and Research. p. 30–31; 2002.

Role of Manufacturer/Distributor

Because of their responsibility to protect the public consumer, manufacturers or distributors typically implement *voluntary recalls* when a marketed drug product needs to be removed from the market. This method of recall is more efficient and effective in ensuring timely consumer protection than an FDA-initiated court action or seizure of the product. Recall notices are sent in writing to pharmacies by the manufacturer of the product or by drug wholesalers. These notices indicate the reason for the recall, the name of the recalled product, the manufacturer, all affected lot numbers of the product, and instructions on how to return the product to the manufacturer. On receipt of the recall notice, a pharmacy staff member, usually a pharmacy technician, will check all pharmaceutical inventory stores to determine if any recalled products are in stock. If none of the recalled products are in stock, a note indicating "none in stock" is written on the recall notice and filed in a recall log to document that the recall was properly addressed. If a recalled product is in stock, all products should be gathered, packaged, and returned to the manufacturer according to the instructions on the recall notice. The package should be reviewed by the pharmacist in charge before returning it to the manufacturer. If patients have received a recalled product, the pharmacist in charge must take the recommended action. On completion of all activity regarding the product recall, a summary of actions taken should be documented on the recall letter and filed in the pharmaceutical recall log. The FDA has been known to request documentation of all recall activities to ensure compliance and, ultimately, patient safety. The technician should keep in mind that it may be necessary to order replacement stock to compensate for recalled items that were removed from stock. In some instances, the recall may encompass all products, and it will be impossible to order replacement stock. The pharmacist in charge should be notified in this case because he or she will need to decide which, if any, alternative products may be required to place into inventory as therapeutic alternatives to the out-of-stock items.

Drug Shortages

Occasionally, manufacturers will be unable to supply a pharmaceutical because of various supply and demand situations. This may involve the inability to obtain raw materials, manufacturing difficulties related to equipment failure, or simply the inability to produce sufficient quantities to stay ahead of the market demand for the pharmaceutical. Although unfortunate, drug shortages are a reality that must be dealt with to avoid compromising patient care. As with drug recalls, the pharmacist in charge should be notified so he or she can communicate drug shortages and recommend alternative therapies effectively to prescribers.

Ordering and Borrowing Pharmaceuticals

Pharmaceutical Purchasing Groups

Most health-system pharmacies are members of a group purchasing organization (GPO). Health systems and hospitals join together in a purchasing group to leverage buying power collectively and take advantage of any lower prices manufacturers offer to large groups that can guarantee a significant volume of orders over long periods of time (typically 1 to 2 years). Retail, chain pharmacies also are able to negotiate better pricing based on volume. Contracts may involve sole-source or multisource products. Sole-source products are products available from only one manufacturer, whereas multisource products (frequently termed *generic* products) are available from numerous manufacturers. Sole-source products may be produced from only one manufacturer; however, the product may be included in what is known as a competitive market basket (i.e., proton-pump-inhibitors, such as omeprazole and lansoprazole), where competing brand-only products are on the market.

GPOs negotiate purchasing contracts that are mutually favorable to members of the group and to manufacturers. In addition to lower prices, pharmacies also benefit because this reduces the time staff spend establishing and managing purchasing contracts with product vendors. A GPO guarantees the price for pharmaceuticals over the established contract period, which may be 1 year or more. With the purchase price predetermined, the pharmacy can order the product directly from the manufacturer or from a wholesale supplier. Occasionally, manufacturers are unable to supply a given product that the pharmacy is buying on contract, which may require the pharmacy to buy or substitute a competing product not on contract at a higher cost. Most purchasing contracts will include language to protect the pharmacy from incurring additional expenses in the event this occurs. Generally, the manufacturer will be liable to rebate the difference in cost back to the pharmacy when this occurs. Therefore, it is important that the pharmacy technician documents any resulting off-contract purchases and shares these with the pharmacist in charge for reconciliation with the contracted product vendor.

Direct Purchasing

Direct purchasing from a manufacturer involves the execution of a purchase order from the pharmacy to the manufacturer of the drug. The advantages of direct purchasing include not having to pay handling fees to a third-party wholesaler, the ability to order on an infrequent basis (e.g., once a month), and a less demanding system for monitoring inventory. Some disadvantages include the following: a large storage capacity is needed; a large amount of cash is invested in inventory; the pharmacy's return/credit process becomes more complicated; and staff resources required in the pharmacy and accounts payable department to prepare, process, and pay purchase orders to more companies is increased. Other disadvantages have to do with the likelihood that the manufacturer's warehouse is not local in relation to the pharmacy, which creates a dependency on the shipping firms used by the manufacturers to ship products reliably. In addition, the delivery schedule is often unpredictable or not available on weekends, and there may be delays in delivery.

For most pharmacies, the disadvantages of direct ordering outweigh the advantages. As a result, most pharmacies primarily purchase through a drug wholesaler. Some drugs, however, can be purchased only directly from the manufacturers. These products generally require unique control or storage conditions.

Consequently, most pharmacies will have a combination of direct purchases from manufacturers and drug wholesalers.

Drug Wholesaler Purchasing/Prime Vendor Purchasing

Purchasing from a drug wholesaler permits the acquisition of drug products from different manufacturers through a single vendor. When a health-system pharmacy agrees to purchase most (90 to 95 percent) of its pharmaceuticals from a single wholesale company, a prime vendor arrangement is established, and, customarily, a contract between the pharmacy and the drug wholesaler is developed. Usually, wholesalers agree to deliver 95 to 98 percent of the items on schedule and offer a 24-hour/7-day-per week emergency service. They also provide the pharmacy with electronic order entry/receiving devices, a computer system for ordering, bar-coded shelf stickers, and a printer for order confirmation printouts. They may also offer a highly competitive discount (minus 1 to 2 percent) below product cost/contract pricing and competitive alternate contract pricing. Some wholesalers will offer even larger discounts to pharmacies that may prefer a prepayment arrangement. In these situations, the wholesaler monitors the aggregate purchases of the pharmacy (e.g., a rolling 3-month average) and bills the pharmacy this amount in advance (prepayment). This may be attractive to both the wholesaler and the pharmacy because it creates larger cash flow and investment capital for the wholesaler while saving the organization money on its pharmaceutical purchases.

These wholesaler services make the establishment of a prime vendor contract appealing and result in the following advantages: more timely ordering and delivery, less time spent creating purchase orders, fewer inventory carrying costs, less documentation, computer-generated lists of pharmaceuticals purchased, and overall simplification of the credit and return process. Purchasing through a prime vendor customarily allows for drugs to be received shortly before use, supporting the just-in-time ordering philosophy mentioned earlier in this chapter. Purchasing from a wholesaler is a highly efficient and cost-effective approach toward pharmaceutical purchasing and inventory management.

Borrowing Pharmaceuticals

No matter how effective a purchasing system is, there will be times when the pharmacy must borrow drugs from other pharmacies. Most pharmacies have policies and procedures addressing this situation. Borrowing or loaning drugs between pharmacies is usually restricted to emergency situations and limited to authorized staff. Borrowing is also limited to products that are commercially available, thus eliminating items such as compounded products or investigational medications. Most pharmacies have developed forms to document and track merchandise that is borrowed or loaned (see **Figure 16-9**). These forms also help staff document the details imperative to error-free transactions.

The pharmacy department's borrow and loan policies and procedures should provide detailed directions on how to borrow and loan products, which products may be borrowed or loaned, sources for the products, and reconciliation of borrow-loan transactions (the pay-back process). Securing the borrowed item may require the use of a transport or courier service or may include the use of security staff or other designated personnel. This information is vital for pharmacy technicians to understand and fulfill their responsibility when borrowing and loaning products.

Products Requiring Special Handling

Most pharmaceuticals will be handled and processed in the inventorying and purchasing systems described above, with the exception of controlled substances, investigational drugs, compounded products, repackaged drugs, and drug samples.

Controlled Substances

Controlled substances have specific ordering, receiving, storage, dispensing, inventory, record-keeping, return, waste, and disposal requirements established under the law. The *Pharmacist's Manual: An Informational Outline of the Controlled Substances Act of 1970* and the *ASHP Technical Assistance Bulletin on Institutional Use of Controlled Substances* provide detailed information on the specific handling requirements for controlled substances.

The pharmacy technician should know two principles regarding controlled substances: (1) Ordering and receiving Schedule II controlled substances requires special order forms and additional time (1 to 3

Community Pharmacy
555-3779

Borrowed From: ________________ Lent To: ________________
Drug: ________________
Amount: ________________
(# of vials, tablets, etc. and bulk or unit dose packaging)
Date: ________________ By: ________________
****
Date ordered: ________ From: ________ By: ________
Date returned: ________ By: ________
Date in Loan Book: ________ By: ________
Value: $________

Figure 16-9. Borrow/loan form.

days), and (2) these substances are inventoried and tracked continuously. This type of inventory method is referred to as a perpetual inventory process, whereby each dose or packaged unit, such as a tablet, vial, or ml of fluid volume, is accounted for at all times. In some pharmacies, pharmacy technicians work with pharmacists to manage inventory and order, dispense, store, and control narcotics and other controlled substances (see Chapter 6).

Investigational Drugs

Investigational drugs also require special ordering, inventorying, and handling procedures. Generally, the use of investigational drugs is categorized into two distinct areas: (1) in a formal protocol approved by the institution, and (2) for a single patient on a one-time basis that has been authorized by the manufacturer and the FDA. In both cases, the physician may be responsible for the ordering, and the pharmacy staff handles the inventory management of the investigational drug. Some pharmacies associated with academic affiliations or institutions conducting clinical research may have formally organized investigational drug services managed by a pharmacist principally dedicated to pharmaceutical research activities. In these cases, the investigational drug service pharmacist may be responsible for the ordering, dispensing, and inventory management of investigational drugs according to the research protocol. Pharmacy technicians often prepare or handle investigational drugs and participate in the required perpetual inventory record-keeping system. Again, pharmacy technicians must learn the department procedures for investigational drugs and be competent in the proper handling, storage, dispensing, and inventory systems involved.

Compounded Products

Compounded pharmaceuticals are another type of product handled by pharmacy personnel, and, unlike drugs ordered from an outside source, compounded products are extemporaneously prepared in the pharmacy as indicated by scientific compounding formulas. These products may include oral liquids, topical preparations, solid dosage forms, or sterile products.

The use of these products requires that prescribing patterns and expiration dates be monitored closely. Compounded products typically have short expiration dates ranging from days to months. Because pharmacy technicians likely will identify usage patterns and determine stock and product needs, procedures for monitoring patient use, product expiration dates, and additional stock needs must be well known and adhered

to by technicians to prevent stock shortages. Specific pharmacy technicians may initiate compounding activities, but this may vary according to departmental procedures (see Chapter 13).

Repackaged Pharmaceuticals

Although manufacturers supply many drugs in a prepackaged unit dose form, the pharmacy staff is responsible for packaging some products. These items are generally unit-dose tablets and capsules, unit-dose oral liquids, and some bulk packages of oral solids and liquids. Each pharmacy establishes stocking mechanisms for these products and relies on pharmacy technicians to identify and respond to production and stock needs. Generally, designated technicians coordinate repackaging activities, but some pharmacies may integrate repackaging with other pharmacy technician responsibilities. Knowledge of the department's procedures for repackaging is required to prevent disruptions in dispensing activities (see Chapter 13).

Nonformulary Items

Nonformulary items also require special handling. No matter how much planning is devoted to formulary management, some patients will still need medications not routinely stocked in the pharmacy. The pharmacist usually determines when a nonformulary medication should be ordered into stock. However, the pharmacy technician is often in the best position to monitor the supply and determine when and if additional quantities should be ordered. Nonformulary medications generally are not mixed into the shelving system of formulary products in the pharmacy; they fall outside normal inventorying mechanisms. Often, manual tracking mechanisms and computer system queries of active nonformulary orders are the two most common techniques used to monitor and order these products.

Medication Samples

The last products requiring special handling are medication samples. Traditional inventory management and handling practices do not work well with medication samples for two reasons. First, medication samples are not ordered by the pharmacy—they are usually provided to physicians on request by the drug manufacturer free of charge. This often occurs without the pharmacy's knowledge. Second, samples are not usually dispensed by the pharmacy. These factors make it difficult to know whom to contact if a medication sample is recalled and to ensure that medication samples are not sold. Because of difficulties in controlling samples, organizations may allow samples to be stored and dispensed in ambulatory clinics only after being registered with the pharmacy for tracking purposes. These difficult logistical and control factors have led many organizations to adopt policies that simply disallow medication samples altogether.

If an organization does allow samples, they will probably be stored outside the pharmacy and require that pharmacy personnel register and inspect the stock of medication samples. Pharmacy technicians are sometimes involved in inspecting medication sample storage units. These technicians are often responsible for determining if a sample is registered with the pharmacy, stored in acceptable quantities, labeled with an expiration date that has not been exceeded, and, generally, stored under acceptable conditions. The technician should review the department's policies and procedures regarding medication samples to learn the role of the pharmacy technician in this regard. Many hospitals strive to maintain compliance with the standards of the Joint Commission on Accreditation of Healthcare Organizations (JCAHO). Its standards on medication management are intended to promote consistently safe practices related to the procurement, storage, dispensing, and administration of pharmaceuticals and the use of sample drug products that fall into this standard.

Proper Disposal and Return of Pharmaceuticals

Expired Pharmaceuticals

The most common reason drugs are returned to the manufacturer is because they are expired. The process for returning drugs in the original manufacturer packaging is relatively simple and not particularly time-consuming when done routinely. Returning expired products to the manufacturer or wholesaler prevents the inadvertent use of these products while enabling the department to receive either full or partial credit for them. Some wholesalers limit credit given on returns of short-dated products. Generally, wholesalers will not give full credit on returns of products that will expire within 6 months. To return products, pharmacy personnel must complete the documentation required by the product's manufacturer or wholesaler and package the product so it can be shipped. Many wholesalers have implemented electronic documentation systems to further simplify the return process. Technicians often perform these duties under the supervision of a pharmacist. Some pharmacies contract with an outside vendor that completes the documentation and coordinates the return of these products for an agreed on fee. In that case, the pharmacy technician

need only assist the returned goods vendor with the location and packaging of expired pharmaceuticals.

Pharmaceuticals compounded or repackaged by the pharmacy department cannot be returned and, for safety reasons, must be disposed of after they have expired. Proper disposal prevents the use of subpotent products or products without guaranteed sterility. The precise procedure for disposal depends on the type and content of the product. Some products, such as expired repackaged solids, can be disposed of using the general trash removal system, whereas others, such as expired compounded cytotoxic products, must be disposed of according to hazardous waste removal procedures. Each pharmacy has detailed procedures for hazardous waste removal, and the pharmacy technician should be familiar with these procedures. Disposal of expired compounded or repackaged pharmaceuticals by the pharmacy technician should be completed under the supervision of the pharmacist.

Other products requiring disposal rather than return are chemicals used in the pharmacy laboratory. Most pharmacies will stock a supply of chemical-grade products used in extemporaneous pharmaceutical compounding. Examples of chemical products include sodium benzoate or sodium citrate (preservatives), lactose or talc (excipients), buffers, and active ingredients, such as hydrocortisone, triamcinolone, neomycin, or lidocaine powders. When such products expire, they should be disposed of in accordance with the pharmacy's hazardous waste procedures.

Expired controlled substances are disposed of uniquely. These products may not be returned to the manufacturer or wholesaler for credit. They must be destroyed, and the destruction must be documented to the satisfaction of the DEA. The DEA provides a specific form, titled "Registrant's Inventory of Drugs Surrendered" (Form 41), for recording the disposal of expired controlled substances (see **Figure 16-10**). Ideally, the actual disposal of expired controlled substances should be completed by a company sanctioned by the DEA or by a representative of the state board of pharmacy. In other cases, the DEA may allow the destruction of controlled substances by a pharmacy, provided the appropriate witness process is followed and documented. The DEA disposal of controlled substances form should be completed properly and submitted to the DEA immediately after the disposal. A copy of the record of disposal form will be signed by a DEA representative and returned to the pharmacy, where it is kept on file. Previously, the DEA allowed

U. S. Department of Justice / Drug Enforcement Administration

REGISTRANTS INVENTORY OF DRUGS SURRENDERED

PACKAGE NO.

The following schedule is an inventory of controlled substances which is hereby surrendered to you for proper disposition.

FROM: *(Include Name, Street, City, State and ZIP Code in space provided below.)*

Signature of applicant or authorized agent

Registrant's DEA Number

Registrant's Telephone Number

NOTE: CERTIFIED MAIL (Return Receipt Requested) IS REQUIRED FOR SHIPMENTS OF DRUGS VIA U.S. POSTAL SERVICE. See instructions on reverse (page 2) of form.

NAME OF DRUG OR PREPARATION	Number of Containers	CONTENTS (Number of grams, tablets, ounces or other units per container)	Controlled Substance Content, (Each Unit)	FOR DEA USE ONLY		
				DISPOSITION	QUANTITY	
Registrants will fill in Columns 1,2,3, and 4 ONLY.					GMS.	MGS.
1	2	3	4	5	6	7
1						
2						
3						
4						
5						
6						
7						
8						
9						
10						
11						
12						
13						
14						
15						
16						

FORM DEA-41 (9-01)   Previous edition dated **6-86** is usable.   *See instructions on reverse (page 2) of form.*

Figure 16-10. DEA form 41 (Registrants Inventory of Drugs Surrendered).

Source: Drug Enforcement Administration http://www. deadiversion. usdoj. gov/21cfr_reports/surrend/41/41_blank. pdf

for shipment of expired controlled substances and the completed disposal form to the regional DEA office, but this practice is no longer permitted.

The usage and disposition of investigational drugs must also be documented carefully. Expired investigational drugs should be returned to the manufacturer or sponsor of an investigational drug study according to the instructions they provide. The pharmacy technician may be responsible, under the supervision of the pharmacist, for the completion of documentation, packaging, and shipment of the expired investigational agents. Investigational drug products that expire because of product instability or sterility issues should never be discarded. These doses should be retained with the investigational drug stock and be clearly marked as expired drug products because the investigational study sponsor will need to review and account for all expired investigational drug products.

Pharmaceuticals that need to be returned because of an ordering error require authorization from the original supplier and the appropriate forms. The Prescription Drug Marketing Act mandates that pharmacies authorize and retain records of returned pharmaceuticals to prevent potential diversion of pharmaceuticals. The pharmacy technician must be familiar with pharmacy department procedures for returning medications to a supplier. Typically, a pharmacy will have a process for returning misordered medications to the prime drug wholesaler on a routine basis, which prevents the need for storage in the pharmacy of overstocked or misordered products. The pharmacy technician may be responsible for relevant documentation, filing paperwork, and packaging returned products under the supervision of the pharmacist.

Summary

The movement of pharmaceuticals into and out of the pharmacy requires an organized, systematic, and cooperative approach. The pharmacy technician plays a vital role in maintaining the functionality of these systems as the medication is ultimately used to provide pharmaceutical care. The pharmacy technician's familiarity with product conditions and uses positions him or her to identify quality and care issues that can strengthen the purchasing and inventory control system.

Recommended Reading

American Society of Hospital Pharmacists. ASHP statement on the formulary system. *Am J Hosp Pharm.* 1983; 40:1384–5.

Wetrich JG. Group purchasing: an overview. *Am J Hosp Pharm.* 1987; 44:158–92.

Bicket WJ, Gagnon JP. Purchasing and inventory control for hospital pharmacies. *Top Hosp Pharm Manage.* 1987; 7(2):59–74.

Yost RD, Flowers DM. New roles for wholesalers in hospital drug distribution. *Top Hosp Pharm Manage.* 1987; 7(2):84–90.

Roffe BD, Powell MF. Quality assurance aspects of purchasing and inventory control. *Top Hosp Pharm Manage.* 1983; 3(3):62–74.

Soares DP. Quality assurance standards for purchasing and inventory control. *Am J Hosp Pharm.* 1985; 42:610–20.

Kroll DJ. The pharmacy technician as a purchasing agent. *J Pharm Tech.* 1985; 1(1):29–31.

U.S. Department of Justice Drug Enforcement Administration. Pharmacist's manual: an informational outline of the Controlled Substances Act of 1970. 8th ed. Washington, DC: DEA. http://www. deadiversion. usdoj. gov/pubs/manuals/pharm2/2pharm_manual. pdf (accessed 2001 Mar).

American Society of Hospital Pharmacists. ASHP technical assistance bulletin on institutional use of controlled substances. *Am J Hosp Pharm.* 1987; 44:580–9.

Hughes TW. Automating the purchasing and inventory control functions. *Am J Hosp Pharm.* 1985; 42:1101–7.

American Society of Hospital Pharmacists. ASHP technical assistance bulletin on use of controlled substances in organized health-care settings. *Am J Hosp Pharm.* 1993; 50:489–501.

Self-Assessment Questions

1. Which of the following methods of maintaining a formulary is more convenient and yields the most current product information in a purchasing and inventory system?
   a. bound formulary book
   b. on-line formulary

2. The formulary contains important information to assist the pharmacy technician in which of the following areas of product information?
   a. identification of trade names of products
   b. identification of product concentration
   c. identification of package size
   d. all of the above

3. Receiving and storing pharmaceuticals is a simple process that should be reserved solely for trainees and other inexperienced staff.
   a. True
   b. False

4. When receiving a shipment of pharmaceuticals, use the packaging slip to check in the order.
   a. True
   b. False

5. Reviewing the product's expiration date is not a part of the receiving process.
   a. True
   b. False

6. When documenting the receipt of pharmaceuticals for which the purchase order or manufacturer's invoice cannot be located, which of the following should be recorded?
   a. product name and amount
   b. product name, strength, and amount
   c. date of receipt, product name, and amount
   d. date of receipt, name of receiver, product name, strength, dosage form, and amount

7. A receiving copy of a purchase order is not required to check in an order if a manufacturer's invoice is available.
   a. True
   b. False

8. Reading a pharmaceutical product label three times is a legal requirement reserved for pharmacists and is a practice pharmacy technicians are not expected to use.
   a. True
   b. False

9. Describe three product-handling issues that a pharmacy technician should monitor to maintain and improve the quality of the inventory management system.

10. A want book ordering system is necessary when a minimum/maximum level system is used in a pharmacy purchasing system.
    a. True
    b. False

11. Describe three patient care situations that might require adjustment of the pharmacy's inventory level on a short-term basis.

12. What is (are) the most important consideration(s) in processing a manufacturer's recall notice?
    a. timely response in checking the inventory
    b. timely response in removing affected products from the inventory
    c. documenting the inspection and any action required
    d. receiving proper credit from the manufacturer
    e. a, b, and c

13. Describe the primary benefits of being a member of a pharmaceutical purchasing group.

14. List two advantages of purchasing pharmaceuticals directly from the manufacturer.

15. List three disadvantages of purchasing pharmaceuticals directly from the manufacturer.

16. List four advantages of a prime vendor arrangement.

17. Effective purchasing and inventory systems make the need for a borrow and loan system unnecessary.
    a. True
    b. False

18. Schedule II medications are ordered in the same manner as all other pharmaceuticals.
    a. True
    b. False

19. Describe two situations in which investigational drugs are used in patient care, and identify who is customarily responsible for ordering investigational drug products.

20. Medication samples are routinely ordered by the pharmacy and dispensed directly to patients as ordered by the physician as a means of reducing

pharmaceutical carrying costs.
a. True
b. False

21. List the necessary data elements to credit a patient for pharmaceuticals.

22. List two situations that necessitate crediting a patient for pharmaceuticals.

23. Schedule II controlled substances that have expired cannot be returned to the manufacturer for credit.
a. True
b. False

24. Investigational drug products that have expired should be discarded by pharmacy staff because they are generally free and there is no charge/credit issued for expired investigational drugs.
a. True
b. False

Self-Assessment Answers

1. b. An on-line computerized formulary is generally more current than printed formularies and can be searched more rapidly.
2. d. The formulary serves as a valuable reference in determining all aspects of product information required in a pharmaceutical purchasing system.
3. b. Receiving and storing of pharmaceuticals is an important process that should be performed routinely by experienced pharmacy staff. However, it is important for trainees and inexperienced staff to learn the receiving and storing process.
4. b. The receiving copy of the purchase order should be used to check in a pharmaceutical order because it documents precisely what was ordered. The packing slip documents the products the supplier shipped and, if shipped in error, may be different than the products ordered.
5. b. Review of the expiration date for all pharmaceuticals received is an important process that prevents short-dated or expired products from entering the pharmaceutical inventory.
6. d. It is important to document essential information about the product, the receiver, and the date of receipt.
7. b. If shipped in error, the manufacturer's invoice may be different from the purchase order. A copy of the purchase order should be available to check in a shipment of pharmaceuticals.
8. b. It is an important practice for pharmacy technicians to read a label carefully when placing the product into inventory or retrieving it for dispensing as a measure to avoid a potentially hazardous dispensing error.
9. A pharmacy technician may contribute positively in the handling of pharmaceuticals by
   ■ identifying look-alike pharmaceutical packaging,
   ■ identifying unclear or misleading labels on pharmaceutical products, and
   ■ suggesting storage locations for products that will minimize selection errors.
10. a. A want book is necessary in a minimum/maximum order system to facilitate timely identification of products that need to be ordered.
11. A pharmacy technician may be able to identify
    ■ increasing inventory requirement for seasonal products, such as asthma medications;
    ■ increasing inventory requirements of a particular patient requiring high doses of a pain medication; and
    ■ decreasing inventory requirements following a period of high use of a particular product by one or more patients.
12. e. The most critical processes in responding to a manufacturer's recall is a review of the inventory for affected products, removal from the hospital's inventory, and documentation of the inspection and any action required.
13. The primary benefits of belonging to a pharmaceutical purchasing group include
    ■ obtaining preferential pricing,
    ■ reducing pharmacy staff time devoted to contract matters, and
    ■ ensuring preferred pricing over a period of 1 year or more.
14. The primary advantages of purchasing pharmaceuticals on a direct basis are
    ■ no handling fees, and
    ■ ordering is required only on a periodic basis.
15. The major disadvantages of a direct purchasing program for pharmaceuticals are
    ■ the need for large storage capacity,
    ■ the reliance on independent shipping firms, and
    ■ the large amount of money invested in the pharmaceutical inventory.
16. The major advantages of a prime vendor arrangement for the purchase of pharmaceuticals are
    ■ reduced order turnaround time,
    ■ lower inventory and carrying costs,
    ■ readily available drug use data, and
    ■ a singular system for processing credits and returns.
17. b. Even highly effective purchasing and inventory systems do not eliminate the occasional borrowing or lending of pharmaceuticals.

18. b. Schedule II medications require the use of a specific order form and require a longer turnaround time for receipt of product.

19. Investigational drugs are used in patient care on a one-time-only basis or as part of an ongoing study to treat multiple patients. The physician or primary investigator is customarily responsible for ordering investigational drugs.

20. b. Medication samples are not routinely ordered by the pharmacy and require a separate system for the pharmacy to monitor drug use and storage.

21. The essential data needed to credit a patient for a pharmaceutical are
    - patient name,
    - patient account number or medical record number,
    - pharmaceutical name or item number,
    - number of units to be credited, and
    - reason for the credit.

22. Two situations that create a need to credit a patient for a pharmaceutical are
    - an incorrect order entry of a pharmaceutical product, and
    - the return of an unused tamper-proof product.

23. a. Schedule II controlled substances must be destroyed and documented according to the requirements of the DEA.

24. b. Expired investigational products should never be discarded and should always be returned to the study sponsor unless otherwise directed by the study sponsor.

Introduction to Drug Information Resources

17

BONNIE S. BACHENHEIMER

Drug therapy has become increasingly complex, and the number of new drug approvals has significantly increased in the past decade. Therefore, pharmacy technicians are frequently challenged with drug information questions throughout the workday and are called on to become more knowledgeable about the handling, availability, and uses of medications. A basic knowledge of the resources available will make the technician more resourceful and better able to assist the pharmacist with certain drug information requests.

Pharmacy reference books and electronic media (including the Internet) that are available in all practice settings often hold answers to typical day-to-day practice-related questions. These resources may also be used as study aids for the technician certification examination or to expand the technician's general knowledge about medications. Therefore, it is essential that the technician understand the basics about frequently used, reputable pharmacy references.

The purpose of this chapter is to classify the various types of drug information requests, to show which questions are appropriate for a pharmacy technician to answer, and to guide the technician in where to look for answers to drug information requests. With time and practice, technicians will be able to find the information they need quickly and efficiently and, in doing so, will become even more valuable members of the health care team.

The Drug Information Request

Before responding to a drug information question, technicians must clearly differentiate questions that fall within their scope of practice, and thus may be answered by a pharmacy technician, from those that must be answered only by a pharmacist. In many situations, the distinction between the two types of questions may not be apparent. When approached with a drug information request over the phone or in person,

Learning Objectives

After reading this chapter, the technician should review the drug information resources available at his or her own practice site and discuss the potential uses of each with a pharmacist. Furthermore, the technician should be able to

1. Classify the drug information request and get appropriate background information.

2. Distinguish between questions that may be answered by a technician and those that should be answered only by a pharmacist.

3. Identify the best resource to use when answering a specific pharmacy-related question.

4. Locate answers to drug information questions at the workplace.

technicians should identify themselves as pharmacy technicians so the person asking the question will know the type of information that may be appropriately conveyed. If there is any doubt about the nature of the question, the technician should defer the question to the pharmacist.

The technician should be sure to establish who the person initiating the request is and to obtain the necessary contact information (phone, fax, pager, etc.) in case the person needs to be called back. The requestor could be another health care professional (pharmacist, technician, nurse, physician, respiratory therapist, etc.) or a patient. The search for and response to drug information requests will be different depending on who is requesting the information. Information about the requestor—his or her training and knowledge of the subject—will have an impact on what the final response will be and how it will be given.

Obtaining background information will help to determine what the requestor needs and will make the search for information more efficient. The goal of obtaining background information is to understand why the requestor needs the information. Background information is especially important to determine if the question pertains to a specific patient or requires interpretation and, therefore, the expertise of a pharmacist. The technician should also determine the urgency of the request and the extent of the information needed so an appropriate amount of time is allotted to answer the request. Often, part of the question can be answered initially (if needed urgently), with the rest answered later when there is time to research the answer and give a more thorough response.

Classifying the Request

After information is gathered about the request and the requestor, the technician should think of the type of question asked and classify the request. Classifying the type of request helps to narrow the search, making it more efficient. Many of the questions technicians face fall into the categories in **Table 17-1**, which lists common types of questions technicians may get with examples of each.

Technicians should not interpret a patient-specific question or provide information that may require

TABLE 17-1. TYPES OF DRUG INFORMATION QUESTIONS FOR PHARMACY TECHNICIANS	
Classification Type	**Examples**
General Drug Information	■ What is the brand name of warfarin?
	■ Do Anaprox® and Aleve® contain the same active ingredient?
	■ Who manufactures Enbrel®?
	■ Is Claritin® available as a generic? Is it a prescription or over-the-counter (OTC) product?
Availability/Cost	■ What dosage forms of Imitrex® are available in your pharmacy?
	■ Is Zoloft® available as a liquid? If so, what size and concentration are available?
	■ What are the prices of Adalat CC® and Procardia XL®?
	■ How long is the shortage of vancomycin oral capsules expected to last?
Storage/Stability	■ Should Lovenox® be stored in the refrigerator?
	■ How long is a flu shot stable after it is drawn up in a syringe?
Calculations	■ How many milliliters are in an ounce?
Preparation	■ How should ampicillin be reconstituted?
Pharmacy Law	■ In what controlled substance schedule is zolpidem (Ambien®)?
	■ Can Tiazac® be substituted for Cardizem CD® (is it AB rated)?
	■ How many times can a prescription be transferred from one store to another?
Miscellaneous	■ Where can I find the phone number for Aventis?
	■ When will the patent for Allegra® expire?
	■ Where can I get more Lovenox® teaching kits?

professional judgment. A simply stated question can actually be a complex patient-specific situation requiring the pharmacist to find out more about the patient's problems and apply clinical judgment to answer the question appropriately. Many times, the person requesting the information may be indirectly asking for a pharmacist's point of view or interpretation of a situation and may require an in-depth analysis and recommendation from the pharmacist. Attempting to interpret or answer such a question could result in miscommunication and delivery of inaccurate information. Both scenarios could be harmful to the patient. Examples of questions that require a pharmacist's interpretation and should not be answered by a technician are provided in **Table 17-2**. The reason it is necessary for a pharmacist to answer is also included.

Conducting the Search: Choosing the Right References

A number of drug information resources are available to the pharmacy technician. The key to answering questions quickly and accurately is knowing where to find the necessary information. Not all references contain every possible answer to every drug information question. At times, it may be difficult to find a reference that contains the information being sought. Pharmacists usually search for information until they exhaust all possible resources. They often use multiple resources to verify the information they find, such as when determining the dose of a medication for a pediatric patient. As part of a systematic search strategy, a pharmacist is taught to consult tertiary references first, then secondary references, and finally primary references.

Tertiary references are general references that present documented information in a condensed and compact format. They may include textbooks; compendia [e.g., *American Hospital Formulary Service Drug Information* (*AHFS DI*), *Drug Facts and Comparisons*]; a computerized system, such as Micromedex® Clinical Information System; review articles; or much of the information found on the Internet. Tertiary references are the most common references used because they are easy to use, convenient, readily accessible, concise, and compact. Disadvantages of tertiary references are that information may not be up-to-date, information could have errors, and specific topics may not contain enough information because of space restrictions.

Secondary references include indexing systems, such as Medline, that provide a list of journal articles on the topic that is being searched. Secondary systems are used when new or very up-to-date information is required or when no information can be found in tertiary references.

Primary references are original research articles published in scientific journals, such as the *American Journal of Health-System Pharmacy (AJHP)* or the *Journal of the American Pharmacists Association (JAPhA)*.

Other resources that can be used include pharmaceutical manufacturers and specialized drug and poison information centers.

If the information cannot be found in a tertiary reference, then the technician should consult a pharmacist who may advise an alternative search strategy or consult a secondary reference. If time permits, the technician should consult as many resources as possible and compare the information.

Common References

There are numerous resources that are especially useful for pharmacy professionals. This section highlights common, reputable drug information resources. A brief discussion of the resource, features, and questions that the reference will help answer is provided. The following discussion may not apply equally to all practice settings and does not include all the available references. Technicians should familiarize themselves with the references in their practice settings to determine which ones best fit their needs.

General Drug Information

General drug information references are found in virtually every type of pharmacy setting. Many general information references are available in a variety of formats, including textbook, CD-ROM, palm, and Internet versions. The following sections describe some of the most common general references that pharmacy professionals use.

Drug Facts and Comparisons (published by Facts and Comparisons) is probably the most widely used reference for pharmacy professionals. It is easy to use and available in regularly updated print and electronic versions. It is a comprehensive general drug information reference that provides complete drug monographs. It is organized by therapeutic class (e.g., antihistamines, topicals) and includes tables that allow quick comparisons of drugs within the same class. Tables compare pharmacokinetic parameters (onset, duration, metabolism), adverse effects, drug interac-

TABLE 17-2. TYPES OF DRUG INFORMATION QUESTIONS FOR PHARMACISTS

Classification	Examples	Rationale
Identification & Availability	What is the alternative to Brevital® during the current shortage?	While it is appropriate for a technician to get technical information about availability (anticipated length/reasons for a shortage), questions that require clinical knowledge, such as therapeutic alternatives, must be answered by the pharmacist.
Allergies	Which narcotic is safe to use for a patient with a codeine allergy?	For allergy questions, the pharmacist must get more patient-specific information, such as a description of the allergy, what is being treated, etc. Clinical judgment is required.
Dosing & Administration	What is the usual dose of propranolol? How long should ciprofloxacin be given for a urinary tract infection? What is the best way to give gentamicin IV?	Dosing and administration questions depend on many things, especially the indication for use and patient-specific information (age, weight, kidney and liver function, etc.).
Compatibility	Is Primaxin® compatible with dopamine?	More information is needed (e.g., doses, concentrations, fluids, type of IV lines, etc.), and the pharmacist must interpret information found in a reference and apply it to the situation.
Drug Interactions	Is it okay to take aspirin with warfarin?	Drug interaction questions are complex and require patient-specific information and interpretation by the pharmacist to apply the significance of a potential interaction to a specific patient.
Side Effects	What are the side effects of Lexapro®? Can Vioxx® cause renal failure?	Package inserts and textbooks provide lists of side effects that are often difficult to interpret and convey. Also, the pharmacist must interpret whether the reason for the request is because an adverse event is suspected with one or more medications.
Pregnancy & Lactation	Is albuterol safe to use in pregnancy? Can I get a flu shot if I am breastfeeding?	Pregnancy and lactation questions are complicated because more information is needed about the patient as well as the stage of pregnancy or age of the infant. The pharmacist must interpret the findings and apply them to the specific situation.
Therapeutic Use	Has clonidine been used to treat opiate withdrawal?	The use of drugs for off-label uses often requires evaluation and interpretation of the literature and clinical judgment.

tions, dosing, and multiple ingredient preparations (lists of individual ingredients of the cough and cold preparations, analgesic combinations, etc.).

The following information may be found in this reference: general drug information (pharmacology, drug interactions, doses, adverse effects, warnings, precautions, etc.); product availability (dosage forms, brand/generic names, manufacturer, etc.); active ingredients and strengths of multiple-ingredient products; controlled substance schedules; whether products are over the counter (OTC) or by prescription; whether products are sugar-free, alcohol-free, or dye-free; drug company phone numbers and addresses; and color-coded pictures that may assist in product identification.

United States Pharmacopeia Drug Information [USP DI] *(published by Micromedex)* is a three-volume set that provides medication information for health care professionals (Volume I) and patients (Volume II). Volume III (*Approved Drug Products and Legal Requirements*) provides information on laws affecting pharmacy practice.

Volume I (*Drug Information for the Healthcare Professional*) provides comprehensive general drug information. The drug monographs are arranged alphabetically, but discuss similar medications in a single section. The monographs provide brief discussions on how medications work, their indications and other uses, adverse effects, potential drug interactions, admixture information, storage requirements, auxiliary label recommendations, and so on.

Volume II (*Advice for the Patient*) provides a more general discussion of the medications in language that patients will understand. This volume answers questions patients may ask, such as how to take the medication; special considerations about whether to take during pregnancy and breastfeeding; and common adverse effects that may occur when taking the medicine. This information may be photocopied and given to patients to reinforce issues that were discussed during patient counseling.

Volume III (*Approved Drug Products and Legal Requirements*) contains the FDA's published list of approved drug products, ***Approved Drug Products with Therapeutic Equivalence Evaluations*** (also known as the *Orange Book*). This volume provides information related to bioequivalence of products, or whether generic drugs can be substituted. Volume III helps the professional to identify a drug's chemical properties, determine if a drug has been discontinued, or select an appropriate

generic substitute for a brand name drug. This volume also includes information about federal requirements regarding product quality, packaging, storage, and labeling.

All *USP DI* volumes contain a section with color-coded pictures that may assist with product identification.

The Physicians' Desk Reference [PDR] *(published by Thomson Medical Economics)* contains manufacturers' package inserts. A package insert is a manufacturer's product information sheet that provides general drug information, such as how it works, indications, adverse effects, drug interactions, dosage forms, stability, dosing information, and so on. The *PDR* is organized according to the manufacturer's products (as opposed to therapeutic class). The *PDR* contains other useful information, such as colored pictures of tablets, capsules, or packaging, that may be used for product identification. Package inserts list active and inactive ingredients, preparation, administration, stability, storage instructions, and availability. The *PDR* also lists phone numbers and addresses of manufacturers and Drug and Poison Information Centers.

The *PDR* is not comprehensive; it contains information only on select brand name drugs. Information about generic medications is not included. The information is written by the manufacturer and approved by the FDA. It offers information only about FDA-approved uses of a drug. It does not provide comparative information of similar medications. Therefore, using the *PDR* to compare products is not as simple as with other reference books.

American Hospital Formulary Service Drug Information [AHFS DI] *(published by the American Society of Health-System Pharmacists, ASHP)* is a detailed, comprehensive, general drug information reference. This textbook provides complete drug monographs that are organized by therapeutic class (e.g., anti-infectives, cardiovascular). It provides detailed information about the use of a drug, its side effects, dosing considerations, and so on. Its coverage is not limited to FDA-approved uses of medications. It offers especially useful preparation and administration instructions for injectable products. *AHFS* is widely used by pharmacists because it provides in-depth, unbiased, evaluative reviews of medications. It is extensively reviewed by editors and contains information from various reputable sources.

AHFS does not provide many tables to allow direct comparisons of agents within a therapeutic class. Nor does it provide extensive product availability information, as *Drug Facts and Comparisons* does. Also, since *AHFS* is peer reviewed, information about new drugs may not be incorporated as quickly as in other references.

Lexi-Comp's Drug Information Handbooks and Clinical Manuals (published by Lexi-Comp) include numerous handbooks that provide drug and disease state information specific to different health care professionals (pharmacists, physicians, dentists, allied health professionals, etc.). The *Drug Information Handbook* and the *Drug Information Handbook for Allied Health Professionals* contain general drug information monographs. They are widely used because they are quick, convenient, and easy to use. The *Drug Information Handbook* is alphabetically organized according to generic name. The monographs in the *Drug Information Handbook* are comprehensive and include pharmacology, dosing, drug interaction and safety, as well as available doses and strengths. The *Drug Information Handbook for the Allied Health Professional* is not as comprehensive as the *Drug Information Handbook*, but may be appealing to technicians because it allows quick access to basic data on the most frequently used medications.

Other Lexi-Comp handbooks that may be of interest to pharmacy technicians include *A Patient Guide to Diseases and Conditions, Psychotropic Drug Information Handbook, Medical Abbreviations,* and the *Pediatric Dosage Handbook*. All the handbooks contain extensive appendixes with helpful charts, abbreviations, measurements, and conversions.

Mosby's Drug Consult (published by Elsevier Science) is a comprehensive general drug information reference. This publication used to be called Mosby's *GenRx,* but the title was changed to reflect changes in the current edition. *Mosby's Drug Consult* contains extensive information about prescription brand and generic products. It provides complete drug monographs that are organized alphabetically by generic drug names. The monographs are fairly extensive and provide information to assist the health care professional in using the drugs clinically. Information in each monograph includes medication names (generic, brand, and chemical names), manufacturer, dosage forms, general uses of agents, clinical trial information when available, adverse reactions and precautions, costs, and therapeutically equivalent products. This textbook is more comprehensive than the *PDR*. A key feature is its indexing system, which allows identification of all drugs within a therapeutic class, schedules of controlled substances, pregnancy categories, and so on.

American Drug Index (published by Facts and Comparisons) is an alphabetical listing of drugs with brief information on each, including drug name (generic, brand, and chemical name), manufacturer, dosage form, strength and packaging information, and general uses (e.g., general anesthetic, narcotic, antitussive). It also contains pharmaceutical manufacturer phone numbers and addresses, weight and measuring conversions, and a list of drugs that should not be crushed. Its extensive cross-indexing is useful for quickly identifying a brand or generic product or determining product availability.

Micromedex® Healthcare Series (published by Thomson Micromedex) is a comprehensive reference system that is accessed electronically by CD-ROM, the Internet, or personal digital assistant (PDA). Depending on the subscription, Micromedex Healthcare Series contains comprehensive drug information, poison information, Material Safety Data Sheets, foreign drug information, tablet and capsule identification, disease and trauma information, herbal information, stability, compatibility, pregnancy information, patient information, and more. Drug information for patients is available in both English and Spanish. Unfortunately, the cost of the subscription prohibits many pharmacy settings from purchasing this system.

Availability/Cost Information

Red Book (published by Medical Economics) contains product information and prices for prescription drugs, OTC products, and medical supplies. It contains National Drug Code (NDC) numbers for all products, available packaging, and therapeutic equivalence ratings (according to the FDA's *Orange Book*), as well as a comprehensive listing of manufacturers, wholesalers, and third-party administrator directories. There are sections with other useful practical information, such as lists of sugar-, lactose-, galactose-, and alcohol-free products; sulfite-containing products; medications that should not be crushed; and color photographs of many prescription and OTC products.

Compatibility and Stability Information

Trissel's Handbook on Injectable Drugs (published by American Society of Health-System Pharmacists, ASHP) is a textbook often used in hospital and home health care pharmacies. It focuses solely on injectable medications. It provides data on the solubility, compatibility, and stability of many different medications. Specifically, this handbook is useful to determine when two medications may be safely mixed together in an IV bag, in a syringe, or at a Y-site on an administration set. This reference also addresses special handling requirements of certain agents (glass vs. plastic containers, light restrictions, filters, refrigeration requirements, expiration, etc.).

King Guide to Parenteral Admixtures (published by King Guide Publications, Inc.) is also useful for determining compatibility and stability of injectable medications. It lists medications and their compatibility with common infusion solutions and, when available, compatibility of medications mixed together in a syringe, by Y-site, or other types of sets. A section discusses reconstitution stability under different conditions and precautions to be taken in preparation and administration. There is also information regarding total parenteral nutrition solutions and total nutrient admixtures.

When assessing questions regarding injectable drugs, careful attention must be paid to the concentrations of all drugs, the admixture solutions, infusion rates and routes, and dosing frequency. It must not be assumed that medications listed as compatible under specific conditions will also be compatible at higher concentrations or in different solutions. Technicians should ask pharmacists to help them learn how to interpret the tables provided in these references and should always consult with pharmacists before applying information learned or before giving another health care professional such information.

Miscellaneous References

Material Safety Data Sheets (MSDS) are information sheets provided by manufacturers for chemicals or drugs that may be hazardous in the workplace. The primary purpose of the MSDS is to provide information about the specific hazards of the chemicals or drugs (i.e., to describe acute and chronic health effects), guidelines for their safe use, and recommendations to treat an exposure or clean up a spill. Materials commonly encountered in pharmacies that require MSDS information include chemotherapy agents (e.g., doxorubicin, methotrexate), hormonal agents (e.g., diethylstilbesterol), and volatile or explosive agents (e.g., isopropyl alcohol, ethyl alcohol).

MSDS contain information that may be used to answer the following types of questions:

- What precautions must be taken when preparing and dispensing Adriamycin®?
- Where should isopropyl alcohol be stored?

- How should an employee exposed to Adriamycin® be immediately treated?
- How should a chemotherapy spill be cleaned?

The Internet

The Internet can be a very useful source for drug information if it is used appropriately. Care must be taken to ensure that the information is current, accurate, and from a reputable source. Generally, Web sites that are sponsored by the government, pharmacy and medical organizations, and medical centers are the most reputable. The availability of the Internet has improved the efficiency of searching for drug information. Many pharmacy settings that are not affiliated with major medical center libraries now have a way to perform literature searches, purchase articles on-line, and view government publications, often at no additional cost. Most pharmacy settings today have access to the Internet, and most hospital settings have high-speed Internet connections, which speeds the process even more. Most of the publishers of the references that have been discussed in this chapter either have developed or are developing Internet versions of their references. Internet versions are advantageous because the user no longer has to purchase updates of the hard copy references, and they can be accessed with a log-in and password from any computer with Internet access. **Table 17-3** lists useful Web sites for obtaining drug information and a brief description of what each site contains.

How to Conduct a Search Using MedlinePlus

The National Library of Medicine (NLM) (www.nlm.nih.gov) is the largest medical library in the world. It maintains MedlinePlus, a database of information for both health professionals and consumers on more than 500 health conditions. The MedlinePlus Web site (www.medlineplus.gov) also features a medical encyclopedia and dictionary, health and drug information in Spanish, drug information on prescription and OTC products, health information from the media, and links to clinical trials. The information is government sponsored and updated daily.

Using the MedlinePlus Web site to find information on diseases or consumer drug information is easy:

1. To search for a specific disease or medical condition, go to http://medlineplus.gov.
2. Click on "Health Topics."
3. Search for diseases and conditions by the first

letter of the topic, by broad group (body location/system, procedure, demographics, or health/wellness), or by frequently requested topics.

4. Search for consumer drug information by clicking on the "Drug Information" tab. There are also links to the FDA (recalls, warnings, safety information), clinical trials listings, and Medline.

5. Click on the first letter of the brand or generic name of the drug or product to access drug information. The source of the drug information on this site is the ASHP MedMaster database and the United States Pharmacopeia Drug Information (USP DI®) Advice for the Patient®.

6. On the MedlinePlus home page, another way to search for a topic is by typing in a key word in the "search" window.

How to Conduct a Search Using Medline/PubMed

Although MedlinePlus has links to recently published health professional articles, the best way to search the science literature is to perform a Medline search.

TABLE 17-3. USEFUL WEB SITES FOR OBTAINING DRUG INFORMATION		
Web Site	**Address**	**Description**
Food and Drug Administration	www.fda.gov	Home page for the FDA; contains numerous useful links for both consumers and health care professionals
FDA Center for Drug Evaluation and Research (CDER)	www.fda.gov/cder	Contains links for consumer and health care professionals regarding drug information, such as new drug approvals, drug shortages, safety information, generic drug bioequivalence (*Orange Book*)
Centers for Disease Control and Prevention (CDC)	www.cdc.gov	Home page for the CDC; contains information about diseases, health topics, vaccines, traveler's health, bioterrorism, etc.
National Institutes for Health (NIH)	www.nih.gov	Home page for the NIH; contains information about health topics, clinical trials, and the various divisions of the NIH
FDA Consumer Information	www.fda.gov/cder/consumerinfo	Contains FDA-approved patient drug information from January 1998 to the present; also contains a link to the manufacturer's package insert
National Library of Medicine/Medline/PubMed and MedlinePlus	www.nlm.nih.gov	Home page for the U.S. National Library of Medicine. Links to Medline Plus (health information for consumers) and Medline/PubMed (references and abstracts from biomedical journals)
American Society for Health-System Pharmacists (ASHP)	www.ashp.org	Home page for ASHP; contains news related to health-system pharmacy and many helpful links for pharmacy professionals
ASHP Drug Shortages Resource Center	www.ashp.org/shortage	Up-to-date information on drug shortages, including which products are affected and why, the anticipated time to resolution, and alternatives
ASHP Consumer Drug Information	www.safemedication.com	Reputable Web site for patient medication information
American Pharmaceutical Association (APhA)	www.aphanet.org	Home page for APhA; contains news related to pharmacy and many helpful links for pharmacy professionals
Institute for Safe Medication Practices (ISMP)	www.ismp.org	Homepage for the ISMP; contains medication error alerts, a section for reporting, products available for purchase, and medication error prevention strategies
Virtual Library Pharmacy	www.pharmacy.org	Contains links to pharmacy associations, pharmaceutical manufacturers, government sites, hospitals, journals and books, and more

Medline is a database containing more than 12 million article references published in more than 4,500 biomedical journals and magazines. PubMed is a free Web-based searching system, sponsored by the NLM, which can be used to access specific Medline journal citations. PubMed also contains links to full-text articles.

Searching in PubMed is relatively easy. An on-line help section explains its features and performs more complicated searches. Basically, the user simply enters search terms into the query box and then either hits the "enter" key or clicks "Go." Multiple terms can be typed into the search box, and PubMed will automatically combine similar terms. For example, if the user types in "vitamin C common cold," PubMed will automatically combine "vitamin C" and "common cold." The terms *AND*, *OR*, and *NOT* can be used to combine sets and narrow a search. For example, typing "vitamin C AND common cold" yields all the citations that have "vitamin C" *and* "common cold" as subjects in the articles. This strategy is the most commonly used to get citations that are pertinent to a specific topic. Typing "vitamin C OR common cold" will get all citations with *either* "vitamin C" *or* "common cold" as the subjects in articles (and many more citations). Typing "vitamin C NOT common cold" will eliminate any citations that have "common cold" as the subjects in articles about vitamin C (and many fewer citations). The term *NOT* is the least used when doing searches, because it may eliminate useful citations. To help to narrow down a search, the user may apply limits, such as *English language, human subjects, age, publication year(s)*, etc. A search can also be conducted by author's name or journal title.

Review of a Sample Search

To search for articles on the value of pharmacy technician certification, take the following steps:

1. Go to www.nlm.nih.gov. Click on "Health Information" and then "MEDLINE/PubMed" to get to the PubMed Web site.

2. In the search window, type "pharmacy technicians AND certification."

3. Either hit the "enter" key or click on "Go."

4. The results of the search contain all the articles that have both pharmacy technicians and certification as subjects in the articles.

5. To view more details of one of the citations, click on the blue hypertext author(s) names (to the right of the number of the citation).

6. To save multiple citations, select citations by clicking the checkboxes to the left of the specific citations.

7. Just above and below the citations, there is a display option, which is set to "Summary," but can be changed to display abstracts and other details. After selecting specific citations you wish to save, select "Abstract" from the display menu, and then click on "Display."

8. The selected citations will show up with the abstracts (assuming there was an abstract available). Using your browser's print function, you can print out the citations with the abstracts.

As illustrated in this example, Medline is useful for searching for practice-related issues, such as the value or role of pharmacy technicians, in addition to clinically focused questions. A Medline search can be useful before expanding a service or evaluating an existing pharmacy service. Fortunately, many publishers have full-text articles available for purchase, enabling practice sites that are miles from a medical or pharmacy library to obtain pertinent articles at the click of a button.

Table 17-4 summarizes common types of drug information requests and the references likely to contain such information.

The Response

After the search for information is complete, all the information gathered must be organized and evaluated before responding. The technician should then give a verbal or written reply stating the question and outlining the response that should be made. Recommendations should be supported by references, if applicable. For example, if a pharmacist asks if a certain product is interchangeable, the technician may need to provide proof that it is AB rated. One of the most important steps in answering a drug information question is follow-up. For example, questioning the requestor about whether the information was useful or if the question was answered will ensure that the response was complete. Asking if further assistance is necessary is also good practice.

Conclusion

Pharmacy technicians are frequently asked drug information questions by consumers, pharmacists, and other health care professionals. Using a systematic

TABLE 17-4. REVIEW OF COMMON DRUG INFORMATION REQUESTS AND REFERENCES

Type of Information Needed	Reference Likely to Have Such Information
Product Availability ■ dosage form ■ product strength ■ brand and generic name ■ manufacturer ■ indication	American Drug Index Drug Facts and Comparisons Drug Information Handbook Internet PDR Micromedex Mosby's Drug Consult RedBook (not indication) USP DI (pharmaceutical manufacturer)
Product Identification ■ dosage form ■ product strength ■ brand and generic name ■ manufacturer ■ colored pictures of tablets/capsules	Drug Facts and Comparisons PDR Mosby's Drug Consult USP DI Micromedex
Drug Uses ■ FDA approved indications ■ other uses of the agent	American Hospital Formulary Service Drug Facts and Comparisons Drug Information Handbook Mosby's Drug Consult PDR USP DI Micromedex
Drug Monographs ■ general drug information ■ pharmacology ■ indications and uses ■ drug interactions ■ admixture information ■ doses ■ adverse effects ■ drug interactions	American Hospital Formulary Service American Drug Index Drug Facts and Comparisons Drug Information Handbook Physicians' Desk Reference (FDA-approved indications only) Micromedex Mosby's Drug Consult USP DI
Injectable Drug Compatibility/Stability Information ■ drug diluent and solution compatibilities ■ drug compatibility ■ states conditions for handling products (i.e., glass vs. plastic container, protection from light, filters, refrigeration, expiration, etc.)	American Hospital Formulary Service Handbook on Injectable Drugs Package inserts PDR Micromedex
Preparation	American Hospital Formulary Service Handbook on Injectable Drugs Micromedex Package inserts PDR
Calculations	American Drug Index Drug Information Handbook
Hazardous Chemicals or Drugs ■ specific hazards of the chemicals or drugs used at the work site ■ guidelines for use ■ recommendations to treat or clean up an exposure	Material Safety Data Sheets Micromedex

cont'd

TABLE 17-4. REVIEW OF COMMON DRUG INFORMATION REQUESTS AND REFERENCES

Type of Information Needed	Reference Likely to Have Such Information
Pharmacy Law ■ Generic substitution (bioequivalence) ■ Federal regulations regarding handling and dispensing	*USP DI Volume III* *Orange Book*
Patient Information	*USP DI Volume I* *Internet (FDA, safemedication.com)* *MedlinePlus* (English/Spanish) *Micromedex* (English/Spanish) *Patient package inserts*

approach when faced with a drug information question will aid in understanding the nature of the request, obtaining pertinent background information, and successfully answering the question. Numerous resources are available to assist with answering drug information requests. Becoming familiar with common resources will make the search process more efficient. It is critical for pharmacy technicians to be able to differentiate between basic drug information questions that can be answered by the technician and questions for which clinical judgment is required and should therefore be answered only by a pharmacist.

Self-Assessment Questions

1. When a drug information call is received, the technician should identify him- or herself as a pharmacy technician and obtain the name and contact information of the requestor, find out whether the requestor is a consumer or health care professional, and establish the general question, but if the question involves professional judgment, it should be deferred to the pharmacist.
   a. True
   b. False

2. A pharmacist needs to identify an over-the-counter, sugar-free, alcohol-free cough formula containing guaifenesin and dextromethorphan. How could this question be classified?
   a. availability
   b. storage/stability
   c. pharmacy law
   d. calculation

3. Drug information questions relating to side effects and drug interactions of medications are best answered by a pharmacist.
   a. True
   b. False

4. Pharmacists should answer any question that is related to a medication shortage.
   a. True
   b. False

5. Examples of tertiary references include which of the following?
   a. *Drug Facts and Comparisons*
   b. Medline
   c. The *American Journal of Health-System Pharmacy*
   d. *American Hospital Formulary Service Drug Information (AHFS DI)*
   e. a and d

6. If a technician is asked, "In what strengths is fluvastatin (Lescol®, Lescol® XL) available?" which references(s) would have this information?
   a. *Drug Facts and Comparisons*
   b. *Drug Information Handbook*
   c. *Physicians' Desk Reference (PDR)*
   d. Novartis, the manufacturer of Lescol®
   e. all of the above

7. The question "What is the generic name of Lexapro®?" could be answered with which textbook(s)?

a. *Drug Information Handbook*
b. *PDR*
c. *Drug Facts and Comparisons*
d. *American Drug Index*
e. all of the above

8. Which reference(s) would provide information to answer the following questions: "What company manufactures Vfend®? What is its phone number?"
   a. *PDR*
   b. *Drug Facts and Comparisons*
   c. *American Drug Index*
   d. *Red Book*
   e. all of the above

9. Which reference(s) would provide information to answer the following questions: "How is injectable amiodarone (Cordarone®) prepared (with what diluent, solution)? How long is it stable?"
   a. *PDR*
   b. MSDS
   c. *AHFS DI*
   d. *Handbook on Injectable Drugs*
   e. a, c and d only

10. Which reference would provide information on drugs or chemicals that may be hazardous in the workplace?
    a. *PDR*
    b. MSDS
    c. *American Drug Index*
    d. *Handbook on Injectable Drugs*

11. Conducting a search using MedlinePlus would help the technician find what kind of information?
    a. Drug stability and compatibility
    b. Cost
    c. General health information
    d. General drug information
    e. c and d

12. A physician calls and says he needs to know the identification of a white tablet with imprint code "M C2." Which reference(s) would provide information to answer this question?
    a. *Micromedex*
    b. *Handbook on Injectable Drugs*
    c. *United States Pharmacopeia Drug Information (USP DI)*
    d. a and c only
    e. all of the above

Self-Assessment Questions

13. If a technician wants to know if nitroprusside (Nipride®) is compatible with normal saline, he or she could consult:
    a. the package insert
    b. MSDS
    c. *Handbook on Injectable Drugs*
    d. a and c
    e. *Drug Facts and Comparisons*

14. Which reference contains information to help with patient education and counseling?
    a. *PDR*
    b. *Drug Facts and Comparisons*
    c. MedlinePlus
    d. *United States Pharmacopeia Drug Information (USP DI)*
    e. all of the above

15. A patient is asking a technician if the pharmacy has a medication that she heard about on the radio. Where can the technician find out if the drug has been FDA approved?
    a. Internet
    b. *Drug Facts and Comparisons*
    c. *PDR*
    d. none of the above

16. Which reference would help answer the following question: "Does Prinivil® have a generic equivalent?"
    a. *Orange Book*
    b. *Drug Facts and Comparisons*
    c. *USP DI Vol. III*
    d. *PDR*
    e. a, b, and c only

17. Which reference will help answer the following question: "What is the controlled substance schedule for Ambien®?"
    a. *Drug Facts and Comparisons*
    b. *Drug Information Handbook*
    c. *PDR*
    d. a, b, and c only
    e. MSDS

18. The answer to the question, "How many milliliters are in a teaspoon?" can be found in the following reference(s):
    a. *Drug Information Handbook*
    b. *PDR*
    c. *American Drug Index*
    d. *Drug Facts and Comparisons*
    e. a and c

19. What is the best place for the latest information on bioterrorism and the smallpox vaccine?
    a. *Drug Facts and Comparisons*
    b. *PDR*
    c. MedlinePlus
    d. *Red Book*

20. Which types of Internet sites are the most reputable for health information?
    a. Pharmaceutical manufacturers
    b. Government (i.e., FDA, NLM, NIH, CDC)
    c. Pharmacy organizations (ASHP, APhA)
    d. a, b and c
    e. Independent

Self-Assessment Answers

1. a. When approached with a drug information request, technicians should identify themselves as pharmacy technicians so the person asking the question will know with whom they are speaking. It is important to know who the person initiating the request is and to get contact information (phone, fax, pager, etc.) in case the person needs to be called back. Knowing information about the requestor—his or her training and knowledge of the subject—will have an impact on what the final response will be and how it will be given. If there is any doubt about the nature of the question, the technician should defer the question to the pharmacist.

2. a. This drug information question is related to product availability. Pharmacy technicians may be asked by pharmacists to help identify specific types of products or formulations to purchase.

3. a. Drug interaction and side effect questions are complex. They involve patient-specific information, interpretation of drug information, and clinical judgment. Therefore, a pharmacist should always answer them.

4. b. Although it is best for the pharmacist to approve alternative agents in the event of a medication shortage, the technician can share general information about the shortage. For example, the technician can give the reason for the shortage, whether other dose forms are available, and how long the shortage is anticipated to last. Resources to assist in shortage information include the drug manufacturer, the FDA (www.fda.gov/cder), and ASHP's drug shortage Web site (www.ashp.org/shortage).

5. e. Both *Drug Facts and Comparisons* and the *American Hospital Formulary Service Drug Information* (*AHFS DI*) are general drug information textbooks that are considered tertiary references. Medline provides a list of journal articles on the topic being searched and so is considered a secondary reference. The *American Journal of Health-System Pharmacy* (*AJHP*) is a scientific journal that contains original articles, and is therefore considered a primary reference.

6. e. All resources provide availability information, and any of the listed references may be used to answer this question.

7. e. The *Physicians' Desk Reference* and *Drug Facts and Comparisons* will provide this information, but the index must be used first to find the page on which the product is listed (and may not be very efficient). The *American Drug Index* and *Drug Information Handbook* list products alphabetically, so this type of information may be found quicker with these references.

8. e. All the references listed provide information about manufacturers, as well as company phone numbers and Web sites.

9. e. The *PDR* (the package insert), *AHFS*, and *Handbook on Injectable Drugs* provide information on preparation of injectable products. MSDS provide information about the hazards of medications or chemicals.

10. b. MSDS provide information about the hazards of medications. They specify hazards of chemicals or drugs used at the work site and provide guidelines for their safe use and recommendations to treat an exposure or clean up a spill.

11. e. MedlinePlus is a government-sponsored database that contains information on more than 500 health conditions and general drug information on prescription and OTC products.

12. d. Resources for product identification (pictures) are not available in the *Handbook on Injectable Drugs* (which discusses injectable drugs only). The *United States Pharmacopeia Drug Information* (Volumes I–III) has photographs that may help to identify this tablet. Micromedex has a tablet identification database.

13. d. The package insert, *Handbook on Injectable Drugs,* and *Drug Facts and Comparisons* provide specific compatibility information for Nipride®. The *Handbook on Injectable Drugs* will generally have more information about compatibility than the package insert. *Drug Facts and Comparisons* has limited compatibility information. MSDS do not provide compatibility information.

14. e. The *United States Pharmacopeia Drug Information* (*USP DI Vol. II*) and MedlinePlus are specifically

developed to be used as aids for patient counseling. They are best used to reinforce information discussed during patient counseling. The package insert and *Drug Facts and Comparisons* contain a section for patient information.

15. a. Although the Internet versions of *Drug Facts and Comparisons* and the *PDR* are more up-to-date than the print versions, there is still a significant lag time until new drugs are included in the database. The Internet is the best place to find very recent information. New drug approvals can be found on the FDA's Web site (www.fda.gov/cder).

16. e. The FDA's *Orange Book*, *Drug Facts and Comparisons*, and the *USP DI Vol. III* all contain information on generically equivalent products. The *Orange Book* and the *USP DI* list the bioequivalence rating. The *PDR* does not contain information on generic drugs.

17. d. Controlled substance schedules can be found quickly in *Drug Facts and Comparisons*, the *Drug Information Handbook*, or the package insert (*PDR*). MSDS do not contain that type of information.

18. e. Calculations such as this one can be found in the appendixes in the *Drug Information Handbook* and in the *American Drug Index*.

19. c. The NLM's MedlinePlus (http://medlineplus.gov) contains information on numerous health topics and drug information in lay terms. Clicking on "Health Topics," then "B," and then "Biodefense and Bioterrorism," or "S" and then "Smallpox" will bring up the latest news and useful links to search for more specific information.

20. d. Information found on the Internet should always be evaluated for credibility, the source, supporting evidence, and timeliness. Pharmaceutical manufacturers often have reputable sites because they should contain only FDA-approved content. Government sites are usually reputable because experts have reviewed the information and there is no conflict of interest (they are not selling anything). Pharmacy and medical organizations also often have their information reviewed by experts in the particular field and are therefore considered reputable. Independent sites can contain erroneous or misleading information, especially if a product is being sold.

Computer Technology

18

CONNIE LARSON

Computer technology is advancing rapidly. Although computers have become more advanced and complex, they have also become easier to use. Using computers to store information has many advantages: They take up less space, enable information to be retrieved rapidly, make more information available to more people more easily, and allow information to be updated and distributed very quickly.

Concern for patient safety topped the list of priorities for information technology (IT) health executives in the year 2003. Implementing technology to reduce medical errors and promote patient safety was the top IT priority for more than half of the responders to an annual survey taken by Superior Consultant Company.[1] Computer technology plays an integral role assisting in the safe and efficient administration of health care.

Pharmacy Computer Systems

Although computers are expensive investments for businesses and improper use can result in damage to the equipment as well as loss of crucial information, they generally improve the efficiency, productivity, and accuracy of our work and reduce the cost associated with common tasks.

To capitalize on the investment and avoid loss of information and damage to equipment, many institutions designate a knowledgeable person to manage the computer system and serve as a resource to staff. Designated personnel also ensure that safeguards are built to avoid accidental access to functions that could jeopardize the system. Pharmacy technicians should know who their staff resource person is and how to contact computer support personnel when they need assistance.

Mainframe- versus Personal Computer-Based Systems

Working with computer systems requires a basic knowledge of, as well as some specific training for, the system used in a technician's workplace. There are different types of computers, and their unique characteristics make each suitable for different situations. *Mainframe* computers are large, expensive, powerful computers designed to process large amounts of data that are shared by numerous people. Because they generate a lot of heat,

Learning Objectives

After completing this chapter, the technician should be able to

1. Describe the differences between *mainframe* and *personal* computer systems.
2. Understand basic computer terminology.
3. Describe how automation impacts the drug distribution process.
4. List the types of computer-generated work lists pharmacies use.
5. Describe the difference between the automation needs of *institutional* and *ambulatory care* pharmacies.
6. List the different types of reports that management and staff can use.
7. Describe how technology is used to monitor the clinical status of patients.
8. Describe the advantages of using automation for inventory control.
9. Describe the features of an automated narcotic control system.
10. List three applications for bar coding in health care.
11. List the disadvantages of touch-screen technology.
12. List the advantages of light pen technology.
13. Describe how a mouse works.
14. Describe the future of voice recognition technology.
15. Describe the difference between decentralized and centralized automated dispensing systems.
16. Describe the limitations of automated dispensing systems.
17. List applications for process control devices.
18. Describe the advantages of paperless charting.

mainframe computers need to be stored in large, temperature-controlled rooms. Institutional pharmacies use mainframe systems to access patient information (e.g., room number, age, sex, weight, and laboratory data). Ambulatory care pharmacies use mainframes to record patient prescriptions and access insurance and billing information.

Dumb terminals are an inexpensive way for a large number of users to access information from a central computer's memory. Dumb terminals are useless unless they are connected to a mainframe system. Dumb terminals allow pharmacies to access patient information, such as patient medication profiles and allergy information.

Minicomputers are smaller scaled mainframe computers. They are commonly used by several people within a small organization or by a department within a large organization. Several minicomputers can be used to form a local area network (LAN). LANs are also commonly used by small groups of people. Pharmacy personnel use minicomputers to access patient information just as they would use a mainframe.

Microcomputers, or *personal computers* (PCs), are stand-alone systems that run software programs and manage data accessed from a larger source, such as a mainframe. Basic PC equipment includes a monitor, a central processing unit (CPU), and a printer. PCs have traditionally been used for word processing, spreadsheets, database management, desktop publishing, and telecommunication programs. With the advent of larger PCs that can be used as central file servers, many PCs can be interconnected in a LAN. This allows PC users to share information as needed, such as with a pharmacy order entry system. In the client/server model, LANs can be connected with other PCs, other LANs, minicomputers, and mainframes. In this scenario, information can be shared among the various systems. Today, PCs are as powerful as early mainframes and are available in desktop models, portable laptops, and handheld models.

Interfaces are connections between two or more computer systems that enable data to be transferred. The interface can be unidirectional, allowing one-way information to be entered or removed, or bidirectional, allowing data to be sent back and forth between systems. Building interfaces can be very complicated and expensive. The interface limits the amount of information that can be received from other departments that have their own system, such as the hospital laboratory. Interface applications, for example, provide patient laboratory data and input of pharmacy medication charges for institutional pharmacies and allow retrieval of patient insurance information and payment processing in ambulatory care pharmacies.

The percentage of pharmacy departments that use computer systems has increased from 63.9 percent in 1990 to 75 percent in 1992, according to two ASHP surveys. The surveys defined a *computerized pharmacy system* as a system that at a minimum maintains patient medication profiles and generates prescription or dispensing fill lists. In the 1992 survey, 86 percent of the pharmacy departments had at least one microcomputer.[2]

As the practice of pharmaceutical care grows and pharmacists' responsibilities become more and more patient focused, the opportunity for technician involvement with computers will increase. Many of the tasks traditionally performed manually by technicians, such as cart filling, floor stock replacement, intravenous (IV) admixing, and prepackaging, are now being modified so that computers can do some of the work.

Microcomputers are used for such pharmacy activities as quality assurance, drug information, drug utilization evaluations, adverse drug reaction reporting, nonformulary drug use, and workload statistics computing. An on-line policy and procedure manual and drug formulary allows frequent updating so the most current information is available. Technicians also play a larger role in the collection, input, and organization of such data into microcomputer systems.

The type of computers an organization or department may require depends on the users' needs, the organization's financial resources, and the systems already available within the organization. Pharmacy systems can be part of an institution's mainframe system or purchased separately as stand-alone systems. Several computer companies offer mainframe systems with pharmacy components; others offer stand-alone pharmacy systems. These systems can be customized to improve the efficiency of a particular pharmacy's operation.

If the basic system is not comprehensive, additional software may be available that can help the pharmacy department meet its operational and informational needs.

Institutional Distribution Functions

Results of a 1992 ASHP survey showed that 90 percent of the responding community hospital pharmacies offered complete unit-dose drug distribution services.[2] Automation can have a significant impact in this area.

The type of computer system the pharmacy uses determines the type of information available to the pharmacy. Data can be entered manually into a stand-alone pharmacy system or transferred into the system via an interface with the hospital's mainframe system. Depending on the complexity of the interface, the information the pharmacy receives through it could be simple demographic information or complete medication orders, lab results, and procedures. When an interface involves demographics only, then the pharmacy must input the patients' medication orders manually.

Databases

The pharmacy department or an information technology specialist is responsible for building the system's database during the installation of the system. For patient medication orders or prescription information to be entered, a database must be in place to accommodate all the information that is unique to the institution or pharmacy, such as room numbers, patient care areas, formulary medications, inventory, and insurance and billing information. Tools that assist drug therapy monitoring by screening patient profiles for drug-allergy, drug-drug, drug-food, drug-disease, and drug-lab interactions, as well as maximum dose, dose range, and duplicate therapy checking, are often included with a system. However, maximum dose and dose range checking may require modifications, depending on the institution's therapeutic guidelines for high-risk medications.

System Security

Access to the pharmacy computer system is controlled by having users log into the system using a user name and a password, which can be letters, numbers, or a combination of both. Biometric access using fingerprints is another method of controlling access to secure devices. For this method, individual fingerprints are initially scanned into the system and then linked with a user ID. To access the computer, the individual places his or her finger on a scanner located on the device. Different security levels can be programmed so that users have access only to information related to their specific job responsibilities; for example, only pharmacists can verify medication orders and only authorized individuals can access certain databases to view information or to run work lists or reports. Once a user is finished working on the system, the user must sign off or log off the system so no one can access or input information under another staff member's code.

Another important security issue is protecting the system against viruses. Many pharmacies are tremendously reliant on their computer systems, and a virus can virtually incapacitate a system in a matter of minutes. Introducing a virus is as simple as opening an attachment to an e-mail. For this reason, individuals using the computer should avoid opening any mail or attachment unless they recognize the sender. It is also essential that the system be protected by antivirus software, which must be updated regularly to scan for new viruses.

Computerized Prescriber Order Entry

Computerized Prescriber Order Entry (CPOE) uses software that allows the input of medication and other orders into an electronic patient medical record. The electronic patient medical record with CPOE capability replaces written orders and clinical notes, which can be difficult to interpret because of poor handwriting or blurred fax copies. A variety of safety organizations (e.g., Institute for Safe Medication Practices) recommend CPOE systems to reduce medication errors. CPOE systems contain information similar to that found in a stand-alone pharmacy system, but more comprehensive. Physicians and other authorized health care professionals input medication orders, lab requests and results, and clinical notes related to the care of the patient directly into the system. All authorized users have access to medications, labs, and clinical notes and can display other types of results and clinical information, including radiology x-rays and reports. Available functionality varies among vendors.

The ideal situation is for the CPOE system to be integrated with the pharmacy dispensing system. If the two systems are not fully integrated, the pharmacy will need to get a printout from the CPOE system and then re-enter the medication order into the pharmacy system. This situation introduces the potential for error during the transcription and product selection process. Even with full integration, the pharmacy often has to manipulate the order to facilitate processing parenteral products that require diluents, concentration, and other specific preparation and administration information necessary for accurate medication label generation.

Medication Order Entry

Pharmacy systems not using CPOE or not fully integrated with a CPOE system require separate entry of medication orders into the system to generate medication labels as well as to establish a medication profile for each patient. The patient profile has sections for demographic and medication information. Medication orders are entered into the system by using predefined commands or menu options to select the type of medication order. Usually, the type of medication order (IV piggybacks [IVPB], syringe medications, large-volume parenterals [LVP], and unit-dose products) determines the data input requirements and type of label that will be printed. Label requirements are different for IVPB, syringe medications, LVPs, and unit-dose products. In a medication section of the entry screen(s), the technician can use short codes or mnemonics for the medication (name, strength, and dosage form), medication and schedule, or groups of medications specific to a medical service or physician. Medication order entry can be time-consuming, but short codes speed the process by minimizing the number of keystrokes needed. The first few letters of a drug name can also be used to search medications, though this approach takes longer than the short-code approach.

Other information that must be entered manually or included in the short code is the medication administration schedule, the medication's start and stop date and time, charging information, label quantity, and any precautions or instructions that may be necessary for a label (e.g., protect from light).

After the medication order is entered, the pharmacy technician should make sure the right medication, dosing schedule, and dose were entered into the correct patient's profile. A pharmacist must verify medication orders entered by a technician before they can be active. Institutions use a variety of methods to identify the orders that are awaiting verification. Some computer systems highlight or use flashing for orders requiring verification. Pharmacy technicians should familiarize themselves with the system used at their institution.

Patient Medication Profiles
Patient medication profiles are usually organized by medication type or by order of input. Active medication orders should be listed first and separated from discontinued medications. Discontinued medications should only be available for review upon entering an appropriate command or at the end of the profile. Sorting capabilities may be available.

If profiles are arranged by medication type, the first section of the medication profile may list all scheduled unit-dose and bulk medications. The second section may list all scheduled IVPBs and syringe admixtures. The third section may list all prn medications. The fourth section may list all

LVPs. Discontinued medication orders would be last and sorted as above. Medication orders within a medication type might be listed alphabetically or from newest to oldest order. Also, it is desirable to have certain medication orders readily identifiable on the patient's profile because of the medication type, such as investigational drugs, restricted drugs, nonformulary drugs, and controlled substances (CS). Identification could be by a variety of means, such as the use of a heading or asterisks or sorting capabilities using the *dispense* category. The profile structure for a sample CPOE system is shown in **Figure 18-1**, and an example of the profile structure in the pharmacy system is depicted in **Figure 18-2**.

Work Lists
Work lists are used to perform a variety of pharmacy tasks. The typical pharmacy work list is used for unit-dose cart fill. The cart-fill work list extracts medication information from the patient profile to be used for dispensing medications for a patient. Work lists are also used for cart-fill updates, IV pick, IV fill, IV fill updates, and labels. Work lists contain patient-specific information, with the exception of pick lists. *Pick lists* contain the quantity of each medication needed to provide multiple patients with a supply of medications for a specified time period (e.g., 12 or 24 hours), including the quantity of IV solutions and additives/medications to meet the needs for small- and large-volume parenterals. Work lists can be printed daily or as often as necessary, depending on the computer software and the pharmacy's requirements. A 24-hour

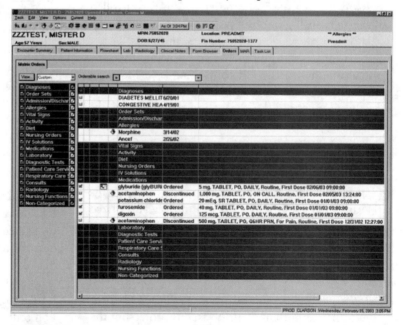

Figure 18-1. Profile Structure for CPOE System.

cart fill is common, but often IV admixtures are produced in batches (e.g., one batch per shift) to decrease waste. Other reports the pharmacy needs are admission, discharge, and transfer (ADT) notices to ensure that patient medications are delivered to the right place. Some pharmacy systems can generate medication administration records (MARs) that are primarily used by the nursing staff.

Ambulatory Care Prescription Functions

Like institutional pharmacies, ambulatory care pharmacies want to streamline workflow, reduce costs, increase efficiency and productivity, and decrease errors. Computers help realize these goals.

Generally, pharmacists struggle with finding enough time to provide the needed level of clinical services, such as patient counseling. Computers allow pharmacists to spend more time providing clinical services (pharmaceutical care). The type of information ambulatory care pharmacies manage is similar to the type inpatient pharmacies manage (e.g., patient drug profile, inventory management). Computer functions important to an ambulatory care pharmacy operation are shown in **Table 18-1**.

An important distinction between ambulatory care pharmacies and institutional pharmacies is that ambulatory care pharmacies are responsible for billing and collecting payment for their products, whereas institutional pharmacies may be responsible for billing, but not collecting payment. Ambulatory care pharmacies need payer and insurance carrier information and third-party billing functions as part of the computer

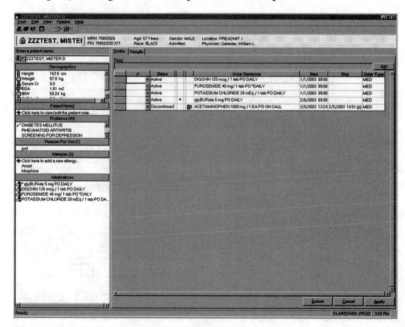

Figure 18-2. Profile Structure for Pharmacy System.

TABLE 18-1. AMBULATORY PHARMACY COMPUTER FUNCTIONS

Database Maintenance

1. Drug file (medications and IV solutions)
   a. Mnemonics
   b. Brand and generic name
   c. Price structure
2. Physician file
   a. Phone number
   b. Address
   c. Drug Enforcement Administration (DEA) number
3. Clinical monitoring
   a. Drug-drug, drug-food, drug-disease, drug-lab interactions
   b. Dose range checking
4. Payer and insurance information

Interfaces with Other Systems

Patient Information

1. Demographic information (age, address, phone, sex)
2. Allergies, weight, height, diagnosis
3. Insurance

Prescription Processing

1. Patient selection by
   a. Name
   b. Patient number
   c. Prescription number
2. Prescription information
   a. Medication name, dose, route, frequency, duration, and expiration date
   b. Quantity of medication and refills if allowed
   c. Comments and special instructions
   d. Patient education material
   e. Receipts
3. Pharmacist verification of orders entered by technicians
4. Label generation
5. Price inquiry

Management Functions

1. Distribution reports
   a. Narcotic use records
2. Financial reports
   a. Billing information
3. Workload data
4. File maintenance

database. These features allow the processing of insurance claims while the patient's prescription is being filled. Because health plans vary with regard to medications covered, copayment, and generic substitution requirements, computers are instrumental in preventing pharmacies from dispensing prescriptions that are not in accordance with the payer's insurance information.

In some cases, an ambulatory care pharmacy may have access to inpatient records of its affiliated organization and vice versa. Sharing information among practice settings promotes continuity of care because pharmacists in both settings can access their patient's drug profile to see what medications the patient was on as an inpatient or outpatient. Care must be taken when a patient is admitted to the hospital, however, because patients often receive their medications from more than one pharmacy. In such cases, the affiliated pharmacy's patient record may be incomplete.

Management Functions

Pharmacy departments are responsible for managing their resources effectively and controlling costs. Computers allow management and staff to generate reports that can help evaluate and improve workflow and medication use. Printed reports give management the opportunity to analyze and interpret data more thoroughly. Some common and valuable reports used by management include monitoring nonformulary drug use, drug usage patterns, drug costs, productivity, workload, and pharmacist interventions. Intervention data can be useful for justifying clinical pharmacist positions or additional resources. The most useful report details the type of intervention (e.g., prevention of medication error), time spent, dollar impact, and significance of the intervention (e.g., life-threatening situation). Unfortunately, most systems do not have built-in reports, so they must be "written" or developed, by the pharmacy department.

Patient-Monitoring Functions—Clinical Decision Support Systems

Basic Patient-Monitoring Functions

Many programs automatically perform some patient-monitoring functions or Clinical Decision Support System (CDSS) checks for therapeutic duplication, drug-allergy, drug-drug, drug-food, drug-disease, and drug-lab interactions and IV compat-

ibility. This functionality provides real-time alerts during the medication ordering process and also in the pharmacy dispensing process. CDSS provides important patient safeguards for medication use.

Therapeutic duplication checking detects patients on drugs in the same American Hospital Formulary Service (AHFS) pharmacologic-therapeutic classification or whether there is more than one order for the same medication.

Drug-allergy interaction checking alerts the user that he or she is attempting to order a drug that is recorded as an allergy in the patient's electronic medical record. The allergy program should provide sufficient detail of the type of reaction so that the prescriber can evaluate the reaction versus the need for the patient to receive the medication. If the detail is missing, further investigation is warranted before proceeding with the order. (See **Figure 18-3**.)

Drug-drug interaction checking identifies drugs in a patient's profile that may cause problems when taken concomitantly. For example, when amiodarone and warfarin are used together, amiodarone may inhibit hepatic metabolism of warfarin, resulting in potentially life-threatening bleeding complications (see **Figure 18-4**). The alert should provide appropriate information to address the interaction, such as a dose modification when one medication increases the elimination of another medication from the body. Some drug combinations cause only minor problems, and the benefit of the combination may outweigh the risks.

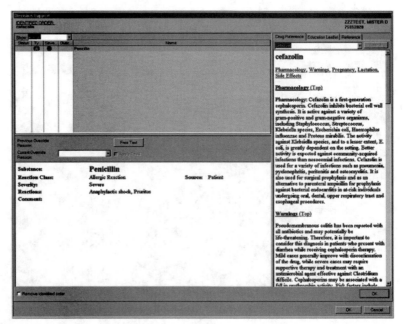

Figure 18-3. Drug-Allergy Alert.

Drug-food interaction checking informs the user that the patient has been prescribed a drug that may cause problems with certain foods. Often, certain foods will decrease the efficacy of a drug or increase the likelihood of an adverse reaction. This interaction notification serves as a prompt for the pharmacist or other health care professional to provide patient counseling or modify the drug regimen to minimize problems.

Drug-disease interaction checking identifies drugs that may cause problems with the patient's medical condition. For example, aspirin can increase the risk of bleeding and is generally contraindicated for patients with hemophilia.

Drug-lab interaction checking detects medication orders that might interfere with certain laboratory tests.

IV compatibility programs check medication orders for potential problems with physical incompatibilities (e.g., precipitation of ingredients or color changes) and stability of components (e.g., greater than 10 percent decomposition of one or more components in an admixture in 24 hours or less).

When a potential problem is detected, the user will receive an alert message. The user will make a determination based on the information presented and the patient's clinical situation and either proceed with the order, which is called *overriding the alert*, or cancel the order. Ideally, a CPOE system will allow the prescriber on the ordering side to document the action taken on the patient's electronic medical record when overriding

an alert. The pharmacist verifying orders on the dispensing side should receive the same alerts and be able to access prescriber reasons for overriding the order. The system may also offer the ability to print the interaction information and view or print a monograph related to the alert information.

Be aware that CDSS not only assists the pharmacy staff in providing quality patient care, as intended, but also has the potential to provide nuisance information. For example, IV incompatibility information programs may alert inappropriately or not provide suitable information. Therapeutic duplication checks often alert for appropriate drug therapy combinations. Sometimes manipulating the database settings in the medication formulary can decrease nuisance alerts. Eliminating nuisance alerts and providing relevant, detailed, patient-specific information will increase the likelihood that the clinician will consider the alert information in planning the patient's medication treatment. CDSS should be customizable by the institution. Alert generation is often customizable based on the severity of the interaction. Typically, interactions are classified as *minor, moderate,* and *severe.* The institution should be able to specify the severity level of the alerts that will be presented to the user, further decreasing the potential for nuisance alerts. Generally, severe alerts should be presented to all users. Some moderate alerts may be appropriate at specific institutions. As time progresses, the quality of these tools should improve as computer software suppliers receive feedback from users.

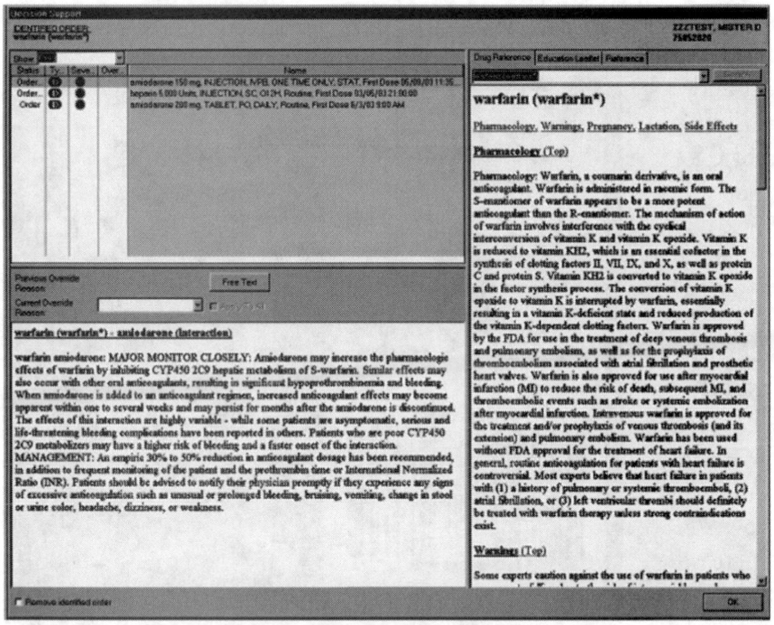

Figure 18-4. Drug-Drug Interaction Alert.

Additional Patient-Monitoring Functions

Other on-line patient-monitoring features include screening doses to make sure they do not exceed maximum dose or dosage range recommendations and screening for drugs that are contraindicated in patients who are pregnant or lactating. Institutions that use uncommon doses as part of protocols can customize dosing guidelines to suit specific populations (e.g., geriatrics, pediatrics, neonatology). Pharmacokinetic monitoring programs are also common. These programs use patient-specific data to generate dose and frequency recommendations.

An important patient-monitoring tool that has grown in popularity is on-line intervention documentation. Newer pharmacy systems are incorporating pharmacists' interventions as part of the order entry process. These systems guide the pharmacist through the pharmaceutical care model. On-line documentation promotes continuity of care by improving communication among staff members. This function may be part of a pharmacy stand-alone system, a mainframe system, or a system using handheld technology. The information can then be downloaded to a PC and incorporated into a spread-sheet or database program for analysis.

Inventory and Narcotic Control

Pharmacy technicians typically play an active role in inventory and narcotic control. Computerization of inventory functions is useful in tracking costs, purchases and usage, wastage, discarded or outdated inventory, and items loaned to or borrowed from other pharmacies. The ability to generate purchase orders when a preset medication-specific reorder point is reached ensures adequate stock. Vendor computer files are useful for keeping records of purchase agreements for minimum order quantity, price, price payment policy, and return goods policy.

Common narcotic control features are reports for daily CS use by patients, quantities dispensed to nursing units or pharmacy areas, and error and discrepancy records. Most systems provide separate controls for Schedule II drugs.

Computerized inventory records allow pharmacies to update their inventory upon receipt and dispersal, record and maintain records on all purchases of CS, and maintain records of expired CS. Appropriate security clearance is important for narcotic control records; access should be limited to the technicians and pharmacists involved with record keeping. Computerized narcotic accounting makes it easier to detect and investigate potential diversion. Automated dispensing systems (described later) can offer more control of CS than traditional lock and key systems. Systems that dispense by dose offer the greatest control.

Current Technology

The pharmacy must weigh all the costs associated with purchasing and implementing new technology against the expected benefits in terms of improved quality, safety, and efficiency, before deciding to put new equipment into practice. These technologies require informed, educated operators who understand how technology can be used. The goal should be to increase quality and reduce errors in the most cost-effective manner. Automation can allow departments to maintain or increase the level of service without significant

changes in staffing. The use of technology is much more likely to change the scope of a technician's responsibilities than result in job elimination. Current computer technology used in health care includes bar coding, touch screens, light pens, voice recognition, medication packagers and unit-dose apportionment systems, automated dispensing systems, process control devices, and paperless charting.

Bar Coding

Bar codes are a unique arrangement of lines (thick and thin) used to identify the item on which they are printed. Bar coding medications identifies the drug name, strength, dosage form, lot number, and expiration date of a particular drug product (see **Figure 18-5**). To translate the bar code, a handheld or fixed-position scanner is needed. Some community and institutional pharmacies use bar codes to save time and promote accuracy when performing tasks such as ordering, distributing, returning inventory, billing patients for drugs dispensed, crediting patients for drugs returned, and filling and checking unit-dose carts.

Bar codes can help health care teams to ensure that the patient receives the correct drug, dose, and dosage form via the correct route and at the correct time. To implement this system in an institutional setting, bar codes are assigned to each nurse, medication, and patient.[3] This process is called *point-of-care* and is considered by many patient safety groups as a major patient safety technology strategy. Before the nurse gives a dose to a patient, the nurse scans his or her bar code, the patient's bar code, and the medication bar

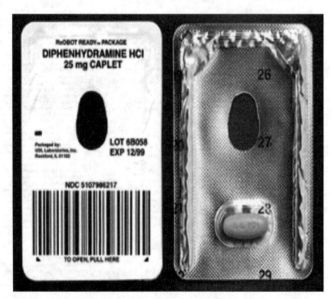

Figure 18-5. Example of a Bar-Coded Medication.

code. The system then verifies that the patient, medication, dose, and time are correct. If a discrepancy exists, such as a contraindication (e.g., allergy) or incorrect medication or patient, the system alerts the nurse. If the system does not identify any problems, the nurse administers the medication, and the system charts it as given.

Bar codes are also used in the ambulatory care setting to verify the accuracy of filled prescriptions. In this situation, the stock medication bottle, the prescription, and the prescription label are bar coded. The bar codes are then scanned to ensure that they match. If they do not, the pharmacist or technician is notified and the error is corrected.

Basically, bar codes present information in a manner that a computer can read. Although bar-coding systems accurately identify medications and patients, pharmacists and technicians should not rely on such systems completely. It is still important for pharmacists and technicians to check their work to ensure accuracy and appropriateness.

A major step forward in the patient safety technology arena regarding standardizing and requiring bar codes on medications was the announcement in March 2003 that the FDA rules will require bar coding for medications. A limitation is that the rule does not require lot number and expiration date be included in the code.

Input Devices: Touch Screens, Light Pens, and Mouse Technology

Touch-screen technology senses the location of a finger as it nears or touches a screen. Touch technology can be difficult for some people to use. It is most efficient in situations that require minimal input to get to the end result. Tools used in touch-screen technology, such as a stylus or pen, facilitate entry of data into small devices, such as handheld computers. Light pen technology is similar to touch-screen technology. A pen that contains a light-sensitive tip is used instead of a finger. Accuracy is similar to using a pen or stylus.

CPOE systems have used light pen technology, but most new systems require keypad input and mouse selections. The mouse allows one to control the computer by moving the mouse and pressing buttons. Traditional mouse devices have a ball made of rubber protruding from the underside, and, as the ball is dragged across a flat surface, the ball movement is sensed and a signal is sent to the CPU to indicate how far and in what direct the mouse has moved. The CPU then causes a pointer to move on the screen, reflecting the

movement of the mouse. It takes practice to be comfortable moving the mouse to the desired spot on the monitor. Buttons on top of the mouse are used to make selections once the pointer is at the desired spot on the monitor. The buttons produce a "click" sound when pushed and released. The terminology "point and click" refers to the process of using a mouse. Using a mouse allows the software to include a huge amount of data available by pointing an item on the screen and then clicking to enable drop-down lists to be viewed. Drop-down lists hide information that the user does not want to access in all situations, allowing the presentation of information on the screen to be less cluttered.

Voice Recognition

Voice recognition technology eliminates the need to use a keyboard to enter data. The goal of voice-input systems is for the system to recognize any person speaking. Currently, most applications must be "trained" to recognize a particular voice and a limited number of words. Voice recognition technology is primarily used by physicians to transcribe patient discharge summaries. Some PC software packages use this technology already, and it could be useful for documenting pharmacists' interventions or patient education in medical records.

Automated Packaging and Unit-Dose Apportionment Systems

Computerization has improved the unit-dose packaging process tremendously. Computers make unit-dose packaging more efficient because they can save templates for medications, thereby reducing variations and increasing safety. In addition, most computer systems used for packaging can produce labels with bar codes and keep records to be used for quality assurance purposes.

System Access

To access the system, employees must enter a code. The menu of options or available functionality accessible to each employee can be controlled to provide the desired level of security. The pharmacy computer system administrator usually assigns options, security, and codes based on the job responsibilities of the pharmacy employees. A variety of functions can be performed on a patient- or unit-specific basis and can be traced to an individual transaction. The actual dispensing of medications may be by single dose, or the system may allow access to limited quantities. Single-dose dispensing devices are less error prone than systems that allow access to multiple drugs.

Technician Roles

Usually, technicians assume most of the responsibilities for operating and stocking the devices, allowing the pharmacist to spend more time on clinical activities. Pharmacists are, however, involved in the checking procedures and often in the quality assurance activities associated with the equipment.

Automated Dispensing Systems—Inpatient

Traditional unit-dose drug distribution systems are very labor-intensive. The use of automation in this area is an important issue for hospital pharmacy departments. Automated dispensing systems, which are storage, dispensing, and charging devices for medications, save time and allow better control and tracking of inventory. The different systems vary in storage capacity, amount of space needed for the device(s), functionality, cost, and the ability to store refrigerated medications.[4] These systems have two broad applications: decentralized (e.g., Pyxis MedStation, Omnicell Sure-Med, McKesson Acudose-Rx) and centralized (e.g., AutoMed Efficiency Pharmacy, McKesson Robot-Rx).

Decentralized Systems

Decentralized systems are located in the patient care unit and usually contain floor stock medication and supplies and CS. The systems are designed to solve medication management problems, such as lost billing charges, pilferage, narcotic diversion, and poor record keeping.[5] Health care professionals use automated dispensing systems to dispense medications, return medications, record medication waste, and generate reports, among other things. For these reasons, these systems could replace or supplement manual unit-dose systems.

Centralized Systems

Centralized systems are located in the central pharmacy and are used to improve the manual unit-dose cart-fill process. Currently, these systems cannot accommodate all dosage forms because of size or the need for refrigeration, so manual cart-fill systems must supplement these devices.

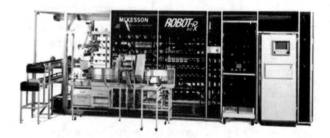

Figure 18-6. McKesson Robot-RX.

The AutoMed ATC produces packaged patient-specific doses of oral solid medications, using bulk medications that are unit-dosed at the time of dispensing. The system will print a pick list for items not stocked in the device and is capable of interfacing to receive patient-specific data. Technicians are primarily responsible for stocking and operating this device.

Robotic Cart Fill

The McKesson Robot-Rx is another type of centralized system that combines bar-code technology, a network system of microcomputers, a conveyor system, and a robot to pick drugs and place them into patient medication drawers or envelopes (see **Figure 18-6**). The cart-fill process for this system has a high degree of accuracy. The system can generate bar-coded labels for patient identification (ID) and medication drawer location. If the patient has moved, the system generates an alert and then prints a new bar-code-printed name label if appropriate. The system will check the patient's profile and request that the drawer be placed on the conveyor if the patient has medications to be refilled. The system scans the patient ID bar code, and then the robotic arm delivers the appropriate medications to the drawer. A manual fill list is generated for items not in the inventory. Return medications can be credited to a patient by scanning the medication and the patient bar code under the credit function.

Technicians typically are responsible for complete operation of the robotic dispensing system, including packaging, stocking, inventory control, cart fill, manual fill, and troubleshooting. **Table 18-2** lists advantages and disadvantages to inpatient automation.

Process Control Devices

Computerized pumps are often used in the IV admixture area of institutional pharmacies to prepare adult and neonatal total parenteral nutrition (TPN). These pumps prepare the base solution and add electrolytes and micronutrients. Other computerized pumps are available to fill batches of syringes.

Technicians are usually involved in the operation of these devices. Some common responsibilities include entering patient orders into the system, setting up the correct medication solutions, setting up log sheets for quality assurance purposes, and operating the device.

Paperless Charting

Paperless charting involves an electronic patient medical record. Documentation consumes an excessive amount of the health care professional's time, and automation of the process should provide caregivers with more time for patient care. Many hospitals have

TABLE 18-2. ADVANTAGES AND DISADVANTAGES OF INPATIENT AUTOMATION

Advantages	Disadvantages
Centralized Automation	
Improved accuracy based on bar-code recognition	Cost of the equipment
Improved efficiency of dispensing functions	May require remodeling and other costs
Cost savings based on purchasing drugs in bulk rather than unit dose	Some systems do not have the ability to stock certain drugs, such as injectables, bulk products, or refrigerated items
Ability to track expiration dates	
Improved inventory management and dispensing activity reporting capability	
Reduced time commitment for pharmacists checking dispensing functions	
Decentralized Automation	
Improved accuracy based on bar-code recognition	Cost of the equipment
Ability to perform dispensing functions in batch mode instead of "on demand," yielding improved efficiency of dispensing	May require remodeling and other costs
Improved inventory management and dispensing activity reporting capability	
Ability to track expiration dates	
Reduced order turnaround time by moving inventory to the point-of-care	

installed bedside terminals for nursing documentation. Also, handheld computers and rolling carts with computer terminals are being used increasingly to facilitate real-time documentation of nursing activities, including medication administration and patient response to medications. The system offers on-line availability of the patient's chart and entire history to any number of people simultaneously. Remote access enhances availability of valuable patient information for physicians who may be called at home or other practice sites. On-line medical records would be ideal for audits, drug use evaluations, and retrospective studies.

Automated Dispensing Systems—Outpatient

The McKesson Productivity Station is an example of an automated dispensing system used in the ambulatory care setting to increase efficiency and improve accuracy in prescription filling and dispensing. Functionality generally includes counting and prefilling prescription vials of common medications. The system uses bar-code technology to verify medication information.

Many of the same advantages and disadvantages of inpatient systems also apply to outpatient technology. Efficiency and accuracy are improved, enabling pharmacists to apply more time to clinical functions and less to routine checking tasks. The systems may, however, be very expensive, and generally a baseline number of prescriptions per day must be processed to make the equipment a cost-effective purchase.

Personal Digital Assistant

A personal digital assistant (PDA) is a computer that fits in the palm of your hand. Other common names are *palm* and *handheld* (see **Figure 18-7**). Their main purpose is to carry your PIM (personal information manager) applications and data: address book, calendar, notes, and tasks. PDAs have touch screens that respond to a stylus, pen, or finger—although touch-screen resolution is often poor. The stylus is used to navigate the screen, enter data using an on-screen keyboard, and enter information using handwriting recognition. Handwriting recognition involves learning how to write letters and numbers so that the PDA will recognize them. Small keyboards are available to attach to the PDA. Software programs are available for the PDA so health care professionals can look at comprehensive drug information just by reaching into their pockets. Internet capability makes PDAs useful for accessing patient records.

Conclusion

Computers are everywhere. Children learn how to use them at an early age, and computer knowledge is a valuable resource for any job. Computer courses are

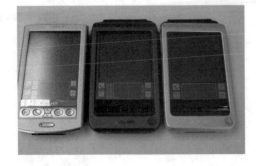

Figure 18-7. Palm PDAs.

available at most community colleges, which often have convenient locations, and some large organizations may offer computer courses for their employees at no cost. In addition to the more traditional responsibilities that technicians perform, they play an important role in managing a variety of computerized systems and automation technologies so pharmacists have more time for direct patient-care activities.

Computers can handle a wide variety of functions. Every year technology will expand to include more applications for pharmacy and health care. Technicians can expect to see their roles change as new technologies are developed in health care.

Recommended Reading

Blissmer RH. Introducing computers—concepts, systems, and applications. New York: John Wiley & Sons, Inc.; 1992–1993.

Kinkoph S et al. Computers—a visual encyclopedia. Indianapolis, IN: Alpha Books; 1994.

References

1. Superior Consultant Company. 14th annual HIMSS leadership survey. February 2003.

2. Crawford SY, Myers CE. ASHP national survey of hospital-based pharmaceutical services—1992. *Am J Hosp Pharm.* 1993; 50:1371–404.

3. Hynniman CE. Drug product distribution systems and departmental operations. *Am J Hosp Pharm.* 1991; 48:S24–35.

4. Perini VJ, Vermeulen LC. Comparison of automated medication-management systems. *Am J Hosp Pharm.* 1994; 51:1883–91.

5. Lee LW, Wellman GS, Birdwell SW, Sherrin TP. Use of an automated medication storage and distribution system. *Am J Hosp Pharm.* 1992; 49:851–5.

Self-Assessment Questions

1. Which of the following describes mainframe computers?
   a. large
   b. expensive
   c. powerful
   d. all of the above

2. Dumb terminals have all of the following characteristics *except* which one?
   a. inexpensive
   b. function as personal computers on their own
   c. useful for a large number of people to access the system
   d. can be hooked up to mainframe systems

3. Personal computers have all of the following characteristics *except* which one?
   a. can be used as a stand-alone system
   b. useful for word processing
   c. cannot run software programs
   d. can manage data from a mainframe

4. An interface is *not* which one of the following?
   a. a connection between two or more computer systems
   b. necessary for the transfer of data between systems
   c. unidirectional only
   d. valuable for receiving information from other systems

5. Responsibilities of technicians that can be enhanced by automation include which of the following?
   a. cartfilling
   b. floor stock replacement
   c. IV admixing and prepackaging
   d. all of the above

6. Which of the following statements is true?
   a. Technicians can gather data for quality assurance activities and use computers to organize and input data.
   b. Only pharmacists can gather data for quality assurance activities and use computers to input data.
   c. Technicians can be responsible for data collection only.
   d. Technicians cannot collect data but can use computers to input data for report generation.

7. Which of the following statements is *not* true?
   a. Pharmacy stand-alone systems must have an interface to the hospital mainframe to display patient demographic information.
   b. Pharmacy systems require a database to input patient data.
   c. Interfaces can supply laboratory results to the pharmacy system.
   d. Manual data input is simplified with the use of mnemonics.

8. Which of the following statements regarding medication entries to a patient profile is *not* true?
   a. Short codes and mnemonics speed up the order entry process.
   b. There are separate pathways to enter different medication types.
   c. Typing in part of the drug name can search medications.
   d. The use of mnemonics prevents the wrong medication from being entered on a patient's profile.

9. Information needed on the patient's medication profile includes all the following *except* which one?
   a. start date of the medication
   b. name and strength of the medication
   c. social history of the patient
   d. route of administration for each medication order

10. Which of the following statements is true regarding technician-entered medication orders?
    a. Technicians are not allowed to enter medication orders.
    b. Technician-entered medication orders are active immediately.
    c. Highlighting or flashing is used to identify technician-entered medication orders.
    d. Once a medication order has been entered by a technician, a pharmacist cannot modify it.

11. Which of the following statements concerning sign-on or access codes is true?
    a. Everyone uses the same code.
    b. Sign-ons identify the individual using the system.
    c. All pharmacy staff have the same level of security assigned to their access code.
    d. A technician need not sign off before someone else uses the same terminal.

12. Which of the following common work lists can be computer generated?
    a. cart fill
    b. IV fill
    c. cart fill pick
    d. all of the above

13. Goals for automation in the ambulatory care setting include all of the following *except* which one?
    a. streamline workflow
    b. increase productivity
    c. increase efficiency
    d. increase costs

14. The information needs of an ambulatory care pharmacy include the following *except* which one?
    a. third-party billing database
    b. price inquiry
    c. copayment amounts
    d. patient room number

15. Which of the following statements regarding management reports is *not* true?
    a. Intervention reports can be used to help justify pharmacist positions.
    b. Report features are always built into the systems.
    c. Data generated from a report could be used to redesign workflow.
    d. Commercially available software is available to simplify the report generation process.

16. Automation can provide on-line clinical monitoring for which of the following?
    a. drug-drug, drug-food, drug-disease, and drug-lab interactions
    b. IV incompatibilities
    c. therapeutic duplication
    d. all of the above

17. The following statements regarding on-line intervention documentation are true *except* which one?
    a. provides continuity of care
    b. allows information to be downloaded for report generation
    c. provides a communication tool for other pharmacy staff
    d. is only available on mainframe systems

18. Inventory control system advantages include all of the following *except* which one?

a. tracks purchases
b. tracks medication usage
c. tracks inventory costs
d. tracks personnel expenditures

19. The following statements concerning narcotic control are true *except* which one?
    a. A separate control system for Class II drugs is not desirable.
    b. Access to records should be restricted.
    c. Record maintenance of narcotic purchases is desirable.
    d. Automated dispensing systems are frequently used for narcotic control.

20. The following statements regarding the use of automation are true *except* which one?
    a. Automation can change the scope of a technician's responsibilities.
    b. Automation requires informed, educated operators.
    c. Automation increases the potential for errors.
    d. Automation can increase quality.

21. Which of the following statements is true regarding the use of bar coding?
    a. Bar codes require the use of a scanner to "read" the bar-code information
    b. Bar codes can identify products only.
    c. Scanners must be in a fixed position.
    d. Bar coding is not useful for inventory control.

22. Touch-screen technology has all of the following characteristics *except* which one?
    a. The technology senses the location of a finger as it nears or touches the screen.
    b. A stylus or pen can be used on touch screens.
    c. Touch-screen technology has a high resolution.
    d. Light pen systems are more accurate than finger systems.

23. Mouse technology includes all of the following characteristics *except* which one?
    a. dragging the device across a flat surface
    b. pressing buttons to select an item
    c. making a "bell ringing" sound
    d. causing a pointer to move on the screen

24. Characteristics of voice recognition technology include all of the following *except* which one?
    a. Most systems accommodate a particular voice only.
    b. The technology recognizes a limited vocabulary.

Self-Assessment Questions

c. Voice recognition could eventually replace manual entry of data.

d. Such technology has no application in health care.

25. What is(are) the advantage(s) of newer automated packagers?
    a. computer-generated labels
    b. programming sets up packaging and labeling
    c. automated labeling can be bar coded
    d. all of the above

26. Characteristics of automated dispensing systems include all of the following *except* which one?
    a. Automated dispensing systems are storage, dispensing, and charging devices.
    b. Decentralized automated dispensing systems are not useful for tracking inventory.
    c. All functions are performed on a patient-specific basis.
    d. The system requires entry of patient medication orders unless obtained from an interface.

27. Disadvantages of a central automated dispensing system using robotics include all of the following *except* which one?
    a. Expired drugs must be manually removed from the system.
    b. Special medication cassettes are required.
    c. A special packager is required.
    d. Special packages are required.

28. Automated dispensing systems using robotics require bar coding for all of the following *except* which one?
    a. patient location label
    b. medications
    c. system operator
    d. patient ID label

29. Advantages of automated dispensing systems using robotics include all of the following *except* which one?
    a. Pharmacist checking of medication cassettes is quick using the bar-code scanner.
    b. Returned medications can be easily credited by scanning the patient ID label and the medication.

c. A high degree of accuracy for filled medications can be achieved.

d. The system restocks itself.

30. Process control devices can do which of the following?
    a. prepare base solutions for TPNs
    b. add electrolytes and micronutrients to TPNs
    c. batch fill syringes
    d. all of the above

31. Features of paperless charting include all of the following *except* which one?
    a. potential to decrease the amount of time the nurse can provide patient care
    b. on-line availability of the patient medical record
    c. ideal for obtaining data for audits
    d. bedside terminals keep the nurse by the patient

Assessment Answers

1. d. Mainframe computers are large, expensive, powerful computers, designed to process large amounts of data.
2. b. Dumb terminals are useless on their own.
3. c. Personal computers are stand-alone systems that can run software programs and manage data accessed from a larger source.
4. c. An interface can be uni- or bidirectional. Unidirectional interfaces send data to another system but cannot receive input back; bidirectional interfaces can send data back and forth.
5. d. Technicians' roles include cart filling, floor stock replacement, IV admixing, and repacking, all of which are enhanced by the use of automation.
6. a. Increasingly, technicians perform a variety of quality assurance activities, which frees pharmacists for clinical activities.
7. a. An interface is not necessary to display this information. If an interface is not present, however, this information must be entered manually.
8. d. The only thing that will prevent the wrong medication from being entered on a patient's medication profile is careful entering and checking by technicians and pharmacists.
9. c. Patients' medication profiles contain medication information, such as name and strength, start date, and the route of the medication. Social history of the patient (e.g., married, single) is included in the patient's medical record.
10. c. Technician-entered medication orders must be identifiable by the pharmacist and highlighting or flashing often identifies such orders.
11. b. It is important that the technician sign off immediately when he or she is finished so that no one else uses his or her code.
12. d. Work lists, such as cart fill, IV fill, and cart fill pick, are used by technicians to identify tasks to be completed.
13. d. Increasing costs is not a goal in the use of automation; however, decreasing cost is one of the goals.
14. d. Patient room numbers are used in institutional pharmacies, not ambulatory care pharmacies.
15. b. Reports usually must be developed by the pharmacy.
16. d. Computers are capable of screening medication orders at the time of order entry for drug-drug, drug-food, drug-disease, drug-lab interactions, IV incompatibilities, and therapeutic duplication.
17. d. Intervention programs can be on mainframes interfaced to PCs or on a pharmacy stand-alone system without an interface.
18. d. Inventory control programs track issues related to medications, not personnel.
19. a. A separate control system for Class II drugs is advisable because of the record keeping required for Class IIs.
20. c. Although errors can occur with any system, manual or automated, automated systems are likely to decrease the potential for errors.
21. a. Scanners are needed to read bar codes and may be hand held or in a fixed position, such as mounted into a tabletop, and items are waved over the top of the scanner to be read.
22. c. Poor resolution is one of the disadvantages.
23. c. Mouse activation makes a "clicking" sound, thus the terms *right-click* and *left-click*.
24. d. Voice recognition technology has very important applications for health care. In the future, technology will be so advanced that a system will be able to recognize any voice input and convert it to the printed word. Health care professionals are likely to use this technology to document information in a patient's medical record.
25. d. Labels previously were prepared manually. Computers can be used to set up packaging and labeling, with provisions for bar coding labels if desired.
26. b. Automated dispensing systems are very useful for tracking inventory. The systems track dispensed medications, returned medications, wasted medications, and individual transactions.
27. a. Expired drugs are removed automatically when the robotic arm reads the medication's bar code.
28. c. During the cart-fill process, bar coding of the medication, patient ID label, and patient

location allow the robot to pick the right medication for the right patient in the right location.

29. a. The bar-code check of the filled cassette is very time consuming. Because of the system's high degree of accuracy, it may soon be possible to eliminate the pharmacist check of machine-filled medications. Manual picks would still require a pharmacist's check.

30. d. Process control devices are computerized pumps that assist in the preparation of IV admixtures.

31. a. Increasing nursing time for patient care is a major advantage.

GLOSSARY

Absorption: The entering of drug into the systemic circulation (the bloodstream), as opposed to the administration of an intact drug formulation into the body.

Accreditation: The process of granting recognition or vouching for conformance with established criteria (usually refers to recognition of an institution).

Additive: Any ingredient introduced into a previously sealed bag or vial; usually a medication.

Addressograph: A raised-letter registration card similar to a credit card and used to imprint patient information on a document.

Admixture: The process of combining ingredients or components in an effort to produce a final product with desired characteristics.

Aerosol: A suspension of very fine liquid or solid particles distributed in a gas and packaged under pressure.

Air Embolus: A phenomenon that results from air entering the body's circulation and obstructing blood flow. Air may enter the circulation as a result of injury, surgery, or intravenous infusion.

Albumin: An important blood protein that binds many medications.

Alcoholic Solution: A nonaqueous solution that contains alcohol but no water.

Antigen: A substance that is capable of causing the production of an antibody.

Apparent Volume of Distribution: The size of a hypothetical compartment necessary to account for the total amount of drug in the body if it were present throughout the body at the same concentration found in the plasma.

Arithmetic Mean: A value that is calculated by dividing the sum of a set of numbers by the total numbers in the set.

Aseptic Technique: The technique and procedures designed to preclude contamination (of drugs, packaging, equipment, or supplies) by microorganisms during processing.

Autoimmunity: A misdirected immune response that happens when the body attacks itself.

Automated Dispensing System: An automated system used to increase efficiency and improve accuracy in prescription filling and dispensing.

Bar Codes: A unique arrangement of lines (thick and thin) used to identify the item on which they are printed.

Batch: A method of grouping like types of work to improve efficiency.

Batch Preparation: Compounding of multiple sterile-product units, in a single discrete process, by the same individual(s), carried out during one limited time period.

Bedside Terminals: Computer access that is available in either a fixed location at the patient's bedside or can be transported to that location for use.

Bi-directional Interface: An interface that allows data to be sent back and forth from system to system.

Biometric Access: The use of biological features such as fingerprints or retinal scans as a method of providing appropriate access to secure devices.

Biopharmaceutics: The study of the relationship of the physicochemical properties and behavior of drugs (under laboratory conditions, not in the body) and drug products on the delivery of the drugs to the body.

Brand Name: A name trademarked by a pharmaceutical manufacturer for their version of a given drug product.

Buccal Route of Administration: A buccal tablet placed inside the pouch of the cheek, where the medication dissolves and is absorbed through the cheek lining into the bloodstream over time.

Capitation: A set payment amount per patient per month or per hospital admission regardless of the health and related expenses associated with the patient's care.

Capsule: A solid medication dosage form in which the drug, with or without inactive or inert ingredients, is contained within a hard or soft gelatin shell.

Care Plan: The treatment plan that is outlined for the patient based upon input from the physician, pharmacist, nurse, patient/caregiver, and other health care professionals as required.

Carrying Cost (also known as **Holding Cost**): All costs associated with inventory investment and storage costs.

Catheter: A hollow tube of variable length and bore, usually having one fluted end and a tip of varying size and shape according to function. It is used to infuse fluids and/or drugs in patients receiving intravenous therapy. Blood may also be withdrawn from it in some cases for laboratory work.

Centralized Automation: A system that is located in the central pharmacy and used to improve the efficiency and accuracy of dispensing functions.

Centralized Pharmacy Services: Centralized pharmacy services, as the name implies, that manage and provide pharmacy personnel, resources, and functions from a central location.

Certification: A voluntary process by which a nongovernmental agency or association grants recognition to an individual who has met certain predetermined qualifications specified by that agency or association. This recognition demonstrates to the public that the certified individual has achieved a certain level of knowledge, skill, or experience.

Chain Pharmacy: One of a corporate-owned group of pharmacies.

Chart: The patient's medical record. This contains a complete record of all of the activities that occur, including a summary of the patient's medication therapy.

Clean Room: A room in which the concentration of airborne particles is controlled and there are one or more clean zones. (A clean zone is a defined space in which the concentration of airborne particles is controlled to meet a specified airborne-particulate cleanliness class.) Clean rooms are classified based on the maximum number of allowable particles 0.5 mcm and larger per cubic foot of air. For example, the air particle count in a Class 100 clean room may not exceed a total of 100 particles of 0.5 mcm and larger per cubic foot of air.

Clinical Decision Support System (CDSS): Patient monitoring functions that provide screening checks for drug interactions and possible errors and suggest alternatives based on pre-defined rules.

Clinic Pharmacy: A pharmacy located in a physician office or clinic building and filling prescriptions for patients' self-use.

Closed-system Transfer: The movement of sterile products from one container to another in which the container-closure system and transfer devices remain intact throughout the entire transfer process, compromised only by the penetration of a sterile, pyrogen-free needle or cannula through a designated stopper or port to effect transfer, withdrawal, or delivery.

Collodion: A liquid preparation of pyroxylin (found in cotton fibers) dissolved in ethyl ether and ethanol. After application to the skin, the ether and ethanol evaporate and leave a pyroxylin film.

Community Pharmacy: Stand-alone business that fills prescriptions, sells a variety of nonprescription products (e.g., cough and cold preparations, toiletries), and counsels patients about proper use of their medications.

Compounding: The mixing of substances to prepare a medication for patient use. This activity would include dilution, admixture, repackaging, reconstitution, and other manipulations of sterile products, as well as a variety of non-sterile preparations.

Computerized Compounding Pump: A tool used to prepare total parenteral nutrition (TPN) and fill batches of syringes.

Computerized Prescriber Order Entry (CPOE): Software that allows the input of medication and other orders into an electronic patient medical record by the prescriber.

Coring: Introducing particulate matter (in the form of a plastic or rubber "core" or plug) into a sterile fluid through the process of penetrating the outer seal of a vial or bag with a needle.

Cream: A semisolid emulsion that may or may not contain medication.

Creatinine: A bodily product found in the blood when muscle is broken down.

Creatinine Clearance: The clearance of creatinine from the blood by the kidneys that can serve to estimate the clearance of medication also filtered by the kidneys. This value may be measured directly from the amount of creatinine in urine over a 24-hour period or estimated using a formula and based on a single measurement of creatinine in the serum.

Credentialing: The process of formally verifying and assessing professional or technical competence through a voluntary, non-governmental method.

Critical Site: An opening providing a direct pathway between a sterile product and the environment or any surface coming in contact with the product or environment.

Critical Surface: Any surface that comes into contact with previously sterilized products or containers.

Database: A store of computerized information organized in such a way to facilitate information searches and the creation of reports.

Decentralized Automation: An automated system located in the patient care area that improves the efficiency of drug and supply distribution by housing the inventory in the area where it is used.

Decentralized Pharmacy Services: Pharmacy services provided from within a patient care area. The most common form of decentralized pharmacy is a pharmacy satellite. A pharmacy satellite is a designated area where drugs are stored, prepared, and dispensed for a segment of the total patient population.

Diastole: The heart muscle is relaxed and the chambers are filling with blood; the pressure is at the lowest point in the normal heart, represented by the second number in a blood pressure reading.

Digestion: The process whereby ingested food is broken up into smaller molecules by chemical or mechanical means.

Dispense as Written (DAW): A designation on a prescription or medication order that obligates the pharmacist to dispense the exact brand written for in the order.

Douche: A solution that is directed into a body cavity or against a part of the body to clean or disinfect.

Drug-allergy Interaction Checking: A computerized system of identifying medications that are recorded as an allergy in the patient's electronic medical record and comparing that information against newly ordered medications to provide alerts during order entry.

Drug-disease Interaction Checking: A computerized system of identifying medications that may cause problems with the patient's medical condition as recorded in the electronic medical record and providing alerts during order entry.

Drug-drug Interaction Checking: A computerized system of identifying medications in a patient's profile that may cause problems when taken concomitantly and providing alerts during order entry.

Drug-food Interaction Checking: A computerized system of identifying medications that may cause problems with certain foods and providing alerts during order entry.

Drug-lab Interaction Checking: A computerized system of identifying medications that may interfere with laboratory tests and providing alerts during order entry.

Drug Usage (Utilization) Evaluation (DUE): An organized study or review of medication use. (Also called medication usage/utilization evaluation.)

Drug Wholesaler: An independent wholesale company that provides the pharmacy with various services related to the procurement, scheduled delivery, and inventory management of pharmaceuticals.

Dumb Terminals: An inexpensive way for a large number of users to access information from a central computer's memory through a mainframe system without providing personal computers at each user location.

Economic Order Quantity (EOQ): An inventory management method also known as Minimum Cost Quantity. It is an accounting formula used to determine the order quantity that minimizes order costs and inventory holding costs.

Elimination: The irreversible removal of drug from the body by all routes, whether it be metabolized by the liver or excreted by the kidney.

Elixir: A clear, sweet, flavored hydroalcoholic solution for oral ingestion.

Emulsion: A mixture of two liquids that normally do not mix where one liquid is broken into small particles and evenly scattered throughout the other. The liquid present in small particles is referred to as the internal phase; the other liquid is called the external, or continuous, phase. An oil-in-water (O/W) emulsion consists of small oil globules dispersed throughout water; a water-in-oil (W/O) emulsion is the reverse: water droplets are distributed throughout the oil.

Endocrine: The internal secretion of a substance into the systemic circulation (bloodstream).

Endocrine Glands: Glands that have no ducts, their secretions being absorbed directly into the blood.

Enema: A solution introduced into the rectum to empty the bowel or to treat diseases of the lower gastrointestinal tract.

Expiration Date: The date (and time, when applicable) beyond which a product should not be used (i.e., the product should be discarded beyond this date and time).

Extract: An alcoholic or hydro-alcoholic extractive solution whose potency is two to six times that of the crude drug.

Extractive: A concentrated preparation of active components extracted from dried plant or animal tissue by soaking it in a solvent. The solvent is then evaporated, leaving the active component behind. Tinctures, fluidextracts, and extracts are examples of formulations prepared in this manner and differ from each other only in their potency.

Extravasation: Discharge or escape of fluid from a blood vessel into the surrounding tissue.

Failure Mode and Effects Analysis (FMEA): A systematic review of a system or process to identify steps where errors may occur and where opportunities for improvement can be made.

Fee-for-service: A payment mechanism in which the patient or the patient's insurance carrier pays the pharmacy directly based upon the service provided.

First Pass Metabolism: The metabolism of drugs by the liver or intestines before reaching the systemic circulation.

Floor Stock: Medications kept in a secured/controlled space in the patient care area for use as first doses, emergency, or convenience medications.

Fluidextract: An alcoholic or hydroalcoholic extractive solution whose potency is adjusted so that each milliliter of fluidextract contains the equivalent of 1000 mg of crude drug.

Formulary: An organized list of drugs approved for use in an organization, or by a prescription drug benefit plan. Also a list of drugs approved by a third party for reimbursement.

Gargle: A solution that treats conditions of the throat. The gargle is held in the throat as the patient gurgles air through the solution.

Gel: A thick, viscous suspension of undissolved drugs in water similar to a magma or milk except that the suspended particle size in gels is smaller.

Generic Name: A name applied to a unique chemical entity without respect to manufacturer. Portions of the name may indicate the class or type of drug represented by the entity (such as the –olol ending associated with the class of drugs known as beta blockers).

Glycerite: A nonaqueous solution that uses glycerin as a solvent, vehicle, or both.

Gonads: Reproductive organs—testes in the male, and ovaries in the female. Gonads function to produce reproductive cells and sex hormones.

Granule: A powder that has been wetted, dried, and ground into coarse pieces.

Handwriting Recognition: The ability of a personal digital assistant, or other computer input device, to recognize letters and numbers through a touch screen.

HEPA Filter: A high-efficiency particulate air (HEPA) filter composed of pleats of filter medium separated by rigid sheets of corrugated paper or aluminum foil that direct the flow of air forced through the filter in a uniform parallel flow. HEPA filters remove 99.97% of all air particles 0.3 mcm or larger. When HEPA filters are used as a component of a horizontal- or vertical-laminar-airflow hood, an environment can be created that is consistent with standards for a Class 100 cleanroom.

HIPAA: Stands for Health Insurance Portability and Accountability Act. Requires health care providers to maintain the privacy of patients' health information.

Home Infusion Therapy: Administration of various intravenous medications and fluids in the home care setting as opposed to the hospital or institutional setting.

Hormone: A chemical substance produced in the body that controls and regulates the activity of certain cells or organs. Usually, it is a chemical made by a gland for export to another part of the body; it is not active at its site of synthesis.

Hydro-alcoholic Solution: A nonaqueous solution that contains a mixture of alcohol and water.

Implant: A medication pump or device inserted semi-permanently or permanently into the body to treat a chronic or long-term condition or disease. Medication is released from the implant and delivered in a controlled fashion.

Incident Report/Occurrence Report: A confidential report, usually initiated by the first person that discovers a medication error, and containing information regarding the patient name, date, time, location, medication, nature of the error or reaction, treatment, and prescriber.

Infiltrate: The diffusion or accumulation in a tissue of substances that are not normally found there.

Inhalant: A fine powder or solution of a drug delivered as a mist through the mouth into the respiratory tract.

Integrated Health Care Systems: Also referred to as integrated delivery networks or IDNs. With an IDN, various hospitals, institutions, or facilities act in concert as a group to provide care via a system wide approach.

Interfaces: Connections between two or more computer systems that enable data to be transferred.

Intra-arterial (IA) Route of Administration: Medication is administered directly into an artery.

Intra-articular Route of Administration: Medication is injected into a joint, such as a knee or elbow.

Intradermal (ID) Route of Administration: Medication is injected into the top layers of the skin. ID injections are not injected as deep as those given subcutaneously.

Intramuscular (IM) Route of Administration: Direct injection of medication into a large muscle mass where the drug is then absorbed from the muscle tissue into the bloodstream.

Intravenous Push: Administration of intravenous medications using a syringe and given over a predefined time ranging anywhere from 2 minutes up to 15 minutes. Only certain medications may be given by this method.

Intravenous (IV) Route of Administration: Medications are introduced into the body through a needle placed directly in a vein.

Intrathecal Route of Administration: Drugs are injected into the space around the spinal cord.

Inventory Turnover Rate: A calculation used to determine the relative efficiency of the pharmaceutical purchasing/inventory process compared to utilization. It is generally performed using the total drug purchases within a predefined period of time and the aggregate value of pharmaceutical inventory taken at a random time (often at the end of the fiscal year). It is described by the mathematical equation: (Total Purchases/Inventory).

Irrigating Solution: A solution used to wash or cleanse part of the body such as the eyes, urinary bladder, open wounds, or abraded skin similar to a douche but used in larger volumes and over larger areas of the body for a more general cleansing than a douche.

IV Compatibility Checking: A computerized system of identifying medications for potential problems with physical incompatibilities (e.g., precipitation of ingredients or color changes) and providing alerts during order entry.

Jelly: A semisolid solution that contains a high proportion of water.

Keypad Input: Use of a keypad or keyboard to input information into a system.

Legend Drug: A drug that can only be dispensed upon the prescription of a physician or other licensed prescriber.

Licensure: The process by which an agency of government grants permission to an individual to engage in a given occupation upon finding that the individual applicant has attained the minimal degree of competency necessary to ensure that the public health, safety, and welfare will be reasonably well protected.

Light Pen Technology: Technology that senses the location of a handheld pen with a light-sensitive tip as it nears or touches a screen.

Liniment: A medication dosage form applied to the skin with friction and rubbing. Liniments may be solutions, emulsions, or suspensions.

Lotion: A suspension intended for external application that contains finely powdered medications to cool, soothe, dry, or protect the skin.

Lozenge: A hard disk-shaped solid medication dosage form that contains medication in a sugar base. Also known as troche or pastille.

Lumen: The space inside a tubular structure such as a catheter.

Magma (also **Milk**): Thick, viscous suspension of undissolved drugs in water usually intended for oral administration.

Mail Order Pharmacy: Large-scale operations that mail maintenance medications (i.e., medications that patients take on a regular basis) to the patients' homes.

Mainframe Computer: Large, expensive, powerful computer designed to process large amounts of data shared by numerous people.

Mean: See **Arithmetic Mean**.

Median: A value in an ordered set of values below and above which there are an equal number of values.

Medication Administration Record (MAR): A document used by the nurse in an institutional setting to record the administration of medications. Information included on the MAR would include selected patient information, a complete record of all active medication orders, the dates and times medications have been administered, the identity of the person administering the medications, and pertinent details about the medication administration such as an injection site. MARs can be written manually or generated from a computer.

Medication Error: Defined by the National Coordinating Council for Medication Error Reporting and Prevention (NCC MERP) as any preventable event that may cause or lead to inappropriate medication use or patient harm, while the medication is in the control of the health care professional, patient, or consumer. Such events may be related to professional practice, health care products, procedures and systems including: prescribing; order communication; product labeling, packaging, and nomenclature; compounding; dispensing; distribution; administration; education; monitoring; and use.

Medication Order: A written medication request on a physician's order form in an institutional setting.

Medication Usage (Utilization) Evaluation: See **Drug Usage Evaluation**.

Metabolism: The process by which a drug is chemically converted in the body to another substance, called a metabolite.

Microcomputer: See **Personal Computer**.

Milk (also **Magma**): Thick, viscous suspensions of undissolved drugs in water usually intended for oral administration.

Minicomputer: Smaller scaled mainframe computer used by several people within a small organization or by a department within a larger organization.

Mnemonic: A shorthand designation used to access a menu in a pharmacy information system or to type in the contents of a field in a shortened manner to save time for the operator. (Example: the mnemonic for ampicillin 250mg capsules might be amp250c.)

Mouse Selection: The use of a mouse to control a computer by moving the mouse and pressing buttons to make selections.

Mucilage: A thick, viscous, adhesive solution of water containing sticky, pulpy components of vegetable matter.

Nasal Route of Administration: Administration of medication into the nostrils.

Nonaqueous Solution: A solution in which a solvent, such as alcohol (ethyl alcohol or ethanol), glycerin, or propylene glycol, is used in addition to or instead of water.

Number: A total quantity or amount that is made of one or more numerals.

Numeral: A word or a sign, or a group of words or signs that expresses a number.

Ointment: A semisolid medication dosage form intended to be applied to the skin or mucous membranes used to lubricate and soften or as a base (a vehicle that contains a drug) for drug delivery.

Ophthalmic Route of Administration: Delivery of medication into the eye.

Opportunistic Infection: A serious infection with a microorganism which normally has little or no pathogenic (disease-producing) activity but which has been activated by a serious disease or by a method of treatment, or allowed to flourish as a result of a serious disease or treatment.

Oral Route of Administration (PO): Medications are introduced into the body through the mouth.

Osmolarity: A property of a solution that depends on the concentration of the solute per unit of total volume of solution.

Otic Route of Administration: Delivery of medication into the ear canal.

Over-the-counter Drug: A drug that can be purchased without a prescription.

Parenteral Route of Administration: A route of administration that bypasses the gastrointestinal tract.

Pareto (ABC) Analysis: (also known as the **80/20 rule**) A type of analysis useful in determining which among a set of potential variables are the primary issues and therefore where efforts are best directed.

Patent: Open, unobstructed, or not closed.

Pathophysiology: Unhealthy function due to a disease in an individual body system or an organ.

Patient-focused Services: (also called **Clinical Pharmacy Services**) Those services involving appropriate use of medications allowing patients to achieve optimal outcomes and improve patient satisfaction, including pharmacokinetics dosing services, drug information services, and nutritional support services, for example.

Patient Profile: A record keeping system to track patient demographic information and medication history.

Perception: The mental process of becoming aware of or recognizing an object or idea.

Peristalsis: Waves of involuntary muscular contractions of muscle in the digestive tract. In the stomach, this motion mixes food with gastric juices, turning it into a thin liquid.

Personal Computer: Stand-alone system that runs software programs and manages data accessed from a larger source such as a mainframe.

Personal Digital Assistant (PDA): A small handheld computer that is used to carry applications such as an address book, calendar, notes and tasks.

pH: The hydrogen ion concentration in a solution/fluid. The lower the pH, the more acidic the solution and the greater the hydrogen ion concentration; a pH of 7.4 is considered to be neutral with the body fluids.

Phagocytosis: The process by which a white blood cell engulfs other cells and particles such as bacteria, other microorganisms, aged red blood cells, foreign matter, and other materials.

Pharmacodynamics: The study of drugs at a target site, or site of action.

Pharmacokinetics: The study of the absorption, distribution, metabolism, and excretion of drugs.

Physiology: The study of how living organisms function including such processes as nutrition, movement, and reproduction.

Point-of-care Bar Code Recognition: A process in which bar codes are assigned to each nurse, medication, and patient for the purpose of positive identification and medication error prevention.

Prescription: An order for a medication or other treatment that must be authorized by a licensed health care professional.

Product-focused Services: Pharmacy functions relating to the provision of medications directly to patients or other health care providers who care for patients. Responsibilities and functions include several processes, such as ordering, storing, preparing, delivering, administering, documenting, and monitoring.

Professional: A person whose occupation or vocation requires advanced training in a liberal art or science, e.g., a pharmacist.

Quality Assurance: A program that attempts to define standards and measure performance of services through a formalized program within the institution/company.

Quality Control: A process of checks and balances (or procedures) followed during the manufacturing of a product or provision of a service to ensure that the end products or services meet or exceed specified standards (e.g., zero errors, zero problems).

Quality Improvement: [also referred to as **Continuous Quality Improvement (CQI)**] A scientific and systematic process involving monitoring, evaluating, and identifying problems and developing and measuring the impact of the improvement strategies.

Real-time Alerts: Alerts that are provided to the user during a critical process, allowing the user to intervene in a timely fashion.

Recall: Process undertaken by a pharmaceutical manufacturer and/or the FDA to notify pharmacies of their intent to recall a particular product due to situations affecting the product as it was manufactured, packaged, or labeled.

Receptors: A structure on the surface of a cell (or inside a cell) that selectively receives and binds a specific substance.

Rectal Route of Administration: Administration of medication by insertion through the anus into the rectum.

Referral: Term used to describe the process whereby a health care provider supplies information to a home infusion therapy provider to determine whether a patient will be accepted to the home infusion service or not. All of the patient's demographic information, current medical treatment, insurance information, and past medical information is entered on the home infusion therapy provider's referral form.

Registration: The process of making a list or being enrolled in an existing list.

Repackaging: The subdivision or transfer from a container or device to a different container or device, such as a syringe or ophthalmic container, or from a bulk container to unit of use.

Secrete: To form and give off.

Sepsis: Widespread infection with microorganisms; eliciting inflammatory response and physiologic changes that can progress to multiple organ system failure and death.

Solution: An evenly distributed, homogeneous mixture of dissolved medication in a liquid vehicle. Molecules of a solid, liquid, or gaseous medication are equally distributed among the molecules of the liquid vehicle.

Sphygmomanometer: An instrument for measuring blood pressure, particularly in arteries. The two types of sphygmomanometers are a mercury column and a gauge with a dial face. The sphygmomanometer in most frequent use today consists of a gauge attached to a rubber cuff that is wrapped around the upper arm and is inflated to constrict the arteries.

Spirit: An alcoholic or hydroalcoholic solution that contains volatile substances. Because the volatile substances dissolve more readily in alcohol, spirits can contain a greater concentration of these materials than water.

Spray: A solution delivered as a mist against the mucous membranes of the nose and throat.

Standard Deviation: A statistic that tells you how tightly clustered data points are around the mean in a set of data.

Stem Cells: The human body's master cells, with the ability to grow into any one of the body's more than 200 cell types. The cell type from which all other cells are derived.

Sterilizing Filter: A filter that, when challenged with a solution containing the microorganism *Pseudomonas diminuta*, at a minimum concentration of 107 organisms per square centimeter of filter surface, will produce a sterile effluent.

Stock Rotation: The process of rotating products with shorter shelf lives (expiration dates) to the front of the shelf to ensure they are used before products with longer shelf lives.

Subcutaneous (subQ) Route of Administration: Medication deposited in the tissue immediately under the skin.

Sublingual Route of Administration: A sublingual tablet placed under the tongue so medication dissolves and is absorbed into the bloodstream through the underlining of the tongue.

Suspension: A mixture of fine particles of an undissolved solid distributed through a gas, liquid, or solid.

Syrup: A concentrated mixture of sugar and purified water. The high sugar content distinguishes syrups from other types of solutions. Syrups may or may not contain medication or added flavoring agents.

Systole: The heart muscle contracting and ejecting blood from the chambers of the heart; the pressure is at the highest point in the normal heart, represented by the first number in a blood pressure reading.

Tablet: A compacted solid medication dosage form that may be molded or compressed. Types of tablets include: oral, sublingual, buccal, effervescent, chewable, and vaginal.

Technician: A person skilled in the practical or mechanical aspects of a profession and who assists professionals in routine, day-to-day functions that do not require professional judgment.

Temperatures: Temperature ranges for the storage of drugs as defined by the United States Pharmacopeial Convention are: Frozen is defined as between –20 and –10 °C (-4 and 14 °F); Refrigerated is defined as between 2 and 8 °C (36 and 46 °F); Room Temperature is defined as between 15 and 30 °C (59 and 86 °F).

Therapeutic Duplication Checking: A computerized system that detects drugs of the same pharmacologic-therapeutic classification or an order for the same medication and provides alerts during order entry.

Third-party Programs: Insurance or entitlement programs that reimburse the pharmacy for products delivered and services rendered.

Three-in-one Total Parenteral Nutrition Solutions: Also referred to as total nutrient admixtures (TNAs) whereby the base components of the parenteral nutrition solution include admixture of the amino acids, dextrose, and lipids all together in one container.

Tincture: An alcoholic or hydro-alcoholic extractive solution whose potency is adjusted so that each milliliter of tincture contains the equivalent potency of 100 mg of crude drug.

Tolerance: A state of unresponsiveness or diminished response to a substance to which a person is normally responsive.

Topical Route of Administration: Application of medication to the surface of the skin or mucous membranes.

Touch Screen Technology: Technology that senses the location of your finger as it nears or touches a screen.

Transdermal Route of Administration: Delivery of medication across the skin.

Uni-directional Interface: An interface that allows one-way information to be passed from one system to another.

Universal Precautions: The principles whereby all health care workers are bound to observe and treat all human blood and certain human body fluids as though they were known to be infectious for human immunodeficiency virus, hepatitis B virus, and other blood-borne pathogens.

Vaginal Route of Administration: Administration of medication by insertion into the vagina.

Validation: Documented evidence providing a high degree of assurance that a specific process will consistently produce a product meeting its predetermined specifications and quality attributes.

Venipuncture: Insertion of a needle into a vein.

Venous Access Device: The device used to gain access to the patient's venous system. Specifically, it is the intravenous catheter used to infuse intravenous fluids or medications. This device can be either a peripheral vein catheter or central vein catheter.

Voice Recognition: Technology that inputs data into a system by recognizing spoken words.

Wash: A solution that cleanses or bathes a body part, such as the eyes or mouth.

INDEX

American Hospital Formulary Service Drug Information (AHFS DI), 379, 381-82

American Journal of Health-System Pharmacy (AJHP), 379

American Pharmaceutical Association (APhA), 9

American Pharmacists Association, Code of Ethics, 108, 109

American Society of Health-System Pharmacists (ASHP), 267, 328, 381, 382
  certification, 9, 10
  computerized pharmacy system, 394
  Guidelines on Preventing Medication Errors in Hospitals, 324
  Guidelines on Quality Assurance for Pharmacy-Prepared Sterile Products, 53, 267, 296, 305-22
  Task Force on Technical Personnel in Pharmacies, 4, 9
  Technical Assistance Bulletin, 294
  Technical Assistance Bulletin on Handling of Cytotoxic and Hazardous Drugs, 285
  Technical Assistance Bulletin on Institutional Use of Controlled Substances, 367
  Technical Assistance Bulletin on Single Unit and Unit Dose Packages of Drugs, 261

American Society for Parenteral and Enteral Nutrition (A.S.P.E.N.), 305

Amikacin, 49, 235, 237

Amiloride/HCTZ, 218

Amino acids, 79, 82, 290

Aminoglycerides, 46, 199, 202, 235, 328

Aminophylline, 84, 209, 270

Amiodarone, 222, 223, 333

Amitriptyline, 211, 214

Amlodipine, 220

Amobarbital, 103

Amoxicillin, 80, 225, 234, 324, 331

Amoxicillin with clavulanic acid, 234

Amphetamine, 103

Amphotericin, 49, 83

Amphotericin B, 238-39

Ampicillin, 78, 80, 82-83, 84, 149, 150, 234, 335, 378

Ampicillin/sulbactam, 47

Amprenavir, 238

Ampules, 282-83

Amrinone, 333

Anabolic steroids, 103

Anafranil, 211

Anakira, 51

Analgesics, 126, 227-28

Anaprox, 378

Anatomy
  of cardiovascular system, 173-74
  of endocrine system, 179
  of gastrointestinal system, 181-82
  of heart, 174
  of immune system, 186-87
  of musculoskeletal system, 177-78
  of nervous system, 171-72
  of reproductive system, 185-86
  of respiratory system, 175-76
  of sensory nervous system, 189
  of urinary tract system, 184-85

Anbien, 214

Ancef, 131, 234

Anemia, 177

Angina pectoris, 220-21

Angiotensin converting enzyme (ACE) inhibitors, 218, 219, 221

Angiotensin receptor blockers (ARBs), 219

Ansaid, 227

Antacids, 120, 223, 224

Antagonists, 202

Anthralin, 244

Anti-inflammatory agents, 226-27

Antibiotic therapy, 47-48

Antibiotics, 123, 324

Anticholinergics, 208, 209

Anticoagulants, 223

Anticonvulsants, 215-16

Antidepressants, 211-12

Antidiarrheals, 223, 225

Antiemetics, 240

Antiepileptics. *See* Anticonvulsants

Antifungals, 238-39

Antihistamines, 210, 241-42

Antihyperlipidemic agents, 216-17

Antihypertensives, 218-20

Antineoplastic drugs, 285

Antiparkinson drugs, 216

Antipsychotics, 212-13

Antipyretic agents, 226-27

Antiseptic throat solutions, 115

Antitubercular drugs, 236-37

Antitussives, 210, 211

Antivirals, 237-38

Anxiolytics, 213-14

APCS. *See* Ambulatory Payment Classification System

APhA. *See* American Pharmaceutical Association

Apothecary system, 75, 332

Appendicitis, 184

Approved Drug Products and Legal Requirements, 381

Approved Drug Products with Therapeutic Equivalence Evaluations, 381

Aquachloral, 214

Aqueous solutions, 115

Arabic numerals, 71

Aranesp, 51

ARBs. *See* Angiotensin receptor blockers

Aredia, 332

Aripiprazole, 213

Aristocort, 244

Arithmetic mean, 86

Aromatic ammonia spirits, 116

Aromatic elixir, 116

Arrhythmia, 175, 222-23

Arrow International, Inc., 60

Arthritis Strength BC Powder, 121

Arthrotec, 227

Artificial tears, 241

ASAP (as soon as possible), 147

Aseptic Preparation of Parenteral Products, 267

Aseptic technique, 267-68, 276-85
  answer key, 301-4
  equipment, supplies, 279-81
  glossary, 317-18
  handwashing, 279
  personal attire, 279
  test, 298-300

ASHP. *See* American Society of Health-System Pharmacists

Asparaginase, 240

Aspart, 229

Aspartame, 256

Aspirin, 24, 103, 217, 221, 225, 227

Astelin, 243

Astemizole, 331

Asthma, 176, 209-10

Atacand, 219

Atarax, 210

Atenolol, 202, 219

Ativan, 103, 214, 215

Atorvastatin, 217

Atracurium, 228

Atrial fibrillation, 222

Atrial flutter, 222

Atropine, 209, 225

Atropine sulfate, 81, 82

Atrovent, 208

Attapulgite, 225

Attire, 279

Atypical agents, 212-13

Augmented betamethasone diproprionate, 244
Augmentin, 234
Autoimmune disease, 188
Automated compounding devices, 57-58
TPN solutions and, 292-93
Automated dispensing systems, 156-57
inpatient, 402-3
outpatient, 403
Automated oral solid systems, 259
Automated packaging systems, 260
Automated syringe filling equipment, 284-85
Automation, 23, 40, 338, 341
inventory management, 363-65
AutoMed Efficiency Pharmacy, 402
Automix, 40
Automix 3+3, 58
Automix 3+3/AS, 58
Avandamet, 230
Avandia, 230
Avapro, 219
Avelox, 51, 236
Aventis, 378
Avoirdupois system, 75
Axid, 224
Azathioprine, 328, 329
Azelastine, 241, 243
Azepam stem, 213
Azithromycin, 47, 235, 334
Azlocillin, 234
Azmacort, 208
Azopt, 241
Azreonam, 235
AZT, 238, 328

B

B. Braun Medical, 58
B. Braun Medical Perfusor, 54
Bachelor of science (B.S.), 3, 10
Bacitracin, 244
Bacitracin/polymixin B, 333
Baclofen, 228
Bactine First Aid Antiseptic Anesthetic, 121-22
Bar coding, 148, 341, 400-401
Barbital, 103
Bard Access Systems, Inc., 60
Base components, 289
Batch repackaging, 258
Baxa, 58
Baxa MicroFuse Dual Rate Infuser, 54
Baxa MicroFuse Extended Rate Infuser, 54

Baxa MicroFuse Rapid Rate Syringe Infuser, 54
Baxter Auto Syringe AS50 Infusion Pump, 54
Baxter Healthcare Corporation, 58
Baxter InfusO.R., 54
Baxter SureMed, 40
Baxter's Intermate Elastomeric Infusion System, 54
BC Powder, 121
BCPS. *See* Board Certified Pharmacy Specialist
Beclomethasone, 208
Beclomethasone diproprionate, 243
Beclovent, 208
Beconase, 243
Bell curve, 86
Ben-Gay Original Ointment, 116
Benadryl, 210
Benazepril, 219
Benicar, 219
Benign prostatic hypertrophy (BPH), 232
Benzalkonium chloride, 242, 282
Benzathine, 123
Benzethonium chloride, 242
Benzodiazepines (BZDs), 103, 213-14, 215
Benzphetamine, 103
Benztropine, 216
Benzyl alcohol, 282
Beta-2 agonists, 208-9
Beta-blockers, 219, 221, 222
Beta-blockers, 241
Beta-lactam antibiotics, 234-35
Betagan, 241
Betamethasone, 101, 228
Betamethasone diproprionate, 244
Betamethasone valerate, 244
Betapace, 219
Betaxolol, 241
Betoptic, 241
Bevel heel, 280
Bevel tip, 280
Bextra, 227
Beyond-use labeling, 102, 252, 261-63
Biaxin, 235
Biguanides, 229
Bile acid sequestrants, 217
Binders, 119
Bioavailability, 198-99
Biological response modifiers, 51
Biological safety cabinets (BSCs), 278, 286-87, 289

Biopharmaceutics, 195-98
answer key, 206
test, 205
Biperidin, 216
Biphasic pills, 231
Biphosphonates, 232
Bipolar disorder, 213
Bismuth subsalicylate, 225
Bisocodyl, 226
Bisoprolol, 218, 219
Bisphosphonates, 232
Blackheads, 244
Bleeding, IV therapy, 269
Bleomycin, 240
Blister oral solid equiment, 259
Blister systems, 258-59
BlisterGard, 116
Blocadren, 219
Blood thinners, 223
Board Certified Pharmacy Specialist (BCPS), 10
Body Surface Area (BSA), 77, 83
Bolus, 124
Bolus injections, 294
Boric acid, 81, 82, 242
Borrowing pharmaceuticals, 366-67
BPH. *See* Benign prostatic hypertrophy
Brand name prescription, 22, 106, 131
Branded generic drugs, 106
Brandy, 116
Bretylium, 222-23, 270
Brinzolamide, 241
Bromocriptine, 216
Bronchitis, 177
Bronchodilators, 208-10
Broviac catheters, 275
BSA. *See* Body Surface Area
BSCs. *See* Biological safety cabinets
Buccal, 127
Buccal agents, 197
Buccal tablets, 119, 123
Budesonide, 208, 243
Buffers, 369
Bulk-forming laxatives, 226
Bumetanide, 218
Bumex, 218
Bupivacaine, 51
Buprenex, 103
Buprenorphine, 103, 227
Bupropion, 211, 212
Buretrol, 271
Buspar, 214
Buspirone, 214
Busulfan, 240
Butorphanol, 103, 227

Butterfly, 275
BZDs. *See* Benzodiazepines

C

CADD-Legacy, 56
CADD-Legacy Plus, 56
CADD-TPN, 56
Caffeine, 98
Caladryl, 118
Calamine lotion, 118
Calan SR, 220
Calcipotriene, 244
Calcitonin, 232
Calcium, 232, 246
Calcium acetate, 232
Calcium carbonate, 224, 232
Calcium channel blockers, 220, 221, 223
Calcium chloride, 232
Calcium gluconate, 290, 292
Calcium lactate, 232
Calcium phosphate, 232
Calculation
    answers, 92-93
    errors, 327-28
    practice, 87-89
Campath, 51
Cancidas, 51
Candesartan, 219
Candida albicans, 49
Cannula, 276
Capitation, 20
Capitation plans, 18
Capoten, 219
Capreomycin, 237
Capsules, 118, 120, 256
Captopril, 202, 219
Carbachol, 242
Carbamazepine, 199, 213, 215
Carbamide peroxide, 243
Carbapenems, 234-35
Carbenicillin, 234
Carbidopa, 216
Carbohydrates, 289
Carbon dioxide, 224
Carboplatin, 240
Cardene SR, 220
Cardiac glycosides, 221-22
Cardiovascular system, 216-23
    anatomy of, 173-74
    pathophysiology of, 175
    physiology of, 174-75
Cardizem, 220
Cardizem CD, 378

Cardura, 220
Care plan, 45
Caregiver, home care role, 47
Carisoprodol, 228
Carmustine, 240
Carteolol, 219, 241
Cartrol, 219
Cascara sagrada fluidextract, 118
Case manager, 44
Caspofungin, 51
Castor oil, 117, 226
Catapres-TTS, 126
Catapres-TTS patch system, 220
Catechol-O-methyltransferase (COMT) inhibitors, 216
Cavedilol, 219
CBC. *See* Complete blood count
CDSS. *See* Clinical Decision Support System
Ceclor, 234
Cefaclor, 234
Cefadroxil, 234
Cefazolin, 147, 234
Cefazolin, 35, 47
Cefixime, 234
Cefoperazone, 47
Cefotaxime, 234
Cefotetan, 47
Cefoxitin, 234
Cefpodoxime, 234
Cefprozil, 234
Ceftazidime, 358
Ceftin, 234
Ceftriaxone, 47, 234
Cefuroxime, 234
Cefzil, 234
Celdinir, 234
Celebrex, 227
Celecoxib, 227
Celexa, 211
Cell killer, 285
Cellulitis, 48
Centers for Disease Control and Prevention, 236, 237, 284, 305
Centers for Medicare and Medicaid Services (CMS), 36
Centigrade, 76
Central catheters, 275
Central nervous system, 171
    disorders, 211-16
Central pharmacy, 32
Central venous catheter (CVC), 61
Centralized computer systems, 402
CEO. *See* Chief executive officer
Cepacol, 115
Cepacol Throat, 120

Cephalexin, 234, 325
Cephalosporins, 47, 234, 235
Cephalothin, 80
Cerebyx, 215
Certificate of Medical Necessity and Plan of Treatment, 45
Certification, 4
Certified pharmacy technician (CPhT), 9
Cerubidine, 335
Cetirizine, 210
CFO. *See* Chief financial officer
CFR. *See* Code of Federal Regulation
Chain pharmacy, 19
Charge only entries, 156
Checklists, 338
Checkpoints, 263
Chemotherapeutic agents, 239-40, 285
Chemotherapy, 50
Chemotherapy order form, 339-40
Chepacol Sore Throat, 115
Chewable tablets, 120
Chibroxin, 241
Chief executive officer (CEO), 32
Chief financial officer (CFO), 32
Chief operating officer (COO), 32
Chlor-Trimeton, 210
Chloral hydrate, 103, 214
Chlorambucil, 240
Chloramphenicol, 78-80, 242, 244
Chlordiazepoxide, 103, 214
Chlorothiazide, 218
Chlorpheniramine, 210
Chlorpromazine, 213, 329
Chlorpropamide, 230
Chlorthalidone, 218
Chlorzoxazone, 228
Cholecalciferol, 245
Cholestyramine, 101, 217
Chromium, 290
Chronic obstructive pulmonary disease (COPD), 208, 209-10
Cillin stem, 234
Ciloxan, 241
Cimetidine, 50, 202, 224
Cipro, 236
Ciprofloxacin, 49, 202, 236, 237, 241, 242
Cisplatin, 240
Citalopram, 211
Cladribine, 240
Claforan, 234
Clarinex, 210
Clarithromycin, 49, 225, 235

Claritin, 210, 378
CLAVE, 61
Clean rooms, 52-53, 277
Clearance, 201
Clemastine, 210
Cleocin, 236
Clindamycin, 34, 236, 245
Clinic pharmacies, 19
Clinical Decision Support System
    (CDSS), 398-99
Clinical pharmacy, 18
Clinical pharmacy services. *See* Patient-
    focused services
Clinical practitioner, 33
Clinoril, 227
Clobetasol, 244
Clofazimine, 237
Clofazine, 49
Clofibrate, 217
Clomiphene, 231
Clomipramine, 211
Clonazepam, 103, 215
Clonidine, 202, 220, 333
Clorazepate, 103, 214
Closures, 284
Clotrimazole, 244
Clozapine, 213
Clozaril, 213
CMS. *See* Centers for Medicare and
    Medicaid Services
CMV. *See* Cytomegalovirus
Coal tar, 244
Cocaine, 81, 103, 329
Coccidiomycosis, 49
Cockroft-Gault equation, 201
Code of Federal Regulation (CFR), 97,
    100, 102, 104
Codeine, 98, 103, 211, 227
Colace, 120
Cold storage, 359
Colesevelam, 217
Colestid, 217
Colestipol, 101, 217
Collodion, 116
Color coding, 334-35
Colorants, 119
Combivent, 208
Comedones, 244
Communication skills, 20
Community college, 2
Community pharmacy, 10, 18-19
Compazine, 329
Complete blood count (CBC), 50
Compliance errors, 325
Compound W, 116

Compounded products, 252-53, 367,
    368
Compounding, 23, 52-58, 99
    environment, 252
    errors, 335-36
    good practices, 252
    log, 23
    nonsterile, 251-57
    nonsterile answer key, 266
    nonsterile equipment, 253, 255
    nonsterile test, 265
    processes, 253
    records, documents, 253
    responsibility, 252
    stability of preparations, 252
Compounding Sterile Preparations, 267
Compressed tablets, 119
Computer security, 395
Computer systems, 393-400
    answer key, 408-9
    test, 405-7
Computerization, 338, 341
Computerized pharmacy system, 394
Computerized Physician/Prescriber
    Order Entry (CPOE), 341, 395-96
COMT inhibitors. *See* Catechol-O-
    methyltransferase inhibitors
Comtan, 216
Concentration, 79-85
    expressed as percentage, 79-80
    expressed as ratio strength, 80-81
Conjugated estrogens, 232
Conjunctivitis, 241-42
Constipation, 184
Contac 12-Hour Capsules, 121
Containers, 258
Continuous infusion, 124, 270, 294
Continuous quality improvement
    (CQI), 36. *See also* Quality improve-
    ment
Controlled Substance Act, 97, 98, 102-
    6
Controlled substances, 367-68
    expired, 369
    ordering, 103-4
    schedules, 103
Controlled-release infusion system
    (CRIS), 273-74
Conventional antipsychotics, 212
Conversion between systems, 76-77
COO. *See* Chief operating officer
Cook Critical Care, 60
Copayments, 21
COPD. *See* Chronic obstructive
    pulmonary disease
Copper, 290

Cordarone, 333
Coreg, 219
Corgard, 219
Cormax, 244
Corticosteroids, 208, 209, 228-29,
    242, 244
Cortisporin, 241
Cough, 210
Cough formulations, 115
Coumadin, 223
Course dose, 332
Covera HS, 220
Cozaar, 219
CphT. *See* Certified pharmacy
    technician
CPOE. *See* Computerized Physician/
    Prescriber Order Entry
CQI. *See* Continuous quality improve-
    ment
Creams, 122, 255-56
Creatinine clearance, 201
Credentialing, 9
Crestor, 217
CRIS. *See* Controlled-release infusion
    system
Critical area, 278
Crixivan, 238
Crohn's disease, 49, 184
Cromolyn sodium, 208, 243
Cross-sensitivity, 234
Cushing's syndrome, 178, 228
Customer service, 20
CVC. *See* Central venous catheter
Cyanocobalamin, 245
Cyclobenzaprine, 228
Cyclophosphamide, 50, 240
Cycloserine, 237
Cyclosporine, 201
Cycloxygenase-2 (COX-2) inhibitors,
    227
Cylert, 103
Cytarabine, 240, 329
Cytomegalovirus (CMV), 49, 238
Cytotoxic drug preparation, handling,
    285-89

D

D.U.E., 132
Dacarbazine, 240
Dactinomycin, 240
Daily dose, 332
Dalmane, 103, 214
Dalteparin, 223
Darbepoetin alfa, 51
Darvocet-N, 228

Drug-food interaction, 399
Drug-lab interaction, 399
Drug-receptor complex, 202, 203
Dumb terminals, 394
DUR. *See* Drug use review
Durable medical equipment (DME), 19
Duragesic, 126
Duration, 243
Durham-Humphrey Amendment, 17
Duricef, 234
Dwarfism, 181
Dx, 132
Dyazide, 218
DynaCirc, 220
Dyrenium, 218

E

Echothiophate iodide, 242
Eclipse, 275
Econazole, 244
Economic models, 362-63
Economic order quantity (EOQ), 362-63
Edecrin, 218
Edrophonium, 228
Education, 338
Efavirenz, 238
Effervescent tablets, 119
Effexor, 211
EID. *See* Elastomeric infusion device
80/20 rule, 362-63
Elastomeric balloons, 54-55
Elastomeric infusion device (EID), 274-75
Elavil, 211
Electrocardiogram, 133
Electrolytes, 290
Electronic balance, 253
Electronic controlled pressure systems, 55
Eligibility verification, 20
Elimination, 201, 202
Elixirs, 116
Elocon, 244
Elsevier Science, 382
Emadine, 241
Embeline, 244
Emedastine, 241
Emollient laxatives, 226
Emphysema, 176
Empty bag method, 292
Emulsion base, 122
Emulsions, 114, 117, 123

Enalapril, 155, 156, 202, 219
Enalapril maleate, patient information sheet, 162-64
Enbrel, 378
End-product evaluation/testing, 263, 296
Endocarditis, 48
Endocet, 106
Endocrine system, 229-33
    anatomy of, 179
    pathophysiology of, 181
    physiology of, 179-81
Enemas, 115
Enoxaparin, 223
Entacapone, 216
Enteral nutrition therapy, 51
Enteric-coated tablets, 119
Enzyme inducers, 200-201
Enzyme inhibitors, 201
EOQ. *See* Economic order quantity
Ephedrine, 103, 209
Epidural administration, 294
Epinephrine, 80, 81, 202, 209, 336
Epivir, 238
Epogen, 51
Eprosartan, 219
Equipment, 295
    maintenance, 263
Equivalencies, 76, 85
Ergocalciferol, 245
Ertapenem, 51
Erythrocyte sedimentation rate (ESR), 48
Erythromycin, 83, 101, 201, 235, 244, 245
Erythropoietin, 51
Escitalopram, 211
Esmolol, 222
Esomeprazole, 225
Esophageal disorders, 183
Esophagus, 181-82
ESR. *See* Erythrocyte sedimentation rate
Estazolam, 214
Estraderm, 126
Estradiol cypionate, 231
Estramustine, 240
Estrogens, 101, 151, 231, 232
Ethacrynic acid, 218
Ethambutol, 49, 236, 237
Ethanol, 115
Ethchlorvynol, 103
Ethics, 107-8
    answer key, 111
    test, 110
Ethinamate, 103

Ethinyl estradiol, 231, 232
Ethionamide, 237
Ethopropazine, 216
Ethosuximide, 215
Ethotoin, 215
Ethyl alcohol, 115, 383
Etidronate, 232
Etodolac, 227
Etoposide, 240
Eureka infusion pump, 55
Exacta-Mix, 58
Excelsior ESP Infusion System, 54
Expectorants, 210, 211
Expiration dating, 58-59, 102, 325
Expired drugs, 369, 371
Extemporaneous repackaging, 258
Extended Stability for Parenteral Drugs, 58
Extended-release dosage, 118, 120-21
    common abbreviations, 120
External education programs, 3
Extractives, 114, 118
Extracts, 118
Extrapyramidal symptoms, 213
Extravasation, IV therapy, 269
Eye dryness medications, 242
Ezetimibe, 217

F

Facts and Comparisons, 379, 382
Fahrenheit, 76
Failure mode and effects analysis (FMEA), 337
Failure mode effect and criticality analysis (FMECA), 337
Famciclovir, 237
Famotidine, 202, 224
Famvir, 237
Fat emulsion, 290
Fat-soluble vitamins, 245
Fats, 289-90
Fatty acid, 256
FDA. *See* Food and Drug Administration
FDAMA. *See* Food and Drug Administration Modernization Act
FDCA. Food, Drug, and Cosmetic Act, 97
Fee-for-service, 20
Felbamate, 215, 216
Felbatol, 215
Feldene, 227
Fellowship, 3
Felodipine, 220

Sublimaze, 103
Sublingual, 127
  agents, 197
  tablets, 119, 123
Sucralfate, 223, 224
Sucrase, 101
Sucret Sore Throat, 120
Sucrose, 256
Sular, 220
Sulf-10, 241
Sulfisoxazole, 235
Sulfonamide, 235, 242
Sulfonamide sulfamethoxazole and
    trimethoprim, 235
Sulfonylureas, 229
Sulindac, 227
Summer's Eve, 115
Superior Consultant Company, 393
Supplies, disposal of, 284
Suppositories, 118, 256
  molds, 255
Suprax, 234
SureMed, 364
Sus-Phrine, 123
Suspensions, 114, 117-18, 198, 256
Sustiva, 238
Suvvinylcholine, 228
Sx, 132
Synalar, 244
Synovium, 48
Synthroid, 230
Syringe, 279-80
  infusion system, 54
  pumps, 54, 271
  systems, 271
Syrup, 115
Systemic corticosteroids, 228-29

T

Tablet triturates, 257
Tablets, 118, 119-20
Tagamet, 224
Talc, 369
Talwin-NX, 103
Tamoxifen, 240
Tamoxifen citrate, 262
Tasmar, 216
Taste, 190
Tavist, 210
Technical college, 2
Technician, 1-2
  certification program, 9-10
  liability issues, 344
  responsibilities, 11, 12
Technology, 11, 13, 30

Tegretol, 215
Telmisartan, 219
Temazepam, 103, 214
Temovate, 244
Temperature conversion, 76
Tenofovir, 238
Tenormin, 219
Terazol 3, 126
Terazosin, 220, 232
Terbinafine, 244
Tetracaine, 329
Tetracycline, 80, 225, 235, 245
Tetracycline hydrochloride, 235
Tetrahydrozoline, 242
Teveten, 219
Theophylline, 208, 209
Therapeutic level, 199
Therapy-specific infusion devices, 56
Thiamine, 245
Thiazide diuretics, 218
Thiazolidinediones, 229
Thioridazine, 213
Thiothixene, 213
Third-party payment programs, 20
Thomson Micromedex, 382
Thorazine, 213
3-in-1 solution, 290
Thyroid disease, 181, 230-31
Thyroid hormone, 230
Thyroid USP, 230
Tiagabine, 215
Tiazac, 220, 378
Ticarcillin, 234
Ticarcillin/clavulanate, 47
Tightly sealed containers, 258
Tilade, 208
Timentin, 47
Timolol, 219, 241
Timoptic, 219, 241
Tinactin, 121-22, 244
Tinctures, 118
Tinzaparin, 223
TNA. *See* Total nutrient admixture
Tobradex, 241
Tobramycin, 235, 241
Tobramycin/dexamethasone, 241
Tobrex, 241
Tocainide, 222
Tocopherol, 245
Tofranil, 211
Tolbutamide, 230
Tolcapone, 216
Tolerance, 214
Tolnaftate, 244
Topamax, 215

Topical administration, 125
Topical corticosteroids, 125
Topical medications, 240-45, 261
Topicort, 244
Topiramate, 215
Toprol-XL, 219
Toradol, 227
Torsades de pointes, 222
Torsemide, 218
Total nutrient admixture (TNA), 58,
    290
Total parenteral nutrition (TPN), 56
    administration of, 293
    automated compounding, 292-93
    gravity fill, 292
    order form 291
    orders for, 290, 292
    preparation of, 292
    solutions, components of, 289-90
Touch screens, 401
TPN. *See* Total parenteral nutrition
Trace elements, 245, 290, 292
Training, 295, 338
  on-the-job, 2
Tramadol, 227
Tramdolapril, 219
Trandate, 219
Transderm Scop, 126
Transderm-Nitro, 126
Transdermal agents/medications, 197,
    255
Transdermal patches, 125-26
Transport
  hazardous drug, 288
  home care, 59
Tranxene, 103, 214
Tranylcypromine, 211
Trazodone, 211, 212, 214
Treprostinil sodium, 51
Triamcinolone, 208, 228, 244, 329, 369
Triamcinolone acetonide, 243
Triaminic, 115
Triamterene, 202, 218
Triamterene/HCTZ, 218
Triazolam, 103, 214
Tricor, 217
Tricyclic antidepressants, 211, 212
Trifluoperazine, 213
Trifluridine, 241
Triiodothyroxine, 230
Trilafon, 213
Trileptal, 215
Trimethobenzamide, 240
Trimethoprim/sulfamethoxazole, 49
Triphasic pills, 231

Triptyline stem, 212
Trissel's *Handbook on Injectable Drugs*, 382-83
Troches, 120, 257
Truhexyphenidyl, 216
Trusopt, 241
Tuberculosis, 236-37
Tubocurarine, 228
Tums, 120, 224
Tussionex, 103
25-hydroxycholecalciferol, 245
Tylenol, 98, 334

U

Ulcerative colitis, 184
Ulcers, 183
Ultralente, 229
Ultram, 227
Ultravate, 244
Unasyn, 47
Unauthorized drug errors, 324
Underfill method, 292
Unit-dose
   apportionment, 401-2
   distribution systems394-95
   system, 33, 34
Unit-of-use packaging, 257
United States Adopted Names Council (USAN), 207
United States Department of Justice, 97, 102
United States Pharmacopeia, 102, 252, 295, 296, 305, 336
   Convention, 53, 332-33
   Medication Errors Reporting Program, 344
   Standards for Sterile Compounding, 294
United States Pharmacopeia Drug Information (USP DI), 381
Units, 328
Units of measure, 74-77, 132
Univasc, 219
Universal Medical Technologies, Inc., 55
Universal precautions, 61
Upjohn, 106
Urinary tract system
   anatomy of, 184-85
   pathophysiology of, 185
   physiology of, 185
Urofollitropin, 231
USAN. *See* United States Adopted Names Council
USP. *See* United States Pharmacopeia

V

Vaginal administration, 126
Vaginal tablets, 120
Vagistat-1, 126
Valaciclovir, 237
Valdecoxib, 227
Validation, 155
Valium, 103, 214, 215, 327
Valproic acid, 199, 213, 215-16
Valsartan, 219
Valsartan/HCTZ, 218
Valtrex, 237
Vancenase, 243
Vanceril, 208
Vancomycin, 46, 47, 199, 202, 236, 378
Vanilla extract, 118
Vantin, 234
Vaseline, 122
Vasopressin, 232, 233
Vasotec, 219
   patient information sheet, 162-64
Vecuronium, 228
Vehicle, 113
Venlafaxine, 211
Venous access devices, 60-61, 275-76
Ventolin, 121, 208
Ventolin Rotacaps, 120
Ventricular fibrillation, 222
Ventricular tachycardia, 222
Verapamil, 196, 220, 223
Verbal orders, 331
Verelan, 220
Verification, 155
Versed, 103, 214, 334
Verstran, 103
Vertical laminar airflow hood, 277-78
Vial spike systems, 273
Vials, 281-82
Vicactil, 211
Vicodin, 103, 228
Vidarabine, 241, 329
Videx, 238
Vinblastine, 50, 240, 338
Vincristine, 50, 240, 327, 338
Vinorelbine, 240, 338
Vioxx, 227
Vira-A, 241
Viracept, 238, 333
Viral infections, 49
Viramune, 238, 333
Viread, 238
Viroptic, 241
Viscous aqueous solutions, 115-16

Vision, 190
Visken, 219
Vitamin A, 245
Vitamin A, 120
Vitamin B, 217
Vitamin B/1, 245
Vitamin B/2, 245
Vitamin B/3, 245
Vitamin B/5, 245
Vitamin B/6, 245
Vitamin B/12, 245
Vitamin D, 120, 178, 232, 245
Vitamin E, 245
Vitamin K, 290
Vitamins, 50, 99, 245, 290
Vitrasert, 241
Voice recognition, 401
Volmax, 208
Voltaren, 227
Volume, 75, 76
Volume control chambers, 271
Volumetric pumps, 260
Voluntary recalls, 365
Volutrol, 271
Voriconazole, 51

W

W/O. *See* Water-in-oil emulsion
Want list/book, 364
Warfarin, 148, 150, 199, 223, 245, 378
Wash, 115
Waste disposal, hazardous drug, 288-89
Water, 290
Water-in-oil (W/O), 122
   emulsion, 117
Water-soluble vitamins, 245
Weight, 75, 75
Welchol, 217
Well-closed containers, 258
Wellbutin, 211
Westcort, 244
Whiskey, 116
Whiteheads, 244
Whole numbers, 72
Wholesaler services, 367
Work environment, 336
Work lists, 396–97
Wrong administration technique errors, 325
Wrong dosage form errors, 325
Wrong drug preparation errors, 325
Wrong time errors, 324

X

Z